KU-174-982

Biology of Isolated Adult Cardiac Myocytes

Biology of Isolated Adult Cardiac Myocytes

Proceedings of the National Heart, Lung, and Blood Institute-sponsored workshop "Biology of Isolated Adult Cardiac Myocytes," held September 22–25, 1987, at Asilomar Conference Center, Pacific Grove, California, USA

Editors

William A. Clark, Ph.D.

Cardiovascular Institute
Michael Reese Hospital and Medical Center, and
The University of Chicago
Chicago, Illinois, USA

Robert S. Decker, Ph.D.

Department of Medicine, and Department of Cell Biology and Anatomy
Northwestern University School of Medicine
Chicago, Illinois, USA

Thomas K. Borg, Ph.D.

Department of Pathology
University of South Carolina
Columbia, South Carolina, USA

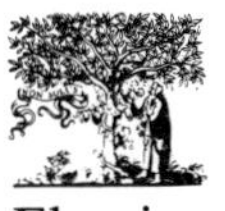

Elsevier
New York • Amsterdam • London

Elsevier Science Publishing Co., Inc.
52 Vanderbilt Avenue, New York, New York 10017

Sole distributors outside the United States and Canada:
Elsevier Science Publishers B.V.
P.O. Box 211, 1000 AE Amsterdam, the Netherlands

Library of Congress Cataloging-in-Publication Data

Biology of isolated adult cardiac myocytes.
Includes indexes.
1. Heart—Muscle—Congresses. 2. Human cell culture —Congresses. I. Clark, William A. II. Decker, Robert S. III. Borg, Thomas K. (Thomas Keith), 1943- . IV. National Heart, Lung, and Blood Institute. [DNLM: 1. Myocardium—cytology—congresses. 2. Myocardium—metabolism—congresses. WG 280 B615 1987]
QP113.2.B55 1988 599'.0116 88-3546

ISBN 0-444-01318-0

Current printing (last digit)
10 9 8 7 6 5 4 3 2 1

Manufactured in the United States of America

TABLE OF CONTENTS

Culture and Morphology

PREFACE

Cells in culture have proved to be valuable investigative tools in many areas of biological and biomedical research. It is, therefore, not surprising that scientists interested in cellular aspects of cardiac function have sought to obtain preparations of isolated cardiac myocytes which could be used in a similar fashion.

Early efforts to isolate adult mammalian cardiac myocytes and to maintain them in culture revealed how sensitive they were to their environment, and how easily and unpredictably they could be damaged. The techniques for obtaining viable preparations were so difficult to define that "witchcraft" might rightly have been included as an essential ingredient. Research has subsequently led to a better understanding of isolation and culture procedures. Now the isolated adult cardiac myocyte has become an important experimental model for the study of myocardial function. Ongoing research with this model includes: studies on cellular growth and hypertrophy; myocyte metabolism; electrophysiology, contractility and response to calcium; the interaction of myocytes with extracellular matrix molecules; myocyte protein synthesis and turnover; biology of myocyte receptors; and gene expression. It is also used to study the biology of myocytes in response to ischemia and myocardial disease processes using cells isolated from myopathic hearts.

Many investigators contributed to knowledge which has led to improved preparations of cardiac myocytes. Among them are 11 grantees who received awards through a special program of the National Heart, Lung, and Blood Institute, "Adult Mammalian Cardiac Myocytes." These grantees met each year to discuss problems and share research findings under the chairmanship of Dr. William A. Clark, who served as consultant to the program.

In response to requests from other investigators to join in these discussions, the grantees organized a workshop, "Biology of Isolated Cardiac Myocytes," at the Asilomar Conference Center, Pacific Grove, California, September 22-25, 1987. Almost 100 scientists assembled for this conference and they represented 8 countries. To the extent possible, their deliberations are summarized in this book.

Of course, as old questions are answered, new questions emerge. To some this is frustrating but it is, after all, the essence of research. Once the preparations became uniformly good, it became obvious that apparently healthy cells in a given preparation were not uniform and the reasons for their heterogeneity now need to be investigated. Furthermore, heterogeneity exists not only among cells, but within cells, where apparently similar regions show variations in activity. Moreover, as they are maintained in culture, where they no longer have to "work", their morphology changes, although they remain viable. The unravelling of these and other mysteries of cardiac cell life will undoubtedly increase understanding of cardiac function and hopefully yield insights into new ways to treat cardiac disease.

Acknowledgements

Special thanks are due to Dr. Paul Simpson, whose creativity in making local arrangements contributed greatly to the discussion which flowed freely throughout the meeting and to Drs. William A. Clark, Robert S. Decker, Thomas K. Borg, Page A.W. Anderson, Robert Haworth, Steven R. Houser, Roy L. White, Beatrice Wittenberg, and Radovan Zak, who served on the Organizing and Scientific Advisory Committees.

Constance Weinstein, Ph.D
Cardiac Diseases Branch
National Heart, Lung, and Blood Institute
National Institutes of Health
Bethesda, Maryland

Myocardial Metabolic Methods

Howard E. Morgan
Sigfried and Janet Weis Center for Research, Geisinger Clinic, Danville, PA 17822

INTRODUCTION

Contractile activity, ion channels, receptors in cell membranes, intracellular signalling, regulation of aerobic and anaerobic metabolism, synthesis of macromolecules and gene expression are events that are important for an understanding of cardiovascular function. When a decision is made to study one of these events, it is vital that a hypothesis is clearly stated and questions are framed that will critically test the hypothesis. The next procedure in the investigative process is the choice of an experimental system in which to seek answers to the questions that have been posed. Ideally, answers to questions dealing with cellular and molecular mechanisms of physiological and pathophysiological events should be sought in the heart of man or of intact unaesthetized animals. Practical limitations as to the types of studies that can be performed have forced investigators to use model systems including anesthetized open-chest animals, isolated organs and cells, cellular organelles and purified macromolecules. As the complexity of the system is reduced, the possibility of obtaining an answer at the molecular level is increased but the relevance of this answer to function of the intact heart becomes less certain.

As examples of questions that can be asked as the reductionist approach proceeds, I will state two hypotheses that relate to overall cardiac function.

1) Oxygen consumption of the heart is determined primarily by the intracellular concentrations of free ionized Ca^{2+} rather than ADP or other phosphate components, and

2) Stretch is the mechanical parameter that links increased heart work to more rapid cardiac growth resulting in cardiac hypertrophy.

The purpose of this paper is to consider what can be measured that will prove or disprove these hypotheses in various experimental systems for studies of the heart and what difficulties are encountered. As the reductionist approach proceeds to the cellular and molecular level what important physiological and pathophysiological stimuli become more difficult to mimic. Advantages and disadvantages of these experimental systems have been the topic of recent reviews [1-3].

WHOLE HEART, IN VIVO

The whole heart in vivo is difficult to study except in terms of integrated metabolism. The major technique that has been used is measurement of arteriovenous (AV) differences of substrates and products in response to changes in substrate concentration, hormone availability, drugs, toxins and heart work. These studies can be carried out in man and closed-chested animals. The advent of new measurement techniques such as positron-emission tomography (PET) and nuclear magnetic resonance (NMR) can provide metabolic data on the intracellular handling of substrates and content of metabolic intermediates.

By the AV difference technique, concentrations of substrates and products in arterial blood can be measured but the difference in these concentrations is likely to be small and subject to large errors. Calculations of rates of uptake and release of substances is dependent upon

Biology of Isolated Adult Cardiac Myocytes
William A. Clark, Robert S. Decker, and Thomas K. Borg, Editors

accurate assessment of coronary flow which is also difficult to obtain. Small biopsies of the heart can be obtained at the time of cardiac catheterization and used for measurement of metabolites and enzyme activity, for preparation of cellular organelles, or for assessment of morphology. Metabolite contents are difficult to interpret because of the delay between the time the biopsy is taken and the time metabolic activity can be stopped by freezing of the tissue. Other difficulties arise if drugs affect the contractility of the heart because substrate utilization and product formation are likely to change as a result of the effect of the drug on contractility rather than directly on a step in metabolism. In the intact heart, heterogeneity due to multiple cell types and to unequal rates of perfusion in various layers of the ventricular wall further complicate the search for molecular mechanisms of metabolic regulation.

In regard to the hypothesis regarding regulation of oxygen consumption, what can be measured in vivo that would bear on the question of whether Ca^{2+} or ADP is the controlling factor. Balaban and co-workers [4] have measured tissue contents of ATP, creatine phosphate and inorganic phosphate during systole and diastole _in vivo_ using P^{31}-NMR. Tissue contents of these metabolites do not change during the cardiac cycle. Measurement of cytosolic ADP concentration is not possible, however, because of the low concentration of ADP and the insensitivity of the NMR method. Free intracellular cytosolic Ca^{2+} cannot be measured _in vivo_ in response to increased preload or afterload or to hormones or drugs. As a result, mechanistic questions relating to control of oxygen consumption by cytosolic concentrations of Ca^{2+} or ADP cannot be addressed in vivo in animals or man.

In regard to the hypothesis that stretch of the ventricular wall, as the result of hypertension or aortic stenosis, is the important mechanical parameter that leads to faster protein synthesis and cardiac hypertrophy [5], little can be done to directly assess this hypothesis in vivo. As a result of pressure overload, end diastolic and end systolic volumes are increased and greater intraventricular pressure is developed. Oxygen consumption, substrate utilization and product formation are increased. The plethora of changes that occur in these circumstances prevents identification of the event that is directly linked to faster rates of protein synthesis. Difficulties in measurement of metabolites, such as cytosolic concentrations of Ca^{2+} and cyclic AMP, prevent even correlative studies of metabolite content and protein synthesis rate from being done. Some of the difficulties in measurement of metabolite content can be overcome by use of open-chest dogs, but the overall experimental situation remains quite complex.

ISOLATED PERFUSED HEARTS

Greater experimental control is achieved by use of isolated hearts perfused as Langendorff or working preparations [1] or of the intraventricular septum perfused via the arterial supply. Bicarbonate buffer containing substrates, hormones and oxygen are used for perfusion via the normal vascular bed. Contractile activity can be arrested with tetrodotoxin or elevated potassium and the ventricle drained while maintaining aortic pressure and coronary flow with a peristaltic pump. The major advantage of the intraventricular septum is the thinness of the preparation that allows for measurements of uptake and release of radioactive compounds on a continuing basis and for assessment of redox state by spectrofluorometric methods.

The metabolic events that can be measured in isolated perfused hearts include 1) consumption of substrates and oxygen or production of metabolites, 2) intracellular metabolites and enzyme activities at a single point in time by rapid freezing of the tissue and assay of metabolites and enzyme activity by spectrophotometric, fluorometric, or immunologic methods. The use of radioactive substrates for assay of metabolites or enzyme activity increases the sensitivity of the assay. These methods do not suffer from the insensitivity of NMR when used for determination of metabolites and intracellular signalling molecules that occur in low concentration within cells. Isolated hearts can be perfused in an NMR spectrometer to continuously measure contents of metabolic intermediates, for example ATP, creatine phosphate and inorganic phosphate in response to a pressure load.

Rates of synthesis of triglycerides, proteins and RNA can be measured using radioactive substrates with simultaneous determination of the specific radioactivity of the immediate precursor pool. The volume of perfusate that must be recirculated per mg of heart tissue is approximately the same as the volume of culture medium that must be used per mg of heart cells, allowing for radioactive labelling of specific proteins to high levels. The perfused heart has the advantage over isolated cells that sufficient tissue is present to allow for measurement of the specific radioactivity of the immediate precursor while cells have the advantage of the ease of repetitive measurements from a single cell preparation.

Difficulties with use of isolated perfused hearts include the heterogeneity of cell type, stability of the preparation for only 3-6h, and expansion of extracellular volume due to use of perfusion medium with low osmotic pressure.

In regard to the hypothesis that changes in cytosolic free Ca^{2+} may modify mitochondrial function by increasing mitochondrial Ca^{2+} and the activity of mitochondrial dehydrogenases, an interesting experiment was performed by McCormack and England using perfused rat hearts [6]. In this experiment, hearts were perfused in the presence and absence of ruthenium red, an inhibitor of mitochondrial calcium transport. During the experiment, the concentration of Ca^{2+} in the perfusate was abruptly increased to 6mM. Changes in cytosolic free Ca^{2+} were monitored by effects on cardiac contractility and the activity of phosphorylase a. Intramitochondrial Ca^{2+} was monitored by measurement of the activity of pyruvate dehydrogenase. In the absence of ruthenium red, increased perfusate Ca^{2+} enhanced contractility and raised the activity of phosphorylase a and pyruvate dehydrogenase. In the presence of the inhibitor of mitochondrial Ca^{2+} uptake, contractility and phosphorylase activity still increased while pyruvate dehydrogenase activity was unaffected by elevation of perfusate Ca^{2+}. These studies indicated that changes in cytosolic Ca^{2+} that were the basis for increased contractility and phosphorylase activity also activated a Ca^{2+}-dependent mitochondrial dehydrogenase. Elevation of pyruvate dehydrogenase activity as a result of an increase in perfusate Ca^{2+} indicates that the intramitochondrial Ca^{2+} content of control mitochondria was sufficiently low to allow dehydrogenase activity to be modified secondary to changes in cytosolic calcium in the physiological range. A complicating factor in interpreting the experiment is the increased contractility and ATP consumption that occurred as a result of elevation of perfusate Ca^{2+} in beating hearts. If elevation of perfusate Ca^{2+} could be shown to increase pyruvate dehydrogenase activity in arrested hearts, the argument supporting a role for cytosolic calcium in controlling mitochondrial metabolism would be further strengthened. Interpretation of the ruthenium red experiment as supporting the Ca^{2+} control hypothesis is also dependent upon the specificity of ruthenium red in blocking mitochondrial Ca^{2+} uptake. In any event, the isolated perfused heart has provided support for the hypothesis that changes in intramitochondrial Ca^{2+} concentration controls mitochondrial metabolism.

The isolated perfused rat heart has also provided useful data to support the hypothesis that stretch of the ventricular wall was the mechanical parameter most closely linked to faster rates of protein synthesis [5,7]. Rat hearts were perfused as Langendorff preparations with buffer that contained tetrodotoxin to arrest cardiac contraction and cannulae were inserted both into the aorta and apex of the left ventricle. The ventricular cannulae was allowed either to hang free or was attached to an overflow reservoir that provided 25mmHg intraventricular pressure. This experimental set up allowed the ventricular wall to be stretched either by increased intraventricular pressure or increased aortic pressure in hearts in which contractile activity was absent and oxygen consumption was unchanged by the intervention. An increase in intraventricular pressure from 0 to 25mmHg in hearts perfused with 60mmHg aortic pressure accelerated protein synthesis [Table 1]. Elevation of aortic pressure to 120mmHg in hearts with zero intraventricular pressure had the same magnitude of effect. Elevation of both aortic and intraventricular pressure had no additive effect. These experiments provided strong support for the hypothesis that stretch was the mechanical parameter linking pressure overload to growth and ultimately hypertrophy of the heart.

TABLE I. Effect of intraventricular pressure and aortic pressure on protein synthesis.

Aortic Pressure, mmHg	Intraventricular pressure, mmHg	Protein Synthesis, nmol phenylalanine $\cdot g^{-1} \cdot h^{-1}$
60	0	632 ± 22
	25	892 ± 24*
120	0	871 ± 35*
	25	892 ± 57*†

Values are means ± S.E. *P<0.05 vs. 60 mmHg aortic pressure, 0 mmHg intraventricular pressure. †P>0.05 vs. 120 mmHg aortic pressure, 0 mmHg intraventricular pressure. Adapted from Xenophontos et al. [7].

HEART SLICES AND ORGAN CULTURE

Two other types of cardiac preparations have been used for cellular and molecular aspects of cardiac function, but in my opinion have limited value as compared to perfused hearts and isolated myocytes.

Cardiac muscle can be sliced cutting only a small proportion of cells. However, the slices must be thin and cut free-hand to prevent restriction of oxygen and substrate supply and crushing of the tissue. Slices have no dependence on vascular integrity for substrate supply and washout of metabolites [2]. Metabolic flux rates, metabolite content, and effects of hormones, anoxia and metabolic inhibitors can be studied in slices. Volume regulation, as reflected in total water content and extracellular volume, can be determined as well as effects of interventions on ultrastructure. Difficulties include the fact that the slice is diffusion limited and has a surface of cut myocytes that introduces heterogeneity into the experimental model. Only single measurements can be made with one slice and contractility cannot be assessed. The availability of tissue is restricted because of the necessity for thin slices. Overall, heart slices have little or no place in studies of cellular and molecular regulatory events.

Organ culture of fetal mouse hearts has the advantage over slices that cells are intact, but the preparation is still diffusion-limited [8,9]. The amount of tissue is small, and the preparation is heterogeneous because of the presence of well-oxygenated and hypoxic cells within the preparation. The major advantage as compared to perfused hearts is the time period over which experiments can be performed. In my opinion, organ culture is of limited value in studying cell biology of the heart.

ISOLATED CARDIAC MYOCYTES

The next step in development of preparations for the study of cardiac metabolism was introduction of isolated heart muscle cell preparations [2,3]. The cells are prepared by digestion of the collagenous framework with proteolytic enzymes and a chelating agent to limit Ca^{2+} availability. Myocytes from embryonic or neonatal cells can be maintained in culture while adult cells are most commonly used as fresh preparations, although adult cells have also been cultured successfully. Dedifferentiation, or perhaps more correctly disorganization of cellular structures, during culture of adult or fetal cells complicates interpretation of metabolic data in relation to the heart in vivo. Fibroblast contamination also is a complication, adding heterogeneity to the experimental model.

Parameters of cardiac cell function can be measured in isolated myocytes that cannot be measured in perfused hearts or more complex intact preparations. Rates of ion flux, binding of radiolabeled ligands, and electrical activity of single ion channels can be measured readily. Furthermore, the investigator can localize the metabolites to cardiac muscle cells. Many studies exploiting these advantages of isolated myocytes are reported in this volume.

Specific radioactivity of precursor pools for RNA and protein synthesis can be measured in cultured myocytes, but these determinations are more difficult because of the limited amount of cells available, especially from fetal or neonatal sources. A clear advantage of isolated myocytes is the ability to measure intracellular free Ca^{2+} and intracellular pH using fluorescent indicators. Concentrations of these intracellular effectors can be measured in cell suspensions or cells adherent to coverslips or in individual cells. Ca^{2+} gradients within cells can be estimated by processing of a video image of the fluorescent dye. These advantages of isolated myocytes may be offset if the myocytes are leaky to Ca^{2+} or if the cells are leaky to Na^{+} and accumulate intracellular Ca^{2+} by Na^{+}/Ca^{2+} exchange. Events that too slow for study in perfused hearts, such as effects of steroid hormones or thyroxine can be explored in isolated myocytes.

Difficulties in the use of myocytes stem in large part from the damage that is done during cell preparation. Digestion of cell surface structures and rupture of gap junctions during preparation may account for greater ion permeability. Loss of cellular constituents during preparation, for example carnitine, can modify metabolism of fatty acids. In 5-20% of cells, damage is so extensive that the rod shape is lost and the cells go immediately into a round contracted form. Heterogeneity resulting from cellular damage may lead to artifacts due to release of degradative enzymes from damaged cells.

In regard to the hypothesis that changes in cytosolic free Ca^{2+} may regulate oxidative metabolism, isolated myocytes offer the best opportunity to test this hypothesis. Measurements of intracellular free Ca^{2+}, oxygen consumption and substrate oxidation can be made on the same cell preparation. Rates of oxygen consumption can be varied, for example by addition of Ca^{2+}, hormones or ionophores to the incubation medium that will increase cytosolic Ca^{2+}.

On the other hand the hypothesis that stretch of cells accelerates protein synthesis is difficult to study in isolated myocytes. Earlier studies by Vandenburgh and Kaufman revealed that stretch of filter discs with adherent skeletal myotubes increased rates of RNA and protein synthesis and decreased protein degradation [10,11]. These studies have been extended to isolated cardiac myocytes by Cooper and his associates

[12]. Stretch of adult cardiac myocytes increased RNA and protein synthesis over 3 days in culture. Molecular dissection of the effect will be difficult in this system because of the limitation on availability of cells.

Another issue that must be addressed in regard to control of growth is the extent to which neonatal cells can serve as models of adult cardiac myocytes. Simpson demonstrated that norepinephrine increased cell size and protein content via an α_1-adrenergic mechanism in cultured neonatal rat myocytes [13]. Cooper and Mann report however that norepinephrine inhibits RNA and protein synthesis in cultured adult rat heart cells [14]. These findings indicate that regulatory mechanisms controlling growth of neonatal cells may differ from those involved in adult heart cells. Further work is needed to clarify similarities and differences in these control mechanisms. At present, we are exploring control of the differential rates of growth in the free walls of the right and left ventricles of isolated perfused neonatal pig hearts to determine the nature of intracellular signalling in this immature heart [15].

HOMOGENATES AND CELLULAR ORGANELLES

Finally, broken cell preparations can be used for preparation of intact cellular organelles such as nuclei, mitochondria and lysosomes or for preparation of membrane systems such as sarcolemma and sarcoplasmic reticulum. Studies of the integrated metabolism of glucose and fatty acids are possible in homogenates, but difficult to interpret because of dilution or generation of cofactors, substrates or allosteric effectors of flux-generating reactions. Flux rates, metabolite concentrations and enzyme activities can be measured and cofactors and substrates can be added. Once the tissue is homogenized, enzyme activity cannot be localized to a specific cell type. In some instances, enzymes redistribute to other cellular structures such as the mast cell protease, chymase, binding to myofibrils [16].

In regard to the hypothesis that cytosolic Ca^{2+} concentrations can control mitochondrial oxidative metabolism, isolated mitochondria have been used as the experimental system. Isolated mitochondria allow for measurement of substrate and oxygen consumption, redox state and ATP production. Transport of materials across the mitochondrial membrane can be assessed by rapid separation of mitochondria from the incubation medium. Difficulties with use of mitochondria relate to their purity and to damage that occurs during preparation. Substances such as cytochrome C can be easily lost and mitochondria can become loaded with Ca^{2+} during their preparation. Until recently, most of the mitochondria that were studied had accumulated sufficient Ca^{2+} during their preparation to obscure control of mitochondrial metabolism by extramitochondrial Ca^{2+}. As a result, one of the most important factors in control of mitochondrial function, the activities of pyruvate dehydrogenase phosphatase, isocitric dehydrogenase and oxoglutarate dehydrogenase in response to increased calcium in micromolar concentrations were obscured from study [17].

Calcium concentrations in the range from 0.1 to 1μM increase activities of these three mitochondrial enzymes approximately 4 fold [18,19,20]. In the case of pyruvate dehydrogenase phosphatase, covalent modification by dephosphorylation results in less enzyme is in the phosphorylated form. However, Ca^{2+} is an allosteric activator of isocitric dehydrogenase and oxoglutarate dehydrogenase. Calcium decreases the Km for isocitrate only in the presence of ADP, an activator of the enzyme. Addition of calcium or ADP alone had no appreciable effect on the affinity of isocitric dehydrogenase for isocitrate. In the case of oxoglutarate dehydrogenase, calcium decreases the Km for oxoglutarate when added alone.

Hansford [17] as well as Denton and McCormack [18,19,20] have proposed a model for energy generation during increased muscular work that is based on the following conditions.

1. Intramitochondrial enzymes catalyzing flux-generating steps are activated by Ca^{++}.

2. Cardiac work and other conditions that require higher rates of energy transduction in the mitochondrion increase free calcium concentrations in the cytosol.

3. Transport processes exist in the mitochondrial membrane for a net inward flux of Ca^{2+} across the mitochondrial membrane, which must reverse when the change in cytosolic calcium concentration reverses.

4. Mitochondrial calcium content in vivo must be in the range that elicits changes in activity of the flux-generating mitochondrial enzymes.

These conditions have been met and the hypothesis that free ionized Ca^{2+} in the cytosol is an important determinant of myocardial oxygen consumption has strong support.

SUMMARY

Isolated perfused hearts, isolated myocytes, properly prepared mitochondria, and purified enzymes have been experimental tools that have provided significant information regarding the role of calcium in controlling the activity of mitochondrial enzymes and oxidative metabolism. Isolated myocytes should be particularly valuable in completing the evidence to support this hypothesis because of the feasibility of cytosolic free Ca^{2+} measurements. The hypothesis that membrane stretch is the mechanical parameter that activates myocardial protein synthesis is supported primarily by studies in perfused hearts and to a limited extent in isolated myocytes. Further exploration of the intracellular signal transducing stretch into faster protein synthesis will benefit from use of isolated myocytes, but the situation may be complicated if the signalling mechanisms are different in adult and neonatal cells. The central feature of a successful experimental outcome is statement of a testable hypothesis and choice of the most appropriate experimental system.

REFERENCES

1. H.E. Morgan and D.L. Siehl in: Methods in Diabetes Research, J. Larner and S. Pohl, eds. (John Wiley and Sons 1984) pp. 211-224.
2. R.B.Jennings and H.E. Morgan in: The Heart and Cardiovascular System, Vol. 1, H. Fozzard, E. Haber, R. Jennings, A. Katz and H. Morgan, eds. (Raven Press 1986) pp. 123-137.
3. A.M. Watanabe, F.J. Green and B.B. Farmer in: The Heart and Cardiovascular System, Vol. 1, H. Fozzard, E. Haber, R. Jennings, A. Katz and H. Morgan eds. (Raven Press 1986) pp. 123-137.
4. H.L. Kantor, R.W. Briggs, K.R. Metz and R.S. Balaban, Am. J. Physiol. 251, H171-H175 (1986).
5. H.E. Morgan, E.E. Gordon, Y. Kira, B.H.L. Chua, L.A. Russo, C.J. Peterson, P.J. McDermott and P.A. Watson, Ann. Rev. of Physiol. 49, 533-543 (1987).
6. J.G. McCormack and P.J. England, Biochem J. 214, 581-583 (1983).
7. X.P. Xenophontos, E.E. Gordon and H.E. Morgan, Am. J. Physiol. 251, C95-C98 (1986).
8. K. Wildenthal, J. Appl. Physiol. 30, 153-157 (1971),
9. K. Wildenthal, E.E. Griffin and J.S. Ingwall, Circ. Res. (Suppl. 1) 38, I-138-I-142 (1976).
10. H.H. Vandenburgh, J. Cell Physiol. 116, 363-371 (1983).
11. H.H. Vandenburgh and S. Kaufman, J. Biol. Chem. 255, 5826-5833 (1980).

12. D. Mann and G. Cooper, J. Mol. Cell. Cardiol. (Suppl. IV) 19, S26 (1987).
13. P. Simpson, Circ. Res. 56, 884-894 (1985).
14. G. Cooper and D.L. Mann, J. Mol. Cell. Cardiol. (Suppl. IV) 19, S25 (1987).
15. C.J. Peterson, H.E. Morgan, V. Whitman and M.H. Klinger, Fed. Proc. 45, 1040 (1986).
16. C.J. Beinlich, M.G. Clark, E.E. McKee, J.A. Lins and H.E. Morgan, J. Mol. Cell. Cardiol. 13, 23-36 (1981).
17. R.G. Hansford, Rev. Physiol. Biochem. Pharmacol. 102, 1-72 (1985).
18. J.G. McCormack and R.M. Denton, Biochem. J. 190, 95-105 (1980).
19. R.M. Denton, D.A. Richards and J.G. Chin, Biochem. J. 176, 899-906 (1978).
20. J.G. McCormack and R.M. Denton, Biochem J. 180, 533-544 (1979).

METHODS FOR THE ISOLATION AND PREPARATION OF SINGLE ADULT MYOCYTES

TREVOR POWELL
University Laboratory of Physiology, Parks Road, Oxford OX1 3PT, U.K.

INTRODUCTION

The major aim of this chapter is to analyze in rather a brief and incomplete manner the techniques available for the isolation of intact cells from the adult mammalian heart. Already one restriction has been included, that of considering hearts from only mammals, this is simply because the author has had direct experience in this particular aspect of the field, but as will be discussed later, this restriction does not seem to preclude the application of experimental procedures described here to heart tissue obtained from any source. As is inevitable, this account will be highly personal in nature and is not in any manner to be viewed as a source reference for the many approaches which have been used for the dissociation of adult cardiac tissue. Although the choice of references cited is of course my responsibility, any omissions should be taken as due to the pressure of brevity and not as any censure or comment on the work concerned. I shall also cover only the isolation of ventricular myocytes, which again is within the remit of my direct experimental experience.

Even given all of the restrictions cited above, it would be pertinent to ask why yet another account should be presented of cell isolation techniques, when a comprehensive review of myocyte characteristics has been published [1,2] (although written more than half a decade ago), and an account given of particular experimental procedures considered important for the successful dissociation of heart tissue [3]? The major reason is quite simple. Even though I have been concerned with single myocytes for more than fifteen years, it is still the case that I am contacted frequently by others entering the field who have had disastrous results from their efforts to obtain single cells. In the case of enquiries concerning my own published work it is invariably the situation that the anxious laboratory had either not followed my protocols <u>exactly</u> or had made some "minor" changes which "did not seem important". I suspect that a similar situation occurs when unsuccessful attempts are made to reproduce procedures published from other sources. In this chapter I shall address the deceptively simple question of identifying the major factors that I consider important for the regular and reproducible preparation of calcium-tolerant ventricular myocytes, <u>in sufficient number</u> to be useful for a wide spectrum of scientific investigations.

ORGAN PERFUSION

I make no apology for starting my analysis with comments about retrograde (or Langendorff) perfusion of the whole heart. It is an absolute essential requirement that this be achieved in a satisfactory manner, since the whole of the isolation procedure depends upon unrestricted access to the tissue vasculature. For those not initiated in the surgical procedures involved, it is advisable to read the clear account presented by Ross [4], on which I have commented previously [3], or to visit a laboratory where Langendorff perfusions are carried out routinely. Following this, it is also advisable to perform retrograde perfusions using standard calcium-containing physiological salt solutions (preferably of the same composition as that to be used in the isolation procedure, but without added enzymes and calcium included at 1.8-2.5 mM) and to measure heart-rate and cardiac output (monitored conveniently by

Biology of Isolated Adult Cardiac Myocytes
William A. Clark, Robert S. Decker, and Thomas K. Borg, Editors

collecting the perfusate descending from the apex of the heart). When stable values are obtained routinely for 1-3 hours, it should be the case that the actual physical cannulation of the organ will not prove the decisive factor in the production of single myocytes.

PERFUSION SOLUTIONS

Those colleagues and associates who have known me during the development of single-cell technology have commented, quite correctly, on my almost paranoic concern with the source and quality of the distilled water which is used for making up the perfusion solutions for myocyte isolation. The reason for this is simple; in the very early days, when there were so many variables which could possibly influence cell yield, I soon noticed that the source of distilled water had a dramatic influence, so much so that for many years in London there was one particular water-still in my laboratory which was used only for producing water for cell-isolation solutions. My concern was not that this should be the case, but rather a failure over the years to detect what characteristics were so important about the water from this particular source. It was certainly not due to the contamination level of calcium or the measured conductivity, or the detectable presence of some trace metals, since analyses of water from many sources showed no marked differences between samples. Fortunately, although this question has never been settled, the availability of membrane water-purifying systems seems to have solved the problem. This contention is based on the many occasions when laboratories have contacted me concerning the fact that their cell yields are minimal or even zero, followed my advice to obtain water from a Milli-Q^R water system (which I have) or an equivalent, and then reported a dramatic increase in cell availability. This is also the first major hurdle to be overcome, obtaining myocytes just once in the laboratory. Even a solitary success indicates that there is no fundamental reason why more successful experiments cannot be accomplished, once protocols have been controlled further.

The basic composition of solutions for cell isolation is simply that of a Krebs-Ringer physiological saline. For rat heart we have used (in mM): NaCl 118.5, $NaHCO_3$ 14.5, KCl 2.6, KH_2PO_4 1.18, $MgSO_4$ 1.18, glucose 11.1; to which fatty acid free bovine albumin is added at 1 mg/ml after the medium had been gassed for at least 30 min with a mixture of O_2 (95%) and CO_2 (5%). For other mammalian hearts (see below), we have also experimented with a Hepes-buffered saline of (also in mM): NaCl 144, KCl 5.4, NaH_2PO_4 0.3, $MgCl_2$ 1.0, glucose 5.6; titrated to pH 7.35 with NaOH and equilibrated with 100% O_2. I have often been asked why a K of about 3.8 mM was used for rat tissue and the reason is simply that this level of K was determined by flame photometry in blood samples taken from the animals used in the experiments. Chemicals used in making up the solutions should be of good quality and particular note should be taken of NaCl, since variations of cell yield can occur when changing from one bottle to another. Likewise, each new batch of albumin should also be checked for effects on cell yield, although we have not resorted to dialysis as further treatment of the powders.

DISSOCIATION PROCEDURES

This section is obviously the most important of the chapter and the most difficult to write. It would be quite straightforward to refer to the numerous research papers or reviews in which our experimental protocols have been detailed and blithely state that, certainly for the last seven years at least, we have never had a failed experiment. While true, this would not be very informative for those urgently requiring a routine preparation of ventricular myocytes. Further, considering the vast activity at present in this field and to the author, who is of course personally biased, too many "new" cell preparation protocols which are merely minor variations of what should now be standard procedures, it would be impossible and rather a misuse of experimental time to check and analyze the suitability of each published variation. I have therefore chosen what for me was the most difficult and potentially dangerous option of conducting a few experiments using variants of the standard protocol to illustrate useful hints on myocyte preparation in general. In doing this I would emphasize yet again that omission of other variations is simply due to arbitrary choice on my part, based on my long experience and the importance of certain central features of all successful techniques.

To do this, I shall concentrate on guinea-pig, rabbit and cat hearts, for when isolating rat ventricular myocytes the method published in 1976 [5,6] still gives cell yields and purities within the published experimental variability [3,5]. The same approach can be used for these other hearts, but I shall now describe the variations we have tested over a small series of experiments. The dissociation solution comprised the Hepes-buffered Ringer described above, to which had been added 20 mM taurine [7], 10 mM creatine [8] and 80 uM $CaCl_2$ (a variation of [3,5,6]). The enzymes used were pre-screened [1,3,5,6] collagenase (Worthington Type 1, 1 mg/ml) and 0.1 mg/ml protease [9-11] (Sigma Type XIV, but Type VII gives similar results). Elastase (10 units/ml) has also been used instead of the protease [10] with no apparent change in yields (for the guinea-pig) compared to those reported here.

Hearts from guinea-pig, rabbit or cat were pre-perfused for 4 minutes [5,6] with Hepes solution to which no calcium had been added (for the guinea-pig 0.1 mM EGTA has also been used [10]) on the same perfusion apparatus developed for rat cells [3,5,6]. After this period the dissociation solution is perfused for 10 minutes and the heart then taken down, sliced and placed in 5 ml of fresh dissociation medium containing 10 mg/ml bovine serum albumin [3,5,6] (Fraction V, Miles Laboratories). This is stirred slowly at 37 °C for 10 minutes, the solution decanted off and replaced with fresh medium and the procedure repeated. The supernatant is centrifuged at low speed [3,5,6] and the cells washed in enzyme-free solution containing the same concentration of albumin and 0.5 mM CaCl2 [3,5,6]. Myocytes are finally resuspended in Dulbellco's MEM (Gibco; with 25 mM Hepes, 1 g/l glucose and 5% (v/v) mycoplasmic-screened horse serum) and stored at room temperature.

These experiments were carried out on hearts taken from 206- 243g guinea-pigs, 0.8-2.0 kg rabbits and 2.0-2.5 kg cats. Heart wet weights were 1-2 g for the guinea-pigs, 3.8-5.8 g for rabbits and 8.3-11.9 g for cats. Yields of cells, given as 10^6 cells per g wet weight of tissue (mean ± s.e.m. (n)), were 2.26 ± 0.20 (17) for the guinea-pig, 3.61 ± 0.71 (7) for the rabbit and 1.32 ± 0.19 (6) for the cat. The purity of cell yields, as measured by the percentage of rod cells counted in quadruplicate in a haemocytometer, is given in Table I.

TABLE I. Proportion of intact cells in successive incubations.

	Incubation 1	2	3	4
Guinea-pig	57.8 ± 2.4(17)	61.1 ± 3.0(16)	61.6 ± 2.1(16)	35.5 (2)
Rabbit	74.3 ± 4.8(4)	78.0 ± 3.9(4)	72.8 ± 4.6(6)	59.7 ± 7.6 (6)
Cat	75.0 ± 3.9(4)	70.8 ± 3.9(4)	66.8 ± 8.1(4)	80.0 (2)

All results given as % rod cells (mean ± s.e.m) with n in brackets.

It must be emphasized that no attempt was made to maximize yields, indeed for the cat there was much tissue remaining at the end of the fourth incubation and the yield as measured in terms of initial heart wet weight can obviously be improved.

What do these results show? In one sense not a great deal, since we do not suffer failed experiments in my laboratory, in any event. However, they demonstrate that it is possible to make variations in protocols and still obtain useful preparations. If only collagenase is used and creatine and taurine are omitted, then cells are still obtained. I included these two compounds through their reported beneficial effects on maintenance of intracellular high-energy compounds, but suspect that control of extracellular calcium during the isolation procedure is still a crucial factor in the successful isolation of cells. Indeed, we have never resorted to the use of post-isolation "recovery medium" [12] and it is interesting to note that the pioneers of this latter approach are now controlling isolation solution levels of calcium at even higher levels than used here to avoid the use of such "power soups" [11]. Another approach is to pre-perfuse the organ with standard calcium-containing saline in order that "recovery" from anoxia induced during removal from the animal be achieved. I have not adopted this for two reasons. Firstly, it is not clear how efficient a simple physiological solution will be for this purpose, since some are of the view that only perfusion with whole blood can preserve function adequately. Secondly and more important, since extracellular Ca is so important, great care needs to be taken to ensure that the isolation solutions are not contaminated by the initial solution containing mM concentrations of this ion. Furthermore, the simple changes made here are more involved than our basic procedures but not as complex as other published protocols (see, e.g. [13]).

CELL VIABILITY

The assessment of "cell viability" depends entirely on the purpose for which the preparation was obtained. In my laboratory we have used isolated myocytes in a wide range of investigations [1-3] and aim to have at least 105 rod-shaped cells in 40-50 ml of final suspension. Of these, only a few ml are required for a day's electrophysiological experiments, the remainder being used for structural and other biophysical studies. In my experience, quiescent rod-shaped calcium-tolerant myocytes offer distinct advantages for a wide range of studies on ventricular mechanisms. The mechanical robustness of the cells is important for electrophysiological studies, with suction pipettes producing the most trauma [14], conventional microelectrodes less [6] and patch-clamp techniques [15] minimal damage to a single cell [17]. The stability of preparation composition and improvement of the percentage of intact cells through culture techniques [8] are of prime importance for transport and biochemical studies.

Any further discussion of techniques for the examination of cell viability within the framework of a particular field of investigation does not seem pertinent here, since many aspects have been covered previously [2,3,13] and additional information is to be found in this volume.

CONCLUSIONS

The preparation of single cells from adult hearts is now a standard procedure in many laboratories. Suspensions containing a high number of intact cells showing good viability require care and good experimental technique and on occasion difficulty has been experienced in some centres in obtaining even minimal yields of myocytes. The cursory examination presented here aims to demonstrate that observation of a few simple rules should alleviate many of the problems and provide isolated cells of sufficient yield and quality for a wide range of cardiac investigations.

REFERENCES

1. J.W. Dow, N.G.L. Harding and T. Powell, Cardiovasc. Res. 15, 483-514 (1981).
2. J.W. Dow, N.G.L. Harding and T. Powell, Cardiovasc. Res. 15,549-579 (1981).
3. T. Powell in: Methods in studying Cardiac Membranes, Vol. 1, N.S. Dhalla, ed. (CRC Press, Boca Raton, 1984) pp. 41-62
4. B.D. Ross, Perfusion Techniques in Biochemistry: A Laboratory Manual (Clarendon Press, Oxford 1972).
5. T. Powell and V. W. Twist, Biochem. Biophys. Res. Commun. 72, 327-333 (1976).
6. T. Powell, D.A. Terrar and V. W. Twist, J. Physiol. 302, 131-153 (1980).
7. R.L. Gao, E.W. Christman, S.L. Luh, J.E. Krauhs, G.F.O. Tyers and E.H. Williams, Arch. Biochem. Biophys. 203, 587-599 (1981).
8. H.M. Piper, I. Probst, P. Schwartz, F.J. Hutter and P.G. Spiekermann, J. Mol. Cell Cardiol. 14, 397-412 (1982).
9. O.T. Bustamante, T. Watanabe and T.F. McDonald, Can. J. Physiol. Pharmacol. 60, 997-1002 (1982).
10. M. Bechem, L. Pott and H. Rennebaum, Eur. J. Cell Biol. 31, 366-369 (1983).
11. Z. Bendukidze, G. Isenberg and U. Klockner, Basic Res. Cardiol. 80, S13-S17 (1985).
12. G. Isenberg and U. Klockner, Pflugers Arch 395, 6-18 (1982).
13. B.B. Farmer, M. Mancina, E.S. Williams and A.M. Watanabe, Life Sci. 33, 1-18 (1983).
14. A.M. Brown, K.S. Lee and T. Powell, J. Physiol. 318, 455-477 (1981).
15. O.P. Hamill, A. Marty, E. Neher, B. Sakmann and F.J. Sigworth, Pflugers Arch. 391, 85-100 (1981).
16. D. Pelzer, G. Trube and H.M. Piper, Pflugers Arch. 400, 197-199 (1984).

CELLULAR ADHESION TO ARTIFICIAL SUBSTRATES AND LONG TERM CULTURE OF ADULT CARDIAC MYOCYTES

THOMAS K. BORG AND LOUIS TERRACIO
Departments of Pathology and Anatomy, School of Medicine, University of South Carolina, Columbia, SC 29208

INTRODUCTION

The extracellular matrix (ECM) of the heart is a complex, three dimensional arrangement of several different classes of macromolecular components [1-3]. These include the interstitial collagen types I, III and V, basement membrane collagen type IV, glycoproteins such as fibronectin and vitronectin as well as the basement membrane glycoproteins, laminin, anchorins and nidogen (entactin), and proteoglycans. In addition to the ECM components, there are also receptors to the specific ECM components found in the plasma membrane of the cardiac myocytes, fibroblasts, endothelial cells and smooth muscle cells of the heart. The individual ECM components and their receptors appear to exhibit both qualitative and quantitative differences during normal development and in certain disease processes such as myocardial hypertrophy [4-9]. Because the ECM is intimately associated with the individual cardiac myocytes, it has been suggested that the ECM may have a functional role in relation to cardiac performance at different stages of development and in disease. However, it is unclear whether the effects of the ECM are a primary or secondary response to various stimuli.

Numerous investigations have shown that when cells are exposed to various types of ECM components _in vitro_, these ECM components have a profound influence on cell function [8,10]. To establish long term cultures of cardiac myocytes, investigators have attempted to duplicate conditions similar to those found _in vivo_. This includes providing the isolated cells with a similar ECM environment _in vitro_ as they are associated with _in vivo_. In order to successfully culture large numbers of adult cardiac myocytes, it appears to be necessary to provide the isolated cells with the proper environment that allows the cells to adapt to culture conditions. Several investigators have now confirmed that there is almost a ten-fold difference in the number of cells progressing into culture when the cells are initially attached to either laminin or type IV collagen which are basement membrane components of cardiac myocytes [8,9]. This chapter will outline the techniques involved in the recognition of isolated cardiac myocytes to various individual ECM components as well as to more complex matrices such as artificial basement membranes and the use of these ECM components to establish high density, long term cultures of adult cardiac myocytes.

EXPERIMENTAL PROTOCOLS FOR CELL ATTACHMENT ASSAYS

Cell isolation

The procedures used in the isolation of cardiac myocytes can affect the number of cells that successfully attach to ECM coated surfaces. The principal reason for this is that the recognition of ECM components is regulated by protease sensitive glycoproteins (receptors) in the sarcolemma [6]. Care should be taken during isolation procedures (which are reviewed elsewhere in this volume) to minimize and standardize the exposure of the cells to proteolytic enzymes found in most preparations of collagenase used for cell isolation. Previous studies have shown that prolonged exposure to

Biology of Isolated Adult Cardiac Myocytes
William A. Clark, Robert S. Decker, and Thomas K. Borg, Editors

collagenase can significantly alter the attachment of myocytes to ECM components [6].

Another critical step in the cell isolation procedure that ultimately affects the number of cells attaching to ECM components is the time the cells are stored prior to plating. This time must be kept to a minimum. Isolated cardiac myocytes do not appear to tolerate being held at temperatures below 30° C. The faster the cells are attached to the substrate, the higher the percentage of cells that will survive in culture. This is especially true for the Ca^{++} stable myocytes. Freshly isolated myocytes that are firmly attached to substrates appear to show a greater tolerance to Ca^{++} than non-attached cardiac myocytes. Myocytes that are rapidly attached to ECM components such as laminin (Ln) or collagen type IV (C-IV) appear to show less spontaneous contraction as well as fewer blebs on the cell surface than those plated on bovine serum albumin (BSA), fetal bovine serum (FBS), or uncoated plastic substrates. This seems to reflect *in vitro* the importance of the basement membrane in myocardial cell structure and function *in vivo*.

Substrate isolation and storage

All of the ECM substrates used for cell attachment are commercially available from a variety of sources. The purity of commercial ECM components is sometimes variable. For example, commercial preparations of laminin contain the glycoprotein nidogen (entactin) and sometimes type IV collagen. For routine attachment and culture these preparations are adequate. If highly purified ECM components are necessary, such as when doing receptor-ligand interactions, then investigators may wish to isolate and characterize the individual ECM component desired. Purification of most of these components has been well described and is beyond the scope of this chapter; however the following references should be helpful: fibronectin [11], interstitial collagens [12], laminin [13], type IV collagen [13], EHS gel [14] and collagen gel [15].

The shelf life of ECM components is variable. Most investigators store ECM glycoproteins such as laminin, fibronectin, vitronectin, and type IV collagen in small aliquots (100 μg) at -80° C and only thaw the amount necessary for current experiments. Interstitial collagens may be stored in 0.5 N acetic acid at 4° C for years. If the ECM component is stored at 4° C for any length of time, sodium azide (0.02%) can be added to prevent bacterial degradation. Caution must be taken to wash plates *very* thoroughly when sodium azide has been used. If the purity of the ECM components is questionable, they can be checked by SDS-PAGE under reducing conditions.

Immobilization of extracellular matrix components

The attachment or immobilization of ECM components, serum or artificial matrices such as collagen gels or tumor basement membranes appear to have different requirements for proper binding to the surface to the culture dish. The choice of plasticware can influence the attachment of the components. Bacteriological grade plastic petri dishes (such as Falcon 1008 from Falcon Plastics) have been used in numerous investigations. Petri dishes have a hydrophobic surface that when coated with purified ECM glycoproteins become hydrophilic. This simple observation allows the investigator to determine that the dishes are properly coated. Tissue culture grade dishes can also be used with the purified ECM components. When collagen gels or artificial basement membranes are used they require tissue culture grade plastic dishes for proper attachment. In general, collagens and glycoproteins such as fibronectin and laminin coat the dishes in a multilaminar manner. This means that binding of the substrate to the plastic does not necessarily show a plateau [16] but will continue to bind to itself even at high concentrations. In practice this does not present a problem since most cells do show attachment plateaus to ECM components usually between 5 to 10 μg/well (Fig. 1).

In general, for isolated cardiac myocytes, glycoproteins such as fibronectin, laminin and collagen type IV should be applied at a concentration of 10 μg/ml of medium or buffer (such as PBS, Hanks' or Moscona's). This operation should be done in the cold, especially with collagens since collagens can easily become denatured even at room temperature. The glycoproteins such as laminin and fibronectin can be used to coat plastic dishes by incubating for a minimum of 30 minutes at 37° C. Most investigators; however, prefer to coat plastic dishes overnight at 4° C. In either case, the dishes should be thoroughly wash (3X) before plating with the cells. It is important to note that if the ECM component has been stored with sodium azide or acetic acid (collagens), the plates must be washed very thoroughly to prevent toxicity to the cells. To prevent non-specific binding, the plates/dishes can be coated with 1% BSA in PBS for 15-30 minutes; however, this procedure has been shown to have little to no effect on attachment of adult cardiac myocytes [9]. When myocytes are going to be used for cell culture the substrate should be sterile if possible and sterile technique used to wash the dishes prior to plating.

When artificial basement membranes or collagen gels are used, it is recommended that tissue culture grade plasticware be used. The basic procedure for formation of collagen gels has been previously described [15] as has the procedure for making gels from basement membrane extracts [14]. The advantage of these types of substrates is that they are believed to mimic the in vivo extracellular environment better than single ECM components. Ultrastructurally and biochemically the tumor basement membranes, such as the EHS gel, contains defined proportions of laminin, type IV collagen, heparin sulfate proteoglycan, and nidogen [14]. The advantage of collagen gels is that ECM components can be added to the polymerization mixture so that the final gel contains ECM components in addition to collagen. This latter procedure allows the investigator to use the structural framework of the collagen gel and also assess the interaction with other ECM components [17]. However, there have been very few investigations in this area and more work is necessary to determine the concentrations of various ECM components added to gels, how these individual components interact with the collagen in the gel, and what affects these components have on adult myocyte structure and function.

Quantitation of cell attachment

The number of cells that attach to the substrate coated dishes can be measured by a variety of procedures including: 1) direct cell counts; 2) enzyme assays; and 3) protein measurements. After plating the cells for a defined time period the dishes are gently washed to remove the loosely bound cells. It is important that the shear force generated by the washing procedure be applied in a consistent manner since the number of cells remaining on the dish can vary with the vigor of the washing process. Cells counts can be done by several different methods. Attached cells can be fixed and the number of cells in a pre-determined number of defined microscope fields can be counted on stained samples or by phase microscopy and the data expressed as cells/mm^2 of culture surface. Alternatively, after washing, cells can also be removed by trypsinization (0.1% trypsin, 1 mM EDTA in PBS at pH 7.4) and counted with a hemacytometer or electronic particle counter. Cell counting methods are labor intensive and require great care to prevent the introduction of error. Possible sources of error include variability from microscope field to microscope field, inherent variability in either mechanical or electronic counters and failure to remove all the cells by trypsinization. However, microscopic cell counts are the best methods if the purpose is to determine the number of cells that progress into culture or to determine the fate of individual cells in response to specific stimuli.

Enzymatic assays are probably the most accurate or at least the most reproducible. Measurement of the cytosolic enzyme, lactate dehydrogenase (LDH), has been used to determine the number of cells for both neonatal and adult heart cells [6,8]. Following washing of the attached cells, they are lysed with a solution containing Triton X-100 and BSA in PBS. The lysates are combined with NADH and pyruvate, the decrease in absorbance at 340 nm is measured with a spectrophotometer and the values compared to the standards made by lysing a known number of cells [6,8]. The details of this assay have been clearly described for hepatocytes [18] and for cardiac myocytes [6,8]. The LDH assay is only sensitive and accurate when the numbers of cells per dish is large (1×10^6) and is somewhat time consuming to run. This is not always feasible for assaying the number of adult cells where the number of cells per heart can be somewhat low especially when using small animals. A more sensitive enzymatic assay has been successfully applied to a wide variety of cells including both neonate and adult cardiac myocytes [19,20]. This assay is based on measurement of the enzyme hexosaminidase and utilizes microtiter plates that can be directly measured in a spectrophotometer. This assay can be used with far fewer cells than the LDH procedure with no sacrifice in sensitivity. Although the assays for cell adhesion can be done in microtiter plates, it is more convenient to use 24 well multiwell plates for heart cell attachment assays. The principal reasons for using 24-wells is that they reduce cell-cell interactions and minimize surface tension effects seen in 96 well plates. This assay uses fewer cells (1×10^4) and is much less time consuming than the LDH method. 24-well plates are coated as previously described, the cells are plated and allowed to attach for a given time period. The substrate for hexosaminidase is p-nitrophenol-N-acetyl-B-D-glucosaminide and is prepared by dissolving the substrate at a concentration of 7.5 mM in 0.1 M citrate buffer at pH 5. This solution is mixed with an equal volume of 0.5% Triton X-100 in water and stored at -20° C. The standard curve can be constructed by placing a known number of cells in the substrate containing Triton X-100 and then diluting this mixture during the incubation period (see below). Following washing of the cells, 200 ul of the substrate/Triton mixture is added to each well. At this point the plate may be frozen and stored for development at a later time. A given sample (usually 50 or 100 ul) is removed from the each well and added to an individual well of a microtiter plate. The cell suspension of known concentration is added to the same plate by serial dilution for determination of a standard curve based on cell number. For development, the plate is incubated at 37° C in 100 % humidity. The time of development is proportional to the amount of enzyme present and for adult cardiac myocytes we routinely use 4 hr of development. The color reaction is developed and the enzymatic reaction stopped by the addition of 90 ul of 50 mM glycine buffer at pH 10.4. The 96-well plate is read at 405 nm in a Titertech multiscan spectrophotometer and the number of cells determined by comparison of the absorbance to the standard curve.

Recognition of artificial substrates by isolated cells

The characterization of the receptor-ECM interaction has been well documented by several laboratories and recently reviewed [21]. There appear to be some species differences in the ability the myocytes to attach to different ECM components; however, these differences may be due to the variability of the isolation procedure (different collagenases, time of exposure to the collagenase, etc) rather than a difference in the number of receptors for a specific ECM component.

One consistent observation throughout these investigations has been that the basement membrane components, laminin and collagen type IV, show the best attachment as well as the ability to allow the myocytes to progress into culture (Fig. 1 and 2) [8,9,25]. Attachment of adult myocytes to interstitial collagens is usually poor (Fig. 1). This observation is difficult to explain since the macromolecular complex containing the collagen receptor is present on freshly isolated adult myocytes although not in as high a concentration as in neonatal or hypertrophied myocytes [22]. The susceptibility of ECM receptors to proteolytic degradation is well-known and the collagen receptor is more sensitive than the complex for fibronectin or vitronectin [6]. It is also possible that the active site of the receptor is damaged or masked at the time of isolation. What ever the explanation, adult cardiac myocytes do not attach in high numbers to interstitial collagen substrates.

Several reports have shown that adult cardiac myocytes attach in fairly large numbers to serum coated dishes. Presumably the mechanism of attachment is via fibronectin and/or vitronectin receptors; although the latter has not been demonstrated on adult cardiac myocytes at this time. The addition of serum in combination with other ECM components does not have an additive, synergistic or competitive effect. The same is true for the addition of BSA. Attachment to fibronectin seems to be somewhat species-dependent (Fig. 1). In assays using rat cardiac myocytes, attachment to human or bovine fibronectin is relatively poor whereas attachment to rat fibronectin is much better. The rate of progression into culture is also increased on rat fibronectin over human or bovine fibronectin (Fig. 2). However, the attachment to fibronectin is still much less than that observed on laminin or collagen type IV (Fig. 1).

There have been only a few reports of the attachment of isolated cardiac myocytes to collagen gels or basement membrane gels [23]. In general, these substrates do not seem to work as well as the single components. This may be because the "right combination" of components in the gel has not yet been found or that masking of specific attachment sites on individual ECM components by other components such as proteoglycans, may occur. Cardiac myocytes on EHS tumor basement membrane tend to round up and form aggregates rather than a layer of individual cells. Although there is great potential to create a compatible ECM gel, it may have to wait until our knowledge of the precise molecular composition of the adult heart ECM is known.

LONG TERM CULTURE OF ADULT CARDIAC MYOCYTES

Many investigations require the long term maintenance of cardiac myocytes <u>in vitro</u> and there have been numerous attempts to culture adult cardiac myocytes [24]. For long-term culture, care must be taken to minimize contamination of the cells during the isolation procedure. The perfusion apparatus should be autoclaved prior to initial use. After isolation of the cells, the apparatus should be rinsed extensively with sterile PBS containing 100 U/ml penicillin, 100 μg/ml streptomycin followed by 70% ethanol and then with sterile distilled water. If this rinsing procedure is carefully followed and no residual medium is allowed to remain in the system, re-autoclaving is not required between isolations. If one experiences problems with contamination or decreased yield, the system

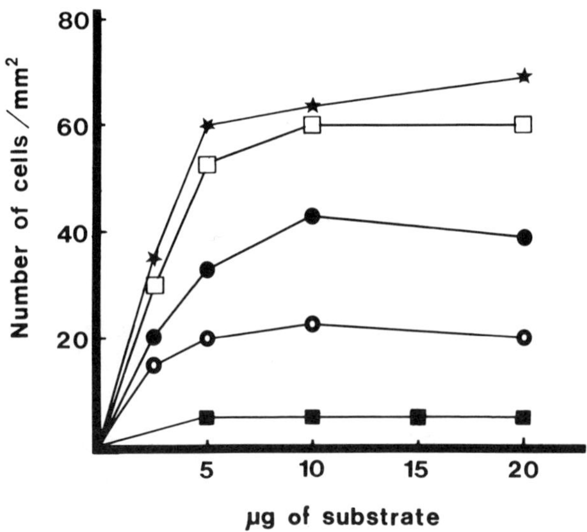

Figure 1. Attachment of adult cardiac myocytes to ECM components. Laminin (★) and collagen type IV (□) result in the greatest number of attached cells. Collagen I (■) essentially does not support attachment. There appears to be a species difference for fibronectin with rat fibronectin (●) supporting the attachment of more cells than human fibronectin (O).

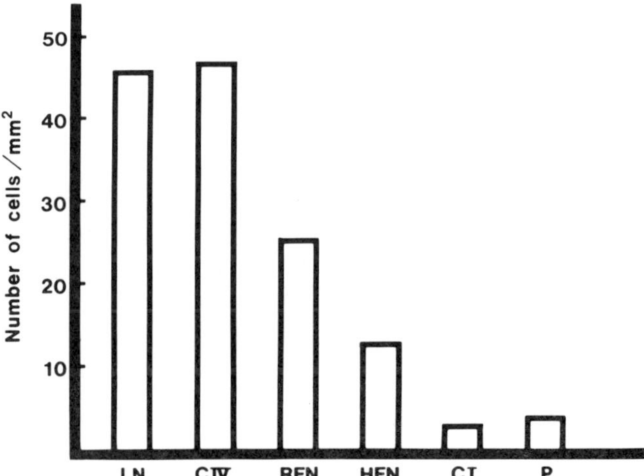

Figure 2. This bar graph represents the number of cells present in culture after 14 days. The cells were initially attached to the ECM substrates and cultured in F12K containing 20% FBS, antibiotics and 10 ng/ml of ARA-C. Laminin (LN), collagen type IV (CIV), rat fibronectin (RFN), human fibronectin (HFN), collagen I (CI), tissue culture plastic (P).

serum (see below), DMEM, F12K, Medium 199, RPMI 1640 and Ham's F12 have all been able to support adult myocytes in high density, long term culture in our laboratory.

Serum appears to be essential for spreading and progression of adult cardiac myocytes into culture. When cells are maintained serum-free attached to laminin or type IV collagen, they maintain their rod-shaped morphology at the light microscope level for up to 10 days in culture. However, there is a constant loss of cells over the 10 day period. Similar results have been reported by Piper using FBS coated substrates [24]. Although chemically defined media does exist for the long-term culture of neonatal cardiac myocytes [28], this type of system has not been perfected for adult cardiac myocytes at this time. Recently it has been demonstrated that after adult myocytes have been attached to laminin and maintained in serum containing medium for 5-7 days, they can be switched to the serum-free medium such as PC1 (Ventrex, Portland, ME) without a loss of cell number or viability [29].

The type and concentration of serum can also play an important role in the culturing of adult cardiac myocytes. We have used FBS, horse serum, newborn bovine serum, adult bovine serum and FBS mixed in various ratio's with each of the other sera to maintain adult cardiac myocytes in long term culture. There is variability from lot to lot of serum and thus serum should be tested for suitability prior to purchase. We routinely test lots of serum for their ability to support adult myocytes in long-term cultures. This involves counting the number of adult cells that progress into culture at 14 days on each type of serum or serum mixtures. Our experience is that routinely FBS (12-20%) or horse serum-FBS (10% each) give superior results to the other sera or combinations of sera. Once a superior lot(s) of serum has been identified we purchase a large volume so that this variable component (type and concentration of sera) can be kept constant for a complete series of experiments.

Isolation of adult heart cells results in a mixture of rod-shaped and round (usually less viable) myocytes and non-myocytes (principally fibroblasts). When establishing a long-term culture of myocytes in the presence of serum, the problem of controlling proliferation of non-myocytes in the cultures must be addressed. Since there is such a large size difference between the myocytes and non-myocytes most of the non-myocytes can be eliminated by density sedimentation before plating [30]. Although single step gradients of Percoll or Ficoll work well, we have found that 5% BSA in culture medium works just as well and may provide a better, non-toxic, environment for the cells. We have found that a 1 minute centrifugation at 50 X g in 5% BSA in F12K repeated 3 times, essentially separates the myocytes from the single non-myocyte cells. The myocytes readily pellet while the non-myocytes remain in the 5% BSA culture medium. Although the sedimented myocytes are highly enriched (greater than 99% by cell counts), a few non-myocytes still remain either by adhering to the myocytes and co-sedimenting or by being trapped among the cellular debris. For long-term culture, additional steps must be taken to eliminate the overgrowth of the cultures by the non-muscle cells.

Since mitosis in adult ventricular myocytes is essentially non-existent, the use of cytosine arabinoside (10 ng/ml ARA-C) [8,31] can be used as a potent anti-mitotic agent. Routinely we add ARA-C to the cultures for 7-10 days, then remove it. Since the cultures are not fully adapted to the culture conditions and not usually used for experiments until 14 days *in vitro*, this allows for the ARA-C to be removed and cleared from the cultures prior to experimentation. The use of ARA-C coupled with density sedimentation virtually eliminates fibroblasts from the long term cultures of adult myocytes. The percentage of myocytes in a culture preparation can be determined by staining with a muscle specific antibody against actin (HHF-35; see chapter on Immunohistochemistry in this volume). Immunofluorescent staining of replicate cultures treated as above, routinely average greater than 98% myocytes.

A number of investigators separate the rod-shaped (viable) myocytes from the less viable round myocytes using gradient centrifugation procedures [32]. However, we have found that only viable myocytes, regardless of shape, will attach to laminin and type IV collagen and spread in culture. Thus there is no need to separate the rod-shaped and round myocytes prior to plating. The non-viable cells will be removed when the cells are washed and fed with the culture medium.

SUMMARY

The following is the routine procedure used in our laboratory to establish long-term cultures of rat ventricular myocytes. Although variations of this procedure work and may be required for different species, this procedure will provide a starting point for those investigators initially trying to culture adult cardiac myocytes.

1. Isolate the cells using the procedures described by Lundgren et al. [7].
2. Wash the cells 3 times in 5 % BSA-DMEM or F12K by centrifugation at 50 x g for 1 min (total spin time including deceleration).
3. Plate the cells in DMEM or F12K containing 0.5% BSA on laminin coated (10 μg/ml) dishes for 60 minutes at 37° C in a humidified atmosphere of 5% CO_2 in air. The plates are coated and washed as described in this chapter.
4. Gently remove the plating medium by aspiration being careful not to leave the cells dry. Wash the dishes with DMEM or F12K containing 20% FBS and 100 U/ml penicillin and 100 μg/ml streptomycin, remove by aspiration and feed the cells with the same medium containing 10 ng/ml ARA-C.
5. The cultures are maintained in an incubator at 37° C in a humidified atmosphere of 5% CO_2 in air and fed every third day with DMEM or F12K, 20% FBS, antibiotics and ARA-C. The ARA-C is eliminated after 10 days *in vitro*.

ACKNOWLEDGEMENTS

The authors would like to thank Evy Lundgren for collaborating in the past and hopefully the future. The authors also would like to thank Willa Gibbemeyer for secretarial assistance. Supported by NIH Grants HL 33656, HL 37669 and HL 24935.

REFERENCES

1. J.B. Caulfield, and T.K. Borg, Lab. Invest. 40, 364 (1979).
2. T.K. Borg, L. Terracio, E. Lundgren, and K. Rubin in: Cardiac Morphogenesis, V. Ferrans, G. Rosenquist, and C. Weinstien, eds. (Elsevier, Amsterdam 1985) pp.69-77.
3. T.F. Robinson, L. Cohen-Gould, and S.M. Factor, Lab. Invest. 49, 482 (1984).
4. T.K. Borg, L.M. Klevay, R.E. Gay, M.E. Bergin, and R. Siegel, J. Mol. Cell. Cardiol. 17, 1173 (1985).
5. T.K. Borg, J. Buggy, T. Sullivan, J. Lax, and L. Terracio, J. Mol. Cell. Cardiol. 18, 247 (1986).

6. T.K. Borg, K. Rubin, E. Lundgren, K. Borg, and B. Obrink, Devel. Biol. 104, 86 (1984).
7. E. Lundgren, T.K. Borg, and S. Mardh, J. Mol. Cell. Cardiol. 16, 355 (1984).
8. E. Lundgren, L. Terracio, S. Mardh, and T.K. Borg, Exp. Cell Res. 158, 371 (1985).
9. E. Lundgren, L. Terracio, and T.K. Borg, Basic Res. Cardiol. 80, 69 (1985).
10. M.J. Bissell, H.J. Hall, and G. Parry, J. Theor. Biol. 99, 31 (1981).
11. S.K. Akiyama, and K.M. Yamada, J. Biol. Chem. 260, 4492 (1985).
12. E.J. Miller, and R.K. Rhodes, Methods of Enzymol. 82, 33 (1982)
13. M.Paulsson, M. Aumailley, R. Deutzmann, R. Timpl, K. Beck, and J. Engel, Eur. J. Biochem. 166, 11 (1987).
14. H.K. Kleinman, M.L. McGarvery, J.R. Hassell, V.L. Star, F.B. Cannon, G.W. Laurie, and G.R. Martin, Biochem. 25, 312 (1986).
15. T. Esdale, and J. Bard, J. Cell Biol. 54, 626 (1972).
16. K. Rubin, A. Olberg, M. Hook, and B. Obrink, Exp. Cell Res. 117, 165 (1978).
17. F.M. Funderburg, and R. R. Markwald, J. Cell Biol.103, 2475 (1986).
18. B. Obrink, Methods of Enzymol. 82, 513 (1982).
19. U. Landegren, J. Immunol. Methods 67; 379 (1984).
20. E. Lundgren, L. Terracio, D. Gullberg, M. Terracio, T.K. Borg, and K. Rubin, J. Cell Physiol. Submitted (1987).
21. R.O. Hynes, Cell 48, 549 (1987).
22. L. Terracio, D. Gullberg, K. Rubin, S. Craig, and T.K. Borg, Anat. Rec. Submitted (1987).
23. L. Terracio, A. Dewey, K. Rubin, and T.K. Borg in: Proc. Ann. E.M.S.A., G.W. Bailey, ed. (San Francisco Press, Inc, San. Francisco 1986) pp. 270-271.
24. S.L. Jacobson, and H.M. Piper, J. Mol. Cell. Cardiol. 18, 661 (1986).
25. J. Haddad, M.L. Decker, L-C. Hsieh, M. Lesch, A. Sammarel, and R.S. Decker, Am. J. Physiol. (Cell Physiol.) In Press (1987).
26. W.C. Claycomb, and N. Lanson, In Vitro 20, 647 (1984).
27. C.F. Meier, G.M. Briggs, and W.C. Claycomb, J. Applied Physiol. 250, H731 (1986).
28. P. Libby, J. Mol. Cell. Cardiol. 16, 803 (1984).
29. L. Bulgasky, and R. Zak, J. Cell Biol. 103, 119a (1986).
30. T. Powell, and V.W. Twist, Biochem. Biophysic. Res. Comm. 72, 327 (1976).
31. E. Lundgren, L. Terracio, D.O. Allen, and T.K. Borg, In Vitro, In Press (1987).
32. B.A. Wittenberg and T.F. Robinson, Cell Tiss. Res. 216:231 (1981).

MORPHOLOGICAL APPROACHES TO THE STUDY OF FRESHLY ISOLATED AND CULTURED ADULT CARDIAC MYOCYTES

Robert S. Decker* **, Marlene L. Decker*, David G. Simpson** and Michael Lesch*. Departments of Medicine (Cardiology),* Cell Biology and Anatomy**, Northwestern University Medical School, 303 E. Chicago Ave., Chicago, IL 60611

The complex organization of the heart and the syncitial properties of its resident myocytes limits the extent to which the biochemical, physiologic and structural characteristics of individual myocardial cells can be garnered in a continually flucuating environment that alters the demands placed on the heart. Another major problem confronting any study of cardiac function is the heterogeneous population of cells present in all myocardial preparations. This diverse cellular population prevents an unequivocal interpretation of "myocytic responses" since it is not presently feasible to dissociate the contribution of the myocytes (which make up 20% of the cardiac cells, but constitute 80% of the myocardial mass) from those of the endothelial and connective tissue cells (which comprise 80% of the heart cells), especially in circumstances that involve pathological changes in the heart [1]. In the past decade the isolation and culture of calcium tolerant adult cardiac myocytes prepared by both enzymatic [2] and physical [3] methods has become an increasingly popular approach to directly study a variety of structure-function relationships in the heart. These calcium tolerant preparations offer unique advantages in the study of myocytic function. They provide a homogeneous population of muscle cells relatively free from other myocardial interstitial cells which frequently contaminate fetal and neonatal cultures. These myocytes can be exposed to a myriad of culture conditions without the uncertainty of capillary and extracellular diffusion processes which operate within the intact heart. Moreover, the isolated cells are free of hormonal and neural influences and, consequently, environmental manipulation is relatively uncomplicated in this paradigm. A preparation of adult cells may also reduce the ambiguities of experimental interpretation; for example, since the observations are retrieved from adult myocytes, they are likely to be directly relavent to the physiologic and/or pathophysiologic state of the heart from which they were derived. As such, cultured adult myocytes represent a novel model system to investigate adult myocardial function at the cellular level.

Freshly isolated, calcium tolerant cardiac myocytes display structural features that are essentially indistinguishable from those of the intact heart [4,5,6,7]. Transmission electron microscopy combined with a morphometric analysis of the relative volume densities of the myofibrillar apparatus, mitochondria, T-tubules and the sarcoplasmic reticulum reveals that freshly prepared myocytes closely resemble their <u>in situ</u> counterparts [5,7]. Nevertheless, the stability of such preparations can vary considerably [8,9,10] and as such, several parameters are judged to be reliable indicators of cell viability and quality. They include the maintenance of (1) high energy phosphate pools [6,10,11,12], (2) electrical excitability [3, 6,10] and (3) rod-shaped morphology [10], with the latter two features being the easiest and most dependable properties with which to monitor the quality of the newly isolated cells. When myocytes from such preparations are explanted into cell culture, a dramatic morphologic transformation attends prolonged culture, regardless of whether the cells are plated directly onto native plastic surfaces [13,14,15,16] or attached to an extracellular substratum such as fetal bovine serum [6,17] or laminin [12,18,19]. In the case of the former, the calcium tolerant myocytes begin to gradually round within a few hours to a

Biology of Isolated Adult Cardiac Myocytes
William A. Clark, Robert S. Decker, and Thomas K. Borg, Editors

few days, losing their rod-shaped configuration and many of their myotypic features [15,16, 20,21]. A reasonable proportion of these rounded myocytes ultimately attach to plastic, spread and reacquire a morphology characteristic of their rod-shaped progenitors [20, 21]. In contrast, myocytes plated onto plastic precoated with either serum [6,11] or laminin [7,18,19,22] rapidly attach as rod-shaped cells and retain this configuration for 1-2 weeks when maintained in serum-free culture media [22]. When such "rapidly attached" [10] cultures are supplemented with serum, the rod-shaped myocytes spread and flatten during the second week of culture [7,18,19]. Such cells appear indistinguishible from those that "redifferentiate" [10] on plastic surfaces [20,21]. If either the "redifferentiated" or "rapid attachment" models [10] are to be employed to further investigate the biological properties of adult cardiac myocytes,a thorough morphological study will be an absolute requisite to any biochemical or physiological experiments conducted on myocardial cell function _in vitro_. Toward this end, we will review a variety of light microscopic and ultrastructural methodologies that can be usefully employed to examine the structural modifications that accompany the isolation and primary culture of these heart cells, and a variety of examples are included to illustrate the value of these morphological approaches.

LIGHT MICROSCOPY

Traditionally, freshly isolated cardiac myocyte preparations are routinely examined by _phase contrast microscopy_. The enhanced contrast created by incorporating a phase plate into the rear focal plane of the objective lens and an annulus into the condenser, diffracts the speciman image one-half wave length out of phase with the

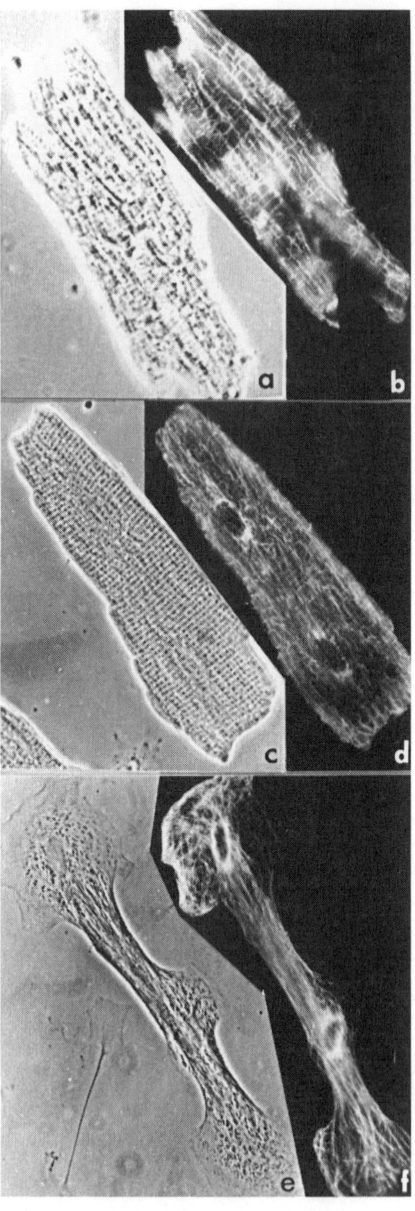

Fig. 1. Phase contrast and fluorescent images of non-overlayed (a,b) and agarose-overlayed (c,d) 1 day myocytes. 7 day cells (e,f) are non-overlayed.b,d and f stained for microtubules

background light and in this way, ordinarily invisible phase retarding objects (i.e., subcellular organelles) produce a dark, clear image in focus. However, by its very nature, phase halos are generated at the cell-medium interface and "optical noise" is produced in the image plane by out-of-focus objects. While these negative features don't seriously detract from the final image of extensively spread cultured cells (e.g., fibroblasts, endothelial cells or spreading myocytes [14]), they become a major concern when examining freshly isolated adult myocytes which range in diameter from 10-30 um [10]. Images of such cells reveal pronounced phase halos and a significant amount of interference [Fig. 1a] is generated by out of focus organelles above and below the plane of focus. This added depth may also interfer with the resolution of <u>fluorescent</u> images [Fig. 1b] whether viewed via epiilluminated or transmitted light. Again the inability to resolve scattered fluorescent signals at different depths in the cell, dramatically increases the optical noise of the final image. Recently, however, Fukui and associates [23] demonstrated that over-laying cells with a thin [0.15mm] layer of 2% agarose and removing culture medium by blotting the agarose with filter paper, gently compresses the myocytes and markedly improves their phase image [Fig. 1c]. Such flattened cells can then be fixed and studied by immunofluorescence microscopy as well. Figure 1d illustrates the enhanced resolution this protocol affords in assessing the distribution of microtubules in freshly prepared myocytes (compare 1b with 1d). As the myocytes spread in culture the requirement of over-laying diminishes and excellent phase [Fig. 1e] and fluorescent [Fig. 1f] images can be obtained without difficulty.

Many of the problems created by phase contrast microscopy can be circumvented by using <u>differential interference contrast(DIC)</u> microscopy. The contrast of the DIC image is produced by a gradient of optical paths created by Wollaston beam splitting prisms. Thus, in both Smith (Leitz) - or Normarski (Zeiss)- type DIC, the image has a shadowcast appearance that is reminiscent of a three-dimensional reconstruction of the myocyte [Fig. 2a, c]. Not only is the DIC image "natural," but the Wollaston beam splitting prisms produce an "optically sectioned" profile that is remarkably shallow, creating excellent depth of field discrimination. Moreover, unlike phase contrast, the DIC image is free of halos and disturbances from objects above and below the focal plane; therefore, DIC produces an image of pleasing contrast, neatly sectioned and isolated out of a complex three-dimensional phase object. Conventional Smith-or Normarski-DIC optics generate good contrast with the condenser iris diaphragm partly stopped down. However, using a 1.32-NA (numerical aperature) rectified condenser coupled with a Plan APO (100/1.32NA) oil immersion objective, DIC profiles of excellent contrast and resolution can be obtained. From such DIC profiles, for example, far more accurate morphometric measurements can be obtained than from corresponding phase contrast images.

Because DIC optics employ rectified, stress-free lenses with high numerical aperatures (NA) arranged for Koehler illumination, the DIC microscope can be rapidly converted into a <u>polarizing microscope</u> by simply replacing the objective lenses with Wallaston prisms with stress-free, brightfield achromatic lenses of high NA. Visualizing isolated myocytes at cross polars illustrates the highly birefringent properties of their contractile apparatus [Fig. 2b,d]. Polarized light microscopy has been used to study the assembly, function and disassembly of the mitotic spindle [24] and Fuseler <u>et al</u>, [25] have demonstrated its utility in the study of cultured neonatal heart cells. With achromatic objective lenses of high NA and matched condensers, an image resolution of slightly better than 0.2um can be achieved free of anomalous diffraction interference. Since a marked reorganization of the myofibrillar apparatus attends prolonged culture of isolated myocytes [20,21], polarizing microscopy in combination with DIC microscopy should provide a useful approach to study the reorganization of birefringent contractile elements in these cells [Fig. 2a-d].

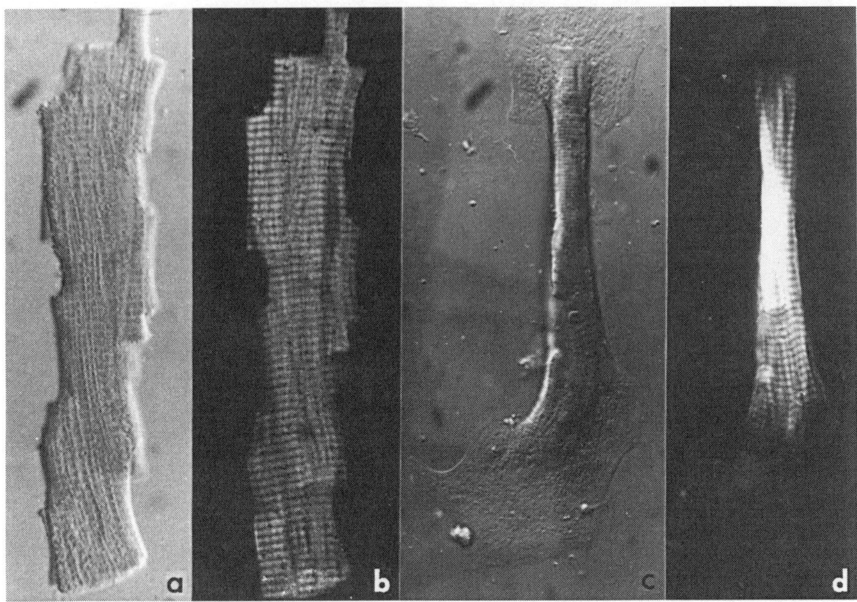

Fig. 2. DIC (a,c) and polarizing (b,d) images of freshly isolated myocytes (a,b) and those cultured for one week (c,d).

Of major concern to all of us that are culturing adult myocytes is the progressive detachment and loss of cells during prolonged culture [10,11,12]. In an attempt to determine why some cells lose contact with the substratum and detach while others do not, myocytes maintained on coverslips were examined with <u>interference reflection microscopy (IRM).</u> Several years ago Curtis [26] and Izzard and Lochner [27,28] demonstrated that the interference patterns observed in reflected light at a high numerical aperature (NA>1) originated from a thin film of medium between the cell and the substratum. Based on the intensity of these interference patterns and a comparison with DIC images, focal contacts of 10-15nm and close contacts of about 30nm cell-substrate separation could be recognized in living chick heart fibroblasts [27,28]. Both classes of contacts have subsequently become associated with firm cell-substrate attachment and active cell spreading [28]. Like DIC and polarizing microscopy, live or fixed cells can be studied by IRM. Coverslips are placed in Rose chambers and inverted on a Zeiss Photomicroscope II equipped with a type II C vertical illuminator, a reflector insert carrying an aperature stop and a 100/1.25 NA epiplanachromat POL oil immersion objective lens. Epiilumination is supplied by a Zeiss 75W xenon source and a 546nm interference filter. Both the xenon and tungsten light sources are used with Calfex heat-reflecting filters which are inserted between each light source to minimize damage to living cells. IRM observations on adult cardiac myocytes reveal that two distinct patterns of focal contact develop during the first and second weeks of culture. In the distal spread zones of, perhaps, half the cardiac myocytes, a black punctate interference pattern develops which can easily be distinguished from the classical low intensity elongate focal contacts seen in the adjacent cardiac fibroblast [Fig. 3a]. Other myocytes display reflection patterns similar to those observed in fibroblasts [Fig. 3b]. These provocative results are consistent with the notion that myocytes which fail to assemble elongate, fibroblast-like focal contacts as they spread may not make sufficient contact with the substratum and, thus, detach as the cells round-up or during the exchange of medium. Examination of such cells with DIC microscopy further illustrates that these regions lack stress fibers that are closely associated with focal adhesions [28]. Future ultrastructural investigation is required to determine whether such myocytes fail to establish focal contacts, because they are unable to elaborate stress fibers which have been previously associated with the development of adhesive contacts in neonatal cardiac myocytes [29]. IRM and DIC microscopy provide a powerful approach to study such relationships.

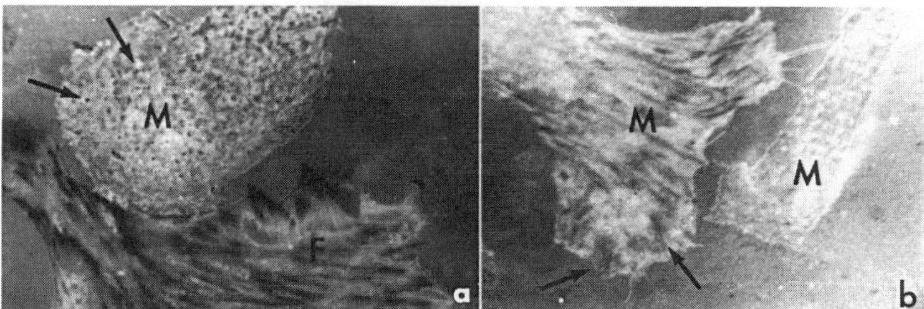

Fig. 3. IRM images of 7 day myocytes (M). Many cells display punctate (arrows) focal contacts (a), while others (b) exhibit adhesive sites (arrows) similar to those seen in fibroblasts (F) (a).

TRANSMISSION (TEM) AND HIGH VOLTAGE (HVTEM) ELECTRON MICROSCOPY

Two approaches are usually employed to culture calcium tolerant cardiac myocytes. The freshly isolated rods are either explanted onto native plastic surfaces or allowed to attach to a variety of substrata, including fetal bovine serum, laminin or type IV collagen [10,17]. On uncoated surfaces the quiescent rods gradually round-up before respreading into flattened, contractile cells [13-16, 20,21]. Myocytes attached to a substratum gradually transform into a spread configuration after approximately two weeks in culture [10,7,12,18,19]. Since considerable controversey surrounds whether the cultured myocyte retains its adult structural properties as it adapts to its new two-dimensional environment [10], numerous TEM studies have been conducted to identify those events that accompany the subcellular reorganization of the myocyte during its adaptation to in vitro life. In the succeeding paragraphs, several preservation, sectioning and staining protocols will be reviewed and discussed in terms of their advantages and disadvantages in the study of freshly isolated as well as cultured cardiac myocytes.

Preservation of isolated myocytes appears to vary considerably from one laboratory to another and the only guiding principle appears to be that fixation protocols employ either isotonic or hypertonic fixatives composed of glutaraldehyde alone or in combination with freshly prepared paraformaldehyde. Routinely, freshly isolated cells are fixed in suspension with 2-4% glutaraldehyde buffered in 0.1M sodium cacodylate (pH7.4) after which the myocytes are gently pelleted in microfuge tubes. Preservation can be conducted at either room temperature (i.e., 22°C) or in the cold (4°C) for periods of at least 1- hr to as long as 24 hrs

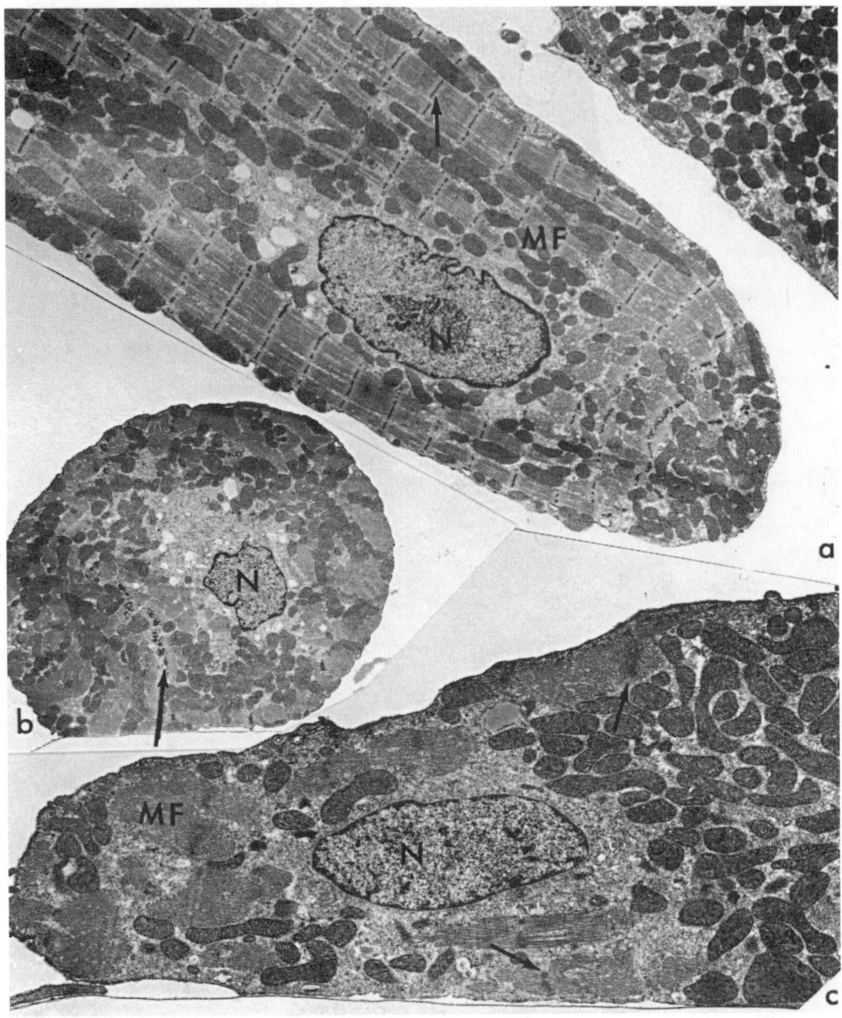

Fig. 4. TEM micrographs of en face (a), transverse (b) and sagital (c) sections of one week old myocytes. N, nucleus; MF, myofibrils; (arrows), Z-disc.

[4,5,6,9,11,15,16,20,21]. The pellets are then thoroughly rinsed in at least three changes of 0.1M sodium cacodylate buffer (pH 7.4) plus 7.5% sucrose (included to maintain tonicity) over a period of 1-24 hr to remove residual glutaraldehyde that might interfer with post-fixation in osmium tetroxide. Secondary fixation to immobilize lipids is conducted with either 1% or 2% osmium tetroxide buffered in 0.1M sodium cacodylate buffer, pH 7.4, which is frequently supplemented with 5% sucrose to maintain isosmolal conditions. Post-fixation should be conducted in the cold (4^oC) for 1-2 hrs. Following osmification, pellets are rapidly rinsed in double distilled water (3 changes) to remove residual traces of

OsO_4 and stained en bloc with 0.5% uranyl acetate to enhance cell membrane contrast. While most investigators employ an aqueous 0.5% uranyl acetate solution, we believe that more consistent cell membrane staining can be achieved if the cells are stained at a mildly acidic pH (6.0); therefore, myocyte preparations are stained en bloc in 0.5% uranyl acetate in 50mM acetate-veronal buffer (pH 6.0) plus 4% sucrose for 1 hr at room temperature [30]. Such en bloc staining frequently removes all traces of glycogen deposits from the myocytes, so caution is warrented if the subcellular distribution of this complex carbohydrate is an important aspect of a study. Pellets are then cut from microfuge tubes, dehydrated in a graded series of ethanols (50-95%, 10 min each) followed by 3 changes of absolute ethanol (10 min each) and propylene oxide (10 min each). The cell pellets are infiltrated with a 50% epoxy resin: 50% propylene oxide mixture for 4-8 hrs at room temperature, drained and then exposed to 100% epoxy resin overnight before being placed in the apex of Beem capsules which are filled with fresh resin. The preparations are then polymerized at 60°C for 48 hours.

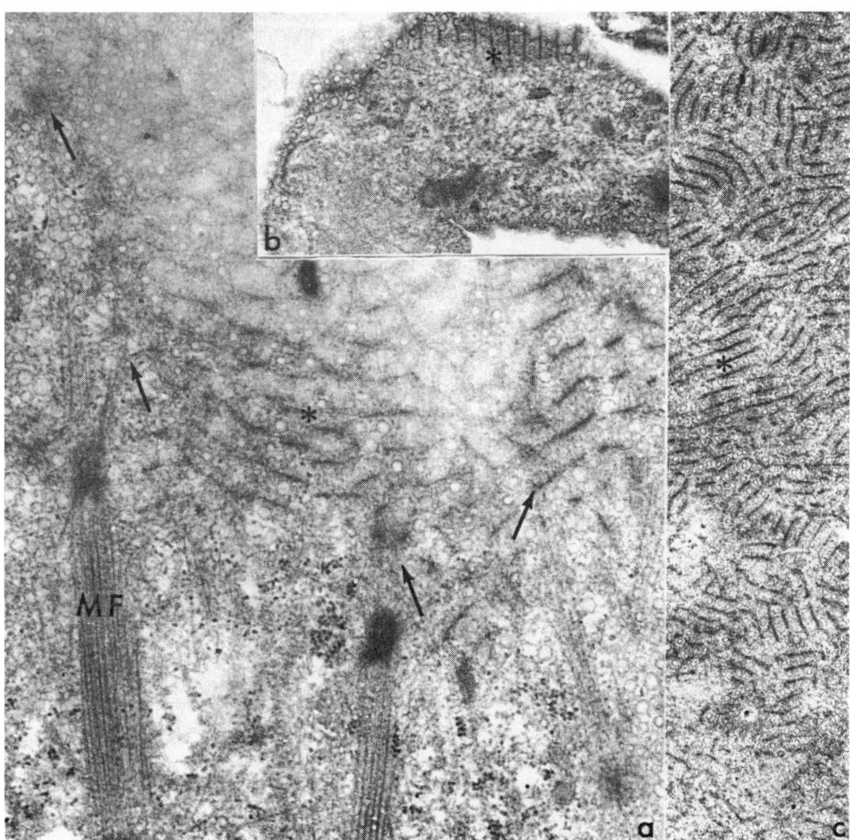

Fig. 5. TEM images of membrane associated leptomeres(*) from one month old myocytes (a,b,c). En face profiles (a) suggest myofilaments (MF) terminate at these sites (arrows) and other sections (b,c) illustrate their distribution.

If the cardiac myocytes are to be cultured, then the preparations should be preserved in situ so that the cell-cell organization can be retained. Fixation and dehydration schedules are identical to those described above except that propylene oxide, which solubilizes culture plastic, is replaced by several changes (at least 3 times, 10 min each) of absolute ethanol to ensure the removal of water which is not miscible with epoxy resins. The cultures are then infiltrated in an absolute ethanol-epoxy mixture (50:50) overnight at room temperature, followed by an additional 24 hr period of infiltration in 100% epoxy. After infiltration, the dishes are drained and the cylindrical portions of the Beem capsules are placed randomly over the surface of the petri dishes, filled partially with fresh epoxy resin and allowed to polymerize for 24 hrs at 22°C. The next day the capsules are filled completely with resin and placed in a 60°C oven for 24 hrs. After the resin is cured, the plastic petri dishes can be broken away from the Beem capsules with a pair of long-nose pliers, leaving fields of myocytes ready for trimming and thin-sectioning.

Examination of cell pellets provides a variety of random sections through myocytes that are positioned rather haphazardly after mild centrifugation. Conversely, en face sections can be obtained from flat embedded specimans that yield uniform profiles of myocytes arrayed longitudinally. These linear images not only provide considerable structural information about the myocyte, itself [Fig. 4a], but also ensure that valuable data on the organization and extent of the intercalated disc is available to the viewer. Such images are also extremely useful in quantitating the volume and surface densities of various subcellular organelles by morphometry. Broad views of the region just immediately above the basal sarcolemmal surface of the myocyte can also be obtained from flat embedded specimans. For example, in the first few thin sections of cells cultured for one month, electron dense leptomeres are observed interspersed between elements of the smooth endoplasmic reticulum which surround the caveolae [Fig. 5a,b,c]. The apparent termination of myofilaments in these structures (adhesion sites?) [Fig. 5a] suggest that they represent membrane associated Z-material and may be the site of assembly of new myofibrils. If sagital or transverse profiles of such myocytes are required, the end of the block is cut off with a jewelers saw and tipped on-end to produce transverse sections [Fig 4b] or rotated 90° for sagital sections [Fig. 4c]. Sections are then stained with lead citrate and aqueous 2.5% uranyl acetate just prior to viewing. Transverse sections provide excellent views of the myofibrillar apparatus and adjacent junctional and non-junctional elements of the sarcoplasmic reticulum, while sagital sections illustrate the intimacy of the basal cell surface and the substratum, for example.

The protocol outlined above represents our standard approach for studying the substructure of freshly isolated myocytes and those cultured for extended periods. En bloc and thin section staining provide the required contrast to visualize the contractile apparatus and various intracellular membraneous compartments. In addition to our routine procedures, several different fixation and en bloc staining procedures have been devised and modified by ourselves and others [20,21] to enhance and delineate sarcolemmal membranes, the T-system, the Golgi apparatus and junctional and non-junctional elements of the sarcoplasmic reticulum in cultured myocytes. These protocols are outlined in Table 1 for the purpose of convenience. Horseradish peroxidase [31], lanthanum chloride [32], colloidal lanthanum [33] and tannic acid [34] have all been employed to label the T-tubular system since such tracers penetrate these invaginations of the sarcolemma. Moses and Claycomb [20,21] have

Table I. Additional Fixation and In Situ Staining Protocols for Cultured Cardiac Myocytes +

Tracer or Stain	Pre-incubation	Fixation-1	Wash-1	Fixation-2	Wash-2$^{\pm}$
Horseradish^{o} Peroxidase (31)	1mg/ml in media 2-6hr at 37°C	2%GA and 1%PA in buffer^{+} 1 hr at 4°C	3x buffer^{+}+ 7%sucrose 1hr at 4°C	1%OsO_4 in buffer^{+} +5% sucrose 1 hr at 4°C	3x dH_2O^{*} 10 min at 22°C
Lanthanum Chloride (32)	5mM $LaCl_3$ in media 1 hr at 37°C	"	"	"	"
Colloidal Lanthanum (33)	none	1pt 4%Ga+1pt 3%$La(NO_3)_3$ 4-8hr at 22°C	"	"	"
Tannic Acid (34)	none	2-4%GA in buffer^{+} 2-4hr at 4°C	"	"	4%Tannic Acid in buffer^{+} 2hr at 22°C
Osmium Ferrocyanide (36)	none	4%GA in buffer^{+} +5mM $CaCl_2$ 2-4hr at 4°C	3x buffer^{+} +5mM$CaCl_2$ 2-4hr at 4°C	1%OsO_4+ 0.8%$K_4Fe(CN)_6$ in buffer^{+}+ 5mM$CaCl_2$ 2hr at 4°C	3x dH_2O^{*} 30 min at 22°C

+, in all instances the buffer refers to 0.1M sodium cacodylate, pH 7.4

o, following the primary wash, cells are incubated in 1mg/ml diaminobenzidine and 0.01% H_2O_2 in buffer for 15-30 min at 22°C

GA, glutaraldehyde; PA, paraformaldehyde

*, dH_2O, double distilled water

±, after wash-2, some cells were "en bloc" stained with 0.5% uranyl acetate (pH6.0) +4% sucrose 1 hr at 22°C

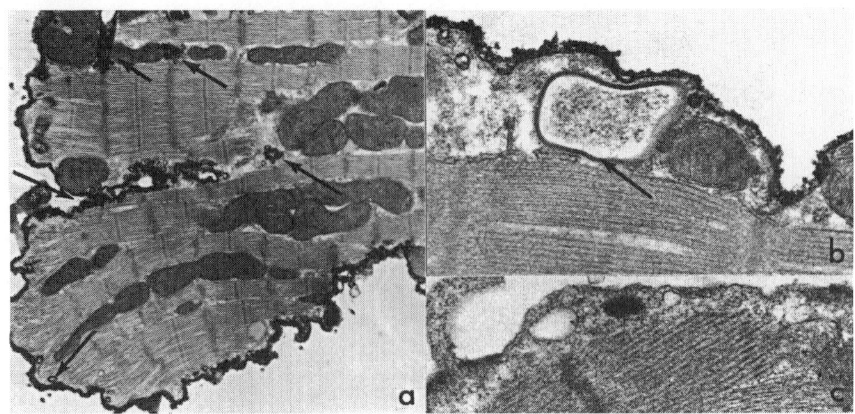

Fig. 6. Distribution of peroxidase (a,b) and cationized ferritin (c) in freshly attached myocytes. Peroxidase permeates T-tubules (arrows) and some vesicles (a), but does not penetrate internalized junctions (b). Ferritin can be found in endosomal-like vesicles but not in caveolae (c).

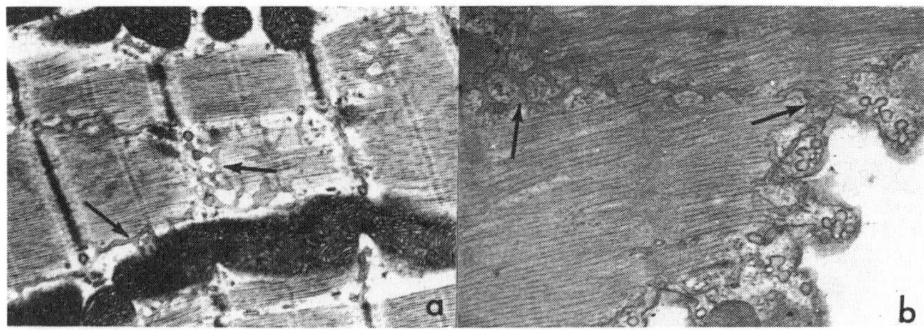

Fig. 7. Non-junctional elements of the sarcoplasmic reticulum (arrows) stained en bloc with uranyl acetate (a) or osmium ferrocyanide (b).

successfully used lanthanum chloride and tannic acid to stain the sarcolemmal glycocalyx and caveolae in addition to T-tubules. In our laboratory horseradish peroxidase seems to be a tracer that diffuses more uniformily through the T-system [Fig. 6a] than the other probes. In this regard, peroxidase [Fig. 6b] and cationized ferritin [Fig. 6c] are also useful probes to label the plasma membrane when used at low concentrations [35]. The use of such tracers cannot be underestimated for they are the only approach to thoroughly investigate the modification of the T-system during culture [7,20,21]. Similarly, reduced osmium ferrocyanide deposits, which enhance the contrast of the sarcoplasmic reticulum [36], reveal quite clearly its reticular or plexiform pattern. Moses and Claycomb [20,21] have elegantly demonstrated its promise in visualizing the sarcoplasmic reticulum in cultured myocytes. Similar images are also readily apparent when myocytes are stained en bloc with uranyl acetate [Fig. 7a]. Although osmium ferrocyanide is principally used to stain the sarcoplasmic reticulum [Fig. 7b], its property of understaining sarcomeric Z-lines accentuates the distribution of 10nm intermediate filaments located at this site [37] and may be useful in future studies investigating desmin's role in myofibrillar organization [38]. Conversely, tannic acid enhances the contrast of many filamentous proteins and is particularly useful in studying the structure of the myofibril and the intercalated disc [20]. This battery of fixation and staining protocols reveals that the structural organization of cultured adult myocyte closely resembles its in situ counterpart and, furthermore, demonstrates that implementing such staining protocols in combination with immunocytochemical techniques will facilitate our future elucidation of myocyte structure.

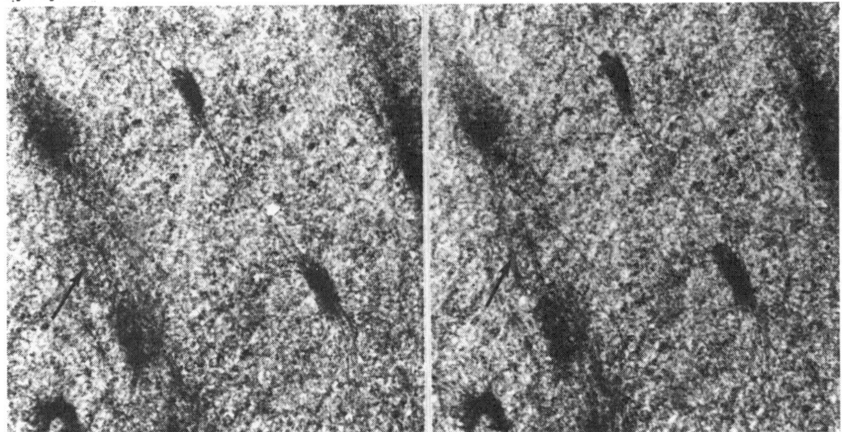

Fig. 8. Stereo pair of an en face thick section viewed with the HVTEM. Note that the Z-like dense structures (arrows) are closely associated with the sarcolemma and myofibrils.

Thin section TEM provides a rather selective and limited view of a myocyte's interior organization and, although crucial in studying sub-structure, a three-dimensional picture of the myocyte can only be achieved by serial sectioning and then reconstructing micrographs, a laborious and time consuming task. High voltage transmission electron microscopy (HVTEM) offers a means of acquiring this third dimensional look by examining thick sections (0.25-0.50um) or whole cell mounts [39]. Since the high accelerating potential of HVTEM (500-1000kV) allows electrons to penetrate thicker sections, depth can be added to the normal two dimensional image derived from conventional TEM. For those routinely viewing thin sections, the same specimans can be employed for HVTEM. Thick sections displaying blue or green interference colors (250nm) are cut with glass knives and then mounted on 300 mesh uncoated grids. The sections are then stained with 5% uranyl acetate in 70% ethanol for 45 min to ensure penetration of the heavy metal and then counterstained with Sato's triple lead stain [40] for 20 min. The thick sections are then carbon-coated on both sides to stabilize them and viewed in the JEOL 1000. Figure 8, illustrates a high voltage en face image of an adult rabbit cardiac myocyte maintained in culture for one month. The stereo images reveal the filamentous organization of the cytoplasm just above the basal plasma membrane. Well organized myofibrils appear to develop just above the caveolar zone. Such observations suggest that HVTEM may play an important role in studying the assembly of myofibrils at the cell surface.

SCANNING ELECTRON MICROSCOPY (SEM)

The dramatic changes in shape that transpire when calcium tolerant rod-shaped myocytes are placed in vitro are ideally suited for study in the scanning electron microscope. The SEM provides an elegant look at the cell surface morphology of the isolated myocyte and Claycomb and Palazzo

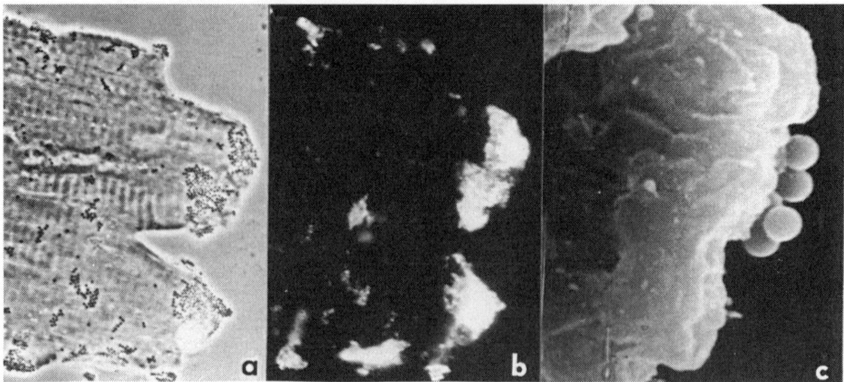

Fig. 9. Phase (a), fluorescent (b), and SEM (c) distribution of anti-laminin coated latex spheres on freshly isolated myocytes.

[14] have described the shape changes that myocytes pass through when plated on plastic surfaces. More recently Piper etal (6) and Lundgren et al [18] have depicted the early phases of attachment and spreading when myocytes are plated onto an adhesive substratum. Piper's group also employed this microscopic mode to follow changes in myocyte surface architecture in response to anoxia and reoxygenation. Although the SEM is primarily employed to investigate cell surface structure, the instrument can also be used as an analytical tool to study the distribution of a variety of cell surface receptors in addition to unraveling the location of various glycocalyx components. For example, the distribution of cell surface-bound laminin can be investigated with the SEM by employing 0.5um fluorescent, latex spheres to which anti-laminin antibody has been conjugated with cyanogen bromide. Cultured myocytes grown on circular 18mm coverslips can then be incubated with relatively low concentrations of spheres (10ug/ml) and prepared for phase [Fig. 9a], fluorescent [Fig. 9b], and scanning electron microscopy [Fig. 9c]. To prepare such preparations for SEM, the coverslips must be fixed in cacodylate buffered 2% glutaradehyde for at least 1 hr at 4°C. The coverslips are then thoroughly rinsed in 0.1M cacodylate buffer plus 7% sucrose in the cold and then postfixed in 1% OsO_4 for 1 hr at room temperature. At this juncture it is preferable to stabilize the myocytes by washing them in 1% tannic acid solution for 1 hr at room temperature. This step is believed to strengthen delicate cell processes [Fig. 10] that might fracture during the critical point drying phase [41]. The cells are then dehydrated in a graded series of ethanols [10,30,50,70%], treated with 2.5% uranyl acetate in 70% ehtanol to further stabilize the cells and thoroughly dried in 3-5 changes of absolute ethanol. The coverslips are then critically point dried from ethanol, perhaps the most crucial aspect of speciman preparation. At this stage its absolutely essential that all the ethanol is evaporated away, otherwise cell processes will be damaged. After drying, the coverslips are attached to scanning stubs with silver paint and gold is evaporated onto the surface of the preparation. This four step fixation protocol minimizes much of the shrinkage that normally accompanies the traditional glutaraldehyde-osmium fixation for SEM [42] and, consequently, preserves many of the delicate processes that mediate contact between the myocyte and the substratum [Fig. 10] and putative junctional complexes that develop between adjacent myocytes. Tannic acid and uranyl acetate en bloc staining also increases the conductivity of the specimens [43], thereby permitting the preparations to be scanned at

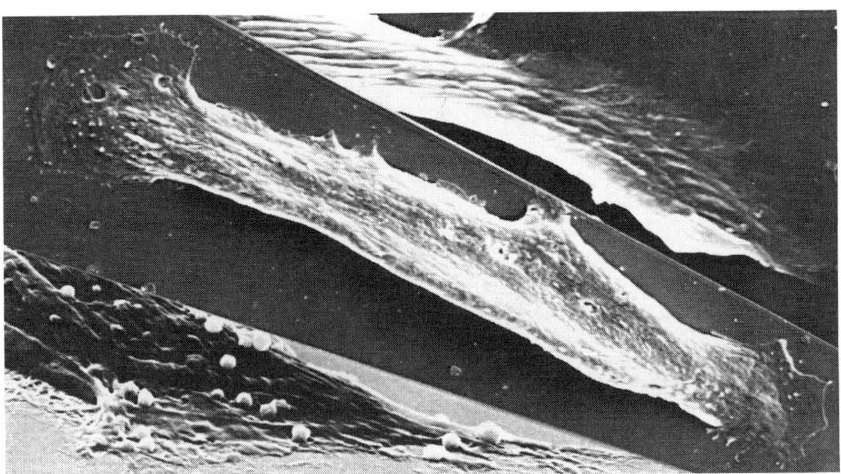

Fig. 10. SEM micrographs of attachment processes of 7-day cultured myocytes.

voltages of up to 5kV without prior coating with gold, if desired. Satisfactory images can be obtained in low and medium magnification ranges with such preparations. The four step fixation procedure also allows us to investigate the distribution of laminin on the freshly isolated myocyte [Fig. 9c] by effectively stabilizing cross-linked antibody-labeled latex spheres to the cell surface. Such a protocol should provide exciting new information about the make-up of the myocyte cell surface, especially when it is applied to other sarcolemmal surface receptors.

FREEZE FRACTURE-FREEZE ETCH MICROSCOPY

Perhaps the most informative way to examine sarcolemmal topography and subcellular organization is to freeze-fracture and/or freeze-etch either freshly isolated [4,5,] or cultured myocytes [44]. Fracture planes produced in membranes at very cold temperatures (-110°C) are believed to pass through the hydrophobic tails of the phospholipid bilayer, revealing the inner aspects of the protoplasmic (P-face) and exoplasmic (E-face) portions of the cell membrane [45,46]. By its very nature, freeze-fracturing creates vast fields of membrane for study, providing opportunities to investigate intramembrane particle (IMP) distribution under a variety of different physiologic and pathophysiologic states, the location and change in caveolae and alterations in the structural organization of gap junctions [Fig. 11] and desmosomes, just to name a few. A significant disadvantage of this approach is that it only permits observations on the internal halves of the sarcolemma and other organellar membranes; the inner or outer surfaces of the myocyte can only be visualized if the ice is sublimated (etched) away after fracturing the cells. Similarly, the intimate associations of contractile proteins, intermediate filaments, microtubules and the like, can only be appreciated in freeze-etched preparations.

Successful freeze-fracturing requires that freshly isolated myocytes be briefly fixed (15-30 min in 2% buffered glutaraldehyde) and pelleted prior to cryoprotection, while cultured myocytes should be grown on small coverslips and preserved in situ. After standard fixation both preparations are cryoprotected with (0.1M) cacodylate buffered glycerol in three stages (10 min in 6% glycerol; 10 min in 12.5% glycerol and one hour in 25% glycerol). Cell pellets are then transferred either to gold alloy holders or can be blotted onto small (3mm) cardboard discs and then frozen quickly in Freon 22 cooled in liquid nitrogen. Coverslips are frozen similarly and mounted on a special Balzers holder designed for cultured cells. The specimens are then mounted in a Balzers apparatus, fractured at $-115^{o}C$ in a vacuum of $5x10^{-7}$mbar and shadowed with platinum at a 45° angle and stabilized from above with carbon. The replicas can then be floated either onto a bleach solution or be cleaned with 40% chromic acid, rinsed in distilled water and mounted on formvar coated 200 mesh copper grids. This technique yields excellent views of cell membranes [Fig. 11].

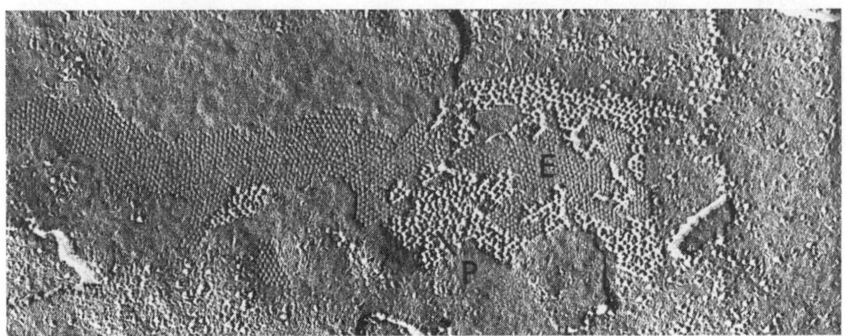

Fig. 11. Freeze-fracture replica of a gap junction found between adjacent cultured myocytes. E-face and P-face components are illustrated.

Conversely, freeze-etching [45] is a more difficult protocol to master for it requires freezing cells and tissues quickly enough to prevent ice crystal formation and its associated cell damage; for environmental water cannot be easily removed from the surface of a cell or subcellular structure in the presence of a cryoprotectant like glycerol. However, Heuser and colleagues [47,48] have developed a rapid freezing technique which permits cultured cells to be "instantly" frozen to liquid helium temperatures in the presence of a volatile cryoprotectant like methanol (10%). The ice crystals that form are so small (50nm) that little intracellular or membrane damage is apparent. When such preparations are dried (i.e., etched) at $-95^{o}C$ for 30-60 min and then rotary shadowed with platinum and carbon, images of fine detail and great resolution are obtainable. In the future, Heuser's rapid freezing technique combined with rotary shadowing will be of great value in elucidating the organization of the contractile apparatus and other cytoskeletal proteins in cultured myocytes.

SUMMARY

The principal objective of this chapter is to provide a brief review of morphological techniques that our laboratory finds useful in studying freshly isolated as well as cultured adult cardiac myocytes. Our approach is designed to combine a thorough light and electron microscopic investigation of myocyte structure in an attempt to unravel the complicated events that attend the culture of this highly specialized cell type. Phase contrast microscopy is a useful first step in examining the quality of a freshly isolated preparation of adult myocytes; however, DIC microscopy reveals far more details about the overall structure of these cells for it optically sections these large cells, thereby filtering out unwanted "noise." Polarizing microscopy provides almost as much information about the integrity of the contractile apparatus as does immunofluorescence; moreover, such observations can be conducted on live cells. Similarly, IRM generates an image of cell-substrate interactions and ought to be a principal tool in any study of attachment prior to commencing a time consuming ultrastructural analysis. Each of these forms of light microscopy presents the investigator with distinct approaches with which to gather valuable structural information and evaluate the behavior of the cardiac myocyte _in vitro_. Such preliminary work should produce a solid foundation upon which selected ultrastructural studies can be formulated and initiated.

The electron microscope is almost as versatile an instrument as the light microscope in many respects. Traditional transmission electron microscopy remains the everyday workhorse of those researchers investigating structure-function relationships. TEM coupled with scanning microscopy compliment one-another by providing a three dimensional view of the external surface of the myocyte and an internal depiction of the myocyte's subcellular organization. High voltage TEM compliments thin section TEM by providing a three-dimensional look at the interior of the myocyte and when used in conjunction with rapidly developing immunogold techniques, HVTEM should in the future be useful in elucidating the "macromolecular" organization of the myocyte. Lastly, freeze-fracture and freeze-etch microscopy opens several new avenues to examine the substructure of myocyte membranes as well as providing another novel method of visualizing contractile and cytoskeletal proteins. The continuing development of light and electron microscopic techniques to analyze myocyte structure remains an exciting and fruitful field of endeavor and will remain crucial to our further characterization of the cultured cardiac myocyte.

ACKNOWLEDGEMENTS

The authors express their grateful appreciation to Melissa Green, Monica Behnke and Jack Gibbons for expert technical assistance and to Ms. Debbie Bland and Belinda Berthold-Coichy for preparing the manuscript. This study is supported by Public Health Service grants HL33616 and HL19648. The high voltage EM work was supported by an NIH grant RR-00592 awarded to the University of Colorado's High Voltage facility. We appreciate Ms. Mary Morphew's effort in preparing our HVTEM micrographs. We also wish to thank Mr. Robert Hughes of W. Nuhsbaum, Inc. (Leitz representative) for his continuing interest and technical advice.

REFERENCES

1. E. Morkin, I.L. Fink, and S. Goldman, Prog. Cardiovas. Dis. _25_: 435: (1983).
2. T. Powell, D.A. Terrar, and V.W. Twist, J. Physiol _302_: 131 (1980).
3. G. Bkaily, N. Sperelakis, and J. Doane, Am. J. Physiol. (Heart Circ Physiol) _247_: H1018 (1984).
4. N.J. Severs, A.M. Slade, T. Powell, V.W. Twist, and R.L. Warren, J. Ultrastruct. Res. _81_: 222 (1982).
5. N.J. Severs, A.M. Slade, T. Powell, V.W. Twist, and G.E. Jones, Cell Tissue Res. _240_: 159 (1985).
6. H.M. Piper, I Probst, P. Schwartz, F.J. Hutter, and P.G. Spieckermann, J. Mol. Cell Cardiol. _14_: 397 (1982).
7. M.L. Decker, D.G. Simpson, M. Lesch, and R.S. Decker, Anat. Rec. (1988).
8. J.W. Dow, N.G.L. Harding, and T. Powell, Cardiovasc. Res. _15_: 483 (1981).
9. B.B. Farmer, M. Mancina, E.S. Williams, and A.M. Watanabe, Life Sci _33_:1 (1983).
10. S.L. Jacobson and H.M. Piper, J. Mol. Cell. Cardio. _18_: 661 (1986).
11. J. Eckel, G. Van Echten, and H. Reinauer, Am. J. Physiol. (Heart Circ. Physiol) _249_: H212 (1985).
12. J. Haddad, M.L. Decker, L-C Hsieh, M. Lesch, A.M. Samarel and R.S.

Decker, Am. J. Physiol (Cell Physiol.), In Press (1987).
13. S. L. Jacobson, Cell Struct. Func. 2: 1 (1977).
14. W.C. Claycomb and M.C. Palazzo, Dev. Biol. 80: 466 (1980).
15. T.A. Schwartzfeld and S.L. Jacobson, J. Molc. Cell. Cardiol. 13: 563 (1981).
16. A.C. Nag, M. Cheng, D.A. Fischman, and R. Zak, J. Molc. Cell. Cardiol. 15: 301 (1983).
17. Piper, H.M., R. Spahr, I. Probst, and P.G. Spieckermann, Basic Res. Cardiol. 80 [suppl 2]: 175 (1985).
18. E. Lundgren, T. Borg, and S. Mardh, J. Molc. Cell. Cardiol. 16: 355 (1984).
19. E. Lundgren, L. Terracio, S. Mardh, and T.K. Borg, Exp. Cell Res. 156: 371 (1985).
20. R.L. Moses and W.C. Claycomb, Am. J. Anat. 164: 113 (1982).
21. R.L. Moses and W.C. Claycomb, Am. J. Anat. 171: 191 (1984).
22. G. Cooper, W.E. Mercer, J.K. Hooper, P.R. Gordon, R.L. Kent, I.K. Lanva, and T.A. Marino, Cir. Res. 58: 692 (1986).
23. Y. Fukui, S. Yumura, T-K Yumura, and H. Mori, Meth. Enzymol, 134: 573 (1986).
24. S. Inoue, J. Cell Biol. 91: 131s (1981).
25. J.W. Fuseler, J.W. Shay and H. Feit, Cell Mus. Motil. 1: 205 (1981).
26. A.S.G. Curtis, J. Cell Biol 20: 199 (1964).
27. C.S. Izzard and L.R. Lochner, J. Cell Sci. 21: 129 (1976).
28. C.S. Izzard and L.R. Lochner, J. Cell Sci. 42:81 (1980).
29. B.T. Atherton, D.M. Meyer, and D.G. Simpson, J. Cell Sci. 86: 233 (1986).
30. D.S. Friend and M.G. Farquhar J. Cell Biol. 35: 357 (1967).
31. R.C. Graham and M.H. Karnovsky, J. Histochem. Cytochem, 14: 291 (1966).
32. G.A. Langer and J.S. Frank, J. Cell Biol., 54: 441 (1972).
33. J.-P. Revel and M.J. Karnovsky, J. Cell Biol. 33: C7 (1976).
34. N. Simionescu and M. Simionescu, J. Cell Biol. 70: 608 (1976).
35. W.J. Brown, J. Goodhouse, and M.G. Farquhar, J. Cell Biol. 103: 1235 (1986).
36. M.S. Forbes, B.A. Planthalt, and N. Sperelikis, J. Ultrastruct. Res. 60: 306 (1977).
37. R.L. Moses and J.B. Delcarpio, Cell Tissue Res. 228: 489 (1983).
38. E. Lazarides, Nature 283: 249 (1979).
39. J.J. Wolosewick and K. Porter, Am. J. Anat. 147: 303 (1976).
40. K. Sato, J. Elec. Micro. 17: 158 (1968).
41. D. Schroeter, E. Spiess N. Paweletz, and R. Bernke, J. Elec. Micro. Tech 1: 219 (1984).
42. D.K. Gusnard and R.H. Kirschner, J. Micro. 110: 51 (1977).
43. L.R. Sweney and B.L. Shapiro, Stain Tech. 52: 221 (1977).
44. G.A. Langer, J.S. Frank, T.L. Rich, and F.B. Orner, Am. J. Physiol (Heart Circ. Physiol) 252: H314 (1987).
45. P. Pinto da Silva and D. Branton, J. Cell Biol. 45: 598 (1970).
46. J.D. Robertson, J. Cell Biol. 91: 189s (1980).
47. J.E. Heuser, T.S. Reese, M.J. Dennis, Y. Jan, L. Jan and L. Evans, J. Cell Biol 81: 275 (1979).
48. J.E. Heuser and M.W. Kirschner, J. Cell Biol. 86: 212 (1980).

MORPHOMETRY OF CULTURED MYOCYTES

R.L. MOSES, J.B. DELCARPIO, and William C. CLAYCOMB*
Departments of Anatomy, and Biochemistry and Molecular Biology,*
LSU Medical Center, 1100 Florida Avenue, New Orleans,LA 70119

INTRODUCTION

Although ultrastructural morphometric analysis of intact cardiac muscle tissue [1-7] and isolated cardiac myocytes [8,9] has been routinely utilized by a number of investigators, similar quantitative studies on long-term cultured cardiac muscle cells have not been reported. The current variety of cultured adult mammalian cardiac muscle cells [10-13] makes such quantitative studies particularly attractive. The main reason for this lack of data is that many investigators have viewed the requisite electron microscopy as difficult. Although in situ electron microscopy of cultured cells is somewhat more challenging than conventional electron microscopy, we have found that sufficient data can be reliably obtained for morphometric studies. In this chapter, we shall summarize our techniques which are applicable to long-term cultures.

Most of the ultrastructural studies in our laboratories focus on two questions. First, how faithfully does a cultured myocyte morphologically resemble the cells in the tissue from which it was derived? Second, if a cultured myocyte is treated in a certain manner or manifests an altered functional capacity, is there a morphological response? The answers to these questions are most accurately stated in quantitative terms, since morphological changes are seldom all or none phenomena (Figure 1). It is much more meaningful to ask how much a cultured myocyte resembles cells of the original tissue than to simply ask if there is a morphological resemblance. Similar questions may be asked concerning cells grown under altered culture conditions, treated with functionally active compounds, or derived from animals with hypertrophied hearts.

We have found that per cent-volume (volume fraction) measurements obtained using the conventional point-count method [14-16], combined with electron microscopic techniques and sampling procedures as outlined below, can provide answers to these questions. For reasons discussed below, surface measuring techniques are more difficult to use, but are also applicable.

CULTURE, FIXATION, STAINING, AND EMBEDDING

Most standard disposable cultureware is suitable for in situ transmission electron microscopy (TEM). We routinely use Corning or Falcon 25 cm^2 culture flasks, but in the past we have used both larger and smaller flasks, as well as disposable petri dishes. We find disposable culture flasks far superior to cover slips in terms of ease of handling. Coating growth surfaces with substrates such as collagen or laminin does not interfere with removal of the plastic flask from the specimen (see Figure 2).

Biology of Isolated Adult Cardiac Myocytes
William A. Clark, Robert S. Decker, and Thomas K. Borg, Editors

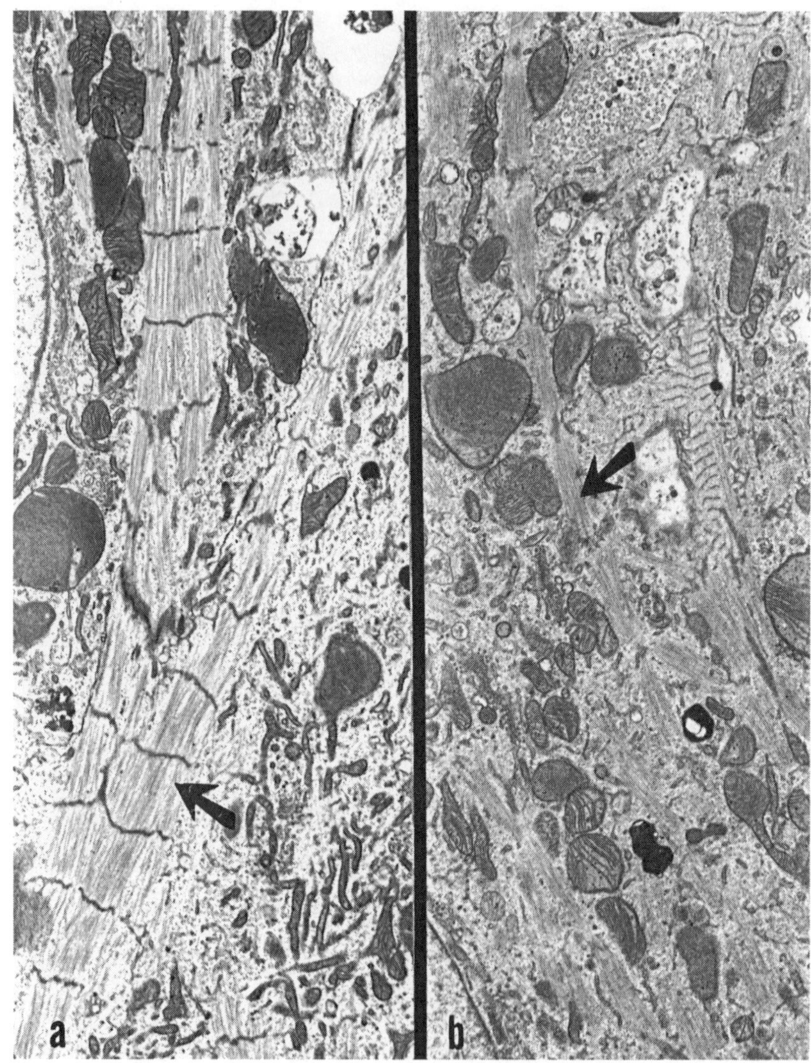

Figure 1. Electron micrographs of control (a) and DAG-treated (b) (see this volume) cultured adult cardiac myocytes. The cells are clearly different, but the difference is best expressed in quantitative rather than qualitative terms. Note that both cells have organized myofibrils (arrows). (a,X 9,700; b,X 10,400)

Although cells may be enzymatically or mechanically removed from the growth surface and processed as a pellet, such treatment is traumatic to the cells, disrupts intracellular morphology, and distorts intercellular relationships. Clearly, in situ methodologies better preserve cultured myocyte morphology. Myocytes should be plated at high enough densities (150,000- 300,000/ml) to ensure easy location.

Our embedding technique is outlined in Figure 2. The cells are fixed in situ using 4.0% glutaraldehyde in 0.1 N sodium cacodylate. Postfixation with either 1.0% osmium tetroxide or 1.0% potassium ferrocyanide is also carried out in situ, as is dehydration in graded ethanols, en bloc staining in 0.5% aqueous uranyl acetate, and infiltration with ethanol-plastic mixtures. Acetone and propylene oxide cannot be used as dehydrating agents since culture flask plastics are soluble in these reagents.

We have used a number of different staining regimens in our ultrastructural studies of cultured myocytes (tannic acid, osmium tetroxide, osmium ferrocyanide, various lanthanum salts) [17]. Our studies have shown that different staining techniques can accentuate different cellular components. For example, osmium ferrocyanide tends to highlight the sarcoplasmic reticulum and T system [18, 19], while, in cells postfixed in osmium tetroxide, the myofilaments are relatively heavily stained (Figure 3). Such differential staining abilities can be taken advantage of in morphometric studies. Caution must be used in morphometrically comparing myocytes stained or postfixed with different reagents since these chemicals may induce differential volumetric changes in cells or organelles. Our results indicate that per cent-volumes for a variety of organelles (mitochondria, myofilaments, T tubes) do not differ between cells postfixed in osmium tetroxide versus those postfixed in osmium ferrocyanide.

The plastic which we use consists of Polybed-812, dodecenylsuccinic anhydride, araldite, and the epoxy accelerator, DMP-30. (Mollenhauer formula, Polysciences). We add about 50% more catalyst than is called for by the recipe. We have found that this plastic works well with a number of different culture vessels. Once components of the kit are opened, they should be used relatively rapidly (within six months).

After exposing the cells to increasing concentrations of plastic (25%, 50%, 75%), we infiltrate with two changes of 100% plastic. While the cells are still covered with the second 100% plastic change, we remove the top of the flask with an electrically heated wire. Care must be taken not to ignite either the plastic or the culture flask. After removing the top, the bottom of the flask is inverted, and the plastic is drained off. The more efficiently the plastic is drained between plastic changes, the greater the likelihood of proper polymerization. Fresh plastic is then added, and Beem capsules with the closed ends cut off are placed flush in the flask bottom. If the cells are to be sectioned en face (parallel to the growth surface) fresh plastic is added to the Beem capsules subsequent to polymerization. If transverse sectioning is to be employed (as is necessary for morphometric studies, see below), the plastic is polymerized and no further plastic is added. In

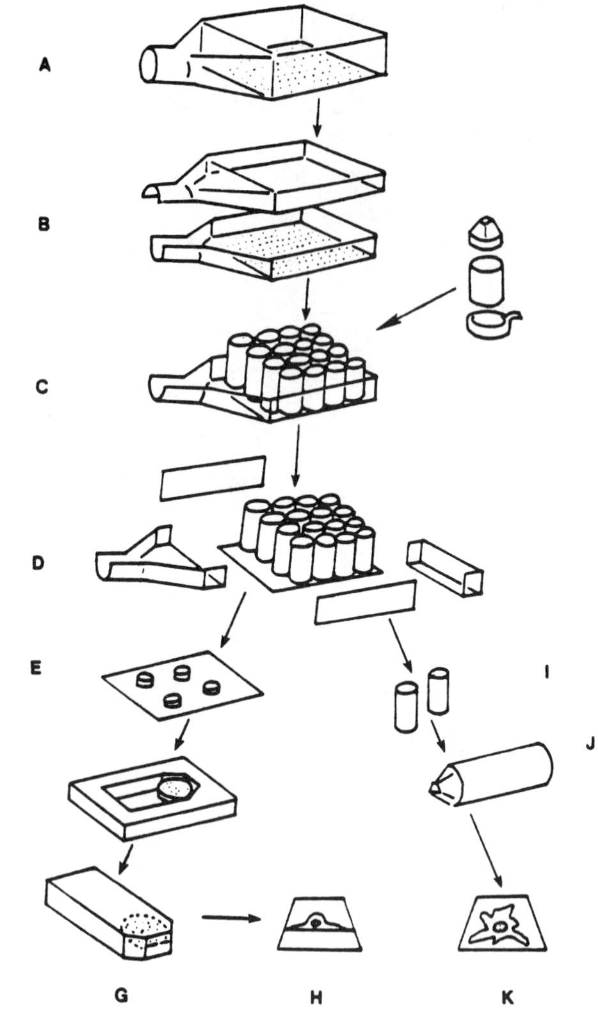

Fiqure 2. Preparation of cultured myocytes for en face and transverse sectioning. Fixation, dehydration, etc. are performed in situ (A). The flask is then cut with a hot wire and drained (B). Cut 00 Beem capsules are then put in place (c) subsequent to addition of fresh plastic. After polymerization and addition of more plastic (for en face specimens), the flask is removed (D). Specimens to be transversely sectioned are reembedded prior to sectioning (E-H), while those to be cut en face are trimmed and sectioned directly (I-K).

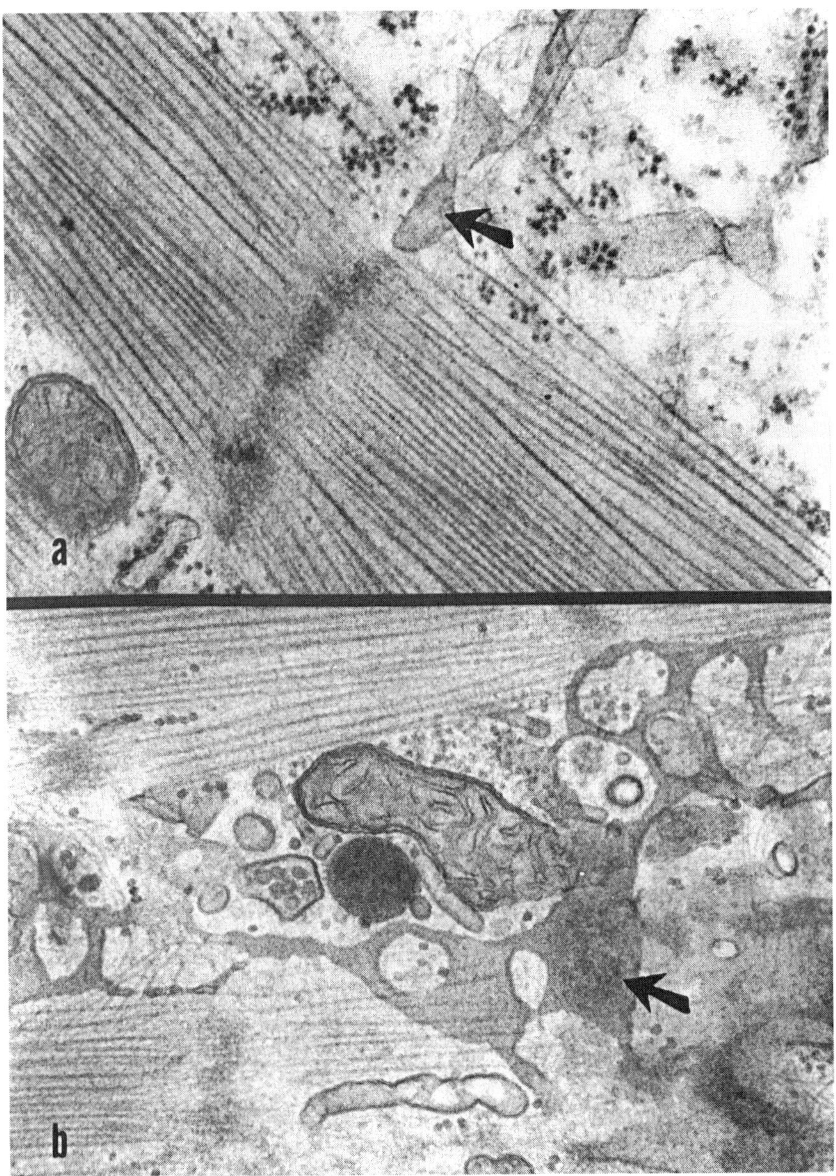

Figure 3. Electron micrographs of cultured adult rat ventricular myocytes postfixed in osmium tetroxide (a) and osmium ferrocyanide (b). Note that the sarcoplasmic reticulum (arrows) is more prominently stained in the cell postfixed in osmium ferrocyanide. (a,X 50,300; b,X 45,700)

practice, we usually prepare cells from a single flask for both en face and transverse sectioning. Cells prepared for en face sectioning can be converted to transverse blocks by sawing off the end of the block containing the cells and reembedding these blocks.

Cells prepared for transverse sectioning can be trimmed and viewed directly if an electron-luscent support film such as formvar is used. A support film is necessary since the bottom edge of the cell also corresponds to the edge of the section and this area is potentially unstable without support in the electron beam. We, therefore, reembed material to be transversely sectioned as illustrated in Figure 2.

The specimens are freed from the flask by breaking off the remaining flask edges with a pair of pliers and then bending the specimen to remove it from the bottom of the flask. We have not found it necessary to use temperature differentials (dry ice, boiling, etc.) to free the specimens. Safety glasses should be worn during these procedures, since the flask plastic tends to splinter.

SECTIONING

We exclusively use transversely sectioned cells for our morphometric studies. Although en face sectioning is less troublesome (sections are usually easier to cut, and no reembedding is necessary), the sample is biased since the basal portions of the myocytes (those portions nearest the growth surface) are usually not retrieved. This is due to unavoidable irregularities in the surface of the block or slight misalignment of the block face relative to the knife edge. These factors lead to "partial" or incomplete initial sections. Since sections subsequent to those initial ones would be routinely examined, possible organellar per cent-volume differences between basal and other regions of the myocyte would be ignored and the resulting data biased. The same reasoning also holds true for the most apical portions of the myocyte, since it would only rarely be sectioned.

Transversely sectioned in situ myocytes are not subject to these biases since both basal and apical aspects of the cell are included within the same section (Figure 4). Although there is lateral variability within myocytes (i.e., subsarcolemmal areas are constructed differently than perinuclear regions), all regions are equally recoverable and should appear at frequencies reflecting their actual occurrence. The only interpretive drawback to transversely sectioned cells is that, on occasion, small isolated processes occur in the sections which are not identifiable as belonging to a muscle versus a nonmuscle cell. In en face sectioned cells such processes are more easily related to the cell of origin.

We orient our transversely sectioned specimens so that the growth surface (i.e. the interface between the layers of plastic) (Figure 4), is either parallel or slightly oblique to the knife edge. This avoids the risk of one bad knife region ruining an entire section.

The interface between the reembedded cells and the subsequently added layer of plastic is weak and may fail, either during sectioning or after exposure to the electron beam. Bonding between the two plastic layers can be enhanced

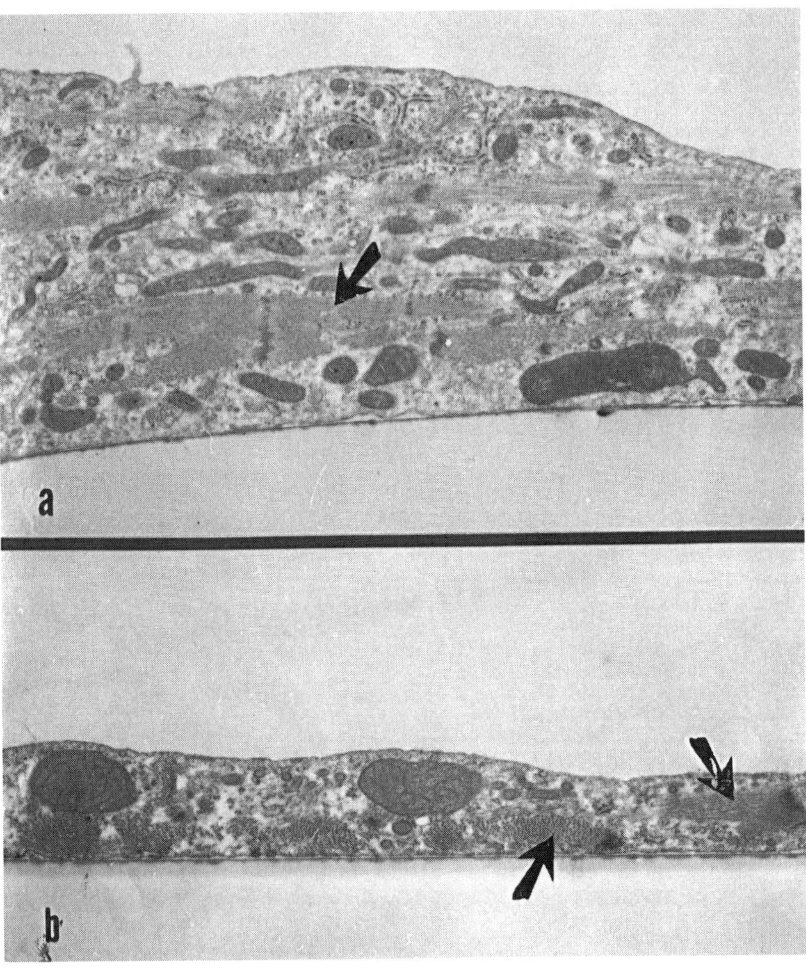

Figure 4. Transversely sectioned adult cardiac myocytes grown in plastic (a) and plastic coated with laminin (b). Note that the cell grown on laminin is much flatter. The growth surface is represented by the dark line subtending each cell. Arrows point to organized myofibrils. (Both micrographs X 11,700)

by "roughening" the original specimen with organic solvents such as absolute alcohol. However, such procedures may also "erase" the basal portions of cells. Electron luscent supports and carbon coating are helpful in stabilizing this interface.

We have found that "white" sections (between silver and gold) are most suitable for morphometric studies. These yield photomicrographs of sufficient contrast with a minimum of superimposition. We retrieve our sections on uncoated 300-mesh copper grids.

SAMPLING

Standardized sampling techniques are critical for accurate morphometric studies. Sampling in culture systems consists of two steps: (1) selection of cells and (2) determination of which part of the cell is to be examined. We assume that there is no difference in cells grown in different areas of the culture flask and retrieve as many myocytes as possible in plastic. Forty to fifty small Beem capsules (00 size) will fit conveniently into a 25 cm^2 culture flask. The only visual selection of cells occurs during block trimming. In order to avoid cutting areas which do not contain cells, the block is trimmed to areas which show a dark line (representing the myocytes) at the junction of the two plastic layers. Once such an area is encountered the block goes through a final trimming and is cut with a diamond knife.

We generally retrieve two or three grids, each containing five to eight sections, from each block. (Cells may be several micrometers in height depending on growth conditions and/or substrate.) However, only one section from one randomly chosen grid (from each block cut) is used in our data pool. The remaining grids are used as a backup and are discarded if not needed.

Once the randomly chosen grid is placed in the microscope, it is necessary to determine the area appropriate for photography. We do this by examining the grid at a low scanning magnification and selecting a section of appropriate thickness which shows a large amount of cellular material. (All sections do not show equal amounts of cellular substance due to the interference of the grid bars.)

Once such a section is selected, all cells on that section are photographed at a standard magnification. This does not result in excessive consumption of film since the cellular layer is relatively thin (Figure 4). The only cells which are not analyzed are those which were cut during trimming, since they may be physically distorted and are at the section's edges where accurate photography is difficult. Likewise, portions of cells under grid bars are not included in the data pool. Exclusion of these cells is a random event and should not influence data.

Thus, rather than systemically photographing a particular area of the grid square [14, 15], we systematically photograph every cell. In this way, we are able to compensate for relative scarcity of tissue in our blocks and the lack of consistent specimen orientation with respect to the support grid lattice.

Typical data pools use twenty different cells taken from at least two (preferably three) different cultures. As with any morphometric analysis, more accurate data is obtained by examining cells from multiple experiments, than by examining many cells from the same experiment [15].

PHOTOGRAPHY

We have standardized our photographic procedures in order to assure consistency in our data. We take all of our micrographs at 7,796X and enlarge them, full frame, to a final magnification of 19,500X. Most intracellular structures can be unambiguously recognized at this magnification. We then make montages out of the micrographs of all the cells within each grid square. Due to lens aberrations inherent in the microscope, there is some mismatching between contiguous micrographs. In transversely sectioned cells this area is negligible. However, in en face sectioned tissue a greater area must be matched.

Photographic procedures must be appropriate for the structures of interest, and higher magnifications may be necessary. Such alterations may, of course, also affect sampling strategies.

MORPHOMETRY

In order to determine per cent-volume of structures within myocytes, we use morphometric test grids. Simplistically, the rationale is to determine the ratio of points which fall on objects of interest to the total number of points falling within the cell. This ratio represents the volume fraction which the structure of interest occupies.

The spacing between points on the test grid must be appropriate for the structures to be analyzed if accurate data is to be obtained [14, 15]. For most structures, test grid spacing should be such that a single organelle is not counted more than once. Point spacing on test grids is determined by the formula

$$d^2 > a \qquad [15]$$

where d is the distance between points and a is the area of organelle (15).

We have empirically determined that, at the magnification which we use, a grid spacing of 1 cm is suitable for volumetric determinations of organelles such as mitochondria. Volume densities of myofibrils are somewhat more problematical, since these are relatively large structures which are often very long in transversely sectioned cultured myocytes. We have also used 1 cm test grids to determine myofibrillar volume densities. A second reason that estimation of myofibrillar volume is difficult is that small, nonmyofibrillar areas may be present between filaments. Although these areas are frequently missed by points in the test grid, their presence may lead to inaccuracies in data. Finally, organized myofibrils are more difficult to detect and interpret in the oblique profiles often observed in transversely sectioned cells (Figure 4).

The transverse tubular (T) system in cultured cardiac myocytes has been a subject of interest in our laboratories for some time. Volumetric determinations of such rare morphological structures present special problems. Since these structures account for less than 1.0% of total cytoplasmic volume in cultured adult ventricular myocytes [20], it is necessary to construct test grids with spacings such that every T tube is counted [14, 15]. Grid spacing for T tubes is determined by the formula

$$d^2 \lesssim a \qquad [15].$$

We have found that test grids with a spacing of 0.5 cm are sufficient for such determinations. In point of fact, volume densities for T tubes determined by use of a 0.5 cm test grid probably underestimate true T tube volume, since small T tubes composed of only a few fused caveolae [11, 12] are not counted. We have opted for conservatism rather than potentially overestimating T tube volume.

We construct our grids by copying the pattern onto overhead transparency film. In order to compensate for errors inherent in xeroxing, final grid spacing is determined after copying. Different grid spacings may be incorporated to make a multifunctional test grid (double coherent test lattice).

Although cultured cardiac muscle cells possess an inherent anisotropy due to oriented myofilaments, this anisotropy is dampened due to random orientation of the myofilaments with respect to the plane of section and to the random location with which test grid points hit various structures. (For further discussion of stereology of anisotropic structures see references 22 and 23).

In our experience, accurate determination of surface density is much more difficult than volumetric measurements. The reason for this is that myocytes have very irregular contours (Fig. 5), and different regions of the cells are specialized for different functions. Many of the surface irregularities are of such small dimensions that collection of large amounts of data points from micrographs of sufficient magnification is prohibitive. When micrographs of lower magnification are used, it is not always possible to determine the precise nature of the membrane specialization.

The test probe system which we employ to determine surface density ratios is a curvilinear grid [24]. This is a test grid composed of semicircles. Curvilinear lines help negate the inherent anisotropy of cells grown on a planar surface. The grid is applied to a photomicrographic montage, and line intersections are counted. The ratio of line intersections with areas of interest to the total number of line intersections with the cell, represents the surface density of the area of interest.

Cardiac myocytes present other problems with respect to surface density determinations since it is often difficult to determine whether a profile is intracellular or an extension of the plasmalemma. Electron dense tracers are of limited value resolving this problem since they are inconsistent in staining efficiency [17]. Our most consistent results have been achieved with osmium ferrocyanide which preferentially stains the surface membrane of the myocyte.

Determination of cell volume of cultured myocytes is also a difficult undertaking. However, such measurements are crucial if reliable in vitro myocardial hypertrophy models are to be developed. Planimetric surface determinations (at the light microscopic level) have been combined with protein

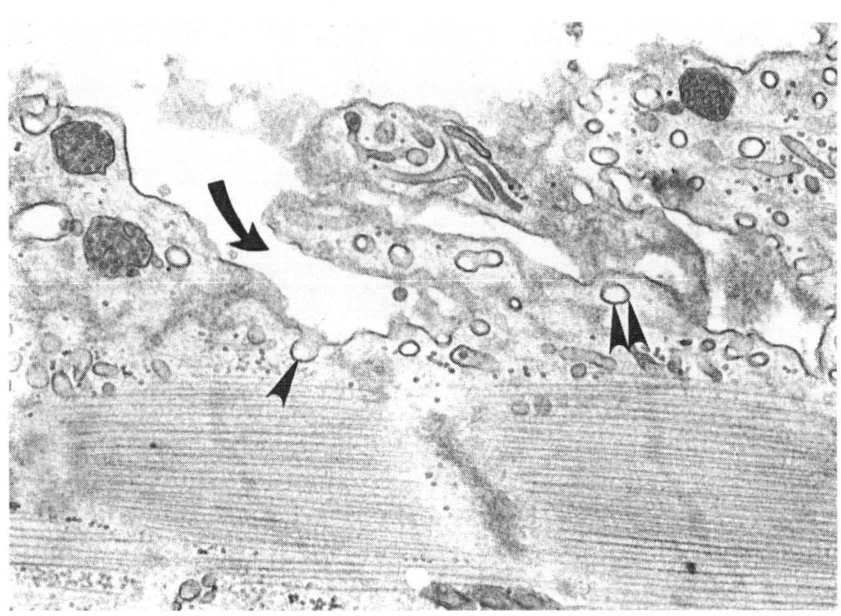

Figure 5. Lateral edge of cultured adult ventricular myocyte. Surface area is difficult to estimate because of irregular T tubes (arrow) and caveolae (arrowhead). Some membrane-bound structures (double arrowheads) are ambiguous with respect to their continuity with the surface. (X 47,000)

determinations (for a given number of cells) to yield an estimate of in vitro hypertrophy [25]. Such studies, however, do not accurately take variability of cell height (Figure 4) [20, 26] into account, nor do they offer the investigator the opportunity to assess volumetric organellar relationships [6]. Likewise, morphometry of cultured cells mechanically or enzymatically removed from the growth surface does not accurately represent the in vitro state, since volumetric relationships may be distorted during retrieval of the myocytes. The most accurate manner to determine the volume of cultured cells is to combine planimetry of the cell outline with ultrastructural morphometry of in situ, transversely sectioned cultured myocytes.

As outlined above, we utilize test grids for our morphometric determinations. In fact, a number of other technologies such as electronic planimetry exist which are capable of generating the same type of data.

CONCLUSION

Morphometric studies of cultured adult and neonatal cardiac myocytes are of obvious value in increasing our understanding of the heart muscle cell. Culture systems provide investigators with a mechanism to study cardiac muscle cells in isolation from the remainder of the organism. Therefore direct and indirect responses of the muscle cells may be studied in the absence of the numerous obscuring factors present in whole organisms. Moreover, since cultured cells may be maintained for weeks or months in vitro [11], developmental studies are possible. Although descriptive ultrastructural studies are useful in characterizing these cultured cells, the subjectivity of such studies diminishes their usefulness as correlates for more precise physiological and biochemical investigations. In addition, morphometric description of cultured myocytes from diseased animals, for example spontaneously hypertensive rats [12], might allow investigators to more accurately correlate maintenance of altered morphology in culture with morphological characteristics of the original tissue. Induction of in vitro hypertrophy is also a fertile area for such studies.

ACKNOWLEDGEMENTS

The authors acknowledge the excellent technical assistance of Sally Guice, Nicholas Lanson, Jr., Elizabeth Underwood, and Kathy Vial.

REFERENCES

1. B.A. Mobley and E. Page, J. Physiol., London, 200: 547-563 (1972).
2. E. Page and C.P. McCallister, Am. J. Cardiol., 31: 172-181 (1973).
3. E. Page, J. Earley, and B. Power, Circ. Res. (Suppl.), 34-35: 12-16 (1974).
4. P. Anversa, L. Vitali-Mazza, and A.V. Loud, Lab. Invest., 33: 696-705.
5. E. Bossen, J.R. Sommer, and R.A. Waugh, Tissue Cell, 10: 733-784 (1978).
6. R.V. Tomanek, Lab. Invest., 40: 83-91 (1979).

7. J. Schaper, E. Meiser, and G. Stammler, Circ. Res., 56: 377-391 (1985).
8. S.P. Bishop and J.L. Drummond, J. Mol. Cell. Cardiol., 11: 423-433 (1979).
9. N.J. Severs, A.M. Slade, T. Powell, V.W. Twist, and G.E. Jones, Cell Tissue Res., 240: 159-168 (1985).
10. W.C. Claycomb and M.C. Palazzo, Dev. Biol., 80: 466-482 (1980).
11. R.L. Moses and W.C. Claycomb, Am. J. Anat., 171: 191-206 (1984).
12. R.L. Moses and W.C. Claycomb, Anat. Rec., 211: 350 (abstract) (1985).
13. W.C. Claycomb and R.L. Moses, Exp. Cell Res., 161: 95-100 (1985).
14. E.R. Weibel, Int. Rev. Cytol., 26: 235-248 (1969).
15. E.R. Weibel, In Principles and Techniques of Electron Microscopy, Vol. III, M.A. Hayat, ed., 237-296 (1973).
16. A.V. Loud, Anal. Quant. Cytol. Histol., 9: 7-12 (1987).
17. R.L. Moses and W.C. Claycomb, Am. J. Anat., 164: 113-131 (1982).
18. M.S. Forbes, B.A. Planholt, and N. Sperelakis, J. Ultrastruct. Res., 60: 306-327 (1977).
19. R.L. Moses and J.B. Delcarpio, Cell Tissue Res., 228: 499-496 (1983).
20. J.B. Delcarpio, W.C. Claycomb, and R.L. Moses, submitted.
21. R.L. Moses and J.B. Delcarpio, Cell Tissue Res., 203: 173-180 (1979).
22. L.M. Cruze-Orive, H. Hoppeler, O. Matheiu, and E.R. Weibel, J. Royal Stat. Soc. Series C., 34: 14-32 (1985).
23. L.M. Cruze-Orive and E. Hunziker, J. Microscop., 143: 47-80 (1986).
24. W.A. Merz, Mikroskop., 22: 132-139 (1968).
25. P. Simpson, Circ. Res., 56 : 884-894 (1985).
26. R.L. Moses, J.B. Delcarpio, and J. Boogaerts, J. Mol. Cell. Cardiol., 14: 52 (abstract) (1982).

IMMUNOHISTOCHEMICAL CHARACTERIZATION OF ISOLATED AND CULTURED CARDIAC MYOCYTES

LOUIS TERRACIO AND THOMAS K. BORG
Departments of Anatomy and Pathology, University of South Carolina, Columbia, SC 29208

INTRODUCTION

One of the foremost goals when using isolated cells is to be able to define the similarities and differences of the isolated cell compared to cells in the intact organ or organism. The criteria for this comparison are not well defined but usually require a series of biochemical as well as morphological characteristics that can be measured in vitro. Where relevant, these criteria should be related to in vivo measurements. Both biochemical and morphological criteria can be expected to change as a function of time in culture. For example, freshly isolated cells have a different morphology compared to cells that have been in culture for 30 days. The amount of protein synthesis would also be expected to be altered in the same example. At the present time there is little data available to determine whether biochemical parameters, such as receptor number, are up or down regulated under in vitro conditions.

The principal methods for determining if isolated and cultured cardiac myocytes have retained a differentiated structure are electron microscopy and immunohistochemistry using antibodies against defined structural components. The electron microscopic characterization of isolated and cultured adult cardiac myocytes are covered elsewhere in this volume. This chapter will deal predominately with the immunohistochemical characterization of freshly isolated and long-term cultured adult myocytes. The advantage of immunohistochemical characterization of the cells is that these techniques are able to bridge the biochemical and functional features with the morphological structure of the cells.

Two time points are of particular interest with isolated adult myocytes: 1) shortly after isolation and 2) after the cells have adapted to culture. Immediately after isolation, it is important to determine that the cells have retained as much of their differentiated structure as possible and that the collagenase digestion has not destroyed the enveloping basement membrane including the sarcolemmal surface glycoproteins. After the myocytes have spread and adapted to the culture environment, a process which requires remodelling of both the cell surface and the contractile apparatus, it is important that the cells re-express their differentiated characteristics.

Those components of critical importance to the structure of the basement membrane include laminin, type IV collagen, nidogen,. fibronectin and proteoglycans [1]. Cell surface glycoproteins which function as receptors for extracellular matrix components (ECM) are apparently also essential to the functions of the cell [2]. Of principal importance within the cell are the contractile proteins as well as the cytoskeletal components. It is interesting to note that an important characteristic of adult cells is that viable cells, when freshly isolated, must have a basement membrane that has not been destroyed by the isolation procedure and that the contractile apparatus with its cytoskeletal connections to the sarcolemma must not be disrupted. These features are in contrast to isolated neonatal and embryonic cardiac myocyte preparations in which the contractile apparatus is completely disassembled. If the adult cells remain relatively quiescent, they will adapt to culture by disassembling the contractile apparatus, reorganizing the basement membrane components,

Biology of Isolated Adult Cardiac Myocytes
William A. Clark, Robert S. Decker, and Thomas K. Borg, Editors

as well as the cytoskeletal components and finally reassemble the contractile components [3,4]. Our knowledge of the coordination of these events is fragmentary but there appears to be a communication between the ECM, cytoskeletal components, and the formation of the contractile apparatus [5,6]. Immunohistochemistry using specific antibodies against cytoskeletal components such as vinculin, talin, desmin, vimentin and alpha-actinin correlated with the ECM specific antibodies against laminin, heparan sulfate proteoglycan, fibronectin, type IV collagen and nidogen as well as antibodies against the contractile proteins will provide essential data for the elucidation of the coordination of process of sarcomerogenesis _in vitro_ [7]. In addition, muscle specific monoclonal antibodies such as HHF-35 (ENZO Biochemical, New York, NY) are essential in determining the purity of long term cultures. This antibody specifically recognizes only muscle actin and does not recognize actin in any non-muscle cells. Thus the percentage of myocytes in replicate cultures can readily be determined using this antibody.

SAMPLE PREPARATION FOR LIGHT MICROSCOPIC IMMUNOHISTOCHEMISTRY

Adult cardiac myocytes can be isolated by a number of procedures as reviewed in this volume and elsewhere [8]. Regardless of the specific method of isolation used to obtain cardiac myocytes, it is important that the procedure be done consistently each time to yield comparable results. We always use the same procedure for the isolation of ventricular rat myocytes [9] as well as the same selected batch of collagenase throughout an experimental series. Once isolated, we have found that attachment of the cells to laminin or type IV collagen (see chapter on cell attachment in this volume) greatly facilitates manipulation of the cells when compared to cell suspensions. Coverslips can be coated with 10 μg/ml of laminin or type IV collagen and freshly isolated myocytes can be attached and cultured. At various times after attachment, the cells can be fixed and processed for immunohistochemistry. Although the choice of fixatives depends on the specifications of the antibodies to be used, it has been our experience that 2.0% paraformaldehyde, freshly prepared, in a buffered solution is almost universally acceptable. The choice of buffer system does not appear to be critical with cardiac myocytes; however, we use Sorensen's phosphate buffered saline. The time of fixation should be kept short (10-30 min) in order to maintain antigenicity, but still adequate to retain cell morphology. Our procedure (Table 1) is to wash the cells with buffer maintained at 37° C followed by addition of the fixative also maintained at 37° C. The cells are then left at 22° C for the remainder of the fixation time. Following fixation, we routinely quench any free aldehydes by treating the cells with 0.1 M glycine in the same buffer as the fixative for 15 min at 22° C. The latter step will prevent interaction of the free aldehydes and the antibodies as well as to reduce non-specific background.

Source of antibodies

Antibodies to most ECM components, cytoskeletal components and contractile elements are available commercially or from the Developmental Studies Hybridoma Bank [10]. However, it is critical to determine if the reagents recognize the antigen of interest in the species of animal that is being investigated. The usual source of antibodies for cytoskeletal components is chicken smooth muscle (gizzard) which sometimes only gives a weak reaction in mammalian cardiac myocytes. The cross reactivity should be checked on sections of heart tissue and/or by Western blots.

Fluorochromes

A number of different fluorochromes are commercially available for use in indirect immunofluorescence staining. These include fluorescein isothiocyanate (FITC), rhodamine, tetramethyl rhodamine isothiocyanate (TRITC), lissamine rhodamine isothiocyanate (LRITC) and Texas red (TR).

Each of these fluorochromes has advantages and disadvantages which need to be considered before choosing the appropriate one for specific experiments. The most commonly used fluorochrome is FITC. Its principal advantage is that the fluorescent signal is very strong with a low background signal. The disadvantages of FITC are that many preparations contain free fluorescein which can increase background and that FITC can rapidly fade during viewing. Both of these disadvantages can be overcome. The problem of free fluorescein can be eliminated by selectively purchasing reagents that have been passed through a molecular sizing column to separate the IgG-FITC from the free fluorescein. The rapid fading of FITC can be compensated for by short photographic exposures or the use of agents that retard the fluorescence fading in the mounting medium [11,12]. The commonly used preparations to retard fluorescence fading are para-phenylenediamine (PPD), n-propyl gallate (NPG) or 1,4-diazobicyclo (2,2,2)-octane (DABCO) [11]. We have found that PPD in polyvinyl alcohol (PVA) at 2 mg/ml is superior to NPG or DABCO in retarding FITC fluorescence fading without quenching fluorescence. However, the disadvantages of PPD in PVA are that it is very viscous, must be prepared immediately before use, and the cells cannot be stored for more than 24 hours after mounting. The latter problem can be overcome by remounting in PVA alone if long-term storage of samples is necessary. Rhodamine, TRITC and LRITC all give a very bright fluorescent signal that is stable for longer times than FITC. However, each of these fluorochromes results in an increase in the overall background fluorescence that can cause problems with certain antigens. This is of particular importance when staining freshly isolated adult ventricular myocytes which can be up to 50 μm in diameter. Any increase in background fluorescence in such large cells can cause problems in resolution of certain antigens such as those of the cytoskeleton. TR does not give as bright a signal as the other fluorochromes but does have the advantage of low background and longer viewing stability. For single antibody stainings, we routinely use FITC or TR.

Double staining for co-localization of two antigens

In order to determine the spatial relationship of 2 substances in a cell it is necessary to perform sequential double stainings. This is easily done if subclass specific monoclonal antibodies are used [13]. If such monoclonals do not exist for the antigens of interest, the cells can still be stained if appropriate controls are performed. We have successfully localized cell surface antigens and cytoskeletal components in the same adult ventricular myocyte. To do so, cells are fixed in 2.0% paraformaldehyde and quenched in 0.1 M glycine in PBS. The cells are incubated with the first primary antibody (such as rabbit anti-collagen receptor), washed and incubated with an appropriate secondary antibody (i.e. goat anti-rabbit) Fab-FITC for 60 min at 37° C. It is important to use the Fab-FITC at a sufficiently high concentration to totally saturate the first primary antibody. Since the Fab-FITC is monovalent, and is used at a saturating concentration, it does not allow for the subsequent "second" primary and secondary antibodies to bind to itself or the first primary antibody. Saturating titers of Fab fragments can be determined by exposing cells preincubated with primary antibody with various concentrations of unconjugated Fab. Then incubating the cells with an appropriate anti-IgG-FITC (i.e. goat anti-rabbit IgG-FITC). The lack of fluorescence indicates a concentration of the Fab sufficient to saturate the primary antibody. Saturation is usually achieved with a 1/20 to 1/15 dilution of the Fab fragments (.15 mg/ml). We routinely use a 1/10 dilution to ensure total saturation since this step is so critical. After the Fab-FITC incubation, the cells are washed (3X for 5 min with PBS containing 0.5% BSA) and permeabilized with Triton X-100 (0.1% in PBS) if the second antigen is to be localized within the cells as with cytoskeletal or contractile proteins. After washing as previously described, the cells are incubated with the second primary antibody for 30 min at 37° C, washed and incubated with the appropriate anti-IgG conjugated to LRITC for 30 min at 37° C. LRITC is used since it does not exhibit any green fluorescence and will not result in false co-localization. The cells are then washed and mounted on slides with PBS:Glycerine or PPD in PVA to retard fluorescence fading. Additional controls consist of substitution of pre-immune IgG, primary antibody preadsorbed with excess antigen (if available) or PBS for the primary antibody. Also to prevent spectral overlap between the LRITC and FITC, an excitation peak of 550 nm should be used for LRITC. This will eliminate the possibility of red FITC fluorescence [14].

IMMUNOHISTOCHEMISTRY AT THE ELECTRON MICROSCOPIC LEVEL

Immunohistochemistry at the light microscope level can provide valuable insights into structure/function relationships in cardiac muscle. However, the lack of resolution cannot provide sufficient detail for the precise location of antigens. This is especially true when investigating the role of cytoskeletal proteins, contractile proteins and/or cell surface receptors in cardiac myocytes. To gain the increased resolution, immunohistochemical techniques must be applied at the electron microscopic level. The preservation of antigenicity is a major obstacle, since most of the procedures in the preparation of samples for electron microscopy have a negative effect on the antigenicity of most proteins. Even when the primary fixative indicates good preservation of antigenicity, the dehydration and embedding procedures often exhibit a detrimental effect on localization of antibodies.

The procedures for immunohistochemistry at the electron microscopic level are summarized in Tables 2 and 3 and relate primarily to freshly isolated and cultured cardiac. Many aspects of the procedures can be applied to tissue samples. A critical decision in the preparation of the sample is the type and duration of fixation. We have found that exposure to the fixative for up to 1 hr at 4° C to be effective since longer times tend to show reduced staining. The fixatives that have been routinely employed for cardiac tissue have been 1.0% freshly prepared phosphate buffered paraformaldehyde, 0.075 M lysine, 0.01 M sodium metaperiodate and 3.0% paraformaldehyde and 0.10% glutaraldehyde in phosphate buffer [15]. In most cases, samples are not fixed with osmium tetroxide. Exposure to the primary antibody can be done at several different times during the sample preparation depending upon the location of the antigen (i.e. cell surface, cytoskeletal, cytoplasmic, etc.). In practice, exposure of the primary antibody can be done after fixation (en bloc) or on thin sections. If the en bloc procedure is used for antigens in the cytoplasm, the cells must be permeabilized with a detergent such as Triton X-100 (0.05 to 0.1% in buffer). Following exposure to the primary antibody, the preparation is thoroughly rinsed in buffer, reacted with a blocking agent such as 1% ovalbumin, then exposed to IgG or protein-A labeled colloidal gold particles. We routinely fix the sample after cytochemical reactions for 15 min with 1% osmium tetroxide in buffer to stabilize the lipid membranes. If the localization of antibodies is combined with either intermediate (IVEM) or high voltage electron microscopy (HVEM), then the en bloc method is preferred in order to visualize the three dimensional staining pattern by stereo-microscopy [16]. For further discussion of HVEM of isolated cells, see the chapter by Decker et al. in this volume. The en bloc procedure is also employed when whole cells are examined by HVEM or IVEM. In these types of preparations, the cells are grown on laminin coated formvar films which lie over gold electron microscopic grids. All procedures can be done on the grids which can then be dehydrated, critical-point dried and examined by HVEM or IVEM [7]. If the specimens cannot be treated en bloc with the primary antibody, then the samples must be dehydrated, embedded and thin sectioned. The thin sections are mounted on gold grids, reacted with the primary antibody followed by a blocking agent such as 1% ovalbumin and reacted with the secondary, labeled ligand. This secondary ligand can be an IgG labeled with ferritin or gold or protein-A coated colloidal gold particles. Thorough washing in between each step cannot be over emphasized. The precise times of staining must be determined for each antibody under investigation.

The limiting factor in the preservation of antigenicity can be the dehydration and embedding procedure. Some investigators recommend dehydration in ethylene glycol and ethanol whereas others use conventional methods such as a graded series of ethanols. Dehydration should be done at 0° C. The embedding media of choice is the acrylate-methacrylate mixture, commercially known as Lowicryl. This embedding media is infiltrated and polymerized at low (-20° C) temperature and appears to minimize loss in antigenicity as compared to conventional embedding media [16]. The procedures for using this medium are summarized in Table 2. The procedures that are summarized in these tables can be altered and changed for each particular antigen.

EXAMPLES OF IMMUNOHISTOCHEMICAL CHARACTERIZATION OF CARDIAC MYOCYTES

As described above, a mixture of cell surface/ECM components and cytoskeletal/contractile components should be demonstrable both shortly after isolation and after the cells have adapted to the culture environment. The following are several examples of the localizations that our laboratory has demonstrated in freshly isolated and cultured cardiac myocytes.

Figure 1 demonstrates the immunofluorescent staining of the cell surface of adult cardiac myocytes for a variety of ECM components. Freshly isolated cells stain positively for laminin (Fig. 1a) and heparin sulfate proteoglycan (Fig. 1b), but do not stain for collagen type IV (Fig. 1c) or for fibronectin (Fig. 1d). An intermediate level of fluorescence was observed using antibodies against chondroitin and dermatan sulfate proteoglycans (data not shown) depending on the individual preparation. The lack of staining for collagen type IV and fibronectin is most likely due to the loss of these antigens during collagenase digestion, since the cells do stain positively for these antigens after 24 hours in culture (Figs. 1e and 1f). An interesting observation is that the staining pattern for laminin shows an increased deposition in a banded pattern indicative of the sarcomere distribution in these cells. Additional studies indicate that this staining pattern is near the Z-line of the cells in the same region where interstitial collagen has been shown to attach to the cell surface [17]. In this same region receptors for the interstitial collagens and fibronectin have also been localized (Figs. 3c and 3d).

After the myocytes have progressed into culture, the basal surface of the cells expresses all the ECM components tested (Fig. 2). The pattern of distribution is different for the individual components. After 14 days in culture the myocytes have flattened and spread out. Laminin staining reveals a dense fluorescent layer that is interrupted by circular non-

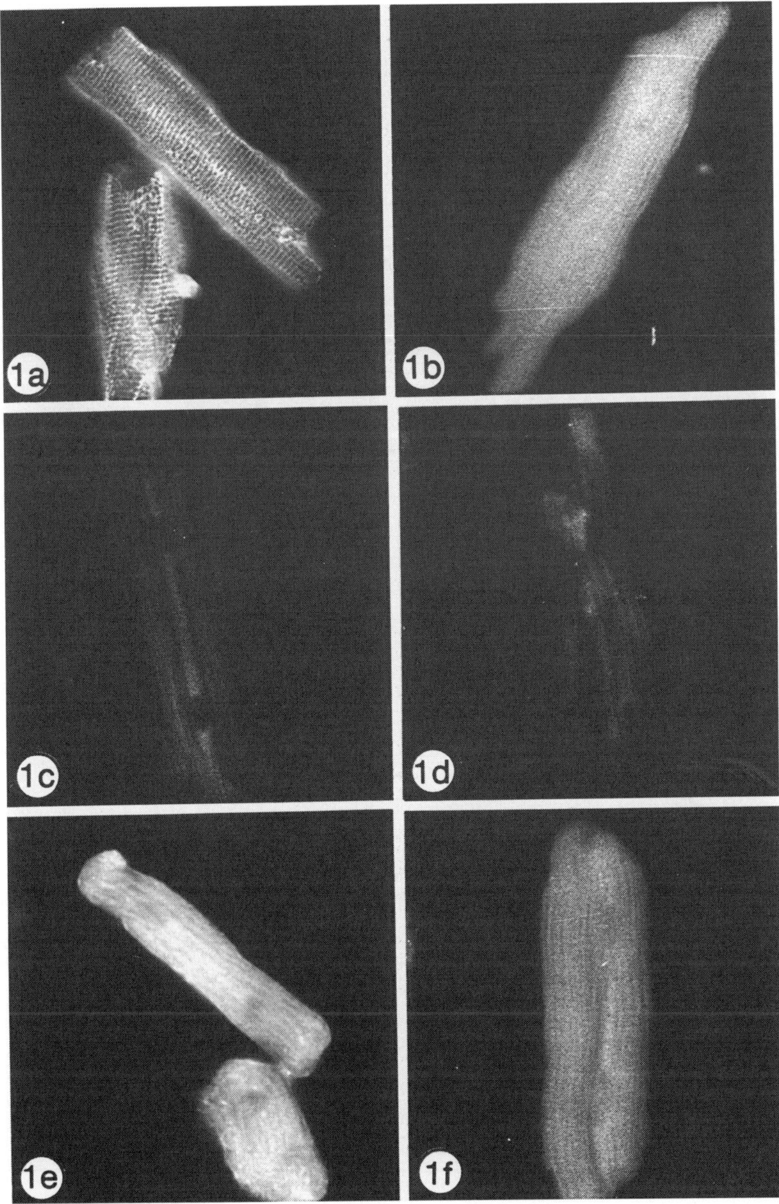

Figure 1. Fluorescence photomicrographs of freshly isolated cardiac myocytes stained for laminin (A), heparan sulfate proteoglycan (B), collagen type IV (C), fibronectin (D). The freshly isolated cells are negative for collagen IV (C) and fibronectin (D) but after 24 hours _in vitro_ they become positive (E and F, respectively).

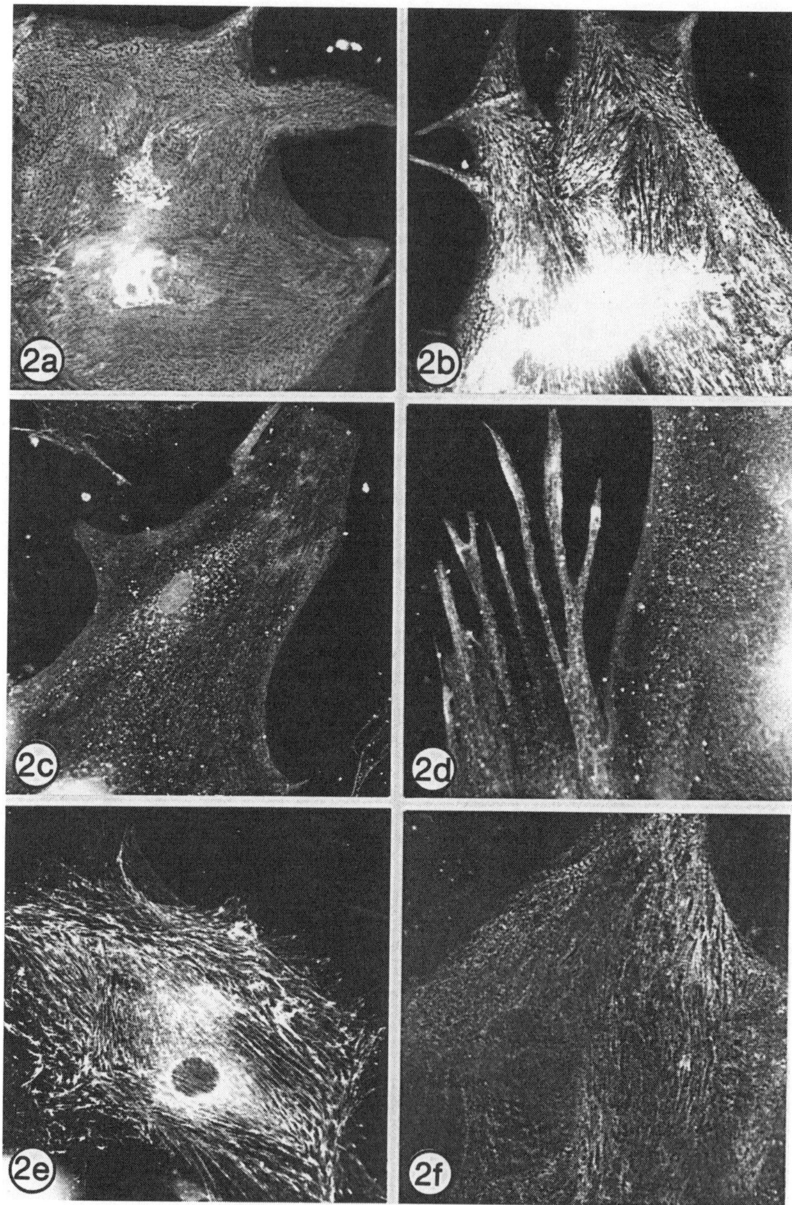

Figure 2. Fluorescence photomicrographs of cells cultured for 14 days stained for laminin (A), heparan sulfate proteoglycan (B), chondroitin sulfate proteoglycan (C), dermatan sulfate proteoglycan (D), fibronectin (E) and collagen type IV (F).

fluorescent areas (Fig. 2a). These non-fluorescent areas are possibly sites of focal adhesions. Heparan sulfate proteoglycan (Fig. 2b), chondroitin sulfate proteoglycan (Fig. 2c), and dermatan sulfate proteoglycan (Fig. 2d) staining results in a moderately dense layer of immunofluorescence beneath the cells. The pattern of heparan sulfate proteoglycan (Fig. 2b) was similar to that for laminin (Fig. 2a), whereas the chondroitin sulfate and dermatan sulfate proteoglycan staining was more diffuse. The staining patterns for fibronectin (Fig. 2e) and collagen type IV (Fig. 2f) were very similar. Both exhibited a linear pattern radiating into the periphery of the cell. In many cases this pattern was similar to the pattern of stress fibers and reorganized contractile elements of these cells.

Freshly isolated myocytes stained for ECM receptors exhibited strikingly similar patterns. When stained with CSAT (the avian fibronectin/laminin receptor) (Fig. 3a), the fibronectin receptor (Fig. 3b) or the collagen receptor (Fig. 3c), the freshly isolated myocytes exhibited a banding pattern indicative of the sarcomere distribution. Electron microscopic localization of the collagen receptor (data not shown) indicates that the receptors are located just lateral to the Z line, at the point where collagen has been shown to attach to the cells in vivo [17]. The localization of these receptors and the ECM components, such as collagen type I and laminin, at a discrete area on the cell surface may reflect a specialized region on the myocyte for cell-ECM interaction.

Complementary to this external ECM site is an internal region of cytoskeletal specialization known as "costameres" [18]. At this region the cytoskeletal components vinculin and talin makes a rib-like structure that are proposed to anchor the sarcolemma to the cytoskeleton. Double immunofluorescent staining of cells with the collagen receptor (Fig. 3e) and vinculin (Fig. 3f) reveals essentially identical banding patterns. This co-localization possibly indicates an ECM-cytoskeletal connection at this site. Such an interaction would have a profound effect on the function of the myocyte and deserves further investigation.

Similar connections were demonstrated in the long-term cultured myocytes. Vinculin (Fig. 4a) and the collagen receptor (Fig. 4b) co-localize in the spread processes of the cell indicating that this association is retained as the cells adapt to the culture environment. This close association of vinculin and the collagen receptor can be demonstrated at the electron microscopic level (Figs. 4c and 4d). The localization of 2 antigens in such close proximity to each other is strong support for the maintenance of the ECM-cytoskeletal interaction in cultured myocytes.

Characterization of the contractile and cytoskeletal elements of the freshly isolated and long-term cultured myocytes is readily achieved by immunohistochemistry. Localization of actin can be visualized by using anti-actin antibodies; however, fluorescently labeled phalloidin (Molecular Probes, Junction City, OR) is an easy, one-step process that is compatible with immunohistochemical double staining. Freshly isolated (Fig. 5a) and long-term cultured myocytes (Fig. 5b) exhibit a typical banding pattern. Antibody staining for other components such as myosin, desmin, vimentin, alpha-actinin (Fig. 5c, and 5d) and tubulin (Fig. 5e) all give typical distribution patterns in myocytes. The use of the muscle specific monoclonal antibody (HHF-35) enables investigators to determine the percentage of myocytes in long-term preparations as this antibody only reacts with muscle actin and thus will not stain fibroblast (Fig. 5f).

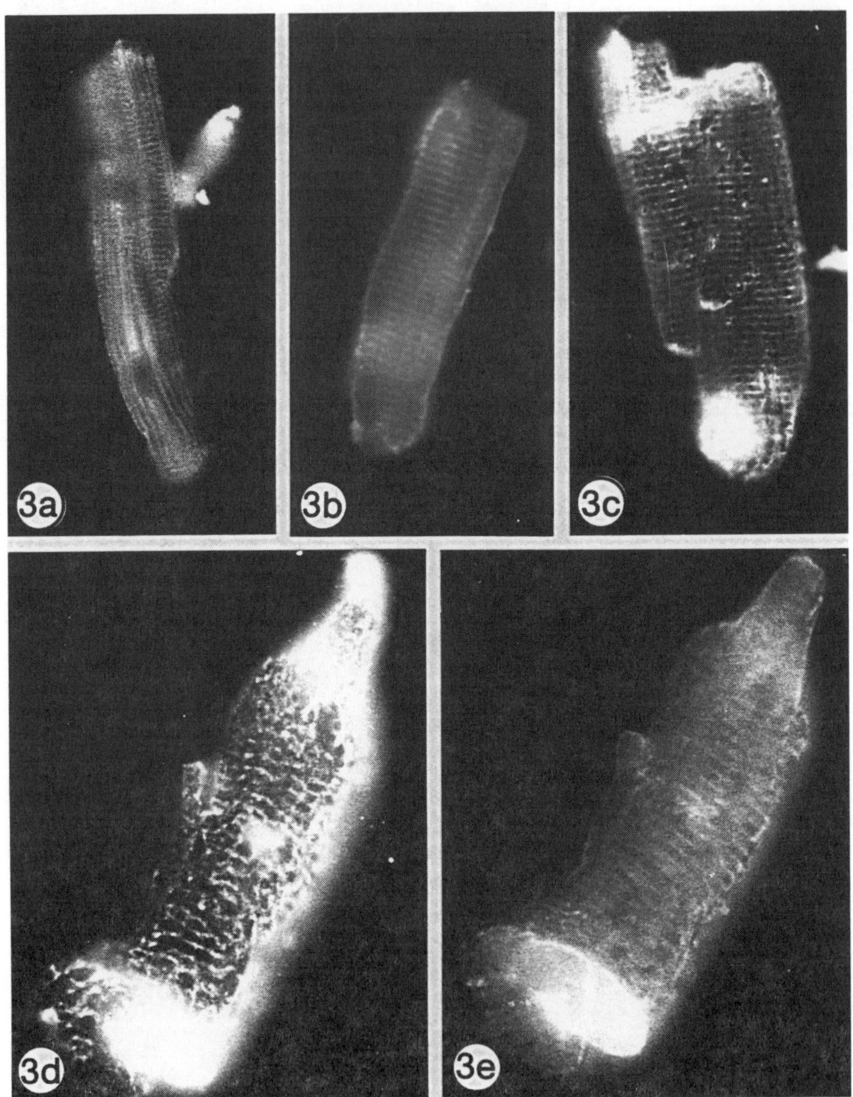

Figure 3. Fluorescence photomicrographs of freshly isolated myocytes stained for CSAT (A), fibronectin receptor (B), collagen receptor (C and D) and vinculin (E). Note that the collagen receptor and vinculin appear to co-localize (D and E).

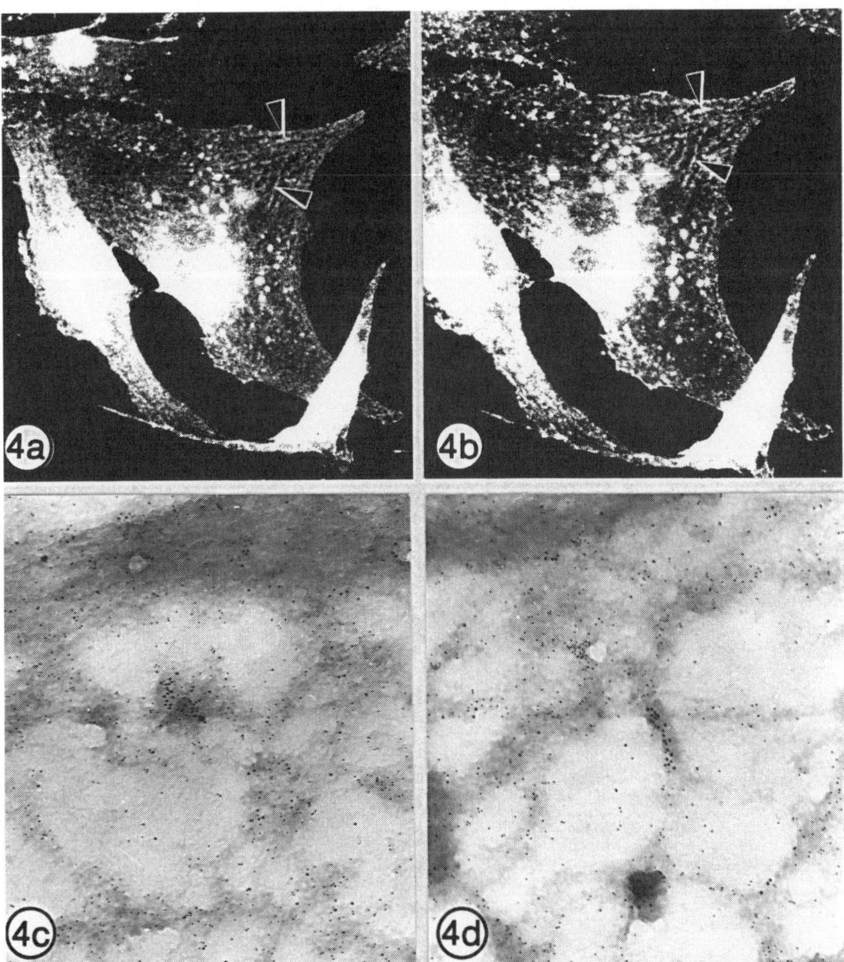

Figure 4. Co-localization of vinculin and the collagen receptor in long term cultured myocytes by immunofluorescence (A and B) and whole mount immunogold staining (C and D). The same discrete fluorescent areas (arrows) can be seen when the cells are stained for vinculin (A) and the collagen receptor (B). When examined by electron microscopy using two different sizes of gold particles (collagen receptor 15 nm and vinculin 5 nm), clusters of gold particles of both sizes are seen in close association with each other (C and D).

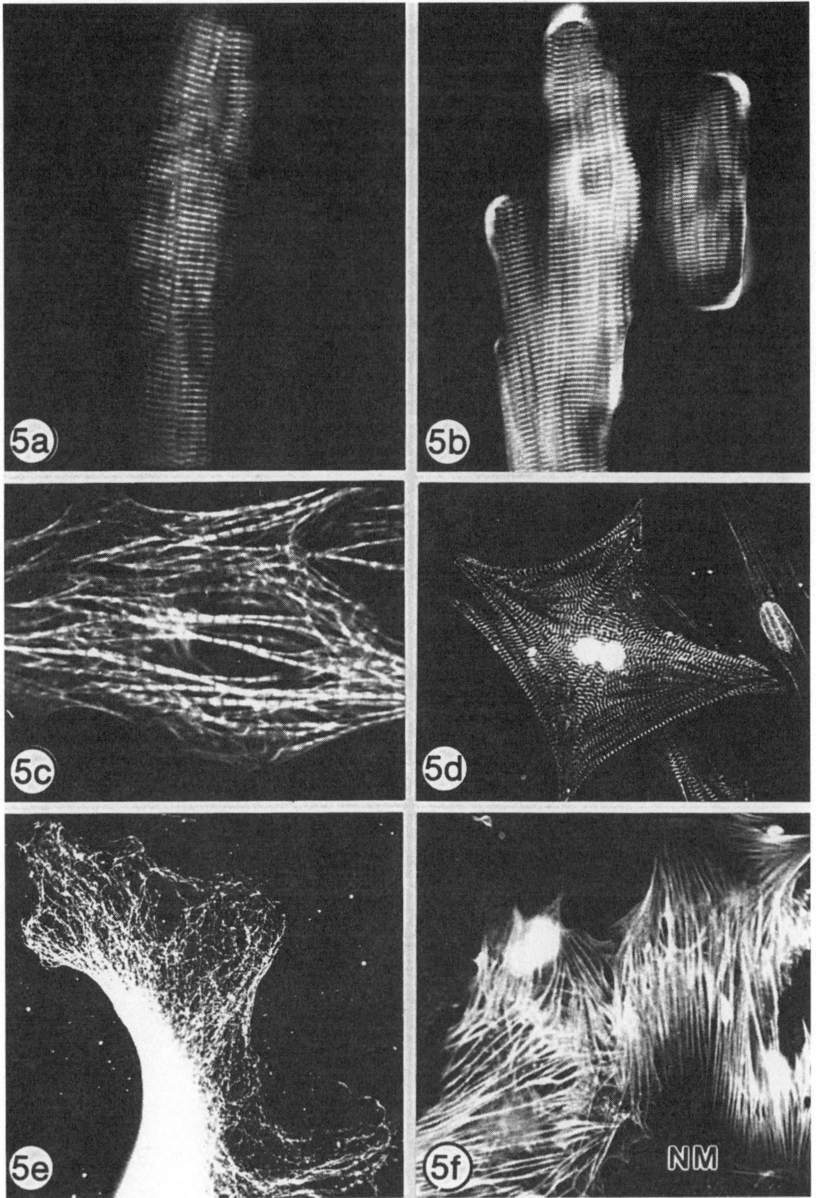

Figure 5. Fluorescent photomicrographs of freshly isolated (A and B) and long term cultured myocytes (C-F). Rhodamine labeled phalloidin (A and C), alpha-actinin (B and D), tubulin (E) and muscle specific actin (F). Non-muscle cells (fibroblasts) do not stain with the muscle specific actin (5F-NM).

TABLE 1

Summary of Procedures for Immunofluorescence

1. Attach or culture cells on 22x22 mm coverslips coated with 10 μg/ml of laminin.
2. Wash the cells 3x with 37° C PBS to remove serum proteins.
3. Fix the cells in 2.0% paraformaldehyde in Sorensen's phosphate buffered saline for 10 to 30 min.
4. Rinse the cells in PBS.
5. Incubate the cells in 0.1M glycine in PBS for 15 min to quench free aldehydes.

5a. If staining for an internal antigen, incubate the cells in 0.1% Triton X-100 for 10 min.

6. Wash the cells 3x for 5 min in PBS containing 0.5% BSA (PBS/BSA).
7. Incubate the cells with the primary antibody diluted in PBS/BSA for 30 min at 37° C or 60 min at room temperature in a high humidity chamber.
8. Wash the cells 3x in PBS/BSA - 5 min each.
9. Incubate the cells in the secondary antibody conjugated to an appropriate fluorochrome (see Discussion in this chapter) for 30 min at 37° C or 60 minutes at room temperature in a high humidity chamber.
10. Wash the cells 3x in PBS/BSA - 5 min each.
11. Mount on glass slides in PBS:Glycerol (1:3) or 2 mg/ml PPD in PVA.

TABLE 2

Summary of Procedures for Fixation and Embedding in Lowicryl

Fixation: 1% paraformaldehyde in Hanks balanced salt solution (HBSS), pH 7.4, 37° C, then cool to 4° C for 60 min

Dehydration and Embedding in Lowicryl K4M:

Rinse twice in HBSS, 10 min each
30% ethanol for 5 min at 4° C
50% ethanol for 5 min at 4° C
70% ethanol for 5 min at -10° C
90% ethanol for 30 min at -20° C
90% ethanol: Lowicryl 1:1, 60 min at -20° C
90% ethanol: Lowicryl 1:2, 60 min at -20° C
100% Lowicryl 60 min at -20° C
100% Lowicryl overnight at -20° C
Embed in Lowicryl (dry gelatin capsules) and polymerize for 5-7 days at -20° C under U.V. light

Sectioning: cut sections 60-90 nM thick and mount on foravar coated, 200 mesh nickel grids

Staining: Float grids on drop of 0.1 M glycine in phosphate buffered saline (PBS), pH 7.4, 3 times, 5 min each

Rinse twice in PBS, 5 min each
Float grid on drop of 1.0% ovalbumin in PBS for 5 min
Float grid on antibody solution for 1-2 hrs in a moist chamber
Rinse grid in PBS 3 times for 5 min
Float grid on 1.0% ovalbumin in PBS for 5 min
Float grid on protein A: gold complex diluted 1:50 with PBS for 1 hr in moist chamber
Rinse grid with PBS followed by distilled water
Post-stain in uranyl acetate and lead citrate

TABLE 3

Summary of Procedures for Whole Mounted Cells for Immunohistochemistry

1. Place 200 mesh gold electron microscope grids on a glass coverslip and coat the grids and coverslip with a thin film of formvar. The grids should then be sterilized by exposure to UV light overnight.

2. Coat the surface of the grids with laminin or type IV collagen at a concentration of 10 μg/ml in sterile culture medium.

3. Place the coverslip in the bottom of the culture dish, plate the cells and culture for an appropriate period of time.

4. Prior to fixation with 2.0% paraformaldehyde, the cells should be washed to remove serum proteins. After fixation the grids can be reacted with antibodies by inverting the grids on a drop of the reagents. The incubation and washing times are the same as described in Table 1 (steps 2-10); however, instead of the standard fluorochrome, the secondary antibody or protein A should be conjugated to colloidal gold.

5. Grids can then be dehydrated in a graded series of alcohols and subjected to critical point drying.

6. A light layer of carbon should be vacuum evaporated on the surface of the grids in order to add thermal stability before viewing by either high or intermediate voltage electron microscopy.

SUMMARY

Immunohistochemical characterization of the isolated and cultured myocytes has enabled investigators to demonstrate that these cells retain their differentiated expression of cytoskeletal, contractile, ECM components, and ECM receptor antigens both immediately after isolation and after long-term culture. These techniques are essential in the investigation of how these cells alter their morphology as they adapt to the culture environment and will be useful tools for evaluating experimental perturbations of cultured cardiac myocytes.

ACKNOWLEDGEMENTS

The authors wish to thank the following individuals for supplying antibodies used in this study: Stefan Johansson, Borje Nordling, Clayton Buck, Kristofer Rubin, Donald Gulberg, Susan Craig, and Keith Burridge. Technical assistance from Tim Sullivan, Bobbie Schneider, Marge Terracio, Nancy Vinson, Art Dewey, X.H. Ma, and Evy Lundgren was greatly appreciated. The authors also wish to thank Willa Gibbemeyer for secretarial assistance. Research was supported in part by NIH grants HL 24935, HL 37669, and HL 33656.

REFERENCES

1. D.R. Abrahamson, J. Pathol., 149:257 (1986).
2. R.O. Hynes, Cell 48, 549 (1987).
3. W.C. Claycomb and N. Lanson, In Vitro 20:647 (1984).
4. A.A. Dlugosz, P.B. Antin, V.T. Nachmias, and H. Holtzer, J. Cell Biol., 99, 2268 (1984).
5. M.J. Bissell, H.J. Hall, and G. Parry, J. Theor. Biol., 99, 31 (1981).
6. L. Terracio, D. Gulberg, K. Rubin, S. Craig, and T.K. Borg, Anat. Rec., Submitted.
7. L. Terracio, K. Robertsson, A.R. Dewey and T.K. Borg, In: Proc. Ann. E.M.S.A., G.W. Bailey, Ed. (San Francisco Press, Inc., San Francisco, 1986) pp. 548-549.
8. S.L. Jacobson, and H.M. Piper, J. Mol. Cell. Cardio., 18, 661 (1986).
9. E. Lundgren, T.K. Borg, and S. Mordh, J. Mol. Cell. Cardiol., 16, 355 (1984).
10. Developmental Studies Hybridoma Bank, T. August, Dept. of Pharmacology and Molecular Sciences. The Johns Hopkins University School of Medicine, Baltimore, MD 21205.
11. K. Valnes and P. Brandtzaeg, J. Histochem. Cytochem., 33:755 (1985).
12. H. Giloh and J.W. Sedat, Science 217:1252 (1982).
13. G.M. Wessel, and D.R. McClay, J. Histochem. Cytochem., 34, 703 (1986).
14. M.W. Wessendorf, and R.P. Elde, J. Histochem. Cytochem., 33, 984 (1985).
15. L.F. Lemanski, D.J. Paulson, C.S. Hill, L.A. Davis, L.C. Riles, and S. Lim, J. Histochem. Cytochem., 33, 515 (1985).
16. J. Roth, M. Bendayan, E. Carlemalm, W. Villiger, and M. Garavito, J. Histochem. Cytochem., 29, 663 (1981).
17. J.B. Caulfied and T.K. Borg, Lab. Invest. 40, 364 (1979).
18. J.V. Pardo, J.D. Siliciano, and S.W. Craig, J. Cell Biol., 97, 1081 (1983).

EVALUATION OF ANOXIC INJURY IN ISOLATED ADULT CARDIOMYOCYTES

HANS MICHAEL PIPER
Physiologisches Institut I, Universität Düsseldorf, Moorenstr. 5, D-4000 Düsseldorf 1, Federal Republic of Germany

1. Models of the hypoxic myocardial cell

Isolated cardiomyocytes allow to investigate the properties of the cardiac muscle cells (i) in a manner specific for the cell type, (ii) with direct control of the extracellular medium, and (iii) with use of sensitive optical or electrophysiological single-cell techniques which are not applicable to a piece of tissue. The use of isolated cardiomyocytes represents a reductionist approach aiming at a deeper analysis of pathophysiological principles on the single cell level. But it may often be the difference between the behavior of isolated cells and cells in tissue that leads to better understanding of causal factors only effective in tissue context.

The reduction of the complex in-vivo situation of ischemia concerns mainly the following circumstances: (i) Cells in suspension or in short-term culture are mechanically isolated from each other and free from the impact of exogenous forces. They are also uncoupled from metabolic influences by other cells. (ii) In general, the extracellular volume will be much larger than the interstitial space in ischemic tissue. And the chemistry of the extracellular fluid will be more stable than in ischemic tissue. (iii) The milieu conditions of ischemia will be reduced to some specified factors. Besides oxygen and substrate deprivation this can be, e.g., acidosis, increased concentrations of lactate or potassium.

There are also a number of caveats in using isolated cardiomyocytes as models of the myocardial cell in tissue. (i) Isolated cardiomyocytes may have altered properties due to the isolation stress. The use of such pre-damaged cells in studies on cellular injury can be misleading. It is therefore advisable to allow the cells to recover before using them. (ii) Isolated cardiomyocytes differ physiologically in some respects from the adult myocardium. Without stimulation they should be quiescent, since they are not driven by pacemaker cells. Consequently, their aerobic energy turnover and their anaerobic energy exhaustion should be slower than in the beating myocardium. (iii) Cells exposed to a certain treatment in the cardiomyocyte model may respond in a way resembling the result of a similar treatment of tissue. But in fact the phenomena may be causally different.

The experimental systems using isolated adult cardiomyocytes for studies of hypoxic injury differ in some important respects:

(i) Most studies have been performed with cardiomyocytes in suspension. In contrast, in several studies by our group surface-attached, short-term cultured cardiomyocytes were used (1).

(ii) In most studies, suspended cardiomyoycytes were mechanically agitated during the experiments. In contrast, surface-attached cardiomyocytes were not exposed to mechanical forces.

(iii) In some studies, hypoxic experiments were performed in nominally Ca^{2+} - free buffers (2-5). Greater pathophysiological interest is directed to studies in which hypoxic injury is studied at physiological Ca^{2+} levels. At low Ca^{2+} concentrations, sarcolemmal permeabilities may be increased (6), but Ca^{2+} influx caused by membrane perforations will be reduced.

(iv) Preparations of suspended cardiomyocytes usually contained 20-40% severely damaged cells. Their presence may have prevented the detection of subtle metabolic changes. From surface-attached cardiomyocyte preparations broken cells can always effectively be removed (1).

Biology of Isolated Adult Cardiac Myocytes
William A. Clark, Robert S. Decker, and Thomas K. Borg, Editors

(v) Cardiomyocytes allowed to recover from the isolation stress under appropriate culture condition have been shown to re-normalize their metabolic properties. Freshly isolated cardiomyocytes in suspension exhibit a number of untypical metabolic features (79).

2. Energy expenditure and energy production in hypoxia

It has been demonstrated that the individual heart muscle cell will not stop mitochondrial respiration and increase glycolytic flux unless exogenous pO_2 has dropped below 0.5 torr (7). This means that the cell as a whole is almost as sensitive to low oxygen tension as the isolated mitochondrion. The cited absolute value for the threshold of the aerobic/anaerobic metebolic transition has been debated. Others found values higher by one order of magnitude in adult rat and in embryonic chick cardiomyocytes (8,9). But this difference has been explained by different energy demands of cardiomyocytes under the chosen experimental conditions (8). Nevertheless, the studies agree in that the range of oxygen tension for the transition from aerobic to anaerobic metabolism is very narrow. Conditions with an oxygen tension below this threshold level are usually referred to as "anoxia". Unlike single isolated cardiomyocytes, the perfused heart responds in a gradual fashion to a reduction of oxygen supply. This is because, the lower the amount of oxygen supplied to the heart per unit of time, the fewer cells along the perfusion path can satisfy their oxyen demand. Therefore, for the perfused heart the more general term "hypoxia" seems appropriate.

The hypoxic and the ischemic myocardium reduce their energy demand immediately after oxygen withdrawal (10,11) In the beating heart the reduction in contractile activity, i.e. mechanical failure, accounts for most of this self-protective mechanism. This, however, is only part of the energy saving mechanism, since myocardium arrested prior to ischemia (11) and quiescent myocytes (12) also quickly reduce their energy demand under hypoxic conditions. Thereby the absolute saving in energy consumption depends on the prehypoxic energy expenditure (11) Except from the energy-conserving effect of early mechanical failure, little is known about the nature of these mechanisms.

In spite of this self-protective reduction of energy demand, anaerobic energy metabolism at the end always falls short of energy needs as indicated by the loss of high-energy phosphates (10). Cultured cardiomyocytes contain elevated amounts of glycogen, and they use glycogen for glycolytic energy production in substarte free anoxia. But when ATP contents have fallen by about 70 %, glycolytic energy production almost stops even though still half of this substrate is left (12). It has been suggested by Kübler and Spieckermann (10) that this inability to use a glycolytic substrate is due to the lack of phosphorylation energy at the phosphofructokinase reaction. In the hypoxic perfused heart (13) and in anoxic isolated cardiomyocytes (12) irreversible injury can be postponed considerably if glycolytic flux is stimulated already at the onset of oxygen deprivation. Since enhanced glycolysis delivers more ATP to the cell, cellular ATP contents decrease at a slower rate. In contrast to the ischemic myocardium, in these systems the waste products of glycolysis, lactate and protons, do not accumulate to the extent as they do in ischemic tissue.

A contribution of mitochondria to the loss of energy in the hypoxic cell is well documented. In the non-respiring state the mitochondrial ATP-synthetase acts in a backward direction, i.e., as an ATP-hydrolase. It was demonstrated by use of the specific inhibitor oligomycin that this mechanism may account for 80 % of ATP breakdown during 20 min of ischemia in the heart (14) and for an equivalent energy saving in isolated heart cells during 40 min exposure to the electron chain blocker rotenone (15). Thus, one major effect by which mitochondria contribute to the aggravation of hypoxic cellular injury consists in the inversion of a normal physiological function.

The functional injury of mitochondria isolated from ischemic and hypoxic myocardium has been the subject of many studies (e.g.,16,17). All these results demonstrate that mitochondrial functions are considerably impaired after a period of ischemia or hypoxia. But these impairments may not be responsible for the functional inability of the heart after reperfusion. This is because even in a working heart at normal work load only part of the total respiratory capacity of normal mitochondria is used, but after an ischemic or hypoxic period functional insufficiency becomes apparent already at low energy demand. This argument applies even more to quiescent isolated cardiomyocytes whose energy demand is much lower than that of the beating myocardium. Indeed, after a period of hypoxia, impairment of mitochondrial metabolism in cardiomyocytes was not found very pronounced when compared with other aspects of metabolic disturbance (18,19). Even in cells rounding up in anoxia, the changes in mitochondrial ultrastructure are relatively moderate.

Other results also indicate that a loss of mitochondrial function determines not the "point of no-return" of hypoxic cell injury. When cytosolic Ca^{2+} just starts to rise in a hypoxic cardiomyocyte, resupply of ATP by resumption of oxydative phosphorylation prevents the impending loss of Ca^{2+} control (20). This indicates that ultimately a shortage of energy primes the cell for death. A cytosolic free Ca^{2+} concentration of 3 μM has been shown to determine the irreversible loss of Ca^{2+} control (20). And it is probably the inability of mitochondria to resume sufficient ATP production at this Ca^{2+} level, defining it as crucial. Since this behavior is based on a normal functional property of mitochondria (21), it does not need specific mitochondrial injury to bring about cell death. In summary, according to current evidence mitochondria are not a "limiting structure" for cell survival.

3. Sarcolemmal integrity of the hypoxic cardiomyocyte

It sounds almost as a trivial truth that cell survival requires sarcolemmal integrity. With holes in the sarcolemma, soluble cell contents will be lost in mass quantity, and Ca^{2+} will rush into the cytosol from outside where Ca^{2+} concentrations are higher by 4 orders of magnitude. In a muscle cell this causes gross disruptions of the cell structures, since at high Ca^{2+} concentrations myofibrils undergo hypercontracture and thereby tear up large parts of the cytoskeleton.

But the rule that cell survival presupposes sarcolemmal integrity, seems to hold only with certain reservations. For heart muscle cells are able to cope with sarcolemmal leaks for brief periods, i.e., the sarcolemma can spontaneously heal over such lesions if they occur in an otherwise healthy cell. Transient sarcolemmal perforations occur, for example, when single cells are impaled by microelectrodes. And the isolation of individual cells from tissue would not be possible if the cells were not able to heal over small membrane defects. For during the course of cell isolation, gap junction complexes are torn out of one of the adjacent cells in toto, allowing in general the enduring cell to survive (22). Therefore, persistent holes in the sarcolemma seem to be a phenomenon secondary to other crucial changes of the cell's condition.

The sarcolemma of hypoxic cardiomyocytes changes physically prior to large disturbances of its phospholipid composition. A very early hypoxic phenomenon in isolated cardiomyocytes is the protrusion of small microblebs (up to about 1 μm in diameter) from the cell surface (23). Microblebs are indicative of small breaks in the connections between the cytoskeleton and the sarcolemma. Other findings also indicate that the structural links between sarcolemma and cytoskeleton are affected already early in the process of hypoxic injury. In isolated cardiomyocytes, it has been demonstrated by the technique of microphotolysis, using a fluorescently labeled lipid incorporated into the sarcolemma, that the lateral diffusion coefficient for such a labeled probe increases by an order of magnitude within 5 min of hypoxia (24) It has been suggested that this increase in membrane fluidity is caused by removing the normal restrictions in lateral diffusion in cardiac sarcolemma. The physical basis of these normal restrictions are supposed to reside in the linkage of the sarcolemma to its cytoskeletal scaffold.

Acid phospholipids of the sarcolemma bind Ca^{2+}. This local pool of Ca^{2+} has been studied in ischemic heart tissue and in isolated hypoxic cardiomyocytes by a histochemical technique, which precipitates structure-bound Ca^{2+} with use of pyroantimonate and, thereby, makes it visible in transmission electron microscopy (25). With this technique it was demonstrated that in the state of progressed hypoxic injury, but prior to detectable sarcolemmal disruptions, the sarcolemma loses its ability to bind Ca^{2+}. In isolated cardiomyocytes this event takes place when myofibrils become ultimately hypercontracted, i.e, at the edge of irrevesible structural injury. Only beyond this time Ca^{2+} was found massively increased at mitochondrial sites, suggesting that influx of Ca^{2+} into the cell has increased. It has been hypothesized that the loss of Ca^{2+} binding to the sarcolemma is due to a change in its phospholipid composition. The observed shift of structure-bound Ca^{2+} from sarcolemmal to mitochondrial sites probably coincides with a rise in cytosolic Ca^{2+} concentration.

In isolated hypoxic cardiomyocytes a rise in cytosolic Ca^{2+} is not the result of large membrane perforations, since it proceeds gradually (20). Furthermore, it can be blocked by divalent cations as, e.g. Ni^{2+}, as it has been demonstrated in cardiomyocytes poisened by 2-deoxyglucose plus cyanide (26). Since this disturbance of Ca^{2+} homeostasis can be reversed by early resumption of oxydative energy production, it seems to be a shortage of energy which primes the heart cell for cell death. The sarcoplasmic reticulum plays a decisive role at the edge of irreversible loss of Ca^{2+} control. Since, when its ability to sequester Ca^{2+} was blocked with caffeine, any recovery of Ca^{2+} control was abolished (20).

4. Release of enzymes from the hypoxic cardiomyocyte

Release of cytosolic enzymes from the hypoxic perfused heart or from hypoxic isolated cardiomyocytes has been demonstrated to correlate with cellular ATP contents in certain experimental models (16,27,28). Already a small reduction in contents of energy-rich phosphates, as it may also occur in physiological stress, leads to a detectable release of enzymes (29,30). Studies on isolated cardiomyocytes in substrate free anoxia have shown that this early enzyme release is due to protein loss from only the cytosolic compartment of cells which are still in the reversible phase of hypoxic injury (16,23,31,-33). Mitochondrial or lysosomal marker enzymes are not so early released, as known also for ischemic myocardium. In fact, release of mitochondrial enzymes seems to be a very late phenomenon in hypoxia indicative of cell necrosis (34-36), and it is characteristic of the "oxygen paradox" (34,35). At the time enzyme release starts in hypoxic cardiomyocytes, half of the phosphocreatine is broken down, but ATP contents have changed only little yet. At this early stage ultrastructural alterations are subtle (23). Large holes in the sarcolemma can be ruled out as causing the protein leakage. The number of hypercontracted cells does not correlate with this early release of cytosolic enzymes. Currently one can only speculate about the nature of the mechanism (37) allowing large molecules to leave an energetically stressed cell without it being freely permeable to much smaller molecules as, e.g., the Ca^{2+} ion, which would immediatly cause hypercontraction.

It might be causally related to the release of proteins from hypoxic cells that the number of subsarcolemmal vesicles increases (23,32), the cell surfaces is protruded into small sarcolemmal blebs (23,32), and the fluidity of the hypoxic sarcolemma rapidly increases by an order of magnitude (24). Leakage of soluble proteins from reversibly energetically stressed cells has also been reported for other cells types (38-41). It has been hypothesized by Spieckermann et al. (30) that the heart cell releases cytosolic enzymes continuously, but at a low rate, and that the release through this unidentified channel is enhanced under conditions of energetic stress.

In infarcted myocardium many cells are lysed. Therefore, a considerable part of the enzyme release from such tissue can be explained by mass loss from broken cells. Indeed, it has been shown that the size of the necrotic area correlates well with the amount of enzymes lost from infarcted myocardium (42). In the clinical setting detection of cardiospecific enzymes in the circulation will generally indicate the occurance of necrotic cells, because the moderate early release of cytosolic enzymes easily remains undetected due to the impeded washout from ischemic areas and the limited sensitivity of the methods in use.

In contrast to surface-attached cardiomyocytes, those in agitated suspension seem to behave in a different way under hypoxic conditions. It has been reported that such preparations release enzymes in parallel to an increase in trypan blue positive cells (2,4,15). There are, however, some reservations concerning the interpretation of theses results:

(i) The amounts of enzymes released were massive in comparison to early enzyme release from surface-attached cardiomyocytes (12). Indeed, such subtle changes were probably impossible to detect in preparations which already under aerobic conditions contain 20-40 % severely damaged cells. In our experience, such preparations have already a considerable enzyme release which makes it difficult to detect small changes.

(ii) The use of trypan blue as a primary criterion for cell viability is also questionable (43). This holds particularly when trypan blue is not used at all as a "vital stain" in its proper sense, but simultaneously with a glutaraldehyde fixation of the cells (2-4). It has been shown in a convincing way that there is no clear relation between severe metabolic injury, ionic imbalances and trypan blue stain (44). On the other hand, hypoxic (5) and cultured cardiomyocytes (45) have been reported to "recover" from positive trypan blue stain.

(iii) In the studies cited a very probable artifact has not been ruled out, namely that in agitated suspensions distorted and blebbed cells are broken by exogenous forces. This could easily explain why hypercontracted cells lose their (cytosolic) enzyme contents in suspensions, but not in the culture model (12) in which they are not exposed to such forces.

5. Contracture of the hypoxic cardiomyocyte

When ATP contents begin to fall, sarcomeres shorten gradually in attached cultured cardiomyocytes (23). Since this shortening is not preceded by an increase of cytosolic Ca^{2+} concentration it is due to a rigor mechanism (20). In isolated cardiomyocytes which are not attached on a substratum and thus completely devoid of any outer mechanical support, these rigor forces cause a sudden, maximal overcontraction (15,20). In regional ischemia rigor bond formation becomes apparent by the increasing stiffness of the tissue. In contrast to the isolated cells, however, the sarcomeres in regionally ischemic tissue become longer than normal, because the stretching from the surrounding contracting tissue is the predominant force. These differences in rigor development may have consequences for hypoxic energy metabolism since rigor bond formation itself can contribute to hypoxic energy depletion by activation of the actomyosin ATPase (see below).

Cultured cardiomyocytes have shortened sarcomeres when cellular ATP levels have fallen to 30 % of their normal aerobic values (23). If anoxic conditions persist, a growing number of cells become ultimately hypercontracted. Then they have a round appearance and large surface blebs. Myofibrils are condensed into homogeneous masses and the structural organization of the interior is widely destroyed. On reoxygenation such cells will not recover. But, in general, even these irreversibly injured cells can retain a closed sarcolemmal surface for some length of time (33). And they are generally also devoid of "flocculent densities", the irregular electron dense deposits in the mitochondrial matrix which have been regarded to be a necessary company of irreversible cell damage (46). Hypercontracted, rounded cells have lost their ability to relengthen (3,15, 23) possibly because the myofibrils are no longer chained together with other cytoskeletal structures. In particular, links between Z-lines and the sarcolemma are broken (23). As a consequence such cells have lost their polygonal appearance and the ordered arrangement of cell organelles. Instead, mitochondria and fragments of the tubular substructures are protruded in large pouches from the cell surface. The factor(s) causing rigor bond formation in the oxygen deficient heart cell are still a matter of debate. Based on the finding by Weber and Murray (47) that, in vitro, rigor bonds between actin and myosin are formed in a Ca^{2+} independent manner if the ATP concentration is below 100 μM, it has been hypothesized that in the hypoxic cell , too, rigor is caused by a lowering of the cytosolic ATP concentration below this level (15,48-53). This reasoning, however, has to cope with the problem that the average ATP concentrations in contractured hypoxic heart tissue can be equal or greater than 1 mM, i.e. tenfold higher than the concentrations causing rigor bond formation in vitro. It has therefore been assumed that the cytosol is not a homogeneous space for ATP but contains a subcompartment next to the myofibrils in which the ATP concentrations can become tenfold lower than in the rest of the cytosol (47,53). So far, no direct evidence has been given for the truth of this assumption. In the following an alternative explanation will be proposed.

In vivo, actin-myosin interaction always proceeds in the presence of ATP <u>and</u> its degradation products ADP and P_i. The thermodynamically "available" energy spend per crossbridge cycle equals the free energy change ΔG of ATP hydrolysis (54):

$$\Delta G = \Delta G_0 + RT \ln [ATP]/[ADP] \times [P_i]$$

(free energy change ΔG_0, universal gas constant R, absolute temperature T, and free cytosolic metabolite concentrations). For the cytosolic compartment of the aerobic beating heart, ΔG values of 60 kJ/ mol ATP have been estimated (55,56). The energy demand of a single crossbridge cycle has been calculated to be 55-60 kJ/mol myosin (57,58).

In the normothermic globally ischemic rat heart, contracture is fully developed after 30 min (59). The average cytosolic ΔG value can be estimated to be about 30 kJ/mol ATP (55). This is approximately the energy needed for loading a rigor complex with ATP and the subsequent separation of actin and myosin (see below). From this the hypothesis can be derived, that contracture is fully developed when the average ΔG value becomes insufficient for untieing a rigor bond.

The rigor states AM and AM-ADP (A, actin; M, subfragment 1 of heavy meromyosin) are supposed to occur as transient states in a normal crossbridge cycle (57,58,60):

```
              ATP
        AM     ┴→  AM+ATP → AM-ATP → A+M-ATP
ADP   ←┤                                    │
        AM-ADP ←┬  AM-ADP-Pi ← A+M-ADP-Pi ←─┘
                ↓
                Pi
```

The net formula of such a cycle is AM + ATP --> AM + ADP + P_i, i.e. the cycle is driven by the energy liberated from ATP hydrolysis. Thereby the steps from (AM + ATP) to (A + M-ADP-P_i), which is the preferred refractory dissociated state in relaxed muscle, account for 30 kJ/mol (57,58). If the energy level is generally lower, persistence of AM and AM-ADP states must be expected since these are of lowest energy content (57).

It is conceivable that single crossbridges remain trapped in the rigor state, if the average ΔG value is too low to allow the cycling of all crossbridges to be completed. In fact, tissue tension in the ischemic rat heart is found to increase after about 10 min (59) at which time a cytosolic ΔG of approximately 45 kJ/mol has been determined (55). The persistence of single rigor complexes can speed up the formation of more such. This is because one rigor bond among the 7 myosin binding sites of an actin molecule activates the actin/tropomyosin complex (61) This becomes apparent in an enhanced affinity of actin for M or M-ADP (61), i.e., rigor bond formation is even more favored. Furthermore, actomyosin ATPase activity is enhanced (61), and this may contribute to the velocity of hypoxic ATP decay. The initial steric structure of rigor complexes is not yet at an energetic minimum (57). A subsequent conformation change leads to force generation and shortening of myofibrils, unless this is prevented by an opposing stretching force as in regionally ischemic myocardium.

In the globally ischemic and hypoxic heart, rigor is accompanied by muscle shortening. This is a gradual process, leading to shortened sarcomeres throughout the tissue. A gradual shortening of the myofibrils is also observed in single isolated myocytes under anoxia if these are attached to a substratum (23). At an average ATP content of about 2 µmol/ g wet weight these cells are in a square, but still polygonal form, the sarcomere length is reduced from the initial 1.9 µm (slack length of sarcomeres) to 1.4 µm (23). At 1.4 µm sarcomere length, myosin filaments are already distorted. This sarcomere length, however, is also observed during forceful contractions in cardiomyocytes and is fully reversible. If the cells in this shortened square form are reoxygenated, they relengthen (23). This behavior demonstrates the reversible nature of this rigor state. In contrast to attached cells, free floating single cells do not shorten in a gradual fashion, but rapidly shrink to a minimal sarcomere length of about 1.1 µm or 60 % their initial length (15,20). This difference of behavior can probably be explained by the complete absence of any force opposing rigor forces in non-attached cells. In surface attached cells, cell adhesion opposes shortening forces. It has been documented in several studies (15,16,20) that such cells are usually unable to relengthen upon reoxygenation although they can regain control of their cytosolic free Ca^{2+} levels (20). Apparently, at 1.1 µm sarcomere length severe disruptions of the cytoskeleton have taken place which normally disable the cells to reassume an elongated shape. As an exception to that rule, it has been reported in two studies that a low number of such shortened cells can still relengthen (5,62) even though not to the full initial length.

There is some apparent contradiction between the results on short-term cultured surface-attached cells and those reported by Stern et al. (62). These authors have reported a behavior of surface attached cells identical to that of free floating cells. They used cells attached on non-treated glas cover slips after 1 h preincubation. In our experience rod-shaped cells attach indeed during 1 h incubation on a glas surface, but the number is small compared to other substrata (1,45,63). But after 1 h on this surface the cells are, in general, fixed only at one of their ends near to the intercalated disc region. If they contract they are apparently unrestrained in their movements. Thus, the case reported by Stern et al. (62) is in fact identical to that of suspended cells under anoxic conditions. Another misleading impression may have arisen from the same report, namely that in a normoxia-anoxia-reoxygenation cycle round cells appear only as a result of reoxygenation. This is neither true for cultured cardiomyocytes nor for

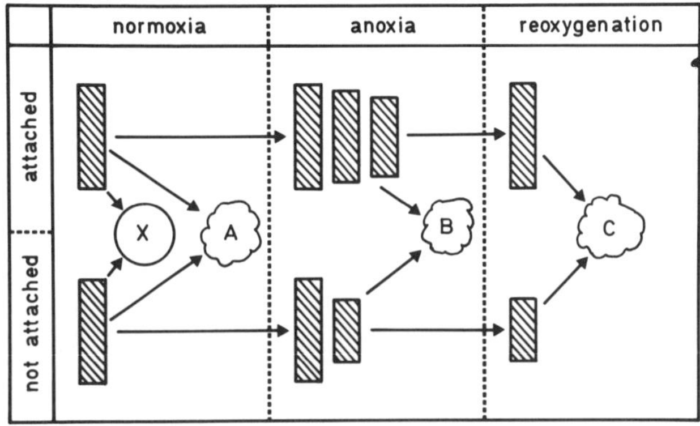

FIG. 1. Schematic representation of possible shape changes of isolated adult cardiomyocytes, attached to a substratum (above) or not attached (below). For a discussion of the forms X, A, B, and C see text.

suspended cells. Round cells have been reported to appear in both preparations under aerobic as well as anoxic conditions (1,3,15,23) (**Fig. 1, A,B,C**). Cardiomyocytes with a round configuration and a smooth surface which dissolve their contractile apparatus are a transitory stage for establishing cardiomyocytes in long-term culture (45) (**Fig. 1,X**).

6. Glycolytic energy production and myocardial cell injury

In studies by Opie and Bricknell (53,64) a beneficial effect of high glycolytic flux rates could be demonstrated for the myocardium under low-flow ischemia. They observed that at low rates of glycolytic flux not only ATP contents decrease more rapidly, but enzyme release and contracture development are more pronounced when compared at a given lowered ATP level. From this the authors have speculated that "glycolytic" ATP is preferentially localized in the vicinity of sarcolemma and myofibrils, thus protecting their integrity.

The results of the cited studies, however, are also compatible with an alternative explanation not assuming a subdivided sarcolemmal space. Under aerobic conditions adenine nucleotides are compartmentalized in cytosol and mitochondria due to the directional specificity of the adenine nucleotide translocator (65). If mitochondria stop respiring as in the case of hypoxia, the mitochondrial membrane potential dissipates and subsequently the directional specificity of the translocator is abolished (65). Therefore, if mitochondrial respiration stands still, assimilation of cytosolic and mitochondrial ATP/ADP ratios and, for other reasons, also of cytosolic and mitochondrial free inorganic phosphate concentrations can be expected (65). Thus, the relative portion of ATP localized in the cytosol should be smaller in hypoxia than under aerobic conditions. But a complete assimilation of ATP/ADP ratios is probably prevented by (i) the compartmentation of anaerobic energy production in the cytosol, (ii) high ATPase activity in the mitochondria (17), and (iii) progressive impairment of translocase activity (16). Thus, dependent on the relative rates of these processes, increased glycolytic flux may lead, at identical average ATP contents of the cell, to a steeper cytosolic-mitochondrial gradient for the ratio (ATP/ADP x P_i) which determines the energy generated by ATP hydrolysis. This means

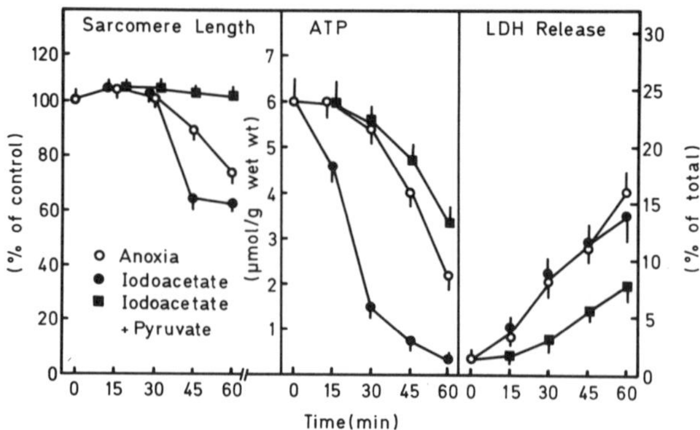

FIG. 2. Sarcomere lengths, ATP contents and release of lactate dehydrogenase of cultured rat cardiomyocytes (i) in substrate free anoxia, (ii) under aerobic conditions with 10 mM glucose and 1 mM iodoacetate, and (iii) as (ii) plus 5 mM pyruvate (31). Mean values ± standard errors of 5 experiments. Sarcomere lengths were determined in each experiment from 20 randomly selected electron micrographs (23). In the individual experiments the variance coefficients were below 15% (for 45 min iodoacetate: 19%). Since fixation causes a small contraction in cardiomyocytes with normal energy balance, the aerobic value, set at 100%, is slightly lower than the subsequent values (23). (From (80) with permission)

that, at a given ATP level, more phosphorylation energy is available in the cytosol.

So far, the dependence of enzyme release and contracture development from changes in the free energy change of ATP hydrolysis have not been investigated. This is because of the difficulties in determing free cytosolic concentrations of ADP and P_i. A comparison of energy depletion of isolated cardiomyocytes by anoxia and by glycolytic blockade, however, indicates the importance of this magnitude for enzyme release and contracture development. As described elsewhere (31) short-term cultured cardiomyocytes were incubated in a saline glucose-free medium either under anoxic conditions or aerobic conditions with presence of iodoacetate. Iodoacetate blocks glycolytic flux on the level of the glyceraldehyde-3-phosphate dehydrogenase reaction and thereby leads to an enormous accumulation of phosphorylated intermediates at the previous steps of the Embden-Meyerhof pathway (31). It is suggested that thus the free cytosolic P_i concentration is lowered under iodoacatate, but increased in anoxia (66). The degradation of ATP to ADP proceeds similarly in anoxia and under glycolytic blockade. Therefore, at a given ATP level, in iodoacetate treated myocytes the (ATP/ADP x P_i) ratio will be higher, i.e., more phosphorylation energy will be available in the cytosol.

It is shown in **Fig.** 2 that contracture develops with a similar time course for anoxia and iodoacetate treatment (statistical difference only for the 45 and 60 min values, $p < 0.01$) even though the loss of ATP is much faster under iodoacetate. The same is true for release of lactate dehydrogenase. The time course for losing this enzyme is identical under both experimental conditions (no statistical differences). This behavior fits the hypothesis that both contracture development and enzyme release depend on the (ATP/ADP x P_i) ratio and not the absolute ATP level.

In cells with glycolytic blockade energy shortage can be relieved by supply of a mitochondrial substrate, e.g. pyruvate. In this case energy depletion is distinctly delayed. It is probably only delayed because iodoacetate is an alkylating agent which interfers also with mitochondrial enzymes and thus prevents fully sufficient oxidative energy production. In fact, with pyruvate, ATP decay proceeds slightly slower than in anoxia, but at 60 min the cells have not shortened and enzyme release is only half that under anoxia. Again, the energetic state of the cells seems to be better when compared to the anoxic situation at corresponding ATP levels.

7. Late reoxygenation of the hypoxic myocardial cell

The paradoxical dramatic aggravation of tissue damage upon reoxygenating myocardium after prolonged periods of hypoxia or ischemia, has been termed "oxygen paradox" (34). It is characterized by abrupt release of cytoplasmic constituents due to the sudden rupture of cell membranes and the unique phenomenon of contraction band formation (67). The latter consists of overcontracted and overstretched adjacent sarcomeres coexistent in the same cell. The mechanism underlying the oxygen paradox is not yet satisfactorily understood.

According to a recently much favoured hypothesis the formation of oxygen radicals causes the sudden tissue deterioration (68,69). A leading role in oxygen radical formation has been ascribed to the xanthine oxidase system (69). This theory could provide an explanation why the oxygen paradox is absent in attached isolated cardiomyocytes since the myocyte, in contrast to the endothelial cell (70), is devoid of this enzyme system (71). It is however questionable whether this is a sufficient explanation since serious doubts about the importance of the xanthine oxidase system for reperfusion injury in heart have arisen (71,72). A more general criticsm applies also to other versions of oxygen radical theories about the oxygen paradox in heart, namely that they are inable to explain why suppression of oxydative phosphorylation in mitochondria protects against the oxygen paradox (67).

It has been hypothesized by Ganote at al. (67) that the oxygen paradox is caused by mechanical forces generated in injured myocardial tissue. In contrast to the isolated cell, a muscle cell in tissue is exposed to the forces of neighbouring cells that resume active contractions or undergo contracture or resist the cell's own shortening. The inhomogeneities arising may account for the formation of overstretched and condensed parts in the myofibrillar apparatus, i.e. of contraction bands. From this mechanical hypothesis follows that the typical signs of the oxygen paradox should be absent in isolated cardiomyocytes and in hearts reoxydized under conditions which prevent resumption of mechanical activity by abolishing aerobic respiratory energy production. Therefore, this hypothesis can cope with both requirements to a theory about the genesis of the oxygen paradox.

In cardiomyoctes not attached to a surface, in which cytosolic Ca^{2+} had become higher than 2-3 µM, reoxygenation was found to cause a rapid rounding of the cells, i.e ultimate hypercontraction, and irregular surface blebbing (20). It may be speculated that this deleterious effect of late reoxygenation is due to a superimposition of a Ca^{2+} contracture on a rigor state, which becomes possible with resumption of even a small ATP production in presence of elevated cytosolic Ca^{2+} levels. The generation of some ATP by oxydative phosphorylation is a necessary prerequisite for this late cell rounding, since it does not occur in the presence of uncouplers or inhibitors of oxydative phosphorylation (73,74).

The similarity of conditions leading to rounding of cardiomyocytes reoxygenated late with the conditions of the oxygen paradox in heart tissue, gives rise to the question whether both have the same principal cause (74). There are, however, a number of facts which do not fit easily such a hypothesis:

(i) The characteristic ultrastructural feature of the oxygen paradox, namely the formation of contraction bands (67), is missing in isolated cells which have rounded upon reoxygenation. Contraction bands indicate the existence of drastic mechanical force inhomogeneities in individual cells. In rounded cells, however, myofibrils are hypercontracted throughout the cell (23). This demonstrates the existence of large tension forces, but not of such inhomogeneities evident in tissue. The impact of grossly inhomogeneous forces on individual cells seems to be specific to cells in tissue.
(ii) Rounding up in hypercontraction is the usual appearance of deteriorated isolated cardiomyocytes, also under aerobic conditions, but contraction bands in tissue are a very specific feature of a hypoxia-reoxydation cycle (67).
(iii) In heart tissue, the development of the oxygen paradox is a sudden event, in which all cells deteriorate simultaneously (34,67). In non-attached isolated anoxic cells, shortening and predisposition for cell rounding develop with a considerable temporal scatter (15,20).
(iv) Isolated anoxic cardiomyocytes round up in response to late reoxygenation only if they are not surface-attached (33). Prior to becoming "oxygen sensitive" they have to shorten (20). It may be the fact that, after prolonged anoxia, non-attached cells shrink to sarcomere lengths below 1.4 µM, whereas surface-attached cells generally do not, which makes them different. It is conceivable that only at such overcontraction of sarcomeres the further imposition of Ca^{2+} contracture forces causes final and crucial cytoskeletal disruptions. But in contrast to isolated myocytes which have to be in this extreme contracture to become "oxygen sensitive", myocardial cells in tissue have not to be in this condition to become susceptible to the oxygen paradox (75).

In summary, the evidence for identity of the oxygen paradox in tissue and oxygen-induced rounding in non-attached cardiomyocytes is not conclusive. In fact, both phenomena seem to be rather different in nature.

8. Summary

From studies on short-term cultured surface-attached cardiomyocytes, which seems to be the most stable system currently available, it is now clear that, in the muscle cell itself, onset of enzyme release, irreversibility of structural cell injury, and cytolysis are separate events. In the heart exposed to ischemia or hypoxia, these events occur in indistinguishable close temporal coincidence, due to a faster progression of metabolic changes and mutual interaction of the muscle cells. Sudden onset of contracture under conditions of anaerobic stress is a phenomenon specific to floating isolated cardiomyocytes. A question yet to be answered is whether this behavior influences the metabolic processes leading to the onset of irreversible injury in a way differing in quality from that in heart tissue or in cultured cells. In respect to the mechanisms leading to loss of Ca^{2+} control in the late stage of hypoxic injury, the various experimental models of the oxygen deprived myocardial cell may not be as different as they seem. The main difference may consist in the velocity of energy depletion. Secondary phenomena as, e.g., mechanical cell-to-cell interactions, differ in importance in the various model systems. But to understand the nature of such secondary phenomena, the comparison of the behavior of the hypoxic cell in models of differing complexity is required. In the isolated cell, a persistent membrane perforation is not the primary cause for structural deterioration. Contracture and gross disruptions of the cytoarchitecture can occur before extracellular Ca^{2+} floods the cell. In the time range of hours these destructions are irreversible, and in tissue context the breaks in the cytoskeletal structure prabably leave the cell too fragile to survive. But it remains an interesting question whether the contracted polygonal and round cells, which are formed in anoxia and have not yet become hyperpermeable, could regain enough metabolic ability to recover also in the structural sense after an extended period of time. Such a hypothesis is not as farfedged as it seems, since in the process of establishing a long-term culture, adult heart cells indeed undergo a very extensive structural reconstruction process.

The exact role of energy metabolism in the process of progressive injury is still an open field for research. So far, in most studies average levels of high energy phosphates and not the free energy change of ATP hydrolysis, i.e. a parameter for the thermodynamically available energy, have been determined. An apparent ATP threshold (1-2 µmol/g wet weight) for resuscitability has been described for ischemic dog myocardium (10,49), ischemic rat hearts (76), and anoxic cultured rat cardiomyocytes (16,23). But it is not definitely clear whether this threshold is a borderline under all circumstances. In energetically poisened cardiomyocytes the ATP concentration may fall to much lower levels, before the cytosolic Ca^{2+} concentrations rises (51). This, however, must not mean that a true recovery from these ATP concentrations is possible before the loss of Ca^{2+} control. It has also been claimed that under certain conditions ischemic hearts can recover from similarly low ATP levels (77,78) But since in the latter studies only some functional parameter for recovery was investigated, they due not prove the possibility of true structural and biochemical recovery from very low energy levels.

Acknowledgment

This study has been supported by the Deutsche Forschungsgemeinschaft, grant Pi 162/2-1.

References

1. Piper, H.M., Probst, I., Schwartz, P., Hütter, J.F., and Spieckermann, P.G., J. Mol. Cell. Cardiol.14, 397 (1982).
2. Altschuld, R.A., Hohl, C., Ansel, A., and Brierley, G.P., Circ. Res. 49, 307 (1981).
3. Hohl, C., Ansel, A., Altschuld, A., and Brierley, G.P., Am. J. Physiol. 242, H1022 (1982).
4. Murphy, M.P., Hohl, C., Brierley, G.P., and Altschuld, R.A., Circ. Res. 51, 560 (1982).
5. Rajs, J., Sundberg, M., Härm, T., Grandinsson, M., and Söderlund, U., J. Mol. Cell. Cardiol. 12, 1227 (1980).
6. Cheung, J.Y., Thompson, I.G., and Bonventre, J.V., Am. J. Physiol. 243, C184 (1982).
7. Wittenberg, B.A., J. Biol. Chem. 260, 6548 (1985).
8. Kennedy, F.G., and Jones, D.P., Am. J. Physiol. 250, C374 (1986).
9. Barry, W.H., Pober, J., Marsh, J.D., Frankel, S.R., and Smith, T.W., Am. J. Physiol. 239, H651 (1980).
10. Kübler, W., and Spieckermann, P.G., J. Mol. Cell. Cardiol. 1, 351 (1970).
11. Spieckermann, P.G., Brückner, J., Kübler, W., Lohr, B., and Bretschneider, H.J., Verh. dtsch. Ges. Kreislaufforsch. 35, 358 (1968).
12. Piper, H.M., Schwartz, P., Hütter, J.F., and Spieckermann, P.G., J. Mol. Cell. Cardiol. 16, 995 (1984).
13. Hearse, D.J., and Chain, E.B., Biochem. J. 128, 1125 (1972).
14. Rouslin, W., Erickson, J.L., and Solaro, R.J., Am. J. Physiol. 250, H503 (1986).
15. Haworth, R.A., Hunter, D.R., and Berkoff, H.A., Circ. Res. 49, 1119 (1981).
16. Piper, H.M., Sezer, O., Schleyer, M., Schwartz, P., Hütter, J.F., and Spieckermann, P.G., J. Mol. Cell. Cardiol. 17, 186 (1985).
17. Rouslin, W., Am. J. Physiol. 244, H743 (1983).

18. McDonough, K.H., and Spitzer, J.J., Proc. Soc. Exp. Biol. Med. 173, 519 (1983).
19. Cheung, J.Y., Leaf, A., and Bonventre, J.V., Am. J. Physiol. 250, C18 (1986).
20. Allshire, A., Piper, H.M., Cuthbertson, K.S.R., and Cobbold, P.H., Biochem. J. 244, 381 (1987).
21. Carafoli, E., J. Mol. Cell. Cardiol. 17, 203 (1985).
22. Bishop, S.P., and Drummond, J.L., J. Mol. Cell. Cardiol. 11, 423 (1979).
23. Schwartz, P., Piper, H.M., Spahr, R., and Spieckermann, P.G., Am. J. Pathol. 115, 349 (1984)
24. Finch, S.A.E., Piper, H.M., Spieckermann, P.G., and Stier, A., Basic Res. Cardiol., 80 (Suppl. 1), 145 (1985).
25. Borgers, M., and Piper, H.M., J. Mol. Cell. Cardiol. 18, 439 (1986).
26. Allshire, A., and Cobbold, P., Biochemical. Soc. Transact., in press.
27. Gebhard, M.M., Denkhaus ,H., Sakai, K., and Spieckermann, P.G., J. Mol. Med. 2, 271 (1979).
28. Higgins, T.J.C., Allsopp, D., Bailey, P.J., and D'Souza, E.D.A., J. Mol. Cell. Cardiol. 13, 599 (1981).
29. Nordbeck, H., Kahles, H., Preusse, C.J., and Spieckermann, P.G., J. Mol. Med. 2, 255 (1977).
30. Spieckermann ,P.G., Nordbeck, H., and Preusse, C.J., in: Enzymes in Cardiology: Diagnosis and Research, Hearse, D.J., and de Leiris, J., eds. (John Wiley, New York, 1979) p. 81.
31. Piper, H.M., Spahr, R., Hütter, J.F., and Spieckermann, P.G., Basic Res. Cardiol. 80 (Suppl. 1), 143 (1985).
32. Piper, H.M., Schwartz, P., Spahr, R., Hütter, J.F., and Spieckermann, P.G., J. Mol. Cell. Cardiol. 16, 385 (1984).
33. Piper, H.M., Schwartz, P., Spahr, R., Hütter, J.F., and Spieckermann, P.G., Pflügers Arch. 367, 129 (1984)
34. Hearse, D.J., Humphrey, S.M., and Chain, E.B., J. Mol. Cell. Cardiol. 5, 395 (1973).
35. Van der Laarse, A., Davids, H.A., Hollaar, L., and Hermens, W.T., Cardiovasc. Res. 15, 11 (1981).
36. Wenger, W.C., Murphy, M.P., Kinding, O.R., Capen, C.C., Brierley, G.P., and Altschuld, R.A., Life Sci. 37, 1697 (1985).
37. Michell, R.H., Coleman, R., in: Enzymes in Cardiology: Diagnosis and Research, Hearse , D.J., and de Leiris, J., eds.(John Wiley, New York, 1979) p. 59.
38. Bütikofer, P., and Ott, P., Biochim. Biophys. Acta 821, 91 (1985).
39. Wilkinson, J.H., and Roinson, J.M., Nature 249, 662 (1974).
40. Zierler, K.L., Ann. NY Acad. Sci. USA 75, 227 (1958).
41. Orrenius, S., Thor, H., Rajs, J., and Berggren, M., Forensic Sci. 8, 255 (1976).
42. Ahmed, S.A., Williamson, J.R., Roberts, E., Clark, R.E., and Sobel, B.E., Circulation 54, 187 (1976).
43. Black, L., and Berenbaum, M.C., Exp. Cell Res. 35, 9 (1964).
44. Cheung, J.Y., Leaf, A., and Bonventre, J.V., Basic Res. Cardiol. 80 (Suppl. 1), 23 (1985).
45. Jacobson, S.L., and Piper,H.M., J. Mol. Cell. Cardiol. 18, 439 (1986).
46. Weber, A., and Murray, J.M., Physiol. Rev. 53, 613 (1974).
47. Katz, A.M., and Tada, M., Am. J. Cardiol. 39, 1073 (1977).
48. Holubarsch, C., Pflügers Arch. 396, 277 (1983).
49. Jennings, R.B., Hawkins, H.K., Lowe, J.E., Hill, M.L., Klotman, S., and Reimer, K.A., Am. J. Pathol. 92, 187 (1978).
50. Altsschuld, R.A., Wenger, W.C., Lamka, K.G., Kinding, O.R., Capen, C.C., Mizuhira, V., Van der Heide, R.S., and Brierley, G.P., J. Biol. Chem. 260, 14325 (1985).
51. Haworth, R.A., Goknur, A.B., Hunter, D.R., Hegge, J.O., and Berkoff, H.A., Circ. Res. 60, 586 (1987).

52. Best, B.M., Donaldson, S.K.B., Kerrick, W.G.L., J. Physiol. (London) 264, 1 (1977).
53. Bricknell, O.L., Daries, P.S., and Opie, L.H., J. Mol. Cell. Cardiol. 13, 941 (1981).
54. Veech, R.L., Lawson, J.W.R., Cornell, N.W, and Krebs, H.A., J. Biol. Chem. 254, 551 (1979).
55. Fiolet, J.W.T., Baartscheer, A., Schumacher, C.A., Coronel, R., and ter Welle, H.F., J. Mol. Cell. Cardiol. 16, 1023 (1985).
56. Kammermeier, H., Schmidt, P., and Jüngling, E., J. Mol. Cell. Cardiol. 14, 267 (1982).
57. Eisenberg, E., and Hill, T.L., Progr. Biophys. Molec. Biol. 33, 55 (1978).
58. Sleep, J.A., and Smith, S.J., Curr. Top. Bioenerg 11, 239 (1981).
59. Hearse, D.J., Garlick, P.B., and Humphrey, S.M., Am. J. Cardiol. 39, 986 (1977).
60. Goody, R.S., and Hohnes, K.C., Biochim. Biophys. Acta 726, 13 (1983).
61. Murray, J.M., Knox, K.M., Trueblood, C.E., and Weber, A., Biochemistry 21, 906 (1982).
62. Stern, M.D., Chien, A.M., Capogrossi, M.C., Pelto, D.J., and Lakatta, E.G., Circ. Res. 56, 899 (1985).
63. Piper, H.M., Spahr, R., Probst, I., and Spieckermann, P.G., Basic Res. Cardiol. 80 (Suppl. 2), 175 (1985).
64. Opie, L.H., and Bricknell, O.L., Cardiovasc. Res. 13, 693 (1979).
65. Klingenberg, M., and Heldt, H.W., in: Metabolic Compartmentation, Sies, H., ed. (Academic Press, London, 1982) p. 101.
66. Gercken, G., and Hürter, P., Pflügers Arch. 292, 100 (1966).
67. Ganote, C.E., J. Mol. Cell. Cardiol. 15, 67 (1983).
68. Zweier, J.L., Flaherty, J.T., and Weisfeldt , M.L., Proc. Natl. Acad. Sci. USA 84, 1404 (1987).
69. Chambers, D.E., Parks, D.A., Patterson, G., Roy, R., McCord, J.M., Yoshida, S., Parmley, L.F., and Downey, J.M., J. Mol. Cell. Cardiol. 17, 145 (1985).
70. Jarasch, E.D., Grund, C., Bruder, G., Heid, H.W., Keenan, T.W., and Franke, W.W., Cell 25, 67 (1981).
71. Kehrer, J.P., Piper, H.M., and Sies, H., Free. Rad. Res. Comms. 3, 69 (1987).
72. Reimer, K.A., and Jennings, R.B., Circulation 71, 1069 (1985).
73. Allshire, A., Piper, H.M., and Cobbold, P.,J. Mol. Cell. Cardiol. 18 (Suppl. 2), 36 (1985).
74. Ganote, C.E., and Van der Heide, R.S., J. Mol. Cell. Cardiol. 18, 23 (1986).
75. Ganote, C.E., and Humphrey, S.M., Am. J. Pathol. 120, 129 (1985).
76. Taegtmeyer, H., Roberts, A.F.C., and Raine, A.E.G., J. Am. Coll. Cardiol. 6, 864 (1985).
77. Ichihara, K., and Neely, J.R., Am. J. Physiol. 249, H492 (1985).
78. Neely, J.R., and Grotyohann, L.W., Circ. Res. 55, 816 (1984).
79. Probst, I., Spahr, R., Schweickhardt, C., Hunneman, D., and Piper, H.M., Am. J. Physiol. 250, H853 (1986).
80. Piper, H.M., Schwartz, P., and Siegmund, B., in: Isolated Adult Cardiomyocytes, Piper, H.M., and Isenberg, G., eds. (CRC Press, Boca Raton) in press.

MEASUREMENT OF SOLUTE UPTAKE AND TRANSPORT IN ISOLATED CELLS

ROBERT A. HAWORTH, ATILLA B. GOKNUR, HERBERT A. BERKOFF
Department of Surgery, University of Wisconsin Clinical Science Center
600 Highland Avenue, Madison, WI 53792, USA

INTRODUCTION

The ability to measure intracellular solute levels is vital to most investigations of metabolism or ion homeostasis in isolated cells. Solutes which are concentrated into cells, like thallium and deoxyglucose, are relatively easy to measure, because the contribution of counts from extracellular solute is small relative to those from intracellular label. Solutes which merely permeate the cells, like 3-O-methylglucose, or are actively removed, like Na, are on the other hand much more difficult to measure. Basically, two approaches have been taken to overcome this difficulty. The first employs a rapid wash with cold medium to remove extracellular label, before the sample is recovered for counting. This procedure has gained favor in studies with neonatal heart cells where the cells are attached to cover slips, facilitating rapid washes [1]. Cell recovery can be quantitated through the use of DNA labelling with ^3H leucine [1]. The procedure has the advantage that the time resolution is just a few seconds, being limited only by the rate at which the uptake medium can be changed for the cold wash medium. A disadvantage is that washing allows the possibility of label redistribution, and any rapidly exchangeable temperature insensitive pools will be lost. For each solute the adequacy of the procedure has to be established, since different solutes may have different temperature sensitivities of efflux. Some idea of the reproducibility of the method can be gained from published data: the standard deviation of measured points is about 40 nmol/mg Na [2] and 0.4 nmol/mg for Ca [1]. These values correspond approximately to the amount of solute in about three hundred picoliters of extracellular medium, and reflect culture to culture variability as well as measurement error. The second approach is to centrifuge the cells through a hydrophobic medium, which separates them from most of the extracellular label, into a layer of perchloric acid [3]. This method naturally lends itself to studies with adult heart cell suspensions, where cells are not attached to a substrate. A problem with such cell suspensions is that a non-viable fraction of cells, whose size can vary from one preparation to another, is invariably present. By incorporating ^3H_2O and a ^{14}C-labelled impermeant solute such as sucrose into the medium at the same time, a measure can be gained of the fraction of pellet water which is external to intact cells [4]. This approach was first used on isolated adult rat heart cells in suspension by Altschuld et. al. [5], to correct their measurements of cell Na made by atomic absorption spectroscopy. We have since used a similar technique to measure cellular levels of 3-O-methylglucose [6] and Na [7], refining it to the point where the standard deviation of uptakes measured on one preparation is of the order of 2% of the pellet volume/mg [6], which corresponds approximately to the amount of solute in fifty picoliters of extracellular medium. The variability observed when results from identical experiments on different cell preparations are pooled arises more from preparation to preparation differences than from random error within any experiment [6]. Thus, even though not all the extracellular solute is removed, the method has a high degree of accuracy. Although the time resolution is not as good as with the wash technique, an advantage is that there is no possible loss of solute through washing. This method, described in detail below, thus also measures any extracellular bound solute.

Biology of Isolated Adult Cardiac Myocytes
William A. Clark, Robert S. Decker, and Thomas K. Borg, Editors

MEASUREMENT OF SOLUTE UPTAKE BY THE DUAL LABEL METHOD

We will describe the procedure for measurement of ^{14}C-sucrose uptake. The procedure is identical for other solutes, substituting the appropriate isotope at a similar specific activity. Any isotope can be used which can be discriminated from ^{3}H by the window settings of the liquid scintillation counter. Cells typically are suspended at 37° in a Krebs Henseleit medium containing 118 mM NaCl, 4.8 mM KCl, 1.2 mM KH_2PO_4, 1.2 mM $MgSO_4$, 1 mM $CaCl_2$, 25 mM HEPES, 11 mM glucose, 1 µM insulin, to pH 7.4 with NaOH. Tritiated water is added (1 µCi/ml). This equilibrates rapidly with the cell water. To measure sucrose permeable spaces we also routinely add 2 mM sucrose as carrier, as in early experiments this was found to improve accuracy and reproductibility. ^{14}C sucrose is then added at time zero. At time intervals thereafter, 0.5 ml aliquots of cell suspension are removed using an Eppendorf disposable pipette tip with the end cut off. Enlarging the hole in this way reduces the shear stress on cells during pipetting. It also reduces the accuracy of the aliquot volume, but this does not matter much, since the ultimate measure is, through the ^{3}H counts, automatically corrected for the amount of cells actually taken. The aliquot is layered on top of 0.5 ml bromododecane, itself layered on top of 0.1 ml 16% perchloric acid, in a 1.5 ml disposable plastic centrifuge tube. To prepare these tubes beforehand, 0.1 ml 16% perchloric acid is placed in the bottom, then 0.5 ml bromododecane is added by running it down the tube wall. by circumnavigating the top of the tube with the pipette tip the entire upper inner wall can be washed free of any trace of perchloric acid, which is important for reproducible results. Once the cell suspension aliquot is layered in the tube, it is centrifuged in a Beckman Microfuge B bench centrifuge for 45 seconds. Brinkmann bench centrifuges also work, even though they have a fixed angle rotor. The cells are all in the perchloric acid layer within five seconds of switching on the centrifuge (pellet volume 2.42 $\pm$ 0.02 µl/mg after 5 seconds, compared with 2.49 $\pm$ 0.18 µl/mg for 40 seconds; mean $\pm$ SD of 3 measurements in one experiment). The tube is immediately removed, to avoid mixing of contents, and kept upright until all aliquots have been taken. At this point the aqueous supernatants are removed with a Pasteur pipette, pooled, and a 50 µl aliquot is added to 3 ml scintillator (Ecoscint). An exception to the pooling is when the solute uptake is sufficiently massive to result in significant solute depletion from the medium. In such cases (as, for example, with ^{14}C-tetramethylphosphonium uptake), an aliquot must be taken from a sample centrifuged after all the solute has been released from the cells by some means. For solutes like 3-O-methylglucose, which merely permeate the cells, the error introduced by ignoring the depletion of extracellular solute by cellular uptake is only 0.2%, for cells suspended at 2 mg/ml. After the supernatants have been largely removed, residual supernatant is removed by a tube connected to a vacuum line. The top portion of the bromododecane layer is also generally removed in doing this. The purpose of this is to allow recovery of the perchloric acid layer without contamination from the supernatant. Such contamination, if present, is evident as an unusually high count in both isotope channels. The purpose of the perchloric acid is to release the cell label and precipitate the protein. This works well for most ionic and hydrophilic solutes, and means that the protein pellet does not have to be recovered. A fraction of the perchloric acid layer (70 µl) is then recovered with an Eppendorf pipette through the remaining bromododecane, and added to 3 ml Ecoscint in a counting vial. Unlabelled perchloric acid (70 µl) is also added to the supernatant counting vial, as the acid does have some quenching effect on the counts. It is not necessary to add 50 µl unlabelled buffer to the vials containing labelled perchloric acid. If it is necessary to recover the entire perchloric acid layer plus pellet, this can be done with a Pasteur pipette, using the tip to break up the pellet before removing the acid layer plus debris. Invariably some bromododecane also is removed; this has no effect on the counts. Activity in the vials is measured in a liquid scintillation spectrometer, counting for 20 min. in two channels optimized for ^{3}H and the solute label. Also counted are a blank with no label, and a vial containing solute label but no ^{3}H. Each also contains unlabelled perchloric acid.

DATA ANALYSIS

All measured counts are first corrected for background by subtraction of the blank. The ^{3}H channel counts must then be corrected for crossover from the solute label channel. If the ratio of counts in the ^{3}H channel to those in the solute channel with is R solute label alone, then the true ^{3}H channel counts from a vial containing both labelled solute and ^{3}H will be the measured ^{3}H channel counts minus R x the measured solute counts. The measured solute counts are the true solute counts, since no crossover from ^{3}H into the solute channel occurs, at least for the solute channel settings we have used. Once the true counts are obtained, the % permeation of the pellet is simply given by the ratio of the pellet solute counts and ^{3}H counts divided by the ratio of the supernatant solute counts and ^{3}H counts, x 100%. This value is independent of the volume of supernatant counted, the number of cells centrifuged, and the volume of the perchloric acid layer retrieved. It is therefore also independent of errors in these quantities, accounting for the high degree of accuracy of the method. Since these quantities are also known, the pellet volume and solute uptake in nmol/mg are also easily calculated.

EXPERIMENTAL VALIDATION

Although it has long been clear to us that solutes like sucrose do not permeate the sarcolemma easily and could therefore by used to delineate the fraction of intact cells in the pellet, we have recently undertaken a more thorough investigation of the relationship between cell condition and their permeation by various solutes. To control the fraction of rod-shaped cells, we mixed freshly isolated rod-shaped cells with various proportions of round cells. The round cells were prepared by placing 10 ml fresh cell suspension in a 15 mm test tube and vortexing it at high-speed (Scientific Industries, model K500-4) for 30 seconds. This treatment almost completely transformed the rod-shaped cells which exclude trypan blue to round cells which stained darkly with trypan blue. Incidentally, this indicates that in any technique for measuring solute uptake, vortexing should be avoided. When a cell suspension containing 50% rod-shaped cells was given ^{14}C sucrose or ^{14}C dextran (MW 20,000) at time zero, the uptake was rapid by part of the cells and thereafter was very slow (Fig. 1). Extrapolation of the slow phase of uptake to time zero allows sucrose-permeable and dextran-permeable spaces to be defined. The % permeability to sucrose was similar to the % rod-shaped cells, while that for dextran was much less (Fig. 1). If the cells were cooled on ice (to inhibit the rate of cellular Na uptake) and ^{22}Na was added, a Na-permeable space was observed similar to that for sucrose (Fig. 1). The slightly higher value for Na is probably caused by some Na binding.

When the fraction of trypan blue permeable cells was varied, the % permeability to sucrose and dextran varied as shown in Figure 2. The difference between sucrose and dextran permeable spaces is largest in permeable cells and, by extrapolation, disappears for intact cells (Fig. 2). A large part of the difference for round cells is probably accounted for by the fact that on exposure to Ca the inner membrane of mitochondria of round cells will become permeable to sucrose [8], but not to dextran, since the molecular weight cutoff for the Ca-activated hydrophilic channel of the mitochondrial inner membrane is around 1000 [9]. Exposure of rod-shaped cells to digitonin (20 μg/ml) also gave

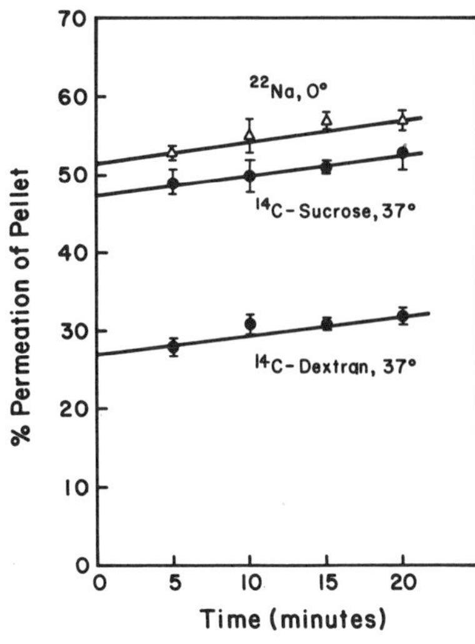

Figure 1 Time course of solute permeation by sucrose and dextran at 37° and by Na at 0°, for cells which are 50% rod-shaped.

round trypan blue permeable cells, and these cells had similar sucrose and dextran permeable spaces to those made permeable by vortexing (data not shown). A significant sucrose-impermeable space of unknown location appears to remain in the round cells (Fig. 2). On average it may be slightly smaller than appearsin the Figure: in data from six vortexed preparations, sucrose permeation was 89.4 $\pm$ 5.6%, while 5.2 $\pm$ 0.4% of cells continued to exclude trypan blue. A significant sucrose-permeable and dextran-permeable space remains in the intact cells (Fig. 2) This would include t-tubules and any intracellular vesicular compartments in rapid equilibrium with the extracellular space. Using bromododecane, all cells

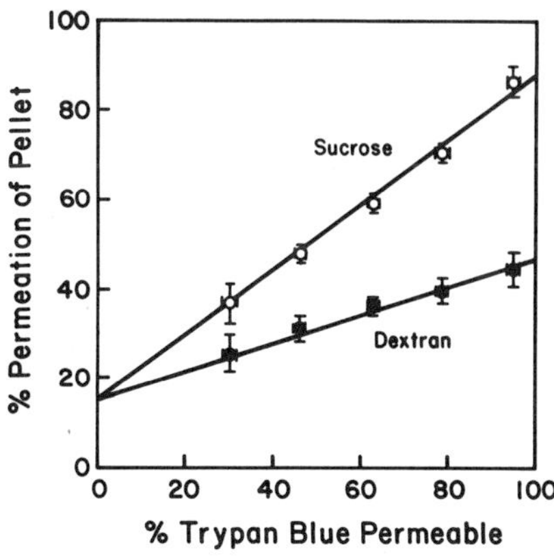

Figure 2 Correlation between % permeation to sucrose or dextran and permeability to trypan blue.

applied appear by visual inspection to end up in the pellet on centrifugation. Prolonged exposure to digitonin can cause some round cells to fail to spin down, and these appear at the interface.

We next investigated the relationship between cell recovery and density of the hydrophobic medium. Density was altered by mixing bromododecane (density 1.038) with bromodecane (density 1.066) in various proportions. Cells (50% rod-shaped) were then centrifuged through these media, and the size of the cell pellet was measured. Figure 3 shows that the pellet size

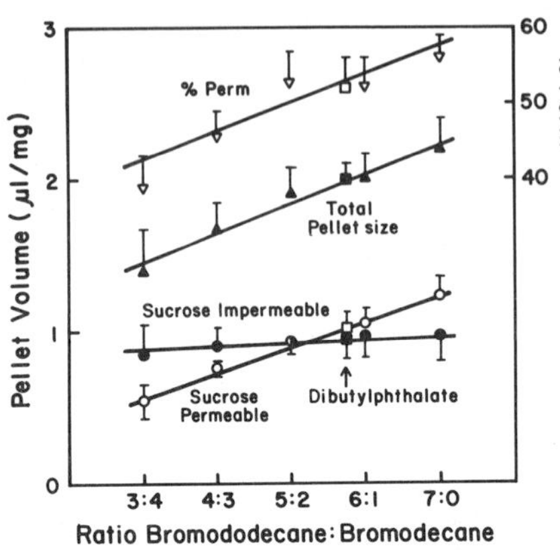

Figure 3 Pellet size found with hydrophobic media of different density. Cells were 50% rod-shaped.

decreased linearly from that achieved with bromododecane, as the density was increased with bromodecane. Moreover, almost the entire decrease was caused by a reduction in the sucrose permeable pellet, with hardly any change in the sucrose impermeable pellet. That is, the permeable cells did not spin down as well in the more dense media, while the impermeable cells did. Residual cell material seen at the supernatant/hydro-phobic medium interface confirmed this interpretation. In media more dense than 3/7 bromododecane plus 4/7 bromodecane, no cells spun down. We also tried dibutylphthalate, which has sometimes been used with other cell types [10]. Cells passed through dibutylphthalate in a manner identical to a mixture of bromododecane and bromodecane of the same density (Fig. 3). Since dibutylphthalate is more viscous and thus harder to handle, and is more toxic than bromododecane, the bromododecane/bromodecane mixture could be preferable. The more dense media can be used to partially discriminate between the intact cells and the permeable cells [10]. From the standpoint of accuracy, however, little is gained by partially excluding the dead cells, and there is some advantage in having as much as possible spin down. We therefore prefer to use bromododecane alone.

In principal the pellet size, in µl, should be proportional to the concentration of cells in the suspension. Figure 4 shows that this is true, up to 8 mg protein/ml, for the sucrose-impermeable pellet, but not for the sucrose-permeable cells. Since solute uptake by the former is the parameter of interest, the method is of use over a wide range of protein concentrations. We generally use 2 to 3 mg/ml. In passing it is noteworthy that the cell volume for intact cells indicated by Figure 4 is 1.46 $\pm$ 0.07 µl/mg for 70% rod-shaped cells, i.e. about 2 µl/mg for 100% rod-shaped cells (N.B. cells lose some protein when they become permeable). This value is much less than that of 7.5 µl/mg reported for neonatal cells [11], which presumably reflects the difference in cell maturity.

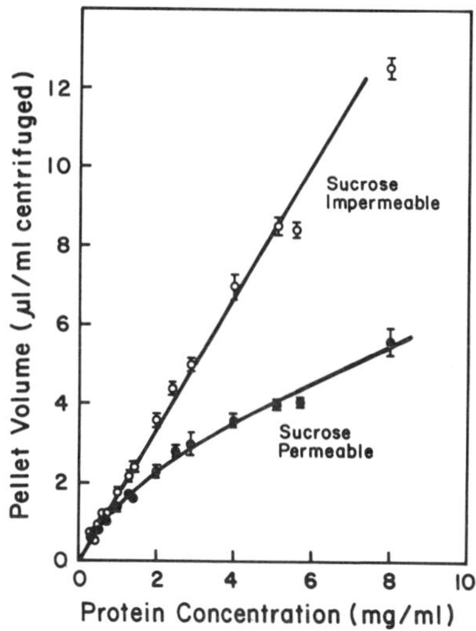

Figure 4
Effect of cell concentration on pellet size per mg protein. Cells were 70% rod-shaped.

To illustrate the use of the method, Figure 5 shows the permeation of cells by ^{14}C-3-O-methylglucose in the presence and absence of insulin, with the uptake inhibited by cytochalasin B (taken from 6), and Figure 6 shows the permeation of cells by ^{22}Na, before and after ouabain treatment, and the effect of the Na channel agonist anthopleurin-A on the rate of Na entry (taken from 7).

Finally, we have compared solute uptake measured by centrifugation, as above, to uptake measured by filtration. Since the filtration method is best suited to solutes which are actively accumulated by cells and which remain inside cells during cold washes, we have used the intracellular Na-dependent uptake of extracellular Ca by Na-loaded cells as a model. Cells were washed in a Ca-free medium either

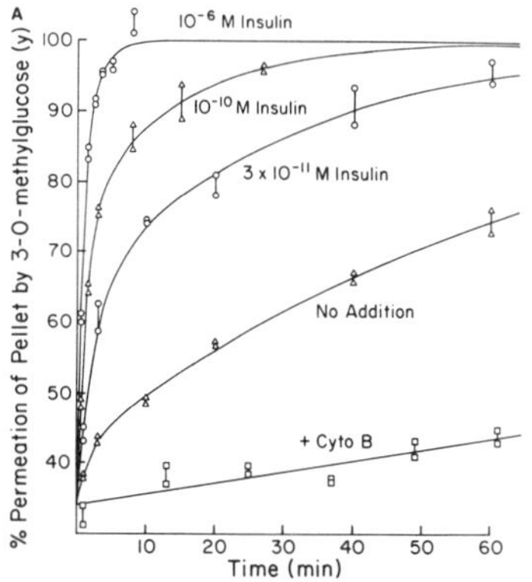

Figure 5
3-O-methylglucose uptake by cells with different concentrations of insulin (see 6 for details; reproduced with permission of Academic Press).

with normal Na or with Na replaced by choline. In the latter medium the cells quickly lost their intracellular Na. They were then exposed to

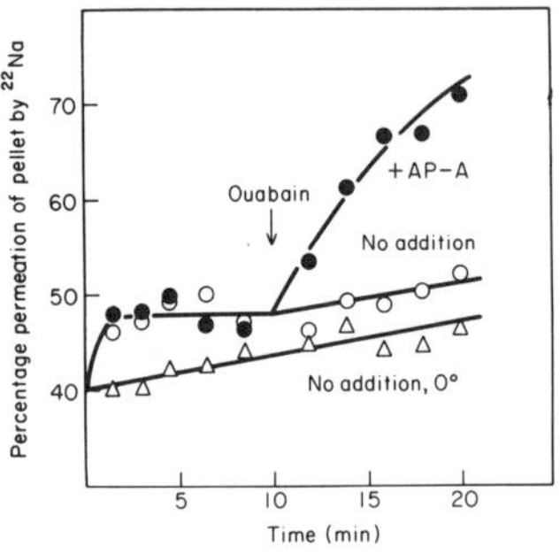

Figure 6 Effect of anthopleurin-A on Na uptake (See 7 for details; reproduced with permission).

ouabain for 30 minutes, during which time the cells in the medium with Na gained Na to the level of 95 mM [12]. ^{45}Ca uptake was then initiated by dilution of the cells into a medium containing normal Na, 1 mM labelled Ca, and 5 µM ruthenium red. In the filtration experiments, cells were 0.12 mg/ml final concentration in 250 µl volume. At the times shown 300 µl ice-cold Na free buffer medium containing excess EGTA was added. A 500 µl aliquot of this was filtered (0.45 µm Millipore filter #HAWP025), and the filter washed twice with 3 ml further cold EGTA medium. In the centrifugation experiments, cells were 1 mg/ml final concentration. At the times shown, 500 µl aliquots were removed and centrifuged as described above. Figure 7 shows the Ca uptake measured by each method. Experiments with quin 2 (unpublished) show that intact cells without Na do not readily take up Ca, presumably because of the lack of intracellular Na for Na/Ca exchange. The ^{45}Ca uptake measured in these samples by centrifugation thus represents Ca binding to the outside of intact cells and to dead cells. This amount is reduced by half in the filtered samples, presumably because of the washing by the EGTA buffer. The difference between the uptake by Na-containing cells and those without Na, on the other hand, represents uptake by intact cells and is the same as measured by either technique. This result thus tends to validate the accuracy of either method under these conditions, in the measurement of cellular Ca

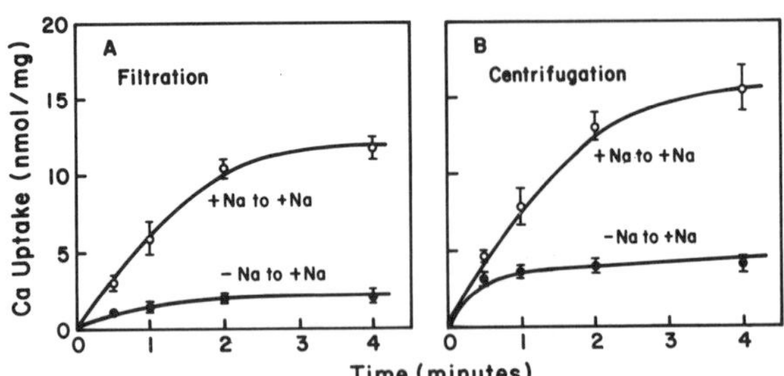

Figure 7 Ca uptake by Na-loaded cells, measured by filtration (A) or centrifugation (B).

uptake. We would caution, however, that the success of the filtration method here may be related to the fact that most of the Ca taken up by cells is sequestered by intracellular organelles and is not so easily released if cells are damaged during filtration and washing. With solutes such as ^{86}Rb we find evidence for such damage: uptakes are lower and much more variable than those measured by centrifugation. We, therefore, do not recommend the filtration technique for most purposes.

SUMMARY

A technique for measuring solute uptake by isolated adult rat heart cells in suspension is described. The technique involves centrifugation of aliquots of cells through a bromododecane layer into perchloric acid. A high degree of accuracy is achieved by incorporation of tritiated water along with the solute label, and expressing results as % permeation of the cell pellet. This eliminates variability from pipetting errors. The method does not require washing of cells and measures all uptake and binding pools. Solute uptake by damaged cells can be allowed for. By extrapolation of data to 100% rod-shaped (intact) cells we conclude that rod-shaped cells exclude dextran to the same degree as sucrose, while damaged cells do not. The technique is applicable to a wide range of protein concentrations and a wide range of ionic and hydrophilic solutes.

ACKNOWLEDGMENTS

This work was supported by grant #HL33652 from NHLBI.

REFERENCES

1. Barry WH, Smith TW, J. Physiol. 325:243-260 (1982).
2. Biedert S, Barry WH, Smith TW, J. Gen. Physiol. 74:479-494 (1979).
3. McCune SA, Harris RA, J. Biol. Chem. 254:10095-10101 (1979).
4. Hunter GR, Brierley GP, Biochim. Biophys. Acta 180:68-80 (1969).
5. Altschuld R, Gibb L, Ansel A, Hohl C, Kruger FA, Brierley GP, J. Mol. Cell. Cardiol. 12:1383-1395 (1980).
6. Haworth RA, Hunter DR, Berkoff HA, Arch. Biochem. Biophys. 233:106-114 (1984).
7. Hunter DR, Haworth RA, Goknur AB, Hegge JO, Berkoff HA, J. Mol. Cell. Cardiol. 18:1125-1132 (1986).
8. Hunter DR, Haworth RA, Southard JH, J. Biol. Chem. 251:5069-5077 (1976).
9. Haworth RA, Hunter DR, Arch. Biochem. Biophys. 195:460-467 (1979)
10. Farris MW, Brown MK, Schmitz JA, Reed DJ, Tox. Appl. Pharm. 79:283-295 (1985).
11. Barry WH, Biedert S, Muira DS, Smith TW, Circ. Res. 49:141-149 (1981).
12. Haworth RA, Goknur AB, Hunter DR, Hegge JO, Berkoff HA, Circ. Res. 60:586-594 (1987).

CHARACTERIZATION OF HORMONE RECEPTORS ON THE ADULT CARDIAC MYOCYTE

IAIN L. O. BUXTON* and LAURENCE L. BRUNTON** *Department of Pharmacology, University of Nevada School of Medicine, Reno Nevada and the **Departments of Pharmacology and Medicine, University of California, San Diego

INTRODUCTION

The adult mammalian cardiac myocyte is a particularly useful model for studies of receptor-signal transduction in cardiac muscle. Over the past several years, we and a number of other investigators have addressed our interest in cardiac muscle receptors to the isolated myocyte. In particular, we have used radioligand binding techniques and studies of second messenger generation to discover the role of the adult cardiac muscle cell in mediating the response of the heart to drugs and neurotransmitters (see Table I). Unlike the use of heterogeneous cardiac membrane preparations, the freshly isolated myocyte can be employed as a reasonably homogeneous population of single cells effectively removing the question of the origin of receptor types. In addition, radioligand binding to the intact myocyte allows one to pose particularly relevant questions of the density of receptors on the myocyte and permits studies of receptor metabolism. While the isolated heart and isolated muscle segments have been the favored preparation for functional studies of heart in the past, the isolated cardiac myocyte is a useful model for these and other studies since it is possible to relate the information one gains from receptor occupancy to biochemical or contractile function in a single cell type. In this chapter we describe the methods required to quantify hormone receptors on the myocyte and discuss specific examples of well characterized receptors and their intracellular responses.

CHARACTERISTICS OF THE ADULT CARDIAC MYOCYTE

It should be of interest to the reader that it is possible to study extracellularly directed receptors for hormones and neurotransmitters on the myocyte at all. This cell, whether isolated with the traditional use of collagenase or a defined mixture of proteases is, after all, a cell that has seen proteolytic enzymes for up to 60 min before further purification. Serial studies of protein recovery during myocyte preparation [I.L. Buxton, unpublished observations] suggest that no more than one-third of myocytes survive as healthy rod-shaped cells. While structural changes may occur [1], it is clear from radioligand binding and functional studies that myocyte receptors do indeed survive. At the outset, however, we offer a caution to the investigator willing to turn his interest in the heart to studies of the myocyte. While it is clearly possible to employ the isolated myocyte for studies of receptor biochemistry, it must be remembered that the cellular heterogeneity existing in the whole heart will be lost. For instance, while it is popular to prepare ventricular or atrial cells there is undoubtedly regional variation in cell characteristics within these boundaries that

Biology of Isolated Adult Cardiac Myocytes
William A. Clark, Robert S. Decker, and Thomas K. Borg, Editors

explains, in part, regional function in the whole heart. If large numbers of myocytes are not needed, this problem can be overcome by dissecting certain regions within the enzyme perfused ventricle from which to prepare cells [2]. In addition to regional distinctions that may be lost in myocyte suspensions, it is possible (though by no means clear) that the myocytes that survive preparation are somehow different than those that do not and thus represent a selected population. This limitation, however, is the limitation that must be applied to any use of the freshly isolated cardiac myocyte. We believe that despite these provisions, the myocyte still represents a significant advantage over the isolated heart for many investigations including receptor biochemistry.

Purity and Yield

These two issues have been raised repeatedly by both advocates and critics of the myocyte preparation. We believe that the procedures for preparation of myocytes detailed in this volume and elsewhere [3] by Dr. Trevor Powell and his colleagues, as well as the work of others [4], are particularly useful and, if followed, will produce both highly purified populations of myocytes as well as large numbers of cells. Our approach to the preparation of the myocyte has been to manufacture a perfusion chamber (plans available from Dr. Buxton upon request) that can perfuse as few as 1 and as many as 12 rat or guinea pig hearts at a time (1-8 rabbit hearts). A simple and rapid method for hanging the hearts, using neoprene O-rings instead of the awkward method of tying the aorta to the canula, has speeded up preparation significantly and improved the reliability of the method in our hands. We are now able to produce 8-10 x 10^8 myocytes from 12 rat hearts (300g animals) with better than 80% viability as measured by counting rod-shaped cells. This yield allows studies of receptors on myocyte membrane fractions or identification of receptor coupling proteins such as the GTP binding protein that couples $beta_1$-adrenergic receptors to stimulation of adenylate cyclase.

The limitations of the preparation can be put in perspective. Our experience with tissue culture cell lines such as the 3T3 fibroblast, the BC_3H1 smooth muscle cell line, the S49 lymphoma cell and numerous others is that even in these model systems, some of them clonally derived, one does not get 100% viability upon subculture (an enzymatic treatment analogous to myocyte isolation). In fact, while the viability of these cell lines varies widely, it is on the order of 90%. This compares favorably with the adult myocyte preparation. Furthermore, like the established cell lines, the difficulty with preparation of cardiac myocytes from adult heart is not in the homogeneity, but rather in the yield of rod-shaped versus rounded-up cells. In other words, selecting for myocytes versus other cell types is easy, what is difficult is preparing living cells. With these observations in mind, the choice of the adult cardiac myocyte for radioligand binding studies can be made by addressing the question to the model. The advantages of employing the myocyte may outweigh concerns about the 20% of cells that are rounded up. For other questions, the model may not offer advantages. For studies of the characterization of receptors and their coupling to response in cardiac muscle, the myocyte is of significant advantage [5,6].

TABLE I. Receptors Found on Adult Cardiac Myocytes

RECEPTOR TYPE	PREVALENCE	ACTION	REFERENCE
Adrenergic			
$Beta_1$	2.2×10^5/myocyte	+ cAMP	7,8
$Alpha_1$	8×10^4/myocyte	- cAMP; + IP_3	5,6,9 39
Cholinergic			
Muscarinic	1.4×10^5/myocyte	- cAMP	10
Histaminic			
H1	5×10^4/myocyte	? cAMP; ? IP_3	11,12
H2	Unknown	??	
Purinergic P1			
A1	6×10^4/myocyte	- cAMP	13
A2	Unknown	??	
Purinergic P2			
P2-ATP	Probable	+ IP_3	14
Serotonergic	Unknown	??	35
Dopaminergic	Unknown	? + cAMP	15
Prostaglandin	Probable	+ cAMP	16
Polypeptide			
Angiotensin II	Probable	+ IP_3	17
Insulin	1.2×10^5/myocyte	+ glucose trans.	18
Glucagon	Probable	+ cAMP	33
Neuropeptide Y	Unknown	? - cAMP	19
ANF	Unknown	??	20
Drug receptors			
Bezodiazepine	Probable	? Cl^- channel	21
Dihydropyridine	Probable	? Ca^{2+} channel	22
Ouabain	7.4×10^5/myocyte	- Na^+/K^+-ATPase	23
Phorbol ester	6.7×10^5/myocyte	+ C-kinase	24

Where receptors have not been directly measured with radioligand binding methods, (such as the dopamine receptor) unknown is listed. If evidence is strong for the presence of the receptor and an intracellular response, from studies in ventricle, probable is listed. For the P2 receptor for ATP, we have measured responses in the purified adult rat myocyte and receptor studies are under way. Data for the insulin receptor were obtained from adult myocytes in culture. The prevalence of phorbol ester receptors was calculated from data of C. Limas (275fmol [^{3}H]phorbol binding/mg protein) assuming 4.4mg/10^6 rat ventricular myocytes [24] and recent unpublished observations [L.A. Speizer, M.J. Watson and L.L. Brunton]. This list of receptors on the adult cardiac myocyte is not intended to be a complete or exhaustive compendium of all receptors or all studies of any single receptor. It does however suggest the state of our actual knowledge of what receptors are on the myocyte. Thus, the table is a useful index of what has been done with the intact myocyte as well as what has not.

RADIOLIGAND BINDING METHODS

The application of radioligand binding methods to studies of the cardiac myocyte is not a difficult task. The equipment one requires is minimal and is generally available to most research laboratories. The basic method involves incubating the myocytes with a receptor-specific agent that is radioactively labeled. After some period of time, the free radioligand is separated from the myocytes and the bound radioactivity quantified by scintillation or gamma counting. Several methods of separating bound and free are possible [25] although filtration using glass fiber filters is the most straight forward. In this way it is possible to relate the binding of radioactivity to the myocytes with the presence of receptors on the myocyte. A number of criteria (see Table II) must be satisfied before it is possible to quantify the binding as the receptor one is looking for.

TABLE II. Receptor Binding Characteristics

a. Specific binding should saturate with increasing radioligand concentration.
b. Specific binding should be proportional to myocyte number.
c. Specific binding should be rapid and reversible.
d. Determination of receptor affinity by kinetic and equilibrium methods should be in close agreement.
e. Competition studies with unlabeled agents should reflect their known rank order of potency.
f. Receptors should demonstrate stereoselectivity in competition experiments employing unlabeled stereoisomers.

Perhaps the most important methodological concern in applying radioligand binding to the myocyte (or any tissue) is the way in which one defines nonspecific binding. Nonspecific binding is the binding of the radioligand to sites other than the receptor of interest and is proportional to radioligand concentration. All radioligands demonstrate nonspecific binding. It is imperative that nonspecific binding be quantified in each experiment. The way to define nonspecific binding is to incubate the myocytes with radioligand and an excess of an unlabeled agent that has known pharmacological specificity for the receptor being studied. In this way, the unlabeled agent saturates the receptor allowing very little, if any, specific binding of the radioligand to receptors. Since nonspecific binding sites do not readily saturate, the radioligand remains bound to them. When bound and free are separated, the remaining signal represents binding to nonspecific sites. This nonspecific signal is subtracted from the signal obtained in the absence of excess unlabeled agent (total binding) and the remaining signal is then the specific receptor binding. The nonspecific binding also includes the background radioactivity which is any binding that occurs to filters in filtration assays or tubes in centrifugation assays so that subtracting nonspecific binding from total binding provides all necessary corrections to the data.

Experimental Approaches

Kinetic determination of receptor affinity In approaching the characterization of a putative receptor on the cardiac myocyte there are essentially three types of experiments that one should undertake. Each of these can be performed with the intact cell and each will provide valuable and distinct information as follows. The first experiment that one should undertake is the kinetic determination of K_D, where the K_D will be the affinity of the receptor for the radioligand. This experiment is demonstrated in Figure 1 for the binding of the alpha$_1$ specific antagonist [^{3}H]prazosin to the intact rat cardiac myocyte.

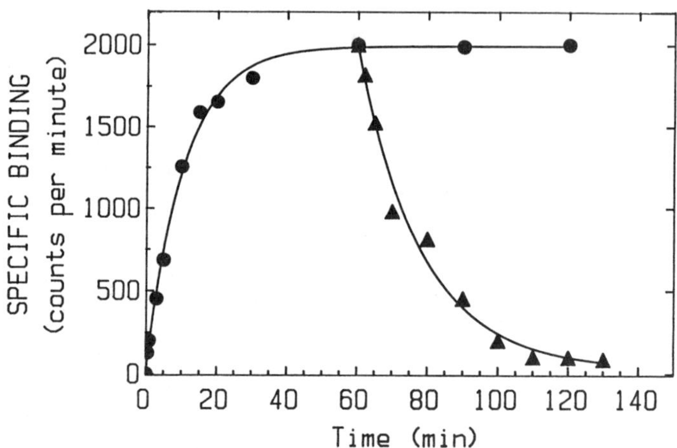

Figure 1. ON AND OFF RATES DETERMINED FOR THE BINDING OF [^{3}H]PRAZOSIN TO THE INTACT CARDIAC MYOCYTE. Approximately 10^5 myocytes were incubated with 36pM [^{3}H]prazosin (80Ci/mmol) at 32° in a shaking waterbath, gassed with O_2 and aliquots withdrawn at selected times. At 60 min, excess unlabeled phentolamine (10uM) was added and the dissociation of [^{3}H]prazosin studied in time. Data are the mean of duplicate determinations in a single representative experiment. The kinetic K_D for prazosin determined in this experiment is 96pM.

The association of radioligand with receptor (on rate) will be a reversible reaction of the type [$R + L \rightleftharpoons RL$] where the receptor (R) and radioligand (L) form a complex (RL) that achieves apparent equilibrium with time. This experiment and its companion, the dissociation of radioligand from the receptor (off rate), are particularly useful experiments that do more than establish the kinetic K_D and thus are recommended to the reader as the first experiment to perform with a new receptor study. In addition to the receptor affinity for radioligand this experiment also allows one to effectively establish conditions suitable to study the binding. For example, what will be the best time to study the equilibrium binding in competition binding studies? This is readily obtained from inspection of the association curve, and should be the earliest time that equilibrium is reproducibly achieved. If sufficient association is not achieved, one can track down several simple potential difficulties.

The incubation temperature may be too high. While 30° is a standard temperature for many receptor studies and cardiac myocytes do well at 32°, some receptors such as the Insulin receptor may require a decreased temperature to diminish internalization and degradation of receptor-ligand complex. Receptor concentration (i.e. myocyte number) must be sufficient to allow a suitable signal, this is a problem with low specific activity ligands and sparse receptor numbers. Some receptor-ligand interactions, particularly dissociation, may occur so fast that it is necessary to modify the incubation conditions (such as temperature) or choose another method of separating bound and free radioligand. In addition to optimizing the conditions for binding of radioligand, it must be remembered at this stage that conditions must be developed at the same time that optimize the viability of the myocytes. This is crucial early on since the incubation of myocytes with antagonist radioligands (antagonist radioligands are preferable in many cases) may not reveal the nature (alive or dead) of the cells. That is, when myocytes die and round-up they may behave like membranes with respect to antagonist radioligands and if one does not count cells following experiments improper conclusions about the characteristics of intact cell binding will be made. Notwithstanding, it is often an advantage to prepare membranes from intact cells in order to investigate the regulation of receptor affinity, as is the case with studies of GTP sensitivity of agonist binding to $alpha_1$ receptors on the adult cardiac myocyte [6].

Both the association and dissociation of radioligand from receptor are exponential functions and can readily be fit to such equations. We employ the computer program GraphPad (H. Motulsky; ISI Press) as this friendly program allows one to fit these and other appropriate equations to the data using non-linear curve fitting routines that are an invaluable aid to the quantification of radioligand binding data [26]. This program also plots data in a readily publishable format.

For the association data, the specific binding can be expressed as the natural logarithm of that binding occurring at equilibrium, ([RL]eq), divided by that occurring at equilibrium minus that at some time prior to equilibrium ([RL]t).

$$\ln \left\{ \frac{[RL]eq}{[RL]eq - [RL]t} \right\}$$

This result is then plotted versus time and a straight line is obtained. The slope of this line is equal to the concentration of radioligand [L] times the on rate (k_1) plus the off rate (k_2) (Eq. 1).

The dissociation data are plotted as the natural logarithm of the specific binding remaining, ([RL]t) versus time. The slope of the line obtained is equal to $-k_2$ (Eq. 2). To derive the kinetic K_D from these data one solves for k_1 (concentration^{-1} x time^{-1}) and k_2 (time^{-1}) and then ratios the two (k_2/k_1) yielding the affinity of the receptor for the radioligand in concentration units. The agreement between this and equilibrium K_D data are often within 20%, but may be acceptable within a factor of two.

$$\text{Equation 1.} \quad \text{Slope} = [L]k_1 + k_2$$

$$\text{Equation 2.} \quad \text{Slope} = -k_2$$

Saturation isotherm The second type of experiment that can be performed is called a saturation isotherm. This experiment, conducted at equilibrium, allows one to determine both the prevalence of a receptor on the myocyte as well as the affinity of the receptor for the radioligand. Figure 2, below, shows such an experiment carried out in order to characterize the myocyte beta-adrenergic receptor.

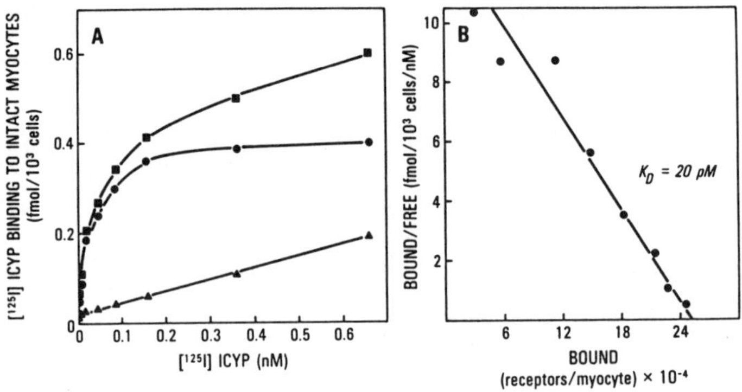

Figure 2. BINDING OF [^{125}I]IODOCYANOPINDOLOL TO INTACT ADULT RABBIT CARDIAC MYOCYTES. Panel A: purified myocytes (2 x 10^3) were incubated with increasing concentrations (5-640pM) of [^{125}I]ICYP (2200Ci/mmol) in the presence (nonspecific binding) and absence (total binding) of unlabeled propranolol (10^{-6}M). Specifically bound radioactivity (●) was determined by subtracting nonspecific binding (▲) from total binding (■). The Hill slope calculated for specific binding = 0.98. Panel B: Scatchard plot of the specific binding.

The saturation isotherm is performed by incubating a sufficient number of cells (less for ligands with higher specific activities; compare legends to Figs. 1 and 2) with increasing concentrations of the radioligand under conditions determined by the successful on and off rate experiments. The concentrations of radioligand to use can be inferred from the literature assuming the receptor of interest has been described elsewhere, but it is best determined under one's own conditions using the kinetic experiments described above. The goal of the experiment is to achieve saturation of specific binding. We employ 8 different concentrations of radioligand and determine total binding in triplicate and nonspecific binding in duplicate. It is usually simple to choose a range of concentrations to employ by using the K_D derived from the kinetic experiments. One may start with 10 times the K_D concentration and generate seven additional concentrations to employ by successive 1:1 serial dilution. Thus if the apparent K_D were 1.0nM, the final radioligand concentrations to use for the saturation isotherm would be 10nM, 5nM, 2.5nM, 1.25nM, 625pM, 312pM, 156pM, and 78pM. Since it is possible to sample the stock radioisotope dilutions and count the radioactivity to calculate radioisotope concentration independently, it is not necessary to worry that these dilutions could be in error. Because the specific binding in this experiment is obtained by subtraction it is a mathematical construct. Thus, it is essential to replicate the points in the experiment several times and to repeat experiments and average the apparent K_Ds obtained. Nonspecific binding will generally be fit by a straight line as it does not saturate due to the very low affinity and practically endless capacity of these sites. The specific binding on the other hand, will be saturable and will be fit by a rectangular hyperbola.

Two parameters can be determined from the specific binding curve. The first, the specific binding at saturation is the B_{max}, and represents the number of receptors present. The second is the apparent affinity, or K_D, which is the concentration of radioligand required to saturate one-half of the receptors. The K_D has the units of concentration. The better the affinity, the lower the K_D. The B_{max} has, at first, units of radioactivity, but must be converted to units such as receptors/number of myocytes by knowing the specific activity of the radioligand (i.e. cpm/fmol), Avogadro's number, and the number of myocytes/vessel. If the receptor distribution is uniform among the cells and each receptor binds a single ligand molecule, then the number of receptors on each myocyte can be determined. Indeed, it is further possible to measure the myocytes and project surface area assuming the myocyte to be a cylinder. While this approach is a simplification (the myocyte has a significant degree of membrane invagination), this approach has the advantage of allowing us to think of receptor responsiveness in terms of the distribution of receptors on cells rather than the less attractive but far more common quantification of receptors/mg of membrane protein. Expression of receptor density on the myocyte is useful when comparisons are to be made between diseased and normal myocytes, or for desensitization or down regulation studies.

While both the B_{max} and the K_D can be obtained from the saturation curve, it is particularly helpful to convert the specific binding data to the ratio of bound/free plotted on the ordinate and bound ligand plotted on the abscissa (Figure 2B). This yields the Scatchard [27] or Rosenthal [28] plot that will more accurately yield the K_D and B_{max} values. As shown in figure 2B, the Scatchard data can directly yield the number of receptor sites per cell from the intercept of the regression line with the abscissa. The K_D is the negative reciprocal of the slope of the line. This approach will yield additional data when the radioligand binds to receptors on the cell with two (or potentially more) affinities. In this situation, as with the insulin receptor on the myocyte, the Scatchard plot will allow one to resolve two linear components, and thus determine two affinity states (or receptor subtypes) and their proportion of total receptor sites. The correct interpretation of these data will require a detailed knowledge of the interactions of agonists and antagonists with receptors, as well as the modulation of receptor affinity states by ions and modifiers such as Mg^{++} and GTP.

Because some radioligands are either very precious or very expensive or both (as with some labeled peptides and monoclonal antibodies) it may be necessary to perform the saturation isotherm with a single concentration of isotope. In this case, one constructs the saturation isotherm with unlabeled ligand that is in all other respects identical to the radioligand and then corrects the binding for dilution of isotope. While this method will magnify the experimental errors, it may be a useful way of conserving radioligand in special circumstances.

Specific binding can also be analyzed by the method of Hill [29] to determine the likelihood that the binding has occurred to a single site rather than co-operative sites, different affinity states or receptor subtypes. For most receptor studies, this approach will not be as useful to distinguish states and subtypes as the competition study described below. A detailed description of the use of the Hill plot is available elsewhere [30].

Competition binding studies The last type of experiment to be discussed here is the competition study. This experiment, too often incorrectly called a displacement experiment (nothing is "displaced" in a competition experiment), yields valuable information on the identity of receptor types, their coupling and regulation and the kinds of drugs that are likely to interact with them. In order to conduct a competition binding experiment one incubates myocytes with a constant amount of radioligand in the absence and presence of increasing concentration of an unlabeled agent that is expected to bind to the receptor being studied. If the unlabeled agent has an affinity for the receptor less and less binding of the radioligand will be measured at equilibrium with higher and higher concentrations of the unlabeled agent. When one plots the binding as a function of the logarithm to the base 10 of the concentration of unlabeled agent, one obtains a sigmoidal curve as shown in figure 3.

There are two features of the competition curve of particular interest. The first is the pharmacologic order of potency. This is frequently expressed as the relative position of the curve, right or left of a standard agent, or the comparison of concentrations required to compete for half of the specific binding (IC_{50}) between two or more unlabeled agents. In radioligand binding studies it is best described as the affinity, or K_D, of the receptor for the competitor. For instance, in the example in figure 3, if the competition had been for $[^{125}I]$ICYP binding to a $beta_2$-adrenergic receptor, the practolol curve would have been right shifted (a lower K_D) and the zinterol curve would have been left shifted (a higher K_D). The second feature of interest is the relative steepness of the competition curve. If there is a single class of sites for a given radioligand on the myocyte, as is the case for the $beta_1$ receptor analysis shown in figure 3, then the competition for binding between 90% and 10% of the specific binding in the absence of competitor occurs over approximately 100 fold concentration of unlabeled agent (81 fold to be precise). This relationship holds only when the radioligand and the unlabeled agent are competing for binding to the same site and both interactions are reversible and reach equilibrium.

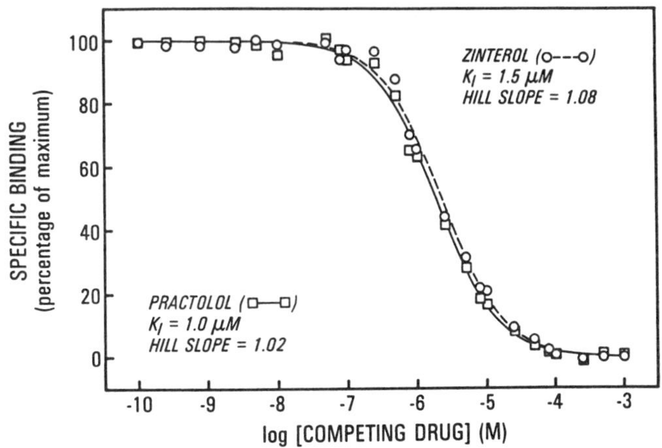

Figure 3. COMPETITION OF $[^{125}I]$ICYP BINDING TO INTACT RABBIT VENTRICULAR MYOCYTES BY BETA-ADRENERGIC SUBTYPE SELECTIVE ANTAGONISTS. Myocytes (3×10^3) were prepared from adult rabbit hearts and incubated at 32° with $[^{125}I]$ICYP (45pM) and increasing concentrations of either practolol (□) a $beta_1$ specific antagonist or zinterol (O) a $beta_2$ more specific antagonist. Data are expressed as the percentage of specific binding occurring in the absence of competitor. Values are the mean of triplicate determinations in a representative experiment. These data indicate that both of the subtype specific antagonists compete for binding with the non-selective radioligand $[^{125}I]$ICYP in a manner consistent with a single class of binding sites (Hill slopes = unity). In addition, the relative affinities of each agent are comparable with binding to a $beta_1$-adrenergic receptor on the myocyte (Zinterol's K_I at a $beta_2$ receptor is approx. 20pM).

When this competition curve is not a single component curve, but rather, is a shallow curve where significantly more that two logarithms of concentration are required to compete for the binding of radioligand (figure 4), then there are probably two binding sites of differing affinity for the unlabeled agent. This may be the result of two different types, or sub-types of receptor present, or it may be the result of interconvertible states of a receptor as seems to be the case with the $alpha_1$ receptor on the rat myocyte [6]. Because it is necessary to carefully measure the apparent steepness of the competition curve, computer methods are invaluable. GraphPad (ISI Press) is particularly helpful in this regard. It is possible to model data to non-linear curve fitting routines that assume single or multiple affinity states of the receptor. Munson and Rodbard [31] have developed LIGAND, a program that is also an invaluable resource. Whether there are one, two, or theoretically, even three receptor states, it is possible to resolve them with non-linear curve fitting methods.

In order to be able to compare the results of competition studies between compounds, experiments, across species lines and perhaps most importantly, from lab to lab, it is necessary to generate a K_I for a given compound (or multiple K_I's) rather than trying to compare IC_{50} values which will only be useful as a comparison within a given experiment. The equilibrium dissociation constant for the unlabeled agent, K_I, is determined by the method of Cheng and Prusoff [32] and is shown in equation 3.

Equation 3. $$K_I = \frac{IC_{50} \times K_D}{[L] + K_D}$$

In this equation, the IC_{50} is the concentration of the unlabeled agent that competes for half of the specific radioligand binding, the K_D is the dissociation constant of the radioligand determined independently and [L] is the radioligand concentration as measured in the individual experiment.

It is very important that the reader recognize that a number of careful assumptions must be made in order to employ computer methods for the analysis of radioligand binding data. For instance, the way in which 100% and 0% specific binding are assigned in the analysis of a competition experiment will greatly affect the non-linear calculations and could result in errors in the affinities and number of sites calculated by the computer method. By the same token, these methods are invaluable since it is not possible to learn the affinities of multiple binding sites or their proportion by simple inspection of the data. We encourage the use of some excellent resources for detailed discussions of the limitations of radioligand binding methods [30,42].

Receptor occupation/activity Radioligand binding studies describe the receptor of interest with respect to those radiolabeled and unlabeled agonists and antagonists employed but do not offer information on receptor function. In this sense, these experiments are purely descriptive. The relationship between radioligand binding and receptor function can be made by relating receptor occupancy by agonist to response in the cell. Whether the measured response is physiological, such as myocyte contraction, or biochemical, such as accumulation of cyclic AMP, these outcomes can be correlated with the number of receptors that have bound agonist. Another approach to understanding receptor coupling to response is to employ pharmacological agents known to bind irreversibly to the receptor, or those that can be photolysed to the receptor (azido derivatives). Thus, removing more and more receptors from being able to interact with agonist may shed light on the spareness of some receptors. Radioligand binding can be used to confirm the proportion of receptors available for agonist binding and parallel studies of biochemistry or physiology can correlate the response.

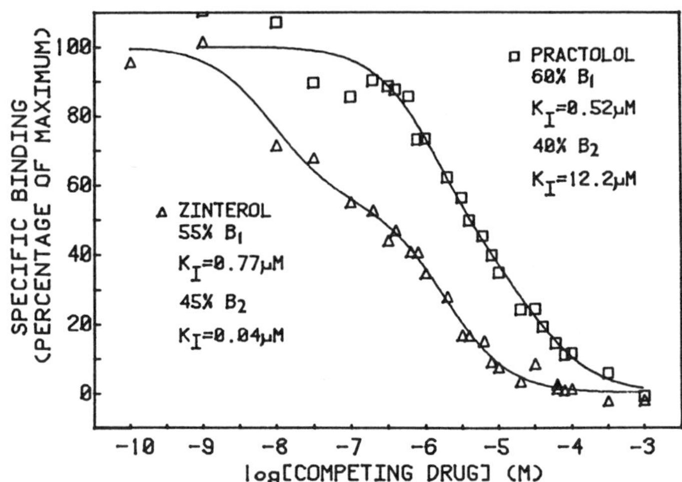

Figure 4. COMPETITION OF $[^{125}I]$ICYP BINDING TO THE NONMYOCYTE FRACTION FROM ADULT RAT HEART. The fractions from the purification of adult rat cardiac myocytes that are normally discarded were saved, pooled and employed in radioligand competition studies. Nonmyocytes were incubated with $[^{125}I]$ICYP (50pM) at 32° in the presence and absence of practolol (□) and zinterol (△). Data are the mean of triplicate determinations in a single representative experiment. Curves are computer generated best fits of the data assuming the presence of two receptor types. Data were fit using LIGAND and assumed 100% specific binding to be that which occurred in the absence of competitor, and 0% to be the value independently obtained in the same experiment by the addition of propranolol (1uM).

EXPERIMENTAL CONDITIONS AND VIABILITY

The issue of viability is not a serious limitation for studies of receptor characterization with radioligand binding methods. The on (k_1) and off (k_{-1}) rates for agonists and antagonists of a wide variety of receptors on the myocyte are such that kinetic determinations can readily be made with freshly isolated cells. Equilibrium binding for those receptors we have studied on the myocyte and others whose presence we predict from studies in ventricular or atrial membranes [33] require only 60 to 240 min of incubation. Because the viability of the isolated myocyte remains within 90% of starting figures for as long as four to six hours following preparation [10], it is possible to study the coupling of many receptors to response within the cell. One can make a clear distinction here between those responses that occur immediately as a consequence of receptor occupation by agonist (e.g. stimulation of adenylate cyclase and production of cyclic AMP) and more distal consequences such as changes in protein synthetic rates that may take many hours to see.

For radioligand binding studies to intact cells it is necessary to consider the environment in which the cell will be placed. The usual method employed for radioligand binding to membranes is not suitable for intact cells. We employ a Krebs bicarbonate buffer containing 1.0mM calcium to which we add BME amino acids (100X concentrate; Gibco). Since the cells need to be kept in suspension during the incubation with radioligand, we add cells to washed glass (siliconized) or plastic scintillation vials and place the open vials in an orbital shaking water bath with a gassing hood. We can then maintain the desired pH by gassing with O_2/CO_2 (95%/5%). While it is also useful to employ organic buffers such as TRIS, it is not always wise as these agents are known to interfere with some receptor types [34].

The incubation volume needed in binding studies must be carefully considered and may change depending on the choice of radioligand. For example, studies of the beta-adrenergic receptor using the iodinated antagonist ligand [^{125}I]iodocyanopindolol ([^{125}I]ICYP) with a specific activity of 3956cpm/fmol (2200Ci/mmol) can be performed in very small volumes as the radioactive signal obtained, even from the presence of relatively few receptors, is robust. This is useful in studies of membranes since it is possible to do experiments in relatively small volumes (250ul) and thus conserve radioligand. In studies of the intact myocyte however, it is not wise to employ less than 1ml incubation volume as it is difficult to maintain a well stirred suspension of high viability. Another practical example of the choice of incubation volume is seen with radioligands of particularly low specific activity such as [^{3}H] on the order of 30Ci/mmol or less. In this case, the receptor concentration (myocyte number) required to see a significant signal (i.e. it is not reasonable to work with less than 1000cpm for competition studies) when placed in 1ml results in a significant bound fraction and thus a reduction in the free concentration of ligand. This complication is avoided by simply increasing the incubation volume for the same number of cells, as we have done recently for studies of the muscarinic receptor on the myocyte [10].

One should consider carefully what additions are made to the incubations with radioligand as some may cause difficulty. Although we routinely employ bovine serum albumin in our incubations, use of more than 0.05% may significantly increase the nonspecific binding of some ligands. The effect is not only to elevate the nonspecific blank, but may alter the calculated free concentration leading to errors in estimates of receptor affinity. This can also be a problem with animal sera. In addition, the investigator should take care to determine viability in control incubations throughout the experiment as some additions to experiments may damage the cells [see ref.10 for details of the effects of Na^+ ionophores in radioligand binding studies of the muscarinic receptor].

COUPLING OF RECEPTORS TO MYOCYTE FUNCTION

Just as the adult mammalian cardiac myocyte is a convenient model for radioligand binding studies, so it is well suited for studies of the coupling of receptors to intracellular response. We have taken particular advantage of the myocyte model for studies of the coupling of receptors to cyclic AMP and inositol phosphate metabolism.

Assessment of Cyclic AMP Metabolism in the Cardiac Myocyte

Both stimulatory and inhibitory receptor coupling to adenylate cyclase can readily be studied in the intact myocyte [10,16]. It is particularly useful to employ the myocyte for studies of receptor regulation of cardiac adenylate cyclase activity because the adult myocyte possesses multiple receptors coupled to both stimulation and inhibition of adenylate cyclase (Table I). There are three experimental approaches to the study of cyclic AMP metabolism in the myocyte. These are, 1) the measurement of total cellular cyclic AMP, 2) [^{3}H]-adenine labeling to measure [^{3}H]cyclic AMP accumulation, and 3) the use of myocyte membranes to measure adenylate cyclase activity *in vitro*.

Total cAMP content Isolated myocytes can be incubated with drugs or hormones and the cell suspension acidified at the desired time with concentrated TCA (trichloroacetic acid) to yield a final concentration of 5-10% TCA. The total cellular cyclic AMP content can be determined by purification of the acid supernatant over Dowex-50 (Biorad) anion exchange columns. The acid pellet can be hydrolyzed in mild base (0.2N NaOH) and the protein content determined with standard dye binding methods. In this way the protein determination will provide a denominator with which to express the result (cyclic AMP/mg protein). The purified sample is then assayed for cyclic AMP content by the protein binding method of Gilman [36]. We have used this method with success [16] and found that as few as 5 x 10^5 myocytes are required for a single cyclic AMP determination. This allows a single myocyte preparation to support an experiment with many different conditions. In this regard, the myocyte is a significant advantage over the isolated perfused heart or heart slices. Using a single isolated perfused heart for a given condition is expensive, and slices, though they provide more latitude than the perfused heart, suffer from their inhomogeneity and poor viability. The cardiac myocyte contains on the order of 5pmol of cyclic AMP/mg protein (unstimulated), and 16-20pmol/mg protein when incubated with maximal beta-adrenergic agonist for three min in the absence of PDE inhibitors.

[^{3}H]Adenine labeling Incubation of myocytes with [^{3}H]adenine (10uCi/ml) for 60-90 min results in labeling of cellular ATP [6,37]. Subsequent treatment of aliquots of labeled cells (2-4 x 10^5) with agonists that stimulate receptors coupled to cyclic AMP metabolism can be assayed as increases or decreases in the accumulation of [^{3}H]cyclic AMP. [^{3}H]Cyclic AMP is purified from TCA extracts in a fashion similar to that for the measurement of total cellular cyclic AMP except that the cyclic AMP peak from the Dowex-50 column is passed over neutral alumina to remove contaminating [^{3}H]ATP. This method may provide advantages because the only [^{3}H]cyclic AMP measured is that accumulated during the labeling period and during experimental stimulation. This approach may help in assessing small changes in cyclic AMP in myocytes that contain 4-5 pmol total cyclic AMP per mg of protein. In addition, the method requires only a single day to obtain results as opposed to two days to obtain results on the total cellular cyclic AMP content of myocytes. We have found this approach invaluable for the *in vivo* assay of alpha$_1$-adrenergic receptor stimulated myocyte cyclic AMP-phosphodiesterase activity [5,11].

Measurement of adenylate cyclase In addition to the methods described above for determination of cellular cyclic AMP in myocytes, it is also possible to use the myocyte as a source of sarcolemmal membrane for the assay of adenylate cyclase [5,10]. We have employed membranes prepared from cardiac myocytes quick frozen in liquid nitrogen and powered in a pre-cooled percussion mortar. This approach allows one to save cells from several cell preparations and combine them as a pooled sample, or to generate large quantities of powder from one or two myocyte preparations and use aliquots of the frozen powder for many studies. We have found that 10^6 adult myocytes yield approximately 2mg of membrane (crude membranes prepared from a simple homogenate by centrifugation at 3000g for 10min) protein. This is sufficient for a 50 tube adenylate cyclase assay (40ug protein/assay tube) assuming a final specific activity of [a-^{32}P]ATP of 30-50cpm/pmol. Although we will not review this assay here, it is well described by Salomon *et al.* [38]. The adenylate cyclase assay is particularly useful in ascribing increases and decreases in cyclic AMP measured in the intact myocyte to the direct regulation of adenylate cyclase by receptors for drugs and hormones.

As well as the measurement of second messenger generation in the myocyte, the consequences of cyclic AMP production, cyclic AMP-dependent protein kinase activation and subsequent protein phosphorylations, can also be studied in the myocyte. Thus, the adult cardiac myocyte is a very useful model for studies of receptor-signal transduction at the cellular level [16].

Measurement of Inositol Phosphate Production

We have investigated the coupling of alpha$_1$ adrenergic and cholinergic muscarinic receptors on the myocyte to the formation of inositol phosphates [9,39,40]. Myocytes can be labeled with [^{3}H]myoinositol (15uCi/ml) for 90-120 min, washed to remove excess label, and stimulated with agonist in the presence or absence of Li^+ to block degradation of inositol-1 phosphate by its phosphatase. Samples containing 2-3 x 10^5 myocytes are acidified with TCA (5%) and extracted with ethyl ether [9] or chloroform:methanol [39] to remove labeled lipids. The aqueous sample is dried, resuspended in neutral buffer and separated on a Dowex-1 (Biorad; formate form) column eluted with ammonium formate buffers. Using this approach we have recently measured [9] significant elevations in inositol trisphosphate production following stimulation of the alpha$_1$ receptor on the adult rat myocyte. The usefulness of the myocyte for studies of receptor coupling to intracellular events is emphasized by our interest in receptor coupling to phospholipase-C activation. While it is not clear that the generation of inositol trisphosphate is an important regulatory event in the release of Ca^{2+} ion from sarcoplasmic reticulum in heart, it is clear that the myocyte is the most useful model of heart in which to carry out this investigation. We can study receptors, their coupling and regulation, the second messengers produced and the subsequent changes in cellular biochemistry produced. It is also possible, with computer assisted digital image analysis, to study both unloaded contraction as well as calcium and pH indicator fluorescence as measures of cellular physiology.

CONCLUSIONS

In the search for the best methods for preparation of viable myocytes, many comparisons have been offered between the isolated cell and the intact heart. Many of the articles in this monograph are, in fact, a tribute not only to the usefulness of the model but also to the homology it bears to the tissue of origin. Much attention has been given in the past to the best method of preparation of the adult myocyte. While many aspects of the preparation of cells still appear more an art than application of science (e.g. what constituent(s) of the collagenase we employ is responsible for successful preparation of myocytes?) it is clearly past time to be concentrating on the preparation of these cells. We believe that a viability of 80% is consistent with the survival of many tissue culture cells following sub-culture and it may not be reasonable to expect to improve the viability much more. The issue of cell origin in the myocyte preparation is, gratefully, never an issue as the persuasive rod-shaped appearance is unmistakably that of a cardiac muscle cell.

Studies of receptors on the adult cardiac myocyte have yielded useful new knowledge about the existence of receptor types and their regulation of cardiac muscle. Perhaps the best studied cardiac receptor system to date is that of the beta-adrenergic receptor. We have found that while both beta-adrenergic subtypes, $beta_1$ and $beta_2$, exist in the rat ventricle, the myocyte possesses only receptors of the $beta_1$ subtype [8]. Thus, the view that the inotropic effects of catecholamines in the heart are mediated via $beta_1$ receptors is confirmed by the myocyte studies. In addition to homologies expected of receptors on the myocyte, there is clear homology in the responses that can be measured in the cell. The agonist specific compartmentation of cyclic AMP action first described in the intact heart [41] can be readily measured in the isolated cell [16]. Studies of myocyte receptors have also led to unexpected results that could not be understood with studies in the isolated heart. For instance, we have found that the $alpha_1$ receptor on the myocyte is coupled to decreased accumulation of cyclic AMP when $beta_1$-adrenergic receptors are concurrently stimulated. This curious result was accompanied by a GTP shift in the affinity of the $alpha_1$ receptor for the agonist norepinephrine [6] suggesting coupling to a GTP-binding protein. Studies of adenylate cyclase eliminated the chance that the $alpha_1$ receptor coupled to inhibition of this enzyme [5]. Studies with pertussis toxin treated myocyte membranes ruled out the involvement of the guanine nucleotide binding protein G_i in the coupling of receptor to response. Our recent data suggest that it is coupling of the myocyte $alpha_1$ receptor to phosphatidylinositol metabolism via a distinct GTP binding protein (G_sP) that explains the GTP shift in agonist affinity in radioligand binding studies [9]. The effects on cyclic AMP metabolism may be due to an effect of IP_3.

These results confirm that the myocyte is not only a model of heart muscle in which one can learn what he expects to learn of heart, but rather, the myocyte offers a unique advantage to learn what we do not yet know about cardiac muscle.

REFERENCES

1. B.I. Terman, and P.A. Insel, J. Biol. Chem. 261, 5603-5609 (1986).
2. S.H. Smith, M. Kramer, S.P. Bishop, and J. Ingwall, in this volume: Biology of The Isolated Cardiac Myocyte (Elsevier, New York 1988).
3. J.W. Dow, N.G. Harding, and T. Powell, Cardiovas. Res. 15, 483-514 (1981).
4. C.J. Frangakis, J.J. Bahl, H. McDaniel, and R. Bressler, Life Science 27, 815-825 (1980).
5. I.L.O. Buxton, and L.L. Brunton, J. Biol. Chem. 260, 6733-6737 (1985).
6. I.L.O. Buxton, and L.L. Brunton, Am. J. Physiol. 251, H307-H311 (1986).
7. I.L.O. Buxton, and L.L. Brunton, Biochem. International 11, 137-144 (1985).
8. I.L.O. Buxton, and L.L. Brunton, Circulation Research 56, 126-132 (1985).
9. I.L.O. Buxton, and K.O. Doggwiler, in this volume: Biology of the Isolated Adult Cardiac Myocyte (Elsevier, New York, 1988).
10. I.L.O. Buxton, D. Rozansky, L.L. Brunton, and H.J. Motulsky, J. Cardiovascular Pharmacology 7, 476-481 (1985).
11. I.L.O. Buxton, Proc. West Pharmacol. Soc. 29, 55-58 (1986).
12. I. Sakuma, S.S. Gross, and R. Levi, Fed. Proc. 46, 962 (1987).
13. K.O. Doggwiler, and I.L.O. Buxton, Fed. Proc. 47, (in press, 1988).
14. I.L.O. Buxton, and K.O. Doggwiler, Fed. Proc. 47, (in press, 1988).
15. M. Sandrini, A. Benelli, M. Baraldi, Pharmacol. Res. Comm. 18, 1151 (1986).
16. I.L.O. Buxton, and L.L. Brunton, J. Biol. Chem. 258, 10233-10239 (1983).
17. K.M. Baker, H.-Q. Han, and H.A. Singer, Fed. Proc. 46, 968 (1987).
18. J. Eckel, G. Pandalis, and H. Reinauer, Biochim. Biophys. Acta 846, 398 (1985).
19. S. Kassis, M. Olasmaa, L. Terenius, and P.H. Fishman, J. Biol. Chem. 262, 3429 (1987).
20. R. Takayanagi, T. Imada, and T. Inagami, Biochem. Biophys. Res. Comm. 142, 483 (1987).

21. M. Holck, and W. Osterrieder, Eur. J. Pharmacol. 118, 293-301 (1985).
22. P. Hess, J.B. Lansman, B. Nilius, and R.W. Tsien, J. Cardiovas. Pharmacol. 8S-9, 11-21 (1986).
23. T. Onji, and M.-S. Liu, Arch. Biochem. Biophys. 207, 148-156 (1981).
24. C.J. Limas, Arch. Biochem. Biophys. 238, 300-304 (1985).
25. M.D. Hollenberg, and E. Nexo, in: Membrane Receptors: Methods for Purification and Characterization S. Jacobs, P. Cuatrecasas, (Chapman and Hull 1982).
26. H.J. Motulsky, and L.A. Ransnas, FASEB J. (in press 1987).
27. G. Scatchard, Ann. New York Acad. Sci. 51, 660-672 (1949).
28. H.E. Rosenthal, Anal. Biochem. 20, 525-532 (1967).
29. A. Levitski, in: Molecular Biology, Biochemistry and Biophysics (Springer-Verlag, New York 1978).
30. H.J. Motulsky, and P.A. Insel, in: Receptor Science in Cardiology (Futura, MountKiosco, New York 1984).
31. P.J. Munson, and D. Rodbard, Anal. Biochem. 107, 220-239 (1980).
32. Y. Cheng, and W.H. Prusoff, Biochem. Pharmacol. 22, 3099-3108 (1973).
33. D.C. Bode, and L.L. Brunton, in: Adult Cardiac Myocytes vol.1 H. Piper and G. Isenberg (CRC Reviews, Boca Ration, Florida in press 1988).
34. K.M.M Murphy, and A. Sastre, Biochem. Biophys. Res. Comm. 113, 280-285 (1983).
35. A.J. Kaumann, J. Cardiovas. Pharmacol. 7S-7, 76-78 (1985).
36. A.G. Gilman, Proc. Natl. Acad. Sci. U.S.A. 67, 305-312 1970).
37. H. Shimizu, J.N. Daley, and C.R. Creveling, J. Neurochem. 16, 1609 (1969).
38. Y. Salomon, C. Londos, and M. Rodbell, Anal. Biochem. 58, 541-548 (1974).
39. J.H. Brown, I.L.O. Buxton, and L.L. Brunton, Circulation Research 57, 532-537 (1985).
40. I.L.O. Buxton, Fed. Proc. 46, 217 (1987).
41. J.S. Hayes, L.L. Brunton, J.H. Brown, J.B. Reese, and S.E. Mayer, Proc. Natl. Acad. Sci. 76 1570-1574 (1979).
42. L.E. Limbird, Cell Surface Receptors: A Short Course in Theory and Methods (Martinus Nijhoff Publishing, Boston, 1986).

MEASUREMENT OF PHARMACOLOGICAL EFFECTS IN ISOLATED MYOCYTES

PAUL C. SIMPSON
Cardiology Service (111-C), Veterans Administration Medical Center and Department of Medicine and Cardiovascular Research Institute, University of California, San Francisco, CA 94121

ABSTRACT

A major important use of isolated myocytes is the investigation of cell responses to pharmacological manipulations. In these experiments, the dose of an environmental variable is titrated and the cell response is measured. This chapter reviews methodological issues in this application of myocyte preparations.

INTRODUCTION

One of the most important applications of isolated myocyte preparations is the investigation of myocyte responses to pharmacological manipulations. Classical pharmacological studies focus on the interaction between drugs or endogenous regulatory molecules and cell receptors, e.g., catecholamines with cell surface adrenergic receptors. However, considered in the broadest sense, these experiments include any which involve titration of the dose of an environmental variable and measurement of the cell response.

A few examples of titrated environmental variables, or "pharmacological agents", include (1) potential or known bioactive molecules, either soluble (e.g., insulin, norepinephrine) or attached to the culture substrate (e.g., laminin); (2) the extracellular nutrient medium or some component of it (e.g., oxygen, glucose); (3) biochemical agents or toxins (e.g., exogenous phospholipase C, adriamycin); and (4) physical factors (e.g., electrical stimulation, stretch). The cell response measured can be (1) morphological (e.g., cell shape, ultrastructure), (2) biochemical (e.g., cAMP, messenger RNA), (3) physiological (e.g.,$^{45}Ca^{++}$ flux), (4) electrophysiological (e.g., calcium channels), or (5) complex, whole-cell responses (e.g., attachment, contraction, growth). The time course of the response can be acute (seconds-hours) or chronic (hours-days). We have used the term "trophic" to distinguish such chronic responses [1]; "developmental" would be an alternate term.

The essential feature of all of these pharmacological experiments is construction of a dose-response curve, i.e., definition of the relationship between the dose of an environmental variable and the selected cell response. In most cases, and perhaps all, a specific receptor will mediate the response of the extracellular agent. Thus pharmacological experiments are the foundation for defining the pathway from stimulus through receptor and post receptor transducing mechanism to cell response.

Elucidation of the nature and mechanisms of myocyte responses to extracellular stimuli is a major goal of research in cardiac cell biology. Isolated myocyte preparations are ideally suited for this work, for two reasons: (1) a single stimulus can be defined and manipulated under controlled conditions; and (2) the response of a homogenous population of heart muscle cells can be studied. These two criteria are difficult if not impossible to achieve in tissue or organ models. In tissue and organ models, neural, hormonal and mechanical interactions complicate definition of the stimulus; and multiple types of cells

Biology of Isolated Adult Cardiac Myocytes
William A. Clark, Robert S. Decker, and Thomas K. Borg, Editors

contribute to the measured response (especially with biochemical assays) or may modify it (through cell-cell interactions).

The aim of this chapter is to review methodological issues that need to be considered if the full potential of isolated myocytes in pharmacological experiments is to be realized. The long-range focus of this work with isolated myocytes is to identify important extracellular stimuli and their intracellular mechanisms, in order to facilitate more precise study in intact preparations.

The following topics will be discussed:

(1) Isolated Myocyte Preparations--cultured and non-cultured cells and their required characterization (number, viability, contamination)
(2) Pharmacological Agents--precautions for use
(3) Experimental Protocols--basic procedures, dose-response, time course, response specificity
(4) Cell Responses--quantitation
(5) Data Analysis--dose-response curves, EC50 and maximum, competitive and noncompetitive antagonists, spare receptors

The author's experience is drawn primarily from work with cultured neonatal cells, but the same principles apply to adult myocytes. Numerous examples of their application are found in the Research Reports of this volume.

ISOLATED MYOCYTE PREPARATIONS

Two classes of isolated adult myocyte preparations are available: "cultured" cells and "non-cultured" or freshly-isolated cells. Operationally, cells can be considered "cultured" if they are maintained for days attached to a culture substrate under sterile conditions. Non-cultured or freshly-isolated cells are typically studied in suspension, although freshly-isolated cells have been used for studies of attachment to laminin and other extracellular matrix proteins [2].

Non-cultured cells are appropriate only for acute pharmacological experiments, with measurement of the cell response over a time span of seconds to a few hours. Cultured cells can be used for both acute and chronic experiments. The latter have response time courses over hours to days.

The following characteristics of both types of preparations should be determined: number and concentration or density of myocytes, cell viability, and contamination by nonmuscle mesenchymal cells ("fibroblasts"). These data define the cells under study.

The **number** of viable cells obtained from each dissociated heart (yield) provides a quality control on the isolation procedure and indicates the representativeness of the cells studied. Equal numbers of viable cells should be allocated to the separate tubes or dishes of control and treated groups, and the **concentration** (cells per ml for non-cultured cells) or **density** (cells per mm^2 for cultured cells) should be the same in all groups and should be specified. The importance of cell concentration or density is that cells can modify neighboring cells and their own extracellular environment, through substrate metabolism, secretion of extracellular matrix proteins, production of autocrine growth factors, and direct cell-cell interactions. These phenomena have not been well studied in isolated myocyte preparations, but can be predicted on the basis of the available data and analogy with other types of cells. These subtle interactions will become apparent through attention to concentration and density effects.

For cultured cells, determination of **plating efficiency** provides an additional useful index of the quality and reproducibility of the preparation. Plating efficiency is the fraction of cells plated per mm^2 that initially attach to the culture substrate, i.e., attached cell density divided by plating density. Typical 100-, 60-, and 35-mm culture dishes have surface areas of 5500-, 2100-, and 800-mm^2, respectively. All plated cells do not attach; higher plating efficiencies indicate better (less damaged) preparations. Further, with the present culture techniques, all cells that attach initially do not remain attached over time, i.e., initial density is higher than final density. The final density at the time of experimentation should be specified, and its relation to initial density is another index of the quality of the preparation.

The numbers of suspended cells can be determined using a hemocytometer or Coulter Counter. Cultured cells can be removed from the dishes with trypsin for counting. Alternatively, the numbers of attached cultured cells can be quantified by direct counting of cells in randomly selected microscopic fields. Knowing the area of the microscopic field for a given objective, one can calculate the cell density and number of cells per dish [3].

A generally accepted **viability** index for freshly-isolated cells is appearance under the phase contrast microscope: rod-shaped with refractile borders and clear cross-striations. The proportion of cells with this criterion should be determined for control and treated groups at the start and end of each experiment. There may be less agreement on the proper viability index for cultured cells. It is the author's bias that cell attachment resisting medium changes may be a reasonable criterion during the early days of culture. A very good index for viability later in culture is cell "flattening", the morphological evidence for adaptation to the culture environment. Thus, in the author's view, determination of myocyte density in culture, at initial and later times, is equivalent to assay of viability. The proportion of cells that remain viable in culture (i.e. flatten) and the rate of flattening appear to depend in part on whether the medium is supplemented with hormones and growth factors (e.g., serum) [4]. Whether cells are studied before or after flattening depends on the purpose of the experiment; for example, one might wish to test the effect of growth factors on the attachment or flattening process.

Attention to **contamination** by nonmuscle cells is an obvious requirement for a defined preparation. For non-cultured cells, the smaller nonmuscle cells appear to be largely removed by sedimentation steps during isolation. There has been little recent published attention to the possibility of nonmuscle cells tightly attached to the myocytes [5]. For cultured cells, some measure to prevent nonmyocyte proliferation must generally be employed. The extent of nonmyocyte contamination can be assessed by counting under the microscope [6].

PHARMACOLOGICAL AGENTS

Using the broad concept of "pharmacological agent" as any potential extracellular stimulus, the essential requirement is that the **dose** be measureable and variable. This requirement may be more simple in concept than in execution. What one adds or applies to the cells should be directly measured if possible. Many bioactive compounds are sensitive to light (e.g., phorbol esters, some calcium channel antagonists), heat (e.g., some peptides), or pH (e.g., catecholamines at alkaline pH). Other compounds are metabolized by the cells (e.g., exogenous diacylglycerols). Many regultory peptides bind to tubes, dishes, or sterile filters. (Parenthetically, some sterile filters contain toxic amounts of detergents and should be rinsed prior to use.) Therefore, for accurate quantitation of dose, and to avoid false-negative results, one should ideally measure the concentration of test substance in the medium at the beginning and end of the experiment. Direct chemical assay or bioassay can be used. We have used both methods to assay norepinephrine added to the culture medium [7,8].

Alternatively, or in addition, in the case of negative results (no response), a **positive control** is useful. For example, one can use another type of cell that does respond to the test substance under the same conditions. This is essentially a bioassay. Cultures of heart nonmuscle cells are a readily available alternate cell type [3,8]. Another useful positive control is a test substance to which the myocytes have been shown to respond. For example, in our work on growth regulation in cultured neonatal myocytes, we always include a group treated with norepinephrine, when testing the response to potential new growth factors. Norepinephrine has been very well characterized in our system and serves as a reference control.

The stock **solution** of a pharmacological agent should be made up in a vehicle in which it is soluble and stable (suppliers often have this information, as well as guidelines for proper storage). For chronic experiments, the stock can be sterilized by filtration, but this should be omitted if not required. The stock is then serially-diluted in buffer or medium prior to adding to the cells. In our studies, solutions are made such that the aliquot added is 1% of the total volume, e.g., 0.010 ml into 1.0 ml. In the case of catecholamines, the vehicle contains 10 mM ascorbic acid as an anti-oxidant and acidifier, which is diluted 100-fold on addition to the cells. In the case of certain potentially-toxic vehicles, such as ethanol or dimethylsulfoxide, final concentrations over 0.1% (vol/vol) should be avoided, as determined by dose-response testing of the vehicle. In any case, all tubes or dishes in a given experiment should receive equal volumes and final concentrations of any vehicle(s), and controls receive vehicle(s) alone.

EXPERIMENTAL PROTOCOLS

The **basic protocol** is simple: vehicle or various doses of the agent are added or applied to the cells, and the response is measured after seconds-hours (acute experiments) or hours-days (chronic experiments). Each separate experiment, including control and treated groups, should be done with cells from the same preparation, and reproducibility over separate preparations should be assessed. In experiments in which the response of a population of cells is assayed, e.g., cAMP content, the smallest experimental unit is a tube or dish containing cells with equal numbers, viabilities and nonmuscle contamination. We typically use triplicate tubes or dishes for each datum point. Care must be taken in aliquoting cells into tubes or dishes from a cell suspension. Cell sedimentation in the suspension or in the transfer pipet can lead to inequalities in cell numbers. There also may be subtle differences between cells aliquoted first or last. We randomly assign cells aliquoted at various times to different groups. In experiments in which single cell responses are assayed, as in electro-physiological experiments, consideration must be given to the adequacy of sampling, to be sure that the entire range of potential responses has been studied.

After the desired time in the presence of test agent or vehicle, cells are harvested for assay, or the end-point data are otherwise collected. Attention to the forgoing considerations of cells, agent, and protocol attempt to isolate variability to the dose of the agent being tested. **Experimental reproducibility** may be enhanced if the following are also noted.

Non-cultured cells used in acute experiments are inherently unstable. For this reason, it may be best to study all groups in all experiments at the same time after cell isolation. Alternatively, one might specifically ask if the response changes as a function of time after isolation. All isolated cells are sensitive to changes in temperature, pH and osmolarity. All experiments, acute or chronic, done in bicarbonate-buffered media at 37°C are subject to variability introduced by the time taken for manipulations outside the incubator. Furthermore, incubators do not equilibrate instantaneously. For example, with the Forma model 3158 water-jacketed CO_2 incubator, the recovery rate after a 20 second door opening is 10, 10, and 30 minutes for temperature, CO_2, and humidity, respectively. Thus frequent or prolonged door opening can markedly change the environment of samples waiting to be terminated. To avoid this source of variability, we alternate among multiple incubators, or use non-biocarbonate buffering and ambient temperature incubations when appropriate. In addition, we routinely use media buffered with Hanks' salts (bicarbonate 0.35 gm/L), rather than Earle's salts (bicarbonate 2.2 gm/L), and maintain incubators with 1% CO_2, rather than 5%. Change in pH outside the incubator is more gradual with the lower bicarbonate. We also terminate one of each triplicate in each group before returning to the second tube or dish, and so on. For similar reasons, and to avoid effects of receptor down-regulation or response desensitization, or other modifications produced by prior agonist exposure (unless these are being studied specifically), we use separate groups of cells for each dose, rather than cumulative dose-response experimental designs.

For complete characterization of a stimulus-response relationship, the following **three types of experiments** are required: (1) dose-response, (2) time course, and (3) response specificity.

Dose-response experiments are often done at the single time point giving a maximum response. Similarly, time course studies typically use a dose producing a maximum response. These two types of experiments can be combined, although the number of groups becomes very large. When beginning work on a novel agent, pilot studies on dose and time course are required.

In constructing a **dose-response** curve, a range of doses or concentrations is required. This range should extend from the dose at which the response is just detectable (threshold) to the point at which it has reached a plateau (maximum). For example, in our work with catecholamines, we use final concentrations that cover three to six log unit dose increments.

Time course experiments generally examine the time over which the response develops. It also may be useful to examine the time course over which the response decays after removal, inactivation, or inhibition of the agonist. Such reversability studies may provide some insight into mechanism. When designing such protocols, one needs to consider that some agents are not easily washed from cells and/or dishes or tubes. For example, lipophilic compounds such as some phorbol esters are difficult to remove from cells.

Experiments on **response specificity** focus on the specific receptor or mechanism responsible for the action of a given agent. Classical pharmacological experiments with receptor agonists employ selective receptor antagonists to show that a response is mediated through a specific receptor.

One can examine the response to a given concentration of agonist (e.g., a maximum dose) in the presence of increasing concentrations of different antagonists. By this means, the IC50 of each antagonist can be determined, the concentration of antagonist that inhibits 50% of the response to a given dose of agonist. The lower the IC50, the more selective the antagonist. A high dose of an effective antagonist will completely inhibit the response. Dose-response studies should also be done with antagonists alone, to ensure that they do not produce nonspecific effects. By definition, a pure antagonist binds to a receptor without altering its function.

In addition, agonist dose-response curves can be generated in the absence and presence of a fixed concentration of each antagonist. Competitive antagonists shift the dose-response curve to the right, but inhibition can be overcome by sufficiently high doses of agonist. More effective antagonists produce larger shifts and are more difficult to overcome with high doses of agonist. Irreversible or noncompetitive antagonists reduce the maximum effect of an agonist, but may not shift the dose-response curve. These concepts are illustrated in the section on data analysis.

In our studies with neonatal cells, we use norepinephrine or epinephrine as agonists. These agents activate $alpha_1$-, $alpha_2$-, $beta_1$-, and $beta_2$- adrenergic receptors. We have employed a variety of selective antagonists, including propranolol ($beta_1$, $beta_2$), yohimbine ($alpha_2$), terazosin or prazosin ($alpha_1$), betaxolol ($beta_1$), and ICI 118, 551 ($beta_2$), to demonstrate that induction of hypertrophy by the catecholamines is mediated through $alpha_1$ receptors and that development of contractile activity requires both $alpha_1$ and $beta_1$ receptor stimulation [8].

In addition to studies with receptor antagonists, several other strategies can be employed to assess response specificity, including selective agonists, inactive analogues, agonist inactivation, and inhibitors. For example, in our studies we have compared the response to norepinephrine with the response to clonidine, an agonist selective for $alpha_2$-adrenergic receptors, and to isoproterenol, an agonist relatively selective for beta receptors[8]. In studies with phorbol ester tumor promoters, we compare the response to alpha-TPA with that to TPA (tetradecanoylphorbol acetate or phorbol myristate acetate, PMA). TPA has a beta-hydroxyl at position 4 and is active in tumor promotion and protein kinase C translocation, whereas alpha-TPA has an alpha-hydroxyl at position 4 and is inactive. The absence of activity produced by the small structural change makes alpha-TPA an excellent agent to assess response specificity. If one is studying an agent that can be inactivated by treatment with heat, pH, proteolytic enzymes, reduction, antibodies, or other means, any of these techniques can be used to further define response specificity. Affinity columns or other means of separation can be employed to remove the putative agonist from a complex mixture. Finally, enzyme or other inhibitors may be useful. For example, in our studies we have shown that breakdown or metabolism of catecholamines eliminates the response to them[8]. In summary, multiple approaches may be required to specify precisely the stimulus responsible for the measured response.

CELL RESPONSES

Construction of a dose-response curve obviously requires that the response be graded and quantifiable. The assumption of gradability is tested by the experiment, and all-or-none cell responses are very rare. Quantitation of the response is generally not an issue in most biochemical and physiological experiments. For certain types of studies, a simple 0-4+ scale may be sufficient to quantitate the response.

Validation of the response assay will be governed by the particular experiment. The general rule is to define what is being measured and to demonstrate that it is in fact being measured accurately and precisely. In biochemical experiments, for example, more than one method of substance identification and determination of recovery are both often required.

DATA ANALYSIS

The following analysis is taken from from classical agonist-receptor pharmacology [9]. However, the same principles can be applied to the broad range of possible studies considered in this chapter.

Response data can be presented as absolute values and examined statistically by analysis of variance. Alternately, treated/control ratios can be calculated for each experiment and summed over the number of experiments. The statistical significance of deviations of ratios from unity can be determined by analysis of confidence intervals [10]. The ratio method is particularly useful for normalizing data from multiple experiments and for graphic presentation of dose-response data. This is particularly true in the case of assays with inherent variability, such as those used in molecular biology[11].

Plotting idealized dose-response or concentration-effect data generates a hyperbolic curve that follows an equation similar to the mass action law:

$$E = (Emax\ C) / (C + EC50)$$

where E is the response at C concentration, **Emax** is the maximum response, and **EC50** is the agonist concentration producing half-maximum effect.

The same relationship holds for ligand-receptor binding in radioligand assays, where E becomes B or concentration of ligand bound to receptors, C is concentration of unbound or free ligand, and EC50 becomes Kd or equilibrium dissociation constant, the free ligand concentration at 50% of maximum binding. The maximum ligand concentration bound at infinitely high concentrations of free ligand (**Bmax**) indicates total receptor number, whereas **Kd** is a measure of affinity (a low Kd signifies a high affinity, and vice versa).

Plotting response on the ordinate versus the logarithm of the dose on the abscissa transforms the hyperbolic curve to a sigmoidal one and improves the presentation. These curves are shown in Figure 1.

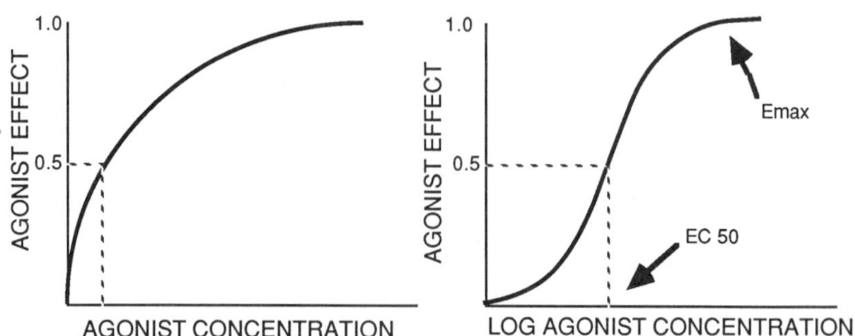

Figure 1. Idealized concentration-effect or dose-response relationship. The EC50 and Emax are indicated.

The EC50 (agonist concentration producing half-maximum response) defines the sensitivity of the response or the potency of the agonist. The EC50 is a function of the number of receptors (Bmax) and their affinity for agonist (Kd) and the efficiency of receptor coupling to post-receptor transducing mechanisms. The magnitude of the maximum response (Emax) is governed by whatever is the rate-limiting step in the overall response pathway. **Full agonists** are capable of producing a maximum response. **Partial agonists** produce a response that is less than maximum, even when all receptors are occupied. The dose-response curve for a partial agonist resembles the curve for a full agonist in the presence of a noncompetitive antagonist. This is shown in Figure 3 below. The molecular mechanisms of partial agonism are not known. Note that the EC50 of a partial agonist can be lower or higher than that for a full agonist; the extent of the maximum reponse is the key distinction.

An experiment with increasing doses of an antagonist in the presence of a fixed concentration of agonist would produce the curve shown in Figure 2.

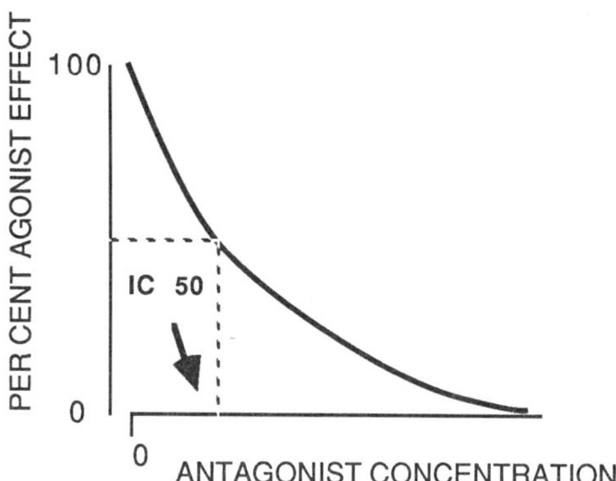

Figure 2. Increasing concentrations of an antagonist reduce the response to a fixed dose of agonist. The response is eliminated at high antagonist doses. (Very high doses may have nonspecific toxic effects, however.) The **IC50** is the antagonist concentration reducing the agonist response by 50%. The IC50 varies directly with agonist dose, e.g., a higher IC50 with a higher agonist dose.

Agonist dose-response curves in the presence and absence of a fixed dose of antagonist are different for competitive (reversible) and noncompetitive (irreversible) antagonists, as shown in Figure 3. Inhibition by a competitive antagonist is reversible by rinsing, whereas an irreversible antagonist is not washed out.

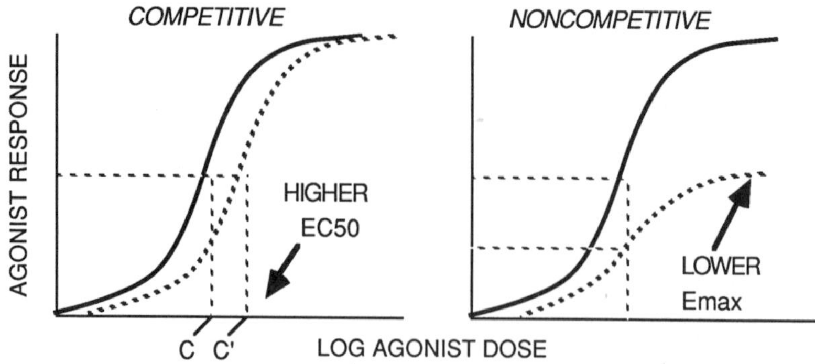

Figure 3. Agonist dose-response curves in the absence (solid line) and presence (broken line) of a fixed dose of a competitive (left) or noncompetitive (right) antagonist. With a **reversible** or **competitive antagonist**, the curve is shifted to the right, and the agonist EC50 is increased. The maximum effect is not reduced but requires a higher agonist dose. (Very high doses may have nonspecific toxic effects, however.) The dissociation constant (**K_I**) of the antagonist can be determined from the Schild equation:

$$C' / C = 1 + (I / K_I)$$

where C and C^1 are the agonist concentrations required to produce the same response in the absence (C) and presence (C^1) of a fixed concentration (I) of antagonist. K_I values determined in this way agree with those from radioligand binding of competitive antagonists.

With a **noncompetitive** or **irreversible antagonist**, the agonist maximum effect is reduced, although the agonist EC50 may not be changed. Antagonists may be irreversible because they have very high receptor affinity or because they form covalent bonds to the receptor. Phenoxybenzamine is an example of an irreversible alpha-adrenoceptor antagonist.

In some cases, the agonist dose-response curve in the presence of low concentrations of an irreversible antagonist remembles the curve in the presence of a competitive antagonist, i.e., the curve is shifted to the right, with no change in Emax. This phenomenon indicates the presence of "spare" receptors. **Spare receptors** are present if the maximum response can be elicited by an agonist concentration that does not occupy the maximum number of receptors (in this case, a portion of receptors are irreversibly bound by the noncompetitive antagonist).

In cells with spare receptors, loss of receptors may be associated only with a right shift of the dose-response curve, without a change in Emax, i.e., similar to the effect of a competitive antagonist. In contrast, in cells with no spare receptors, receptor loss will be accompanied by a decrease in the maximum response, i.e., similar to the effect of a noncompetitive antagonist. The latter situation has been described with reference to beta-adrenergic receptors and responses in human heart failure [12].

Alterations of the agonist dose-response curve analagous to those seen with competitive and noncompetitive antagonists and with partial agonists are seen in a variety of physiologically-relevant circumstances, such as during development (see refs in [6]) or in disease (see [12]). Analysis of dose-response curves may therefore provide the focus for subsequent investigation.

SUMMARY

This chapter reviews the methodology for measurement of pharmacological effects in isolated myocytes. Cultured or non-cultured cells can be used to investigate the nature and mechanisms of myocyte responses to extracellular stimuli, as revealed through the analysis of dose-response curves. Sussessful experiments require characterization of the cells, precautions with the pharacological agents used, and different types of experimental protocols.

REFERENCES

1. P. Simpson, N.H. Bishopric, S. Coughlin, J. Karliner, C. Ordahl, N. Starksen, T. Tsao, N. White, L. Williams, J Mol Cell Cardiol 18 (Suppl 5):45-58 (1986).
2. T.K. Borg, K. Rubin, E. Lundgren, K. Borg, B. Obrink, Develop Biol 104:86-96 (1984).
3. P. Simpson, A. McGrath S. Savion, Circ Res 51:787-801 (1982).
4. S.L. Jacobson, H.M. Piper, J Mol Cell Cardiol 18:661-678 (1986).
5. A.F. Cutiletta, A. Marie-Claude, A. Nag, R. Zak, J Mol Cell Cardiol 9:399-407 (1977).
6. P. Simpson, S. Savion, Circ Res 50:101-116 (1982).
7. P. Simpson, J Clin Invest 72:732-738 (1983).
8. P. Simpson, Circ Res 56:884-894 (1985).
9. H.R. Bourne, J.M. Roberts in: Basic and Clinical Pharmacology, Third edition, B.G. Katzung, ed. (Appleton & Lange, Norwolk, Connecticul, 1987) pp. 9-22.
10. G.W. Snedecor, W.G. Cochran, Statistical Methods, Sixth Edition (The Iowa State University Press, Ames 1967) pp. 32-65.
11. N.H. Bishopric, P.C. Simpson, C.P Ordahl, J Clin Invest 80:1194-1199 (1987).
12. M.R. Bristow, N.E. Kantrowitz, R. Ginsburg, M.B. Fowler, J Mol Cell Cardiol 17 (Suppl 2):41-52 (1986).

MEASUREMENT OF SARCOLEMMAL PERMEABILITY AND INTRACELLULAR pH, FREE MAGNESIUM, AND HIGH ENERGY PHOSPHATES OF ISOLATED HEART CELLS.

Beatrice A. Wittenberg, Jeannette E. Doeller, Raj K. Gupta, and Roy L. White.
Albert Einstein College of Medicine, 1300 Morris Park Avenue, Bronx, N.Y. 10461

The dissociation of adult rat heart into functionally intact, calcium tolerant heart cells in high yields requires that individual cells be freed not only from the extracellular connective tissue framework and blood capillaries but also from neighboring cells which are attached by junctional and non-junctional connections. Many current successful preparations use a Langendorff retrograde perfusion of the heart with collagenase enzyme mixture in a low calcium, well buffered and oxygenated minimal essential medium (MEM).

The decreased calcium concentration is required to loosen cell-to-cell connections [1]. However during the low calcium collagenase perfusion sarcolemmal alterations occur which may induce "leakiness" and calcium overload. These sarcolemmal perturbations must be "healed" by cautiously increasing calcium levels after the "hyper-permeable" period. We have shown [2] that varying the calcium concentration over a narrow range during the collagenase perfusion profoundly affects maintenance of cell-to-cell connections of the isolated cardiac myocyte. Here we describe a procedure currently used in our laboratory to give a high yield of cells with good high energy phosphate levels. We find that the most crucial step in the procedure is the perfusion. This must effectively maintain short diffusion distances for both oxygen and calcium. We describe the intracellular retention of fluorescent dye, the most sensitive assay we have devised to determine the adequacy of the perfusion step.

We also describe the following methods for the measurement of intracellular pH, free magnesium, and high energy phosphate levels:
1) optical absorption spectroscopy which permits simultaneous measurement of intracellular pH reported by 6-carboxyfluorescein and intracellular oxygen levels detected by intracellular myoglobin and cytochromes;
2) ^{31}P NMR which permits simultaneous measurement of intracellular pH, intracellular Mg^{++}, and intracellular ATP and phosphocreatine levels; and
3) ion-specific intracellular electrodes which permit pH measurement in individual cells, so that single cell measurements can be correlated both with electrophysiological measurements and with pH measurements in populations of cells.

I. Preparation of Isolated Heart Cells

Heart cells are prepared by a modification of the procedure of Wittenberg et al., [2,3]. The procedure consists of 3 main steps each using solutions which are supplements of modified commercial MEM Eagle Joklik (K.C. Biological, DMC317). Specific modifications of this commercially prepared medium from the standard MEM are: phosphate is reduced, HEPES buffer replaces most of the bicarbonate, and K^+ is added only as KCl.

1) HEPES-MEM medium is made from K.C. Biological DMC317 which contains: NaCl, 117 mM; KCl, 5.7 mM; $NaHCO_3$, 4.4 mM; Na_2PO_4, 1.5 mM; $MgCl_2$, 1.7 mM; HEPES, 21.1 mM; glucose, 11.7 mM; amino acids and vitamins. We add L-glutamine, 2 mM; taurine, 10 mM; and $CaCl_2$, 10 uM to the commercially prepared medium; pH is adjusted to 7.2 with NaOH. This solution is 285 milliosmolar, and the free calcium activity is 10 uM.

2) HEPES-incubation medium contains: HEPES-MEM supplemented with 0.5 mM calcium chloride and 0.5% dialyzed bovine serum albumin (BSA, Fraction V; see [3]).

Biology of Isolated Adult Cardiac Myocytes
William A. Clark, Robert S. Decker, and Thomas K. Borg, Editors

A. Low Calcium Perfusion

1) Blood Washout. Adult male Wistar rats (350-450 grams) are heparinized and decapitated. The heart is removed rapidly and retrograde perfusion is begun at 32°C with HEPES-MEM gassed with 85% O_2, 15% N_2 and maintained at a fixed perfusion flow rate of 7 ml/min.

In this nominally calcium-free medium the heart beat stops, but beating can be maintained if 1.0 to 1.5 mM calcium chloride is added to the perfusion medium. Blood and calcium washout is complete after 10 ml of HEPES-MEM is perfused through the heart. This fluid is discarded and the heart is enclosed in a water-jacketed chamber of about 100 ml capacity at 32°C.

2) Enzyme Perfusion. Thirty ml of freshly oxygenated HEPES-MEM containing 0.1% collagenase (Worthington Type II) is then recirculated through the heart for 25 minutes at 7 ml/min. Final collagenase activity is near 0.1%, about 150 units/ml, trypsin activity 1-3 units/ml (manufacturer's assay). At the end of perfusion the heart is intact but enlarged, soft and friable. The color is homogeneous and blood vessels are clear of erythrocytes. We find that the cells are more hyper-permeable measured by 6-carboxyfluorescein retention (see below), if the perfusion is suboptimal. Any significant increase in calcium activity during the perfusion suggests excessive cell breakdown or insufficient calcium washout. If the calcium activity in the perfusate at the end of the perfusion exceeds the starting level by more than 5 uM, it is best to start over. The heart is removed from the perfusion apparatus, the ventricles are cut into 8-10 chunks with scissors, and placed in incubation medium which contains 0.5 mM calcium chloride.

B. Mechanical Tissue Dissociation

The tissue chunks are incubated in HEPES-incubation medium containing 0.5 mM calcium chloride and fresh collagenase in 50 ml Erlenmeyer flasks open to room air for 10 minutes at 32°C with stirring by a wrist action shaker. The purpose of the incubation step is to liberate cells from the tissue matrix. Collagenase is added to the HEPES-incubation medium to a final concentration near 0.1%. After 10 minutes, the supernatant cell suspension is removed from the minced tissue. The cells are collected and washed three times with 10 ml portions of HEPES-incubation medium by low speed centrifugation (34xg) at room temperature. The incubations are repeated 1-2 times until the remaining ventricular fragments are totally digested. The cells are then resuspended in HEPES-incubation medium (1.0 - 1.5 x 10^6 cells per ml) containing 0.5 to 1.0 mM calcium chloride.

C. Separation of Intact Cells

Isosmotic Percoll (Pharmacia Fine Chemicals, Uppsala, Sweden; 270 milli-osmolar) is prepared by the addition of one volume of 9.0% NaCl to 10 volumes of Percoll. The pH is adjusted to 7.2, and BSA is added to a final concentration of 0.5% W/V. Cells are suspended in isotonic Percoll diluted with HEPES-incubation medium to a final concentration of 0.1-0.15 x 10^6 cells/ml and 37% Percoll. Ten ml portions of the Percoll cell suspension in Corex centrifuge tubes (length 120 mm, ID= 15 mm) are centrifuged for 5 min at room temperature at 34xg. Intact rectangular cells sediment to the bottom of the tube. Damaged and rounded cells form a distinct layer at the surface. The intact cell pellet is washed twice in HEPES-incubation medium to remove Percoll and dispersed in HEPES-incubation at a concentration of 0.5-1.0 x 10^6 cells per ml. Cells are stored at 30°C in erlenmeyer flasks or culture dishes in HEPES-incubation medium containing 1 mM calcium chloride.

Table I. Characteristics of Heart Cell Preparation after Percoll Purification

YIELD (per heart) cells	protein (mg)	RECTANGULAR CELLS (%)	ATP	PHOSPHOCREATINE
			(nmol/mg cell protein*)	
$10.8^{+}2 \times 10^6$	45.4± 9.0	85±2	29.3±6.3	43.0±14.7

all values are average ± standard deviation n=10
* rectangular cell protein

II. Assessment of Sarcolemmal Permeability with 6-Carboxyfluorescein

The isolation of heart cells from whole, perfused heart requires lowering the calcium concentration in the perfusate. After the calcium and blood have been washed out of the coronary circulation and heart chambers, collagenase is added to the perfusate. After about 25 minutes of perfusion with low calcium collagenase solution, the calcium concentration is raised by incubating the heart tissue in medium containing collagenase with 0.5 mM calcium chloride. This procedure seems to induce a period of hyper-permeability of the heart cell sarcolemma, which occurs during the low calcium collagenase perfusion but before incubation in medium containing millimolar concentrations of calcium chloride.

The magnitude of sarcolemmal hyper-permeability can be easily defined by adding 0.1% 6-carboxyfluorescein during the collagenase perfusion step. Subsequent washes after incubation remove the extracellular dye, leaving only that dye which is trapped in the sarcoplasm of the cells during the re-establishment of normal sarcolemmal permeability. We use fluorescence microscopy to examine the cells after centrifugation through Percoll and subsequent resuspension. We take a 100 ul aliquot of resuspended cells at a concentration of 0.01 x 10^6 cell/ml and disperse them in 1 ml of resuspension medium in a modified tissue culture dish. We fabricate this dish by using a soldering iron to melt a 1 x 1 cm cut out in the bottom of a 35 mm #3002 Falcon tissue culture dish (Becton Dickinson Co., Lincoln Park, NJ). We cut this hole from the inside of the dish while firmly holding the dish right-side up on a heat-proof surface. We then glue a standard #1.5 18 x 18 mm cover slip to the outside bottom of the dish, forming a small well in the dish whose capacity is about 1 ml. We regularly use hot melt glue (Sears catalog #9-80537) as the adhesive to hold the cover slip on and form a water tight seal.

We examine the cells using epi-fluorescence on a Nikon Diaphot microscope with a "B" filter block (excitation peak about 465 nm, emission at 510 nm). We use a 150 W halogen source for the epi-illuminator, 10x fluorite objectives (N.A. = 0.75), and a 35 mm Nikon FG camera with Tri-X film (ASA 400) to record the data. We use a 1 second exposure as our standard. Film is developed for a standard period of time in Microdol.

The degree of dye loading can be judged by eye or for more quantitative studies, a densitometer can be used on the negatives. To control for auto-fluorescence, a sample of cells isolated without dye is examined and photographed at the same settings and exposure. We also regularly take a non-fluorescent light micrograph in the same field to mark the position, sarcomere length, and general viability of the cells. (See Fig. 1 and Fig 2.)

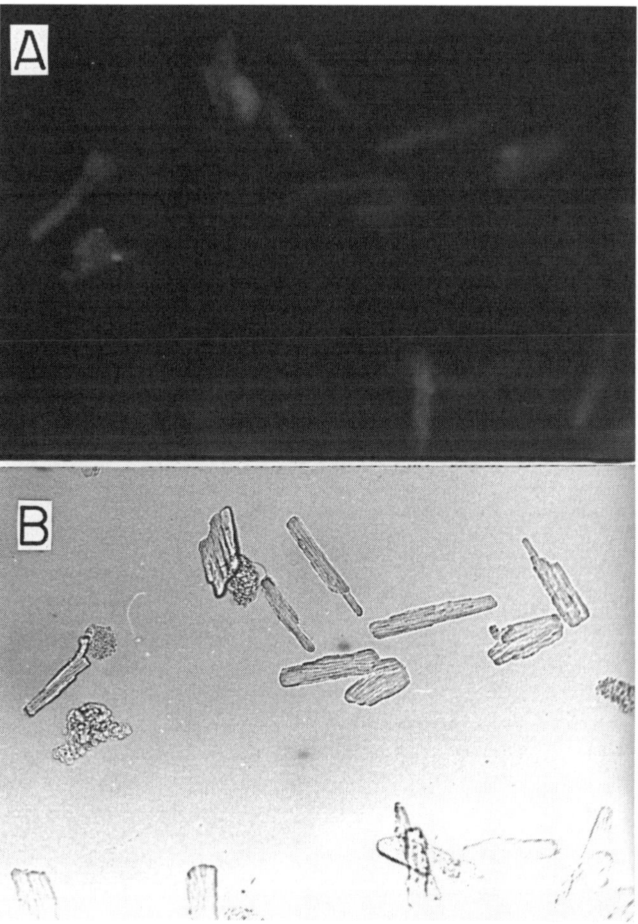

Figure 1. Photomicrograph of well prepared myocytes taken with epi-fluorescence illumination (1A) compared with a photomicrograph of the identical field taken with bright field illumination (1B). 6-Carboxyfluorescein was introduced during the collagenase perfusion. Round and rectangular cells observed in the light micrograph are very faint in the fluorescence micrograph. 19 rectangular cells and 5 round cells are observed in the light micrograph. In the fluorescence micrograph only 14 rectangular cells and 3 round cells are visible.

When 6-carboxyfluorescein is added to the collagenase perfusion during the heart cell preparation, fluorescent labelling is observed in rectangular, clearly striated cells with resting potentials near -50 to -80 mV. After a good perfusion, most rectangular cells are visibly glowing faintly (or not at all) compared to autofluorescence (see Fig. 1A). Figure 1B shows the same field taken with bright field illumination. Figure 2 shows heart cells prepared in the same way except that it took significantly longer to complete the blood washout after decapitation. The rectangular cells are visibly more labelled than in Figure 1. Most round cells have lost their dye and are almost invisible in the fluorescence micrograph. We conclude that brightly labelled cells are those which were either more permeable or permeable for a longer period of time during perfusion than less brightly labeled cells.

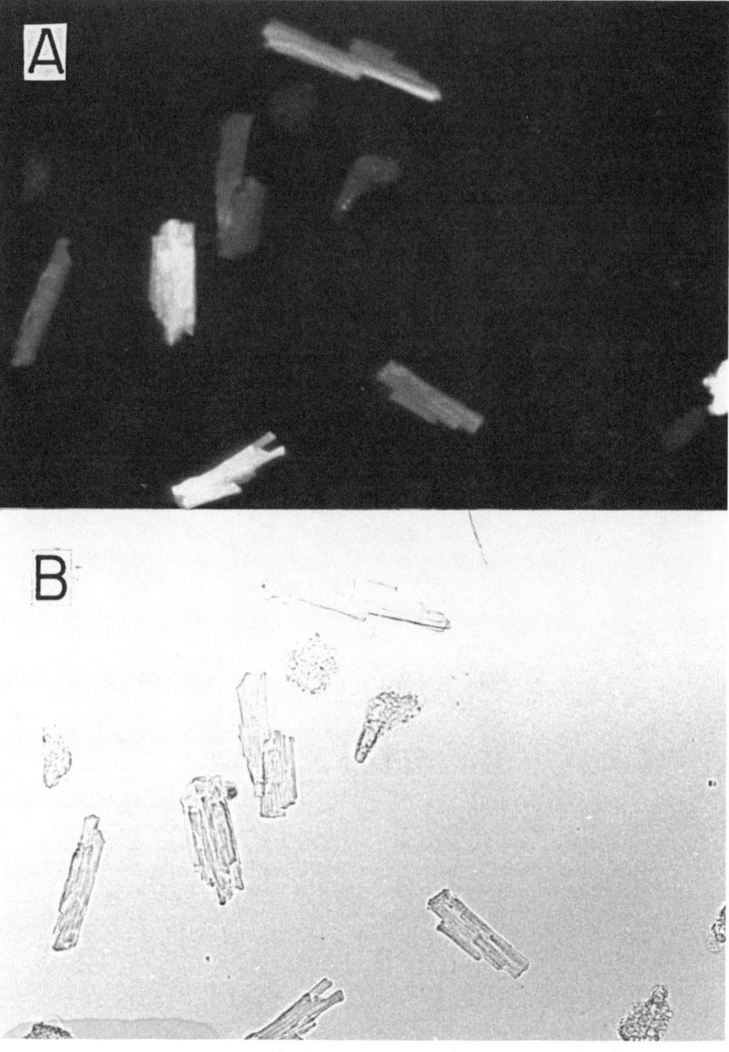

Figure 2. Photomicrograph as in Figure 1 but of heart cells prepared with a long delay between decapitation and beginning of the collagenase perfusion. 6-Carboxyfluorescein was introduced during the collagenase perfusion. Round cells are faint in the fluorescence micrograph, but rectangular cells are much more fluorescent (compared with Fig. 1) demonstrating greater dye uptake and retention. All rectangular cells (6 single and 1 pair) observed in the light micrograph are clearly visible in the fluorescence micrograph.

In order to retain dye when calcium is readmitted in the extracellular medium, the rectangular cells must "heal" or they will lose dye and also become hyper-contracted in response to elevated intracellular calcium. The period when heart cells are permeable to dye and presumably to other low molecular weight molecules is thus rigorously defined. During this period, calcium concentrations in the extracellular medium must be kept to a minimum to avoid calcium overload and irreversible contracture of the cells. On the other hand, it is possible to introduce other low molecular weight compounds including 6-carboxyfluorescein into the sarcoplasm during this period of limited, reversible hyper-permeability. Both brightly labelled and unlabelled rectangular cells demonstrate clear cross-striations, 1.9 um resting sarcomere length, resting potentials of up to -80 mV and active membrane currents for at least 24 hours after preparation.

III. Measurement of Intracellular pH with Intracellular 6-Carboxyfluorescein

We find that the absorption spectrum of intracellular 6-carboxyfluorescein may be used to monitor intracellular pH in populations of stirred cardiac myocytes. The cells may be loaded with 6-carboxyfluorescein during the hyper-permeable period of collagenase perfusion as described above. Alternatively, isolated heart cells may be loaded more reproducibly by incubation with 6-carboxyfluorescein diacetate for 30 minutes at 30°C. After removal of extracellular dye, the visible absorption spectrum of a stirred suspension of dye labelled cells is recorded from 650 nm to 350 nm with a Cary 14 spectrophotometer equipped with a scattered transmission accessory and interfaced to an Aviv Data Acquisition system.

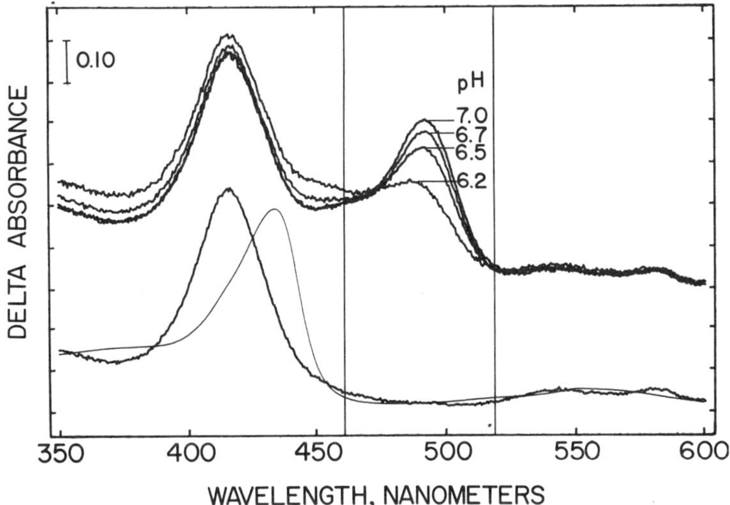

Figure 3. The absorption spectra of oxygenated isolated heart cells with 6-carboxyfluorescein at pH values from 7.0 to 6.2 (upper traces) and oxygenated heart cells without dye (lower dark trace). The heart cell spectrum is dominated by intracellular myoglobin which becomes deoxygenated below 0.2 torr PO_2. The absorption spectrum of deoxygenated myoglobin adjusted to heart cell myoglobin concentration is shown in the lower light trace. Vertical lines delineate the pH sensitive spectrum of 6-carboxyfluorescein in the window of minimal absorption by the heart cells in any state of oxygenation. Intracellular 6-carboxyfluorescein concentration is 500 uM, calculated from the extinction coefficient determined separately, and with a value of 3 ul intracellular water per mg protein.

A suitable dilution of whole milk is used as a light scattering reference for the cell suspension. The milk is diluted with distilled water to adjust the optical density at 650 nm to that of the cell suspension at the same wavelength. The heart cell spectrum is dominated by intracellular hemeproteins and in particular myoglobin [4]. However the myocyte spectrum is fortuitously unfeatured and low in absorbance in the pH-sensitive region of the 6-carboxyfluorescein spectrum from 460 nm to 510 nm (Fig. 3; bottom trace). In the presence of heart cells, the 6-carboxyfluorescein absorption spectrum is sensitive to pH, with an isosbestic point near 465 nm and a pH-dependent maximum near 490 nm (Fig. 3). The ratio of absorbances at 490 nm and 465 nm has a dye concentration independent relationship to pH [5].

To prepare a standard curve, the spectrum of intracellular 6-carboxyfluorescein is obtained from the spectrum of a labelled heart cell suspension in the presence of nigericin (a proton ionophore) after subtraction of a spectrum of the unlabelled heart cells. The peak and isosbestic wavelengths of intracellular 6-carboxyfluorescein are shifted slightly to 495 and 470 nm, respectively (Fig. 4). The ratio of absorbances at 495 nm and 470 nm is plotted as a function of pH. To measure intracellular pH, the spectrum of intracellular 6-carboxyfluorescein is recorded without nigericin (Fig. 4), and the ratio of absorbances at 495 and 470 is referred to the standard curve. The intracellular pH measured with this method in a population of aerated, well stirred heart cells was 7.1. Figure 4 shows that the pH of the intracellular environment is distinctly lower than the pH 7.2 of the standard extracellular medium.

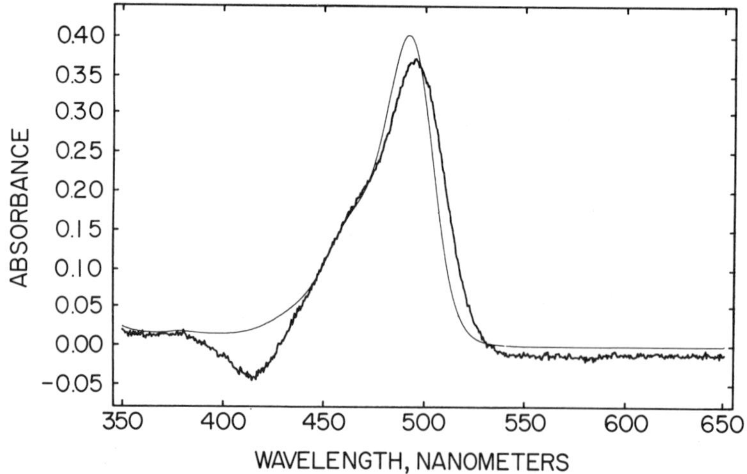

Figure 4. The absorption spectrum of intracellular 6-carboxyfluorescein (dark trace) compared to the spectrum of extracellular 6-carboxyfluorescein adjusted to the same concentration in MEM pH 7.2 (light trace). The spectrum of intracellular 6-carboxyfluorescein is obtained by subtracting the spectrum of unlabelled heart cells from the spectrum of dye-loaded heart cells (see Fig. 3.). The peak wavelength is shifted from 490 nm for dye in MEM to 495 nm for 6-carboxyfluorescein in the intracellular environment. Intracellular pH is 7.1, determined from the ratio of absorption at the peak and isobestic wavelengths (after baseline subtraction), compared to a standard curve obtained with intracellular 6-carboxyfluorescein and nigericin [5].

IV. Measurement of Intracellular pH, ATP, and Phosphocreatine with ^{31}P NMR

We have developed a method for the oxygenation of heart cells by superfusion in a 10 or 16 mm diameter sample tube in the Varian XL-200 multinuclear NMR spectrometer. This method is readily adaptable to other commercial instruments and requires no modifications of the probe or other hardware. The myocyte suspension (6×10^6 cells) is injected into the fiber bores of an 8 or 14 mm diameter bundle of hollow polyamide fibers (Gambro, G.F. 80.m) of 35 mm length. The fiber bundle is sealed at both ends and inserted into the 10 or 16 mm NMR tube which contains superfusion medium and is fitted with inlet and outlet tubes from the perfusion pump. Perfusion with well-oxygenated medium at 10 ml/min is begun immediately. We have demonstrated rapid exchange of substrates across the fiber walls by measuring an equilibrium time of 5 minutes for the Na^+ shift reagent dysprosium tripolyphosphate [6]. The ^{31}P NMR spectrum of a suspension of cells superfused with oxygenated (95% O_2, 5% CO_2) HEPES-incubation medium (without BSA) is shown in Figure 5.

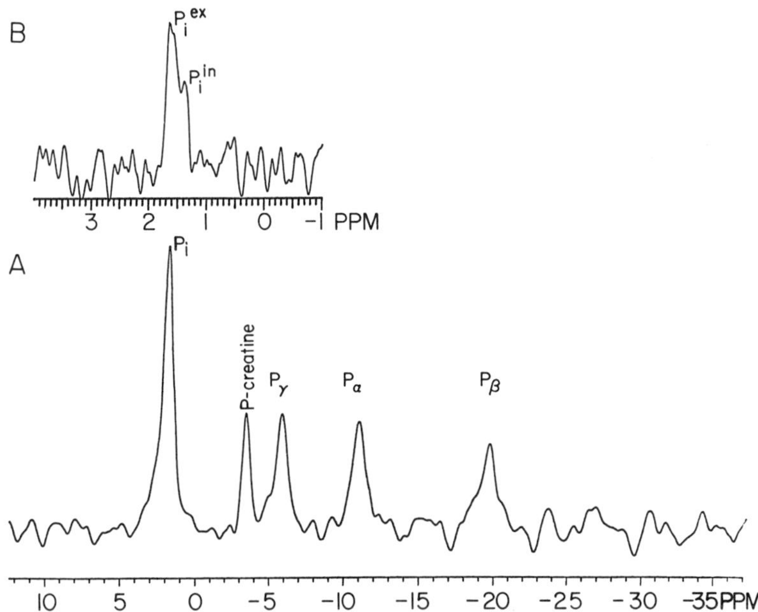

Figure 5A. ^{31}P *NMR spectrum of cardiac myocytes superfused with medium equilibrated with 95%* O_2*, 5%* CO_2 *obtained in 60 minutes on a Varian XL 200 at 81 MHz. The spectrum was stable for at least 6 hours. The inorganic phosphate (*P_i*) peak, phosphocreatine peak and alpha P, beta P, and gamma P phosphate peaks of ATP are clearly identifiable.*

5B. Expanded region of the spectrum showing clearly resolved intracellular and extracellular P_i *resonances. Convolution difference was used to enhance the resolution.*

The myocyte ATP level, 30 nmol/mg protein, and phosphocreatine level, 40 nmol/mg protein, both measured on a separate aliquot by HPLC analysis [7], remained stable in the NMR spectrometer under these conditions for more than 6 hours. The relative concentrations of ATP and phosphocreatine can be measured from the areas under their respective peaks. It is essential to obtain fully relaxed NMR spectra for accurate quantitation. Rapid pulsing which is often used to optimize the signal to noise ratio results in a relaxation time-dependent distortion of resonance intensity. The spectrum in Figure 5 was obtained with a pulse recycle time of 0.8 sec and is thus not fully relaxed. Using the relaxation time for ATP (1 sec) and phosphocreatine resonances (3 sec) we estimate, from the relative areas under the peaks in Figure 5B, a phosphocreatine to ATP ratio of about 1.25. A determination of absolute concentrations requires a knowledge of the fraction of NMR sensitive volume occupied by the cells. This can be obtained by comparing the areas under the dysprosium tripolyphosphate shifted extracellular Na^+ resonance and the resonance of the medium in a fiber bundle identical to that used with the cells. We use that medium with which the cells have been in contact for measurement of extracellular volume to insure the necessary equilibration of cells with medium.

The intracellular pH is measured using the chemical shift of intracellular inorganic phosphate (P_i) resonance relative to that of phosphocreatine [8,9]. We have found it necessary to use the technique of convolution difference to separate overlapped intracellular and extracellular P_i resonances. Figure 5B demonstrates the resolution of intracellular and extracellular P_i resonances in the isolated heart cell spectrum which makes this measurement possible. In the sample shown, intracellular pH was calculated to be 7.1.

V. Measurement of Intracellular Free Magnesium with ^{31}P NMR

The free magnesium in heart cells may be of physiological importance because magnesium is bound to ATP and ADP, and because magnesium and calcium may compete for intracellular binding sites. Intracellular calcium equilibria depend on intracellular magnesium.

We used ^{31}P NMR to determine the fraction of ATP complexed to magnesium and the cytosolic free magnesium in freshly isolated cardiac myocytes [10]. The ^{31}P NMR technique for measuring free magnesium is based upon an accurate measurement of the frequency difference between the alpha P and beta P resonances in the ^{31}P NMR spectrum of intracellular ATP (Fig.5). Because the positions of the ^{31}P resonances of ATP depend on its state of complexation with magnesium (the predominant divalent cation component of the cell), the NMR spectrum allows a direct determination of the fraction of total ATP that exists as the magnesium complex. An accurate knowledge of the dissociation constant of MgATP (K_D^{MgATP}) under simulated intracellular ionic conditions then yields free magnesium directly from the NMR spectral data [10,11].

The myocyte suspension was superfused continuously at room temperature as described above. The chemical shift difference between the alpha P and beta P resonances of cellular ATP was 707 $\pm$ 3 Hz at 81 MHz, corresponding to magnesium-complexation of 89% of the total myocyte ATP. Using a MgATP dissociation constant of 60 uM at pH 7.1 and 22°C, we estimate the cytosolic free magnesium to be 0.5 mM. The free magnesium did not change during a 2 hour period of hypoxia, achieved by superfusion with medium gassed with nitrogen, although ATP and phosphocreatine levels were reversibly diminished to 60% and 15%, respectively, of the aerobic values. The NMR-measured low level of free magnesium in isolated cardiac myocytes is in good agreement with the value of 0.4 mM recently obtained using ion-selective microelectrodes in cardiac ventricular muscle [12].

VI. Ion-selective electrodes

We make ion-selective electrodes by silanizing single or double-barrel glass capillary tubing after pulling to the desired tip configuration with a Kopf electrode puller. We use a 3-5% solution of trimethylchlorosilane (TMCS) in ultrapure CCl_4 for silanization. This solution is placed in the tip of the electrode by backfilling with a (glass!) syringe and 28 gauge needle. For single-barrel electrodes, a very small amount is necessary. For double-barrel electrodes, one barrel is marked and an portion of TMCS solution sufficient to fill the tip of the electrode to the shank is added to the marked barrel. The other barrel is filled to the 1/3 point with water to prevent silanization of that barrel. The electrodes are then baked at 150°C in a vacuum oven (at 24" Hg of vacuum) for 30 minutes to evaporate the CCl_4 and excess TMCS.

We have found it absolutely essential to keep the vacuum oven scrupulously clean to prevent deposition of contaminants on the electrodes. Ovens which are (or were) used to dry histological preparations are particularly bad. We devote an oven exclusively to ion-selective electrode production and invoke the threat of capital punishment on those who would use it otherwise.

After baking we store the electrodes in a dessicator overnight before filling with liquid ion exchanger (LIX). We fill the tip of the silanized electrodes with LIX to the shank, using another glass syringe and 28 gauge needle. An aliquot of resin is aspirated into the needle and forced into the tip. A cat whisker (vibrissae) or a glass fiber from a fiber optic guide which has been cleaned with NaOH is used to tease the LIX to the tip. Gentle heating under a light also facilitates filling.

We back fill the ion-selective electrode or barrel with a solution consisting of 100 mM citrate buffer (pH 6) in a solution of 100 mM NaCl. A silver wire plated with silver chloride completes the electrical connection to the electrode. We seal the back of the electrode with wax. In the case of double-barrel electrodes, we fill the other (voltage recording) barrel with 150 mM KCl. It is essential to break back one of the barrels with forceps so that the barrels are staggered at the back of the electrode. This prevents coupling between the barrels, the most common cause of failure in double-barrel electrodes. Another way to reduce cross coupling is to not back fill the electrodes excessively since inserting the silver wires will displace some of the solution and potentially cause a salt bridge between the barrels. Sealing with wax is essential with these electrodes.

After sealing, we bevel the electrodes on a Sutter electrode beveler. We bevel double-barrel electrodes while monitoring the resistance of the voltage recording barrel. The bevelling of single-barrel ion-selective electrodes can only be done by "feel" and experience, since the resistance is too high to monitor reliably.

The voltage signal from an intracellular ion-selective electrode is the sum of:
1) the potential developed due to the interactions of ions with the LIX;
2) the membrane potential of the cell;
3) any potentials developed in the electrode due to liquid-liquid or liquid-metal junction potentials; and
4) the electrode tip potential.

Tip potentials and junction potentials are constant and factored out during calibration. The cell membrane potential is subtracted from the ion-selective electrode voltage potential by recording differentially between the ion-selective electrode and the voltage recording electrode impaled in the same cell (Fig. 6A and 6B).

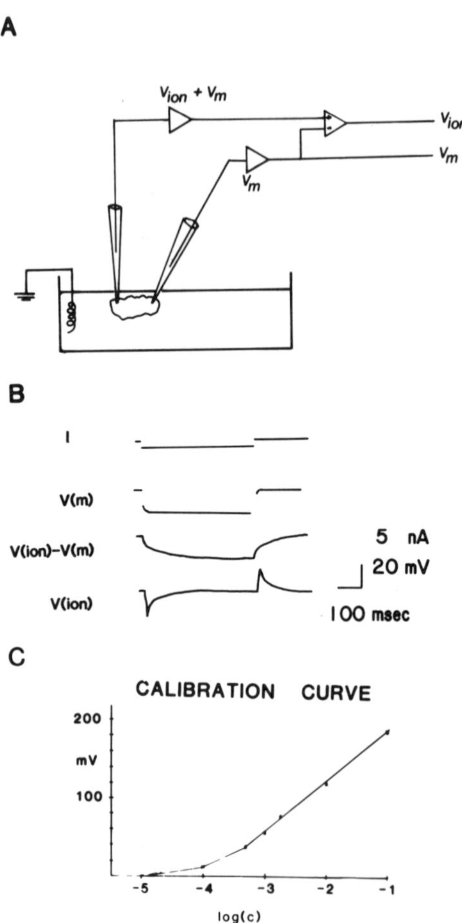

Figure 6A. *Diagram of the electrical connections for recording ionic activities from cells using ion-selective microelectrodes.* V_{ion} *is the difference signal between the ion-selective microelectrode and a (in this case separate) voltage recording microelectrode.*

6B. Illustration of typical records from the apparatus shown above. The top trace is current injected into the cell from a third microelectrode (not shown above). The second trace is the cell membrane potential recorded by the voltage microelectrode. The third trace is the summed potential from the ion-selective electrode, while the bottom trace is the difference signal.

6C. Illustration of a typical calibration curve from an K^+ *ion-selective electrode. The response to increasing* K^+ *concentration was Nernstian (57 mV/decade concentration change) over the range of about 100 uM to 100 mM.*

We calibrate pH microelectrodes with buffered solutions of physiological saline at different pH (usually near pH 6.0 and 7.0). Potassium or sodium selective electrodes are calibrated by constructing standard curves using decade steps of KCl or NaCl from 10 uM to 100 mM. Sodium calibration solutions are made with a constant ionic background concentration of 150 mM by KCl substitution (Fig. 6C).

VII. Summary

We have described the preparation in good yield and the purification of cardiac myocytes dissociated from adult rat heart. We estimate that about 50% of the ventricular cells are recovered. High energy phosphate levels are comparable to those measured in whole heart.

During the isolation procedure, heart cells must be torn from their neighbors. We report that heart cells become transiently permeable to 6-carboxy-fluorescein during the collagenase perfusion.

We describe several methods for monitoring the levels of intracellular H^+, free magnesium, ATP, and phosphocreatine in physiologically intact cells. It is now possible to measure simultaneously: intracellular oxygen, reported by absorption spectra of intracellular components, and intracellular pH reported by 6-carboxyfluorescein; pH, magnesium and high energy phosphate levels using NMR; and measurements of pH, K^+,and Na^+ using LIX ion-selective microelectrodes.

REFERENCES

1. Muir, A., J. Anat. 101, 239-261 (1967).

2. Wittenberg, B.A., White, R.L., Ginzberg, R.D., and Spray, D.C. Circ. Res. 59, 143-150 (1986).

3. Wittenberg, B.A. and Robinson, T.F. Cell Tissue Res. 216, 231-251 (1981).

4. Wittenberg, B.A. and Wittenberg, J.B. J. Biol. Chem. 260 6548-6554 (1985).

5. Thomas, J.A., Kalbeck, P.C., and Langworthy, T.A. in: Intracellular pH: Its measurement, regulation and utilization in cellular function. eds. Nuccitelli, R. and Deamer, D. W. (Alan R. Liss, Inc. NY 1982) pp. 105-123.

6. Gupta, R.K. and Gupta, P., J. Magn. Reson. 47, 344-350 (1982).

7. Harmsen, E., DeTombe, P, Ph., and DeJong, J.W. J. Chromat. 230, 131-136 (1982).

8. Moore, R.D. and Gupta, R.K. Int. J. Quant. Chem. Quant. Biol. Symp. 7, 83-92 (1980).

9. Avison, M.J., Hetherington, H.P., and Shulman, R.G. Ann. Rev. Biophys. Biophys.Chem. 15, 377-402 (1986).

10. Gupta, R.K., Wittenberg, B.A., J. Mol. Cell. Cardiol. 19 supp. IV, S 51 (1987).

11. Gupta,R.K. and Yushok, W.D., Proc. Natl. Acad. Sci. 77, 2487-2491 (1980).

12. Blatter, L.A., and McGuigan, J.A.S., Quart. J. Exp. Physiol. 71 467-473 (1986).

EVALUATION OF RATES OF PROTEIN SYNTHESIS AND DEGRADATION IN ISOLATED CARDIAC MUSCLE CELLS

WILLIAM A. CLARK,* and ALLEN M. SAMAREL**
*Cardiovascular Institute, Michael Reese Hospital and Medical Center, and The University of Chicago, Chicago, IL 60616;
**Northwestern University Medical School, Chicago, IL 60611

INTRODUCTION

All intracellular proteins undergo a continual balanced process of synthesis and breakdown. Processes of growth, atrophy, hypertrophy, remodeling, or differentiation, each involve a shift in the balance between protein synthesis and degradation. Even in apparently normal, stable adult cells which are not undergoing any change, there is a rapid process of protein replacement or turnover that involves an intimate balance between protein synthesis and degradation. It is well recognized that the ultimate regulation of protein synthesis occurs at the level of gene transcription. The availability of mRNA transcripts controls the *type* of protein translated in the cell. In some cases the availability of specific mRNA transcripts also correlates with the rate of synthesis of specific cardiac proteins [1]. However, when viewed from the level of total protein synthesis rates, it appears that it is not mRNA availability which limits the rates of protein synthesis, but rather the availability of ribosomal subunits [2]. Thus, the regulation of specific protein synthesis in an environment not limited by mRNA availability must involve additional regulatory factors such as compartmentation and turnover of mRNA, and rates of chain initiation and elongation [3,4]. As part of an understanding of the total regulation of protein balance in the cell, direct measurement of rates of protein synthesis and degradation may often be necessary.

The basis for most studies on the synthesis and decay of proteins involves the use of radiolabeled amino acids which are incorporated into proteins during synthesis and released from proteins during degradation. A number of significant reviews have described in detail both the theory and practical limitations of this approach [3,5-8]. Most of the complexity involved with use of tracer amino acids derives from significant compartmentation and metabolism of amino acids which influences the manner in which they participate in protein synthesis. Specifically, use of tracer amino acids requires defining the relationship between the appearance (or disappearance) of labeled amino acids in the protein and the underlying process of protein synthesis and decay. The objective of the present review is to discuss how these considerations may be applied in assessing rates of protein synthesis and degradation in isolated cells, with particular reference to the isolated cardiac myocyte in culture.

Proteins are synthesized and replaced in either of two environments: 1) there is no change in the amount of protein, and 2) the amount of protein increases or decreases. While the first case, called the "steady-state", is rarely encountered in cultured myocytes, it will be discussed briefly since it removes a major complexity from the analysis. That is, if there is no net gain or loss of protein then the amount of protein synthesized per unit time must equal the amount removed by protein degradation. Thus, the situation can be fully defined by measuring a single parameter, the fractional synthesis rate, k_s. In the second case, the "nonsteady-state", synthesis and degradation must be treated as

Biology of Isolated Adult Cardiac Myocytes
William A. Clark, Robert S. Decker, and Thomas K. Borg, Editors

independent parameters whose magnitude reflects whether there is net growth or loss in the system[1].

$$k_g = k_s - k_d \quad (1)$$

Equation 1 expresses this relationship in terms of instantaneous fractional rates of growth (g, rate of accumulation or loss), synthesis (s), and decay (d). However, this relation is derived from analysis of a specific pool where a defined quantity of protein is synthesized per unit time, R_s, and reduced to a fractional rate by normalization to the total amount of protein in the pool, P. k_s is thus interchangeable with R_s/P.

The first section of this chapter will deal with problems and techniques for assessing k_s in cultured myocytes, and the second part will address the issue of degradation.

PROTEIN SYNTHESIS IN ISOLATED CELLS IN CULTURE

Evaluation of the fractional rate of protein synthesis during short term pulse labeling in culture essentially depends on solution of the following equation:[2]

$$k_s = \frac{P^*(t_2) - P^*(t_1)}{\int_{t_1}^{t_2} F^*(t)dt - \int_{t_1}^{t_2} P^*(t)dt} \quad (2)$$

where F^* is the specific radioactivity of amino acid in the medium[3] and P^* is the specific radioactivity of amino acid in the protein. While this equation is representative of the general situation in either the steady state or a state of net growth, specific adjustments are possible in culture which make its solution simpler. First, if a single short pulse labeling time is used ($t_1=0$; $t_2=1\text{-}2$ h) then the dilution of the precursor F^* in the medium is minimal (<5%) and F^* remains very much greater than P^*. Thus, the precursor integral can be very well approxi-

----

[1]The notation used in all equations in this chapter is as follows:

Symbol	units	Representation
P	moles	The amount of protein in a specific compartment.
P^*	Ci/mole	Specific radioactivity in protein.
F^*	Ci/mole	Specific radioactivity in free unincorporated amino acid in precursor.
$[P^*]$	moles	The amount of labeled protein in the pool as distinguished from the specific radioactivity P^*.
R_s	moles/ time	The rate of synthesis of protein in pool P.
k_x	$time^{-1}$	The fractional rate of synthesis (s), growth (g) or degradation (d). For example, k_s is the rate of protein synthesis, R_s, as a fraction of the total pool P.

[2]see Zak et al. [6] for derivation and applications of this expression.

[3]see following section for discussion of appropriate selection of precursor compartment.

mated as a constant equal to the mean of the beginning and ending values of F^*. Secondly, during short pulses, the increase of P^* approximates a linear function whose value in the integral in the denominator is $P^*/2$. Third, in practice, $P^*(t_1)$ is usually 0 at the start of a single pulse. Thus, a close approximation of the solution of k_s from Equation 2 can be given by:

$$k_s = \left[\frac{P^*(t)}{\overline{F^*} - P^*/2} \right] / t \qquad (3)$$

The parameters which need to be experimentally determined are simply F^* in the medium and P^* in the protein.

DETERMINATION OF PROTEIN SPECIFIC RADIOACTIVITY, P^*

In order to assess the specific radioactivity of amino acid in a single protein, or mixture of total proteins after labeling in culture, two methods are recommended. The first is to isolate and purify the protein of interest and to determine its specific radioactivity directly by the dansyl chloride[4] derivative method [9,10]. The second method is to evaluate the specific labeling indirectly using the dual isotopic labeling technique described by Clark and Zak [11]. Each method has certain advantages and disadvantages which are described below. The method of choice for a specific experiment depends on methods available for dealing with the specific limitations and disadvantages of each procedure.

Dansyl Chloride Assessment of Protein Specific Radioactivity

The specific radioactivity of leucine, phenylalanine, proline, valine or other amino acid used for pulse labeling protein in a myocyte culture may be determined using the DnCl technique which has been described in detail in [9,10]. In this procedure the protein must be isolated and purified by some method (usually SDS-PAGE). The purified protein fraction is sealed in glass tubes and hydrolyzed by heating at 110 °C in 6 N HCl for a period of 24 h. After hydrolysis the HCl is removed by evaporation or a dowex ion exchange column. Amino acids from the hydrolysate are recovered in a dried form and reacted with [^{14}C]dansyl chloride of a known specific radioactivity. The dansylated amino acid derivatives can then be readily separated on 2-dimensional thin layer chromatography on polyamide coated TLC plates [10]. Amino acid derivatives are located by their fluorescence when viewed under uv illumination. The location of the labeled amino acid is marked and the spot cut out from the TLC plate. The amino acid derivative is then eluted into scintillation fluid for counting. ^{3}H:^{14}C ratios are determined by scintillation counting and the ^{3}H-labeled amino acid specific radioactivity is determined from the isotope ratios and the predetermined specific radioactivity of [^{14}C]dansyl chloride [10]. The amino acid specific radioactivity, P^*, is then compared with the precursor specific radioactivity, F^*, determined in the same manner by isolation of the labeled amino acid from the culture medium. Given the precursor and protein specific radioactivities, and pulse labeling time, k_s of the protein can be computed according to Equation 2 or 3.

Advantages of DnCl: The advantages of the DnCl procedure are that it can be used to evaluate protein k_s *in vivo*, and during any period in

----

[4] 5-dimethylaminonapthalene-1-sulfonyl chloride

culture. It provides a very sensitive and reliable estimate of $P*$ in that derivatized amino acids are readily separated from other labeled contaminants and easily identified under fluorescence by their mobility on TLC. Since there is a stoichiometric relation between DnCl and the amino acid, and the specific radioactivity of the DnCl precursor is known, it is a simple matter to compute $P*$. It is also possible to process protein samples for analysis directly from SDS-PAGE gels by acid hydrolysis of the gel slice containing the protein of interest.

Disadvantages of the DnCl method. Two factors affect the use of this method for analysis of protein from cultured myocytes. First, the necessity to recover microgram quantities of purified proteins limits its use to only the most abundant cell proteins. Secondly, if SDS-PAGE is used as the method of protein purification, the protein must be one that can be well resolved on single dimension electrophoresis and free from contaminating labeled proteins.

Equilibrium-Pulse Method of Analysis of Protein Synthetic Rates

In contrast to the DnCl method, equilibrium-pulse labeling provides an indirect means for determining protein specific radioactivities, which is simpler to conduct and overcomes some of the limitations of the DnCl procedure. The basic principle of this procedure requires that all proteins in the culture be prelabeled to a constant specific radioactivity by continuous incubation in labeling medium prior to initiation of the pulse label. Once the protein reaches a state of constant specific radioactivity it is in equilibrium or at the same specific radioactivity as the precursor amino acid [11]. At this point the second isotopic form of the amino acid may be added to the labeling medium for a short pulse labeling period. After termination of labeling, proteins may be isolated and purified by any standard procedure including 1 or 2 dimension SDS-PAGE, HPLC, immunoprecipitation, affinity chromatography, etc. The specific radioactivity of the pulse label is determined directly from the isotope ratios (typically $^{3}H:^{14}C$) in the precursor and purified proteins. The presence of unlabeled carrier proteins or precipitating antibodies do not directly interfere with the analysis as long as the final isotope ratio can be determined after recovery of the protein of interest.

Advantages of Equilibrium-Pulse labeling. The advantages of this procedure is that it allows for analysis of considerably less recovered protein than the DnCl method. Secondly, processing of the labeled protein is also simpler since, in most cases the recovered protein can be analyzed directly in scintillation spectroscopy for determination of isotope ratios. Protein hydrolysis and derivatization which leads to most of the loss in the DnCl method is eliminated. Thus, it is possible to evaluate a larger number of specific proteins and proteins present in smaller amounts by equilibrium-pulse labeling than by the DnCl procedure. In addition, a greater choice in methods of protein preparation are possible using this approach since non-labeled contaminating proteins do not interfere with the analysis.

Disadvantages of Equilibrium labeling. The major drawback of this procedure is the requirement that prior to initiating a pulse label, equilibrium labeling must be established. This is not always achievable in the case of proteins turning over at very slow rates, or in the case of evaluating changes in protein synthesis rates in the first few days of culture before equilibrium is established. It should also be noted that this method is also not appropriate for use in the intact animal.

DETERMINATION OF PRECURSOR SPECIFIC RADIOACTIVITY, *F**

In assessing the fractional rate of protein synthesis by use of radioisotopic tracers using either the dansyl chloride or equilibrium-pulse method, the specific activity of both *P** and *F** must be determined for use in Equation 2. Considerable attention has been paid towards identifying the proper precursor in a number of studies in both the intact animal and in isolated organs and tissues [12-15]. Since identification of *F** is critical to proper assessment of k_s the following discussion addresses some of the most important issues involved in determination of the precursor specific radioactivity. The diagram shown in Figure 1 is representative of the precursor compartments involved in protein synthesis. The amino acid fluxes between compartments (numbered arrows) change under different experimental conditions and, thus, the proper selection of labeling conditions can have important bearing on the proper precursor specific radioactivity to use in evaluation of either protein synthesis, k_s, or protein breakdown, k_d. The experimental data described below illustrates the basis for the diagram.

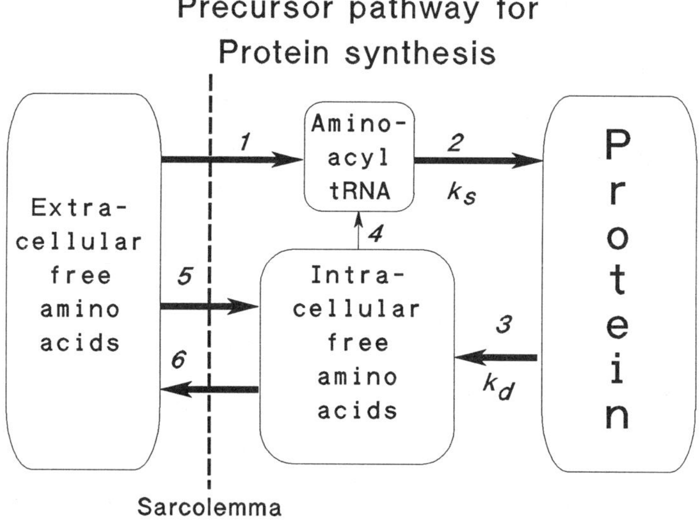

Figure 1. Compartmentation of amino acid precursors in protein synthesis.

Prior to direct measurement of precursor compartmentation, it was generally assumed that pathway 1 (in Fig. 1) did not exist, and that tracer amino acids reached proteins after dilution in a common intracellular free pool of amino acids comprised of extracellular amino acids and amino acids arising from protein breakdown[5]. Thus, the specific radioactivity

----

[5]Endogenous synthesis and metabolism of amino acids also contributes to the intracellular pool when non-essential amino acids,such as proline, are used in protein turnover studies [23].

of the immediate precursor pool in aminoacyl-tRNA would always be lower than that of the extracellular compartment due to the dilution of the intracellular pool by protein breakdown. This dilution is called the "reutilization effect".

Precursor equilibration in the intact heart. Direct measurement *in vivo* of specific radioactivities in the intra- and extracellular free amino acid pools and of that in the aminoacyl-tRNA pool proved not only that a direct pathway existed from the extracellular compartment to the aminoacyl-tRNA pool (pathway 1 in Fig. 1), but that it was the predominant pathway in the heart.

When the equilibration of leucine specific radioactivity in the plasma was compared to that of leucyl-tRNA in the intact heart, complete equilibration was found to occur within a few minutes in both rats [9,16] and rabbits [18]. No difference was noted in equilibration of these compartments using either a single pulse of isotope [16] or continuous infusion of isotope over a period of 30 minutes to 6 h [6,9,18]. Increasing rates of protein synthesis (and degradation) with thyroid hormone also did not affect equilibration of the extracellular compartment with aminoacyl-tRNA [18]. Although the leucyl-tRNA pool equilibrated immediately with the extracellular compartment, there was a significant delay in the equilibration rates of the intracellular pool of free leucine with that of the extracellular compartment when a single pulse of labeled leucine was used [16].

Precursor equilibration in isolated heart and skeletal muscle. Somewhat different findings were observed when the equilibration of the aminoacyl-tRNA compartment was compared with extracellular amino acids in isolated muscle preparations. In the case of both the isolated heart and isolated epitrochlearis muscle, there were limits to the equilibration of aminoacyl-tRNA specific radioactivity with the specific radioactivity of the perfusing solutions. In the isolated perfused working heart, equilibration occurred between the intracellular, extracellular, and phenylalanyl-tRNA pools at perfusate concentrations of greater than 0.35 mM phenylalanine, but not at lower concentrations [19]. This result indicates that the relative flux between pathways 1 and 4 in Figure 1 are influenced by extracellular amino acid concentrations. It is important to note, however, that in the *in vivo* studies cited above, complete extracellular and aminoacyl-tRNA equilibration occurred at much lower plasma leucine concentrations than McKee et al. [19] observed in the isolated heart preparation. This suggests that another factor besides extracellular amino acid concentration might also influence the relative flux rates in pathways 1 and 4. At least one additional factor appears to be the rate of protein breakdown occurring in pathway 3 (Fig. 1). This effect was well illustrated in the studies of Stirewalt and Low [20] in which the extracellular and aminoacyl-tRNA specific radioactivities were compared in protein synthesis determinations using isolated epitrochlearis muscle. In this case, equilibration was not achieved between these two compartments, and increasing extracellular leucine concentrations ("flooding the compartment") to 10 times normal plasma levels still did not bring about equilibration. Unlike muscle *in vivo*, the isolated muscle tissue preparation was in a negative state of nitrogen balance with fractional rates of protein degradation occurring at rates as much as 3 times greater than the rates of synthesis. This state appeared to influence the equilibration of aminoacyl-tRNA with the extracellular precursor.

These results have important bearing on the use of free amino acid specific radioactivities in the culture medium as a valid precursor, $F*$, for computing fractional synthesis rates in isolated cardiac myocytes.

Precursor equilibration in cultured heart cells. The principles discussed above regarding compartmentation of precursor specific radioactivities should apply equally for isolated cells in tissue culture. The option of direct assessment of aminoacyl-tRNA specific radioactivities in culture is considerably more limited for significant technical reasons: First, the size of the aminoacyl-tRNA pool is orders of magnitude smaller than either the extracellular compartment in the medium, the intracellular free pool, or the protein bound pool. Recovering detectable amounts of amino acids from this compartment requires use of radioisotopes of exceptionally high specific radioactivity. However, because of the influence of extracellular concentration on equilibration with the aminoacyl-tRNA compartment, it is not possible to achieve higher specific radioactivities simply by preparing medium without added unlabeled tracer amino acid. Large quantities of high specific radioactivity amino acids must be employed. Second, the half-life of turnover of amino acids on aminoacyl-tRNA is a matter of seconds. Thus, the process of freezing or fixing the culture must occur essentially instantaneously, and without exposing the cells to an amino acid depleted environment to avoid the rapid loss of the state of equilibration of tRNA with its amino acid source pool. Even the briefest rinsing of the cultures with saline prior to fixation might affect the specific radioactivity in the aminoacyl-tRNA compartment. Nevertheless, considering these limitations, several laboratories have reported a comparison of specific radioactivities in medium, intracellular free pools and in aminoacyl-tRNA in cultured cells.

In two studies of cultured skeletal muscle, Schneible et al. [21] and Schneible and Young [22] compared specific radioactivities of leucine in extracellular, intracellular and aminoacyl-tRNA compartments. These studies did not support the model shown in Fig. 1 in that in both studies, the specific radioactivity on aminoacyl-tRNA was less than either extracellular or intracellular free leucine. Furthermore, whereas the intracellular compartment could be "flooded" by raising the extracellular leucine concentration, the specific radioactivity in leucyl-tRNA remained at less than half of the extracellular value. The only way this could occur would be for an additional direct pathway to exist between protein breakdown and acylation of tRNA which did not involve dilution in the intracellular free pool. Similar observations have been reported in other studies in tissue culture using lung fibroblasts and macrophages [23]. However, in a more recent study from Low's group it was reported that in lung fibroblasts leucine in the extracellular compartment equilibrated completely with that in leucyl-tRNA at 0.35 mM leucine in the medium. In this case equilibration did not appear to be dependent on cellular growth (turnover) rates. However, the same study also showed that equilibration of the non-essential amino acid proline reached only 40% to 70% of the extracellular value as the extracellular concentration was raised from 0 to 4 mM proline [24].

Indirect Kinetic Approach for Assessing tRNA Specific Radioactivity

Clark and Zak [11] and Spanier et al. [25] used an indirect kinetic approach, rather than a direct measurement of leucyl-tRNA, to determine the specific radioactivity of leucyl-tRNA in cultured cells. This was accomplished by comparing the fractional synthesis rates, k_s, determined over a short pulse period using the medium specific radioactivity for $F*$, with that obtained using approach to equilibrium labeling kinetics as a means for determining total protein k_s. The basis for the "approach to equilibrium" analysis is the determination that in a steady state, or a positive state of nitrogen balance (i.e. net growth) the rate of change of specific radioactivity in the protein, $dP*/dt$, is directly proportional to the fractional synthesis rate[6]. Thus, when a culture is maintained in precursor held at a constant specific radioactivity, the specific radioactivity of amino acid in protein will increase until it eventually has the same specific radioactivity as the precursor in the medium. The equation describing this equilibration process is:

$$P^*(t) = P^*_{(max)}(1 - e^{-k_s t}) \quad (4)$$

P(max)* is the specific radioactivity of the protein after it has reached equilibrium with the precursor. Solving for k_s in this equation gives the fractional protein synthesis rate. The most important feature of this equation in the present discussion is that it does not make any assumptions at all about the precursor. While this approach to estimation of protein synthesis was first employed by Clark and Zak in a study of protein synthesis in heart cultures [11], it was later employed in a study of protein synthesis in a myeloma cell line using a suspension culture system designed for this purpose [25]. This latter approach was taken for the following reasons. Variables such as changing rates of cell growth, increasing cellular density, depletion of nutrients in the medium, and precise estimates of growth rates in monolayer culture are all difficult to determine and regulate. Each of these parameters might be expected to have an effect on protein synthesis rates during long term culture.

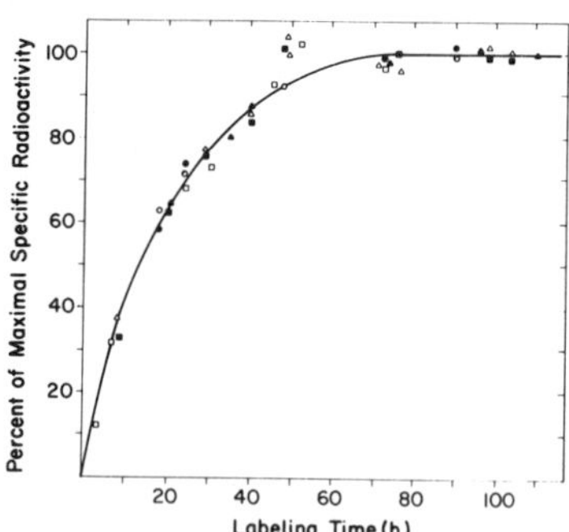

Figure 2. Protein specific radioactivity, *P**, was determined at various times during continuous labeling of cells and expressed as a percent of the maximum value achieved in each culture. Symbols represent different cultures maintained at growth rates ranging from 12 to 28 h doubling times. (Reprinted from Spanier et al. [25], with permission.)

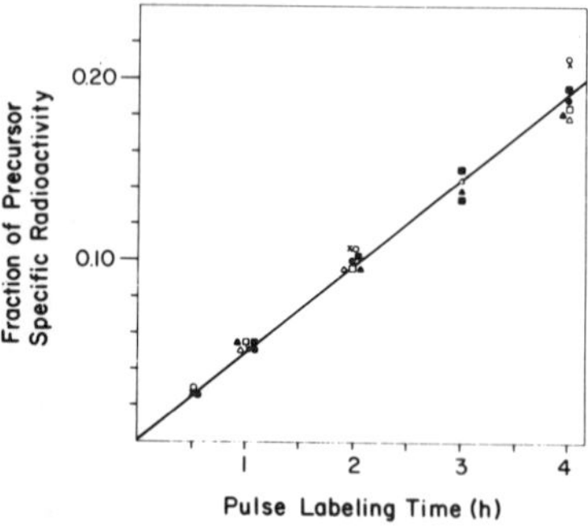

Figure 3. Protein specific radioactivity, *P**, was determined from ^3H:^{14}C ratios in equilibrium- pulse labeled cultures and expressed as a fraction of the isotope ratio of leucine in the culture medium. Symbols represent different cultures maintained at growth rates ranging from 12 to 28 h doubling times. (Reprinted from Spanier et al. [25], with permission.)

---

[6]For a detailed discussion of this concept and for derivation of equations using tracer isotopes for an estimation of protein synthesis rates see Zak et al. [6].

In the suspension culture system described in [25] a precise rate of growth could be maintained indefinitely by constant perfusion of the culture with fresh medium, and constantly withdrawing cells at a rate determined to keep the cellular density constant in the culture vessel. Since this was a fixed volume system, the fractional rate of medium replacement was exactly balanced to match the rate of cell growth. Protein synthesis was measured in this system both by the "approach to equilibrium" method and by standard pulse labeling of proteins for periods ranging from 30 min to 4 h. (Figs. 2 and 3). Fractional synthesis rates determined by both methods were identical [25]. They were also identical when the same techniques were employed in cultured heart cells [11]. Further findings of Spanier et al. [25] significant to this discussion were, first, that "flooding" with increasing concentrations of leucine did not alter observed fractional synthesis rates, and second, measurements conducted over widely differing ranges of protein degradation did not affect protein synthesis rates as measured by either method. The conclusions from these results was that, in both cultured heart cells and the myeloma line in suspension culture, computation of fractional synthesis from the rate of increase in protein specific radioactivity, dP^*/dt, relative to the precursor specific radioactivity in the medium, F^*, did not significantly differ from synthesis rates determined in a manner which did not require determination of the precursor specific radioactivity. Thus, in these studies which were conducted on a stable growing population of cells in culture, the specific radioactivity of free leucine in the culture medium must be very close to the specific radioactivity of the true immediate precursor for protein synthesis, leucyl-tRNA. However, as results from other laboratories have shown, this relationship cannot always be assumed, and may be markedly influenced by changing culture conditions.

Conclusions on Use of Medium Specific Radioactivity for F^*

It is quite possible to make accurate determinations of protein synthesis in isolated myocytes using a variety of isotopes, labeling techniques, and methods for isolating different proteins of interest. However, a number of factors may exist in the culture environment which might effect either the actual rates of synthesis and degradation of specific proteins, or the apparent synthetic rates arising from alterations in the relationship between precursors in the medium and the immediate precursor to protein synthesis, aminoacyl-tRNA. Since direct measurement of this immediate precursor is not always possible, great care must be exercised both in an attempt to evaluate the effective precursor specific radioactivity, and to insure that conditions of the experiment do not alter the balance of amino acid fluxes between various compartments of the precursor pool.

PROTEIN DEGRADATION IN ISOLATED AND CULTURED CELLS

As is evident from previous sections of this review, proteins are not synthesized, and then exist for the life of the cell. Rather, all intracellular protein constituents are in a dynamic state of continual degradation and resynthesis. Protein turnover refers to the replacement of intracellular proteins through a balanced process of synthesis and degradation. Several different experimental approaches have been used in isolated or cultured cells to measure the rate of protein degradation of specific or total cellular proteins. These methods generally involve the use of radioactive amino acids that have been incorporated into previously synthesized proteins. Therefore, as in the case of protein synthesis, thorough understanding of the kinetics and metabolism of tracer amino acids is required prior to interpretation of experimental results.

Kinetics of Protein Degradation

Analysis of protein degradation in living systems is best approached using pharmacokinetic models. In its most simple form, intracellular protein metabolism in general (and protein degradation in particular) can be analyzed by reference to a one-compartment model:

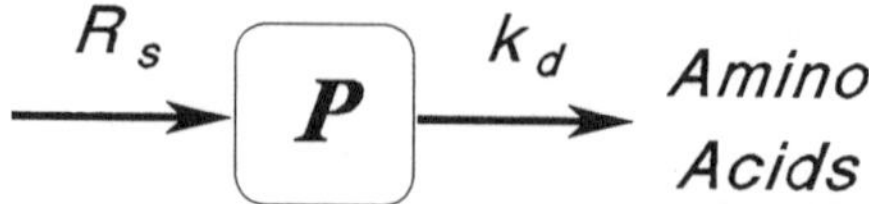

Whereas protein synthesis (R_s) is depicted as a zero order process, protein degradation is represented as a first order process that is dependent only on the amount of protein, P, and the magnitude of k_d, the fractional rate of degradation. A number of assumptions must be verified before application of this simple model. First, newly synthesized proteins in compartment P are indistinguishable from similar, "older" proteins with respect to their susceptibility to proteolysis. Furthermore, no proteins are sequestered in such a way as to make them unavailable for proteolysis. Finally, only one random "branding" or damaging" event is required to target a protein for subsequent rapid degradation. Whereas multiple steps may be required for the ultimate degradative processing of a protein to its constituent amino acids, all subsequent steps are rapid. Based upon this simple one compartment model for protein degradation, the half-life of the protein, $T_{1/2}$, is inversely proportional to k_d:

$$T_{1/2} = (\ln 2)/k_d \qquad (5)$$

Expression of rates of protein degradation in terms of protein half-lives is relevant only in steady-state systems which have been demonstrated to conform to random, single event decay. Thus in the steady state, the protein half-life is a constant representing the equal rates of protein synthesis and decay. In nonsteady state systems, k_d, as well as k_s and k_g (the fractional rates of synthesis and growth, respectively) may all change with time. The expression of experimental data in terms of "instantaneous" k_d (i.e. the fraction of total protein degraded per unit time) is relevant to both steady-state and nonsteady-state systems, and is independent of the kinetic model for protein turnover. In addition, instantaneous k_d values can be meaningfully compared to examine the effect of physiological or pathological interventions on the susceptibility of a particular protein or total protein to proteolysis.

Although this one compartment, "black box" approach to protein turnover is a convenient, and often accurate representation of the kinetics of turnover of cytosolic, short lived intracellular proteins, it has become increasingly apparent that more complex models are necessary to characterize the degradation of other intracellular protein constituents. The failure to conform to this simple model is likely the result of physical or kinetic compartmentation of intracellular proteins, or to the requirement of more than one, random, damaging event necessary to target a protein for degradation. In both situations, decay of labeled protein appears nonrandom (ie. nonexponential). These possibilities will be discussed in subsequent sections of this review.

Regulation of Protein Degradation

Individual cellular proteins "turn over" with half-lives that vary from minutes to days [26]. Furthermore, the half-life of a protein is related in part to its intracellular function [27]. In general, regulatory enzymes whose concentrations fluctuate rapidly tend to be short lived, whereas structural proteins (such as the myofibrillar and cytoskeletal proteins) are much more resistant to proteolysis. This heterogeneity in protein degradative rates demands that the overall process of intracellular protein degradation be selective [28]. However, it should be apparent from the pharmacokinetic model of protein turnover discussed above that the most important factor regulating the degradation of an individual protein is related to physical properties of the protein itself. Certain structural characteristics of intracellular proteins (ie. isoelectric point, molecular weight, hydrophobicity, etc.) are weakly correlated with *in vivo* half-life [29-31]. These characteristics are also related to *in vitro* susceptibility to purified proteases [32]. Although several very rapidly degraded intracellular proteins have been shown to share common amino acid sequences rich in certain amino acids [33], little information is presently available regarding the molecular structures important to the degradation of long lived proteins which comprise the majority of intracellular proteins in mammalian cells.

Furthermore, it is presently unknown what molecular events are responsible for the "branding" of intracellular proteins for subsequent rapid degradation [28]. Based upon the one compartment pharmacokinetic model, these events are entirely random, and can affect a protein irrespective of its age. Once branded, the damaged protein is rapidly and completely degraded. The pharmacokinetic model requires the existence of a degradative machinery capable of reducing a protein to its constituent amino acids at a rate much faster than the branding process. Whereas numerous intracellular proteolytic enzymes (including both lysosomal and nonlysosomal hydrolases) have been described, our knowledge of how they participate in the degradation of specific proteins is at present rudimentary. However, it is clear that the concentration or activity of proteases within the cell is only poorly related to the flux of proteins through the degradative pathway [18]. Except for very unusual circumstances, events preceding a protein's complete proteolytic processing regulate its physiological rate of turnover.

Methods of Assessing Rates of Protein Degradation in Cells in Culture

The rate of degradation of an individual protein, or mixture of proteins, can be measured in isolated or cultured cells with the use of radioactively labeled amino acids. However, these methods must be applied with caution, as both theoretical and technical problems (similar to those discussed above regarding protein synthesis measurements) are frequently encountered. Two methodological approaches are commonly used: (a) an indirect assessment of protein degradation based upon measurements of protein synthesis and accumulation; and (b) a direct assessment of protein degradation based upon the loss of radioactivity from prelabeled protein with time. Both methodological approaches can be applied to steady-state and nonsteady-state systems. Both methods will be analyzed with reference to the pharmacokinetic model outlined above.

Indirect assessment of fractional protein degradation in the steady-state. As discussed in previous sections of this review, the presence or absence of a steady-state markedly influences the complexity of measurements necessary to accurately determine k_d of an individual protein or mixture of proteins. In pharmacokinetic terms, a steady state exists only when the amount of a particular protein does not change with time. Analysis of the compartmental model in terms of the differential equations characterizing entry to and exit from the system yields:

$$dP/dt = R_s - k_dP = 0 \tag{6}$$

$$k_d = R_s/P = k_s \tag{7}$$

R_s/P (total protein synthesized per unit time divided by the amount of protein in compartment P) is identical to k_s, the fractional rate of synthesis. In a steady-state system, $k_s = k_d$. Therefore, the fractional rate of protein degradation in the steady state is best assessed by measurement of k_s using the labeling procedures outlined above. Assuming single event, random decay, k_s can be transformed to yield protein half-life.

Indirect assessment of fractional protein degradation in the nonsteady-state. Although steady-state systems allow for much less complicated solutions of protein turnover kinetics, they are rarely encountered in culture. Furthermore, experiments designed to study growth regulation, or induction or repression of a particular protein or group of proteins in a cell system are not, by definition, in steady-state. Although an indirect assessment of protein degradation can be made in these situations, the analysis of data is more complex. Returning to the description of protein accumulation in the one compartment model:

$$dP/dt = R_s - k_dP \tag{8}$$

dividing both sides of the equation by P, and substituting k_s for R_s/P:

$$(dP/dt)/P = k_s - k_d \tag{9}$$

where $(dP/dt)/P$ is the fractional rate of protein accumulation. Substituting and rearranging the equation yields:

$$k_d = k_s - k_g \tag{10}$$

Thus in the nonsteady-state system, the instantaneous fractional rate of protein degradation, k_d, can be derived as the difference between k_s and k_g.

In these circumstances k_s measurements are best determined using short pulse labeling experiments, especially when studying rapidly degraded proteins. Assessment of k_g, the instantaneous fractional rate of protein accumulation, requires careful measurement of the amount of a particular protein or mixture of proteins over a prolonged time. An example of this procedure as applied to a nonsteady-state cell culture system is described as follows.

In a recently completed study, Mostow, et al. [34] serially examined the fractional rate of total protein degradation of primary cultures of cardiac fibroblasts, in order to determine the contribution of total protein degradation to the rapid growth to these cells following low density subculture. The total amount of total protein per culture was determined at each day following subculture. The data were empirically fit to a sigmoidal function as an estimate of the fractional rate of protein accumulation versus time. Using the same culture dishes as were used to assess total protein fractional accumulation rates, total protein fractional synthetic rates were measured by $[^3H]$leucine pulse labeling at days 1-5, 10, 15 and 21 days following low density subculture. Total fractional protein accumulation rates were then subtracted from average fractional synthesis rates to yield simultaneous fractional rates of total protein degradation (Fig. 4). As is evident from the Figure, k_d values deviated from a relatively constant rate of approximately 40 %/day only during the period of most rapid fibroblast growth (i.e., days 1 and 2 following low density subculture). Thus, enhanced fractional synthesis rates, as well as markedly reduced fractional degradation rates, both contributed to the rapid growth of fibroblasts following subculture.

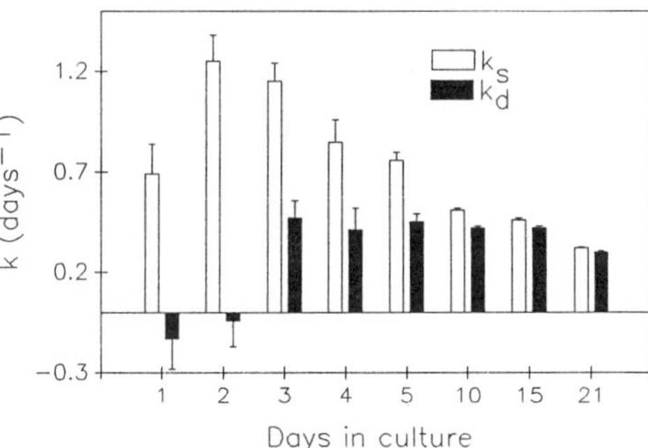

Figure 4. Fractional rates of synthesis and degradation of total protein in cardiac fibroblasts following low density subculture.

Direct assessment of protein degradation in the steady-state. The direct assessment of rate of degradation of an individual protein can be accomplished by examining the loss of radioactivity from prelabeled protein with time. As discussed previously, the kinetics of protein synthesis and degradation can be modeled by reference to the differential equation describing the one compartment model given in Equation 8. If the system is in steady state (i.e. $dP/dt=0$), then the input and output rates of P are equal. If the protein of interest is biosynthetically labeled by incorporation of a tracer amino acid at time=0, then the behavior of the labeled protein $[P*]$ is described by the following equation:

$$d[P*]/dt = -k_d[P*] \tag{11}$$

Rearranging and integrating the differential equation yields the well known equation for exponential decay:

$$[P*](t) = [P*](0)e^{-k_d t} \tag{12}$$

where $[P*](0)$ and $[P*]$ are the amounts of radioactively labeled protein at time=0 and time=t, respectively. In the steady state, the equation can also be expressed in terms of specific radioactivities $P*$ in Equation 12 rather than amount of labeled protein $[P*]$ because of the unique relation between synthesis and degradation in the steady state.

Direct assessment of fractional protein decay rate in nonsteady-state. The direct assessment of the average fractional rate of degradation of an individual protein in nonsteady-state systems can also be analyzed by reference to the differential equation for the one compartment model, given above in Equation 8. If R_s and k_d are constant, but $R_s \neq k_d P$, then the amount of the protein in compartment P will vary with time. However, if a portion of protein P is prelabeled at time=0 (by biosynthetic pulse labeling), then the amount of labeled protein $[P*]$ is still described by the equation for exponential decay, Equation 12. However, the expression of parameters in terms of specific radioactivities (i.e. $P*$) is incorrect, as both the amount of labeled protein and the total amount of protein in the compartment both change with time. Thus in nonsteady-state systems, the fractional rate of a protein's degradation can be directly assessed only by observing the decline in the amount of labeled protein *[P*]* with time. This analysis assumes that the labeled protein is indistinguishable from the entire pool of protein *P* with respect to its susceptibility to proteolysis. Furthermore, k_d is also assumed to remain approximately constant during the time required for measurements. If either assumption proves false, then nonlinear decay curves are obtained [8]. Pulse-chase experiments are conducted as described for the steady state. However, the labeled protein must be quantitatively recovered and analyzed for the amount of remaining radioactivity. Data are plotted as the log of labeled protein, *[P*]*, remaining in the cells versus time. The absolute value for the slope of the best fitting line equals the average value for k_d during the time of observation.

Choice of Methodological Approach

Choosing the best method to analyze the fractional degradative rate of an individual protein or mixture of proteins depends on a number of factors. In a steady-state system, indirect measurement of k_s provides the simplest and most accurate assessment of k_d for both individual proteins, as well as protein mixtures. This approach however, does not provide information regarding the kinetic model that best describes the turnover of a particular protein. In contrast, examination of decay curves for an individual, prelabeled protein by the direct approach (in either steady-state of nonsteady-state systems) allows for the verification of random versus nonrandom turnover, and provides information about the mechanisms involved in protein processing. However, direct assessment of k_d for a mixture of proteins in pulse chase labeling experiments yields data that are very difficult to interpret. In this case, the observed decay curve is a composite of the decay of many proteins that possess differing k_d values. In addition, the extent of labeling of the protein mixture during the pulse markedly affects the rate at which label is lost from the protein mixture. In turn, the extent of labeling is dependent upon both synthetic rates of the individual proteins that comprise the mixture, as well as the length of the pulse labeling period [8]. Therefore, pulse-chase methods are best restricted to studies of individual proteins, where experimental values for k_d can be confirmed by indirect measurements in either steady-state, or nonsteady-state systems.

Future Direction in the Study of Protein Degradation in Isolated and Cultured Cells

Several recent advances in cellular and molecular biology should have a direct bearing on the future study of protein turnover in isolated cell systems. Mass microinjection of in vitro labeled proteins has already provided important information regarding the relationship between protein structure and protein degradation [35]. The ability to transfect and express foreign genomic DNA into cultured cells will undoubtedly influence the experimental approaches used to study protein turnover at the molecular level. These developments, coupled with the ability to produce site specific mutations of individual proteins, will help to reveal many of the important steps involved in protein degradation that, at present, remain elusive. Similar techniques will also prove useful in investigating the proteinases responsible for physiological protein turnover, and in elucidating the role of protein degradation in the regulation of cellular growth.

REFERENCES

1. A.W. Everett, A.M. Sinha, P.K. Umeda, S. Jakovcic and M. Rabinowitz. Biochemistry 23, 1596-1599 (1984).

2. D. Siehl, B.H.L. Chua and N. Lautenbsack-Belser and H.E. Morgan. Am. J. Physiol. 248, C309-C319 (1985).

3. H.E. Morgan , D.E. Rannels and E.E. McKee in: Handbook of Physiology - The Cardiovascular System I, pp. 845-871 (1985).

4. A.W. Everett and R. Zak in: Drug-Induced Heart Disease, M.R. Bristow, ed. (Elsevier, Amsterdam 1980) pp. 63-80.

5. J.M. Reiner. Arch. Biochem. and Biophys. 46, 53-99 (1953).

6 R. Zak, A.F. Martin and R. Blough. Physiological Reviews 59, 407-447 (1979).

7. A.W. Everett and R. Zak in: Degradative Processes in Heart and Skeletal Muscle, K. Wildenthal, ed. (Elsevier Amsterdam 1980) pp. 31-47.

8. J.C. Waterlow, P.J. Garlick, and D.J. Millward. Protein Turnover in Mammalian Tissues and in the Whole Body (North Holland, Amsterdam, 1978).

9. A.W. Everett, G. Prior and R. Zak. Biochem. J. 194, 365-368 (1981).

10. J. Airhart, J. Kelley, J.E. Brayden, R.B. Low and W.S. Stirewalt. Anal. Biochem. 96, 45-55 (1979).

11. W.A. Clark and R. Zak. J. Biol. Chem. 256, 4863-4870 (1981).

12. G.E. Mortimore, K.H. Woodside and J.E. Henry. J. Biol. Chem. 247, 2776-2784 (1972).

13. A. Vidrich, J. Airhart, M.K. Brunno and E.A. Khairallah. Biochem. J. 162, 257-266 (1977).

14. Y. Hod and A. Hershko. J. Biol. Chem. 254, 4458-4467 (1976).

15. B. Poole. J. Biol. Chem. 116, 6587-6591 (1971).

16. A.F. Martin, M. Rabinowitz, R. Blough, G. Prior and R. Zak. J. Biol. Chem. 252, 3422-3429 (1977).

18. M.S. Parmacek, N.M. Magid, M. Lesch, R.S. Decker and A.M. Samarel. Am. J. Physiol. 251, C727-C736 (1986).

19. E.E. McKee, J.Y. Cheung, D.E. Rannels and H.E. Morgan. J. Biol. Chem. 253, 1030-1040 (1978).

20. W.S. Stirewalt and R.B. Low. Biochem. J. 210, 323-330 (1983).

21. P.A. Schneible, J. Airhart and R.B. Low. J. Biol. Chem. 256, 4888-4894 (1981).

22. P.A. Schneible and R.B. Young. J. Biol. Chem. 259, 1436-1440 (1984).

23. J.N. Hildebran, J. Airhart, W.S. Stirewalt and R.B. Low. Biochem. J. 198, 249-258 (1981).

24. R.B. Low, J.N. Hildebran, P.M. Absher, W.S. Stirewalt and J. Arnold. Connect. Tiss. Res. 14, 179-185 (1986).

25. A.M. Spanier, W.A. Clark and R. Zak. J. Cell. Biochem. 26, 47-64 (1984).

26. I.M. Arias, D. Doyle and R.T. Schimke. J. Biol. Chem. 244, 3303-3315 (1969).

27. A.L. Goldberg and A.C. St. John. Ann. Rev. Biochem. 45, 747-803 (1976).

28. R.J. Beynon and J.S. Bond, Am. J. Physiol. 251, C141-C152 (1986).

29. A.L. Goldberg and J.F. Dice. Annu. Rev. Biochem. 43, 835-869 (1974).

30. J.F. Dice and A.L. Goldberg. Arch. Biochem. Biophys. 170, 213-219 (1975).

31. P. Bohley, H.G. Wollert, D.D. Reimann and S. Reimann. Acta Biol. Med. Ger. 40, 1655-1658 (1981).

32. J.S. Bond in: Intracellular Protein Turnover, R.T. Shimke & N. Katanuma, eds. (Academic Press, New York, 1975) pp 281-293.

33. S. Rogers, R. Wells and M. Rechsteiner. Science 234,364-368.

34. W.R. Mostow, A.M. Samarel, R.S. Decker and M. Lesch. J. Cell Biol. 105, 105a (1987).

35. K.V. Rote and M. Rechsteiner. J. Biol. Chem. 261, 15430-15436 (1986).

SPATIAL DISTRIBUTION OF MYOSIN mRNA IN CARDIAC TISSUE BY *IN SITU* HYBRIDIZATION TECHNIQUES.

DAVID J. DIX and BRENDA R. EISENBERG.
Physiology Department,
Rush Medical College,
1750 West Harrison Street,
Chicago, IL 60612.

INTRODUCTION

Detection of mRNA at the cytological level using RNA hybridization probes yields information concerning location, quantity and kind of gene transcripts being expressed [1] and has been used to detect expression of myosin heavy chain (MHC) unique to myogenic cells [2]. Actin gene expression in chicken muscle cultures has been visualized using a biotin-labeled cDNA probe and fluorescent detection [3] and quantified using isotope-labeled probes and autoradiography [4]. Intracellular distributions of mRNAs for the cytoskeletal proteins actin, vimentin and tubulin in chicken myoblasts and fibroblasts have been demonstrated to be non-homogeneously distributed [5]. *In situ* hybridization protocols using isotopic and non-isotopic labelling methods have been optimized for application to both cell cultures and frozen tissue sections [6].

Synthesis of either RNA or DNA hybridization probes complementary to specific mRNAs is possible. RNA probes (riboprobes) have some advantages in that they are transcribed using phage RNA polymerases (SP6, T3 or T7) with high specificity for their respective promoters [7-8]. This allows either the hybridizing or the non-hybridizing riboprobe to be synthesized. The non-hybridizing riboprobe serves as a control for non-specific binding. Uniformity of riboprobe length and labelling density enhance reproducibility of the hybridizations. A good signal-to-noise level is possible: a high signal is achieved because RNA/RNA hybrids have greater thermal stability, Tm, than RNA/DNA hybrids; a low background is obtained because unhybridized RNA can be removed by ribonuclease [9].

Either an isotope-labelled nucleotide or a biotin-labelled nucleotide can be enzymatically incorporated into nucleic acid probes. Biotin-labeled riboprobes have similar hybridization kinetics to unlabelled polynucleotides [8] making them useful hybridization probes. Isotope-labelled riboprobes have been used for *in situ* hybridizations yielding quantitative results on paraffin embedded tissue sections [9-11]. Isotope labels are impractical for three reasons. First, the half-life of the isotope and the degradation effect on the riboprobe prevent long-term storage of probe. Secondly, the track length of emissions in autoradiographic emulsions preclude all but tritium as a viable label for subcellular localization of mRNA. Finally, if tritium is to be used, exposure times are weeks long. Biotin labelling has the advantages of long-term storage, and detection methods which are quick, easy, and provide high spatial resolution, including ultrastructural.

Biology of Isolated Adult Cardiac Myocytes
William A. Clark, Robert S. Decker, and Thomas K. Borg, Editors

METHODS

There are several existing protocols for <u>in situ</u> hybridization which using isotope label [4, 9, 11] but in our hands many practical problems were encountered. Sections had bad structure, non-specific background signal was high, time for an experiment was long, reagents were expensive, and isotope-labelled probe half-life was short. To avoid these shortcomings, we have developed a protocol using biotinylated riboprobes and enzymatic detection on frozen tissue sections. Frozen tissue has the additional advantage of allowing hybridization and immunofluorescence on serial sections. Structural detail of the tissue is retained, allowing fine resolution of the cellular localization of specific mRNAs. The volume of solutions used is kept to a minimum and results are very reproducible. These advantages allow us to perform a greater number of hybridizations with a wider selection of variables. The discussion below outlines the steps in the application of the technique to rabbit cardiac tissue [12, 13].

<u>Riboprobe Production</u>

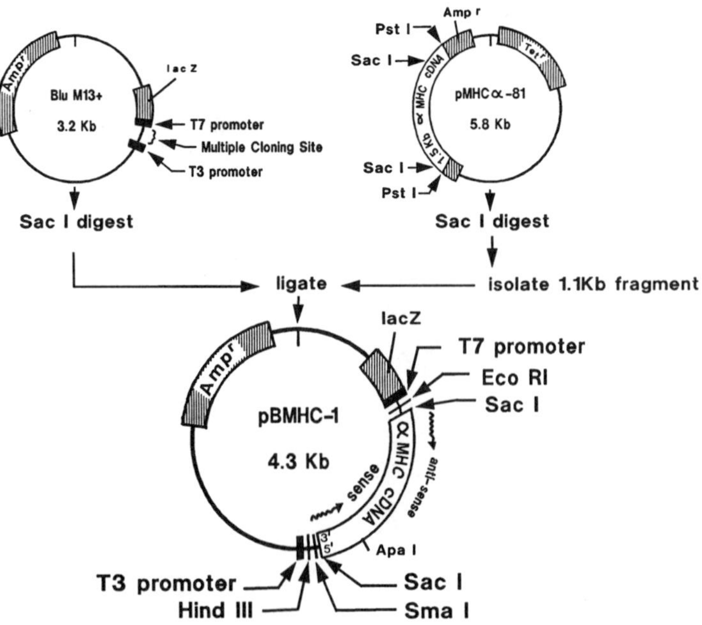

Fig. 1. Subcloning of riboprobe template. The 1.1 kb Sac I fragment of pMHCα-81 is ligated into the transcription vector Bluescribe M13+.

Subcloning and orientation. The initial clone was pMHC-81, a cDNA of rabbit α-MHC [14]. The 1.1 kb Sac I fragment of pMHCα-81 is isolated from a low-melting-temperature agarose gel and ligated [15] into the Sac I linearized transcription vector Bluescribe M13+ (Stratagene Cloning Systems, San Diego, CA) resulting in the subclone, pBMHC-1 (Fig. 1). The bacterial host strain JM 109 is transformed with the subclone plasmid [16]. Recombinant colonies are picked from selective media, plasmid DNA purified, and the recombinant pBMHC-1 identified by restriction digests. Plasmid DNA to serve as a template for transcription is purified on a cesium chloride gradient [17].

Several terms are currently in use to describe the two riboprobes that can be transcribed. One DNA strand encodes the mRNA probe, also termed sense or non-hybridizing probe. The other DNA strand encodes complementary cRNA probe, also termed anti-sense or hybridizing probe. Orientation of the insert of pBMHC-1 with respect to the T3 and T7 promoters was determined by restriction analysis with Sma I and Apa I as shown diagrammatically and in the gel (Fig. 2). The Sma I site is near the T3 promoter yielding a fragment of 250 nt, so T3 polymerase will transcribe the mRNA probe. The T7 promoter will transcribe the cRNA probe. If we had obtained the Sma I to Apa I fragment of about 800 nt the opposite orientation would have been deduced, i.e. T7 would transcribe mRNA.

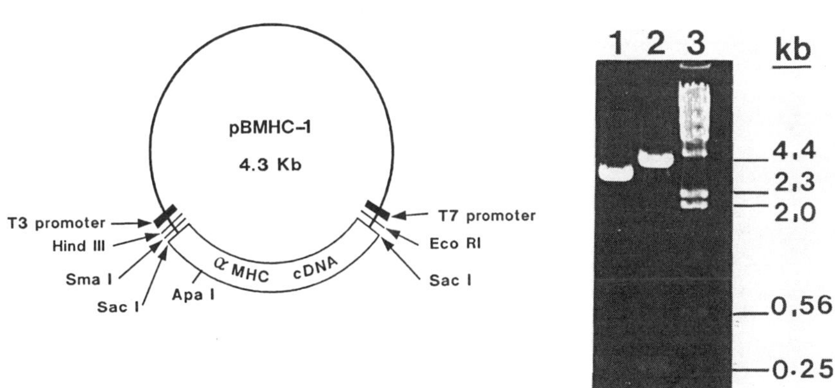

Fig. 2. Orientation of insertion. On left; diagram of Sac I subclone pBMHC-1. On right; restriction digests with Sma I and Apa I of Bluescribe alone (lane 1) and of pBMHC-1 with the 250 nt fragment (lane 2). Lane 3 is a Hind III digest of lambda phage to act as a size marker.

Transcription and biotinylation. The subclone is used as a template for transcription of RNA probes and allows for transcription of the cRNA probe using T7 RNA polymerase and the mRNA probe using the T3 RNA polymerase (Fig. 3). It is essential that the hybridizing cRNA is used for testing the presence of endogenous mRNA and a non-hybridizing mRNA strand is used as a control to test for the numerous artifacts.

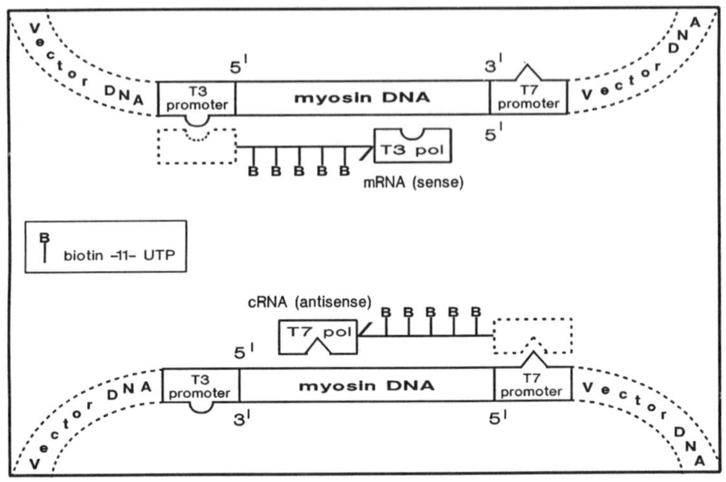

Fig. 3. **Transcription of riboprobes**. The upper part of the figure shows synthesis of the mRNA probe with the T3 polymerase; the lower part of the figure is cRNA transcribed from the other DNA strand by T7 polymerase. Biotin label is incorporated at every uridine residue of both transcripts.

In order to control the length of the transcribed riboprobe and to avoid transcribing vector sequences it is necessary to linearize the template DNA with a restriction endonuclease. The linear template must not contain a protruding 3' end, as this can cause extraneous transcripts from the opposite strand and vector sequences (Promega Biotec, Madison, WI). These requirements are met by use of Hind III for the T7 and Eco RI for the T3 transcriptions (sites shown in Fig. 3).

The labelled biotin-11-UTP (BRL, Gaithersburg, MD) is an acceptable substrate for phage polymerases in the transcription reaction [8] and wholly substitutes for the regular nucleotide in the transcription reaction. A typical transcription reaction is 5 µg template DNA, 1 mM NTP's, 10 mM DTT, 1X manufacturer's transcription buffer, and 200 Units T3 or T7 RNA polymerase (BRL, Gaithersburg, MD) in a total volume of 50 µl. This reaction is incubated at 37°C for 2 hours. Enzymatic removal of the DNA template and column chromatographic purifications have proven unnecessary; several ethanol precipitations with ammonium acetate will suffice.

New transcripts are checked on denaturing sizing gels (Fig. 4) for integrity and length uniformity. In lanes 1 and 2 of Fig. 4 the upper bands are the DNA templates and lower bands are cRNA and mRNA, respectively, confirming that the transcripts are full length (1.1 kb). It has been observed that biotinylated RNA migrates through gels more slowly than unlabelled RNA. The extent of retardation depends on the number of biotinylated uridines incorporated. This explains why the cRNA with 298 uridines does not run as far as the mRNA with only 112 uridines. The specificity of the polymerases for their own promoter was confirmed by reversing the combination of polymerase and linearizing restriction enzyme (not shown) resulting in very short RNA transcripts.

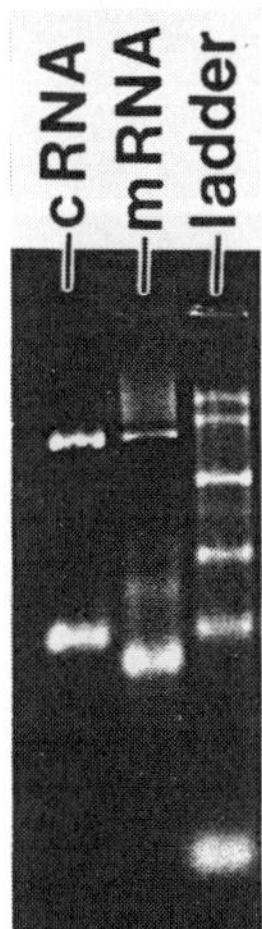

Fig. 4. Transcript sizing gel. 1.5% agarose/ 1 M urea gel run at 8 V/cm for 1 hour.
Lane 1: cRNA; T7 polymerase/ Hind III transcript with biotin.
Lane 2: mRNA; T3 polymerase/ Eco RI transcript with biotin.
Lane 3: RNA ladder. Starting at the bottom of the gel the size markers are 0.24, 1.4, 2.4, 4.4, 7.5, 9.5 kb.

Several laboratories have reported that shorter probe fragments (200-400 nucleotides) yield better signal-to-noise ratios, particularly when using a biotin label [6, 18]. We have not attempted to shorten probe length by alkaline hydrolysis as this would very likely remove the biotin label as well. An alternative to hydrolysis of longer transcripts is to prepare template DNA linearized at restriction sites nearer the promoter, thus yielding shorter transcripts. Our 1.1 kb myosin probe has worked well and it may be that shorter riboprobes are not necessary when hybridizing an abundant mRNA such as myosin.

Because results from the cRNA and mRNA need to be compared it is necessary to standardize concentrations of probe between batches. The T3 polymerase is more efficient in utilizing Bio-11-UTP as a substrate and usually yields more probe than the T7. Concentration can be approximated by UV fluorescence in gels. A better method is to include trace amounts of tritium labelled nucleotide in transcriptions and make scintillation counts of acid precipitated material. Spectrophotometry is not used because differing amounts of biotin incorporated into probes complicates interpretation of results. Transcriptional yields of the 1.1 kb riboprobe from pBMHC-1 have been excellent, 5-10 µg of probe per µg template. Thus large quantities of biotinylated riboprobe can be prepared, aliquoted, and stored in distilled water at -80°C indefinitely.

At all times one should be aware of the threat of RNase contamination of stock solutions and reaction mixes. Gloves should always be worn, glassware should be baked at 180°C, distilled water should be treated with diethylpyrocarbonate (DEPC), solutions and plastic ware should be autoclaved. Always use DEPC-treated water to make up solutions.

Myosin Riboprobe Specificity

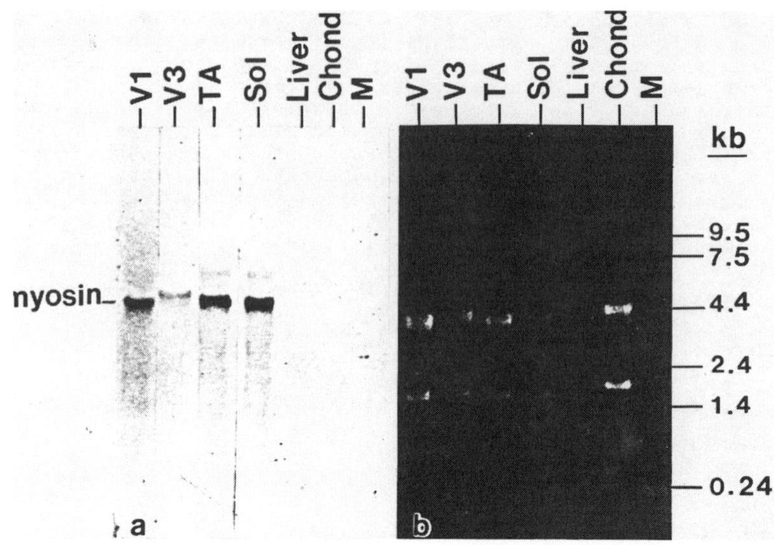

Fig. 5. Northern hybridization. A 1% agarose/formaldehyde gel (panel b) of RNA extracted from various tissues is run, transferred to nitrocellulose and hybridized with cRNA (panel a). All muscle RNA shows hybridization at about 6 kb as expected for myosin. V1 is α-MHC from hyperthyroid rabbit; V3 is β-MHC from hypothyroid rabbit; TA is fast-skeletal muscle from rabbit; SOL is β-MHC from soleus muscle in rabbit; liver from rabbit; Chond from chondrocytes in culture (gift from Dr. L. Sandell); M is a size marker.

The α-MHC sequence being utilized in pBMHC-1 encodes the carboxy-terminus of the light meromyosin (LMM). The α to β sequence similarities in the LMM lead us to expect that the initial riboprobe will be >90% similar to all MHC isoform mRNAs in rabbit muscle. To confirm myosin riboprobe specificity, cellular RNA was extracted from various types of skeletal and cardiac muscle [19]. The initial extraction buffer contained 0.1 mM aurin tricarboxylic acid to limit nuclease activity. These extracts were analyzed qualitatively by gel transfer hybridization with biotinylated riboprobe [7, 20]. Similar amounts of RNA extract were loaded and run on agarose para-formaldehyde gels that transferred to nitrocellulose by capillary action (Northern transfer). Filters were hybridized with biotinylated cRNA or mRNA probes at 55°C overnight. Filters were washed four times in 0.1 X SSC, 0.1% SDS for 20 minutes at 25°C. Detection on the filter was with streptavidin-alkaline phosphatase as recommended (Clontech Labs, Palo Alto, CA). The cRNA hybridized to RNA bands at the location expected for 6-7 kb myosin mRNA extracts from hypo- and hyper-thyroid cardiac and from skeletal slow, mixed and fast muscles. No hybridization was seen to RNA from the non-muscle tissue of liver and chondrocyte. The mRNA probe did not hybridize (not shown), further confirming the orientation of the insert and specificity of the probe. The pBMHC-1 is a myosin heavy chain subclone yielding a riboprobe non-discriminatory of isomyosins as expected. We prefer Northern hybridizations to dot blots which in our hands yield a high non-specific binding due to ribosomal RNA in the total extracted RNA.

Fixation and Hybridization for Light Microscopy

In summary, sections are fixed, prehybridized and carried through the hybridization, wash, and detection steps as outlined in Fig 6. The use of biotinylated riboprobes of various lengths and sequences; tissue fixed and prepared by different methods; enzymatic and non-enzymatic detection methods; and a broad range and abundance of endogenous mRNAs create a need for experimentally determining the optimal hybridization conditions for each research application.

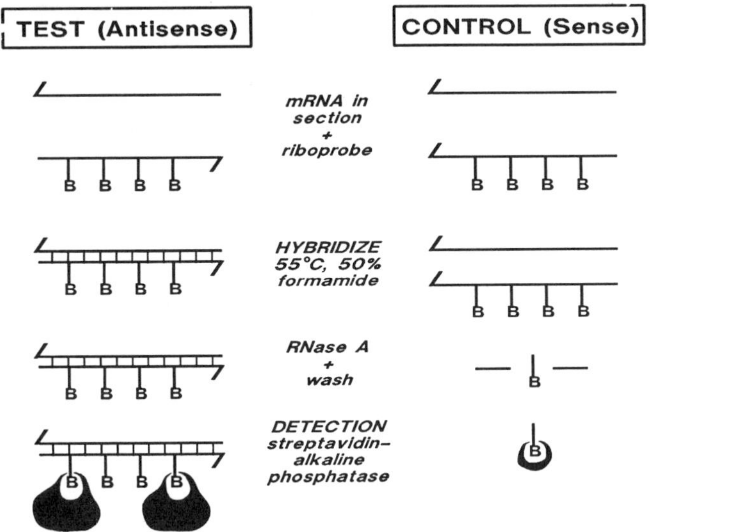

Fig. 6. Hybridization and detection with biotinylated riboprobe. The test hybridization with cRNA probe yields a hybrid resistant to RNase removal, resulting in a dense color signal. The control hybridization with mRNA probe yields no hybrids and little color signal.

The removal of muscle tissue from rabbits and subsequent freezing is far from trivial. The extensive manipulations of the frozen section during <u>in situ</u> hybridization requires minimal freezing damage to the blocks of tissue. The heart is removed from an anesthetized rabbit. Small blocks of muscle are flash-frozen in isopentane cooled by liquid nitrogen soon after removal from the animal (see [11] for a discussion of mRNA autolysis). Frozen sections (6-8 μm) are cut from these blocks, mounted on coverslips coated with poly-l-lysine to prevent detachment and fixed with 4% paraformaldehyde in PBS/5 mM $MgCl_2$ for 15 minutes. Fixation and all subsequent steps involving the sections, unless otherwise noted, are done on 12 mm round coverslips in 24-well tissue culture plates to minimize volume of solutions. We have found it preferable to cut and fix sections the day they are to be hybridized to reduce the risk of sections detaching from the coverslips during processing.

A sufficient quantity of each probe is thawed and 20 µg tRNA and 20µg salmon sperm DNA is added to each, blocking nonspecific binding of nucleotides by the tissue. These probe mixtures are dried down in a vacuum centrifuge. The probes are resuspended in deionized formamide (10 µl per section) at 90°C for 10 minutes in order to fully denature. A prewarmed cocktail of reagents (10 µl per section)is added to the probe such that the final hybridization buffer contains 2X SSC, 0.2% BSA, 10 mM DTT, 10% dextran sulfate, and 50% deionized formamide (see [17]). The optimal probe concentration for the 1.1 kb MHC riboprobe and streptavidin-alkaline phosphatase detection on frozen cardiac sections was determined experimentally to be 1 ng/µl.

The paraformaldehyde fixed sections are treated with 0.2 M tris (pH 7.4)/0.1M glycine for 10 minutes to reduce nonspecific binding of the riboprobe to the section. The sections are heated to 65°C for 10 minutes in 2X SSC/50% deionized formamide to reduce protein binding and secondary structure of cellular mRNA. The sections are then inverted onto 20 µl droplets of probe on parafilm, covered with a second sheet of parafilm, and incubated for three hours at 57°C. Separate sheets of parafilm should be used for each type of probe to prevent diffusion of probes leading to possible misinterpretation.

The probe concentration, time, and temperature for _in situ_ hybridization with isotope labeled riboprobes has been thoroughly examined [9]. Limited alkaline hydrolysis was used to normalize the length of the probes to about 150 nt, this is not possible with biotinylated riboprobes. Cox et al. (1984) found the optimal probe concentration to be 0.2 ng/µl. The maximal signal at that probe concentration was reached after four hours of hybridization. The optimum hybridization rate occurred at the Tm of RNA:RNA hybrids less 25°C. The important point to note is that these results are unique to _in situ_ hybridization with radioactive riboprobes on paraffin embedded sea urchin embryos.

The Tm for a riboprobe/mRNA hybrid can be theoretically derived by the following formula: Tm = (18.5 log [Na]) + (54.8 x fraction GC content of probe) + (79.8°C) - (1°C x % mismatch) + [11.8 (fraction GC content of probe)^2] - [650/probe length (nt)] - (0.35°C x % formamide) [9] We have achieved good results at a hybridization temperature 33°C below the MHC riboprobe/mRNA Tm of 90°C. The manufacturer of the biotinylated nucleotide (BRL, Gaithersburg, MD) claims that biotinylated probes exhibit a 5°C reduction in Tm. This accounts for our need for a lower hybridization temperature than expected from the above equation.

Following hybridization, the sections are incubated at 37°C on droplets of prewarmed 20 ng/µl RNase A in 0.5M NaCl/10mM Tris pH 8.0 to remove unhybridized probe. The negative control hybridization with mRNA riboprobe depends on an adequate RNase A concentration for low background staining of sections. Following digestion of unhybridized probe, the sections are washed in prewarmed 2X SSC/50% deionized formamide at 37°C for 30 minutes, prewarmed 1X SSC/50% deionized formamide at 37°C for 30 minutes, and then three washes of 10 minutes each with agitation in 1X SSC at room temperature.

Detection of Riboprobe

Isotope labelled probe can be detected and quantified by standard autoradiographic methods [21]. Biotinylated hybrids can be detected utilizing the strong affinity of avidin or streptavidin for the biotin label [22]. Streptavidin conjugated to alkaline phosphatase has been used on neuronal tissue sections [23] and streptavidin-peroxidase was used with cultured cells [24, 25]. Silver intensification of streptavidin-colloidal gold has been successful with cDNA probes on brain sections [26]. Hybridization labels can also be detected by primary anti-biotin antibody and visualized by indirect immunofluorescence or immunoperoxidase [24]. Quantitative histochemical results can be achieved with statistical sampling methods, appropriate controls, and densitometry equipment [27].

Detection of riboprobe:MHC mRNA hybrids is currently done using streptavidin-alkaline phosphatase (SAP, Fig. 6). The sections are blocked for nonspecific protein binding by submerging in a pre-warmed buffer (0.1 M tris pH 7.4, 0.1 M NaCl, 2 mM $MgCl_2$, 0.5% triton X-100, 3% BSA) for 10 minutes at 42°C. The sections are then inverted onto droplets of 1 µg/ml SAP in 4X SSC, 0.5% triton X-100, 2 mM $MgCl_2$ for 10 minutes. Three washes of 3 minutes each (with shaking) in the buffer without the BSA is followed by a 2 minute rinse in a third buffer (0.1 M tris pH 9.5, 0.1 M NaCl, 50 mM $MgCl_2$). The sections are then color developed for 1 to 12 hours on droplets of 330 µg/ml nitro blue tetrazolium (NBT) and 167 µg/ml 5-bromo-4-chloro-3-indolyl phosphate (BCIP) in the third buffer. Color development is usually allowed to run overnight in a moist chamber between sheets of parafilm. The enzymatic reaction is stopped by placing the sections into 20 mM tris pH 7.5/5 mM EDTA. Sections are dried through ethanols, cleared with xylene and mounted onto slides with Permount.

RESULTS AND DISCUSSION

Numerous controls are routinely run on serial sections of heart. These include using no probe to rule out endogenous biotin or phosphatase; mRNA probe to rule out non-specific binding; pretreating with RNAse as a negative control to destroy MHC mRNA; and post-hybridization with RNAse A to remove unhybridized probe. An important control hybridization for all poly-adenylated RNAs is biotinylated polyuridine. Photo-biotinylation is rapidly accomplished with a sunlamp, poly-uridine, and photobiotin with a photoactivatable thiol group which binds the polynucleotide.

Effect of cRNA Probe Concentration

Frozen cardiac tissue is fixed in paraformaldehyde and processed for *in situ* hybridization as discussed in methods. In all hybridizations sections are processed without the addition of any riboprobe to test for background staining (Fig 7 a). Zero probe must give a low signal or else the false positive negates interpretation of all other results. Biotinylated riboprobes have the added problems that some tissues have natural biotin (e.g. liver) or endogenous activity of the detection enzyme (e.g. red cells have peroxidase, liver has alkaline phosphatase).

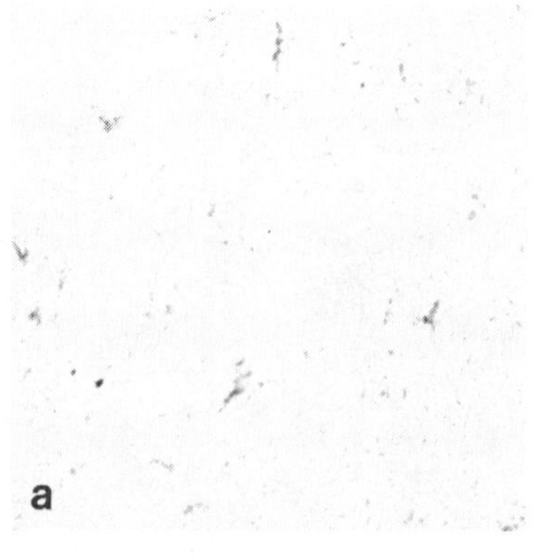

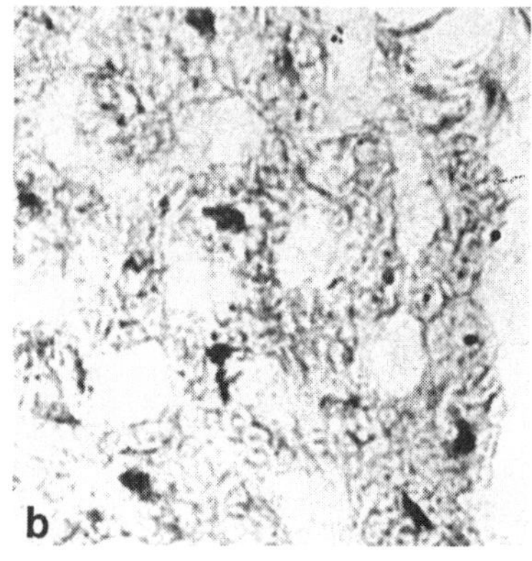

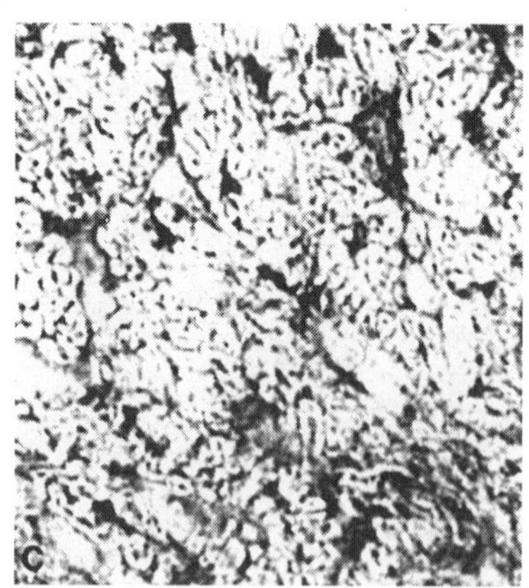

Fig. 7. Effect of probe concentration. Frozen section of adult rabbit ventricle hybridized *in situ* with various concentrations of a myosin heavy chain cRNA probe: (a) no probe, (b) 1 ng/µl, (c) 10 ng/µl. Sections were treated with 20 µg/ml RNase and washed extensively before detection of hybridized biotinylated riboprobe with streptavidin alkaline phosphatase. Increase in probe concentration gives a corresponding increase in hybridization until a maximum is reached (b and c). The choice of optimal probe concentration is determined as the minimum probe at which good hybridization results, typically in the 1 ng/µl range. Magnification X600.

Effect of RNase Concentration for cRNA and mRNA

Nucleotides bind non-specifically to proteins and structural components in sectioned tissue. Unhybridized DNA or RNA probes must be removed by extensive washes so that the signal is a true indicator of endogenous mRNA content. RNA probes have the advantage that unhybridized probe can be removed by RNase A which degrades single-stranded RNA but leaves the double-stranded RNA/RNA hybrid intact. The choice of buffer wash times and RNase A concentration are made empirically to remove non-specific nucleotide binding (Fig. 8). The mRNA serves as the control since it does not hybridize and can be selectively removed by RNase A (Fig. 8 a, b, c). In contrast, cRNA forms a stable hybrid that is not removed by increasing concentration of RNase A (Fig. 8 d, e, f). Under the conditions used here 20 ng/µl RNase removes non-specifically bound nucleotide and decreases background signal.

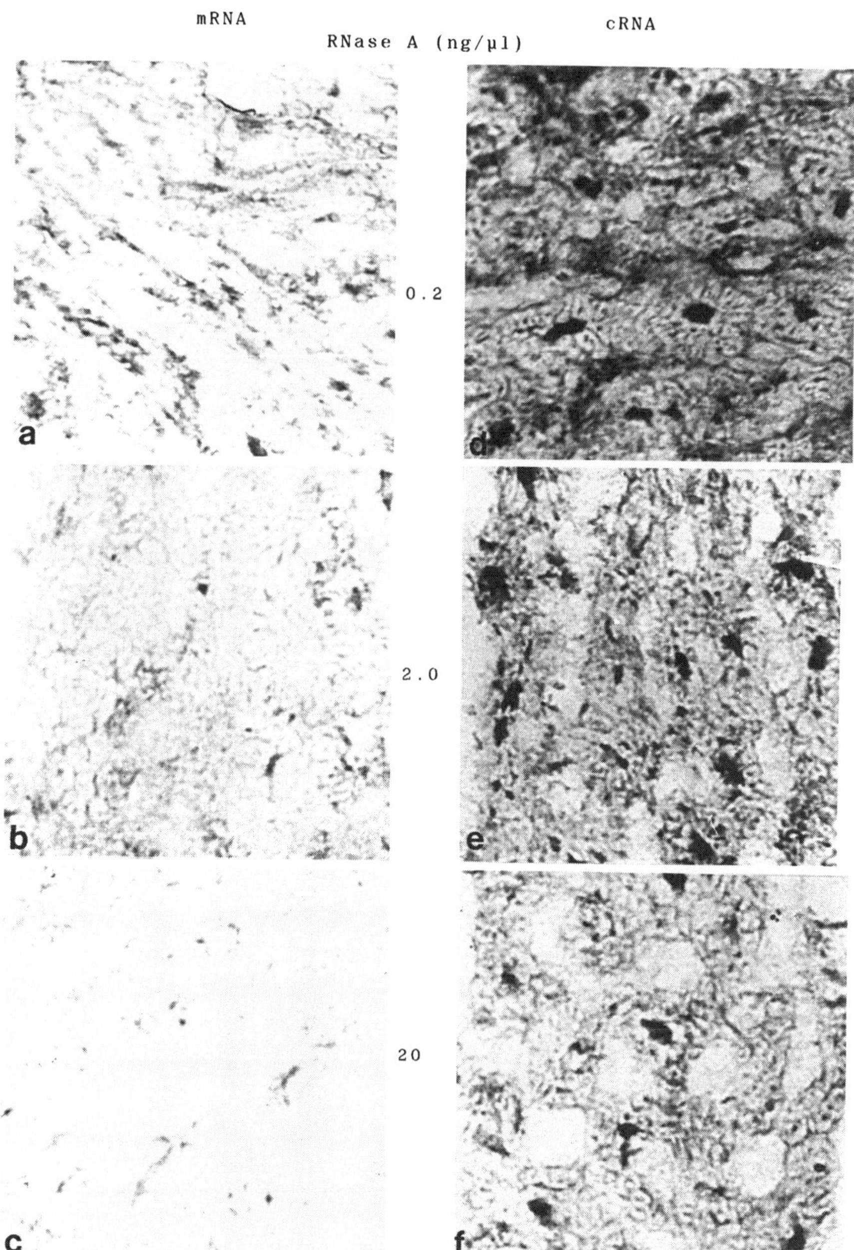

Fig. 8. Effect of RNase A concentration. Frozen sections of rabbit ventricle hybridized with mRNA (left panels) or cRNA (right panels) at probe concentration of 1 ng/µl and RNase concentrations as indicated. Note that the mRNA probe can be removed by increasing the RNase A but the hybridized cRNA probe remains in the tissue and is detected. Mag. X600.

Subcellular Localization of MHC mRNA

Adult rabbit ventricle has been successfully frozen, fixed, hybridized, and detected histochemically for the distribution of myosin heavy chain mRNA within the cells. The pattern of MHC mRNA distribution within the cell can be seen at subcellular resolutions with light microscopy. The MHC mRNA in the cardiac myocytes produce a staining pattern of dense nuclei, radial spokes in cross section through myocytes, and striations in longitudinal sections. The specificity of the cRNA probe, the structural quality of the tissue, and the spatial resolution of the reaction product are all now acceptable. The questions of where the MHC mRNA is and how this pattern relates to the transcriptional and translational state of the cell can now be approached.

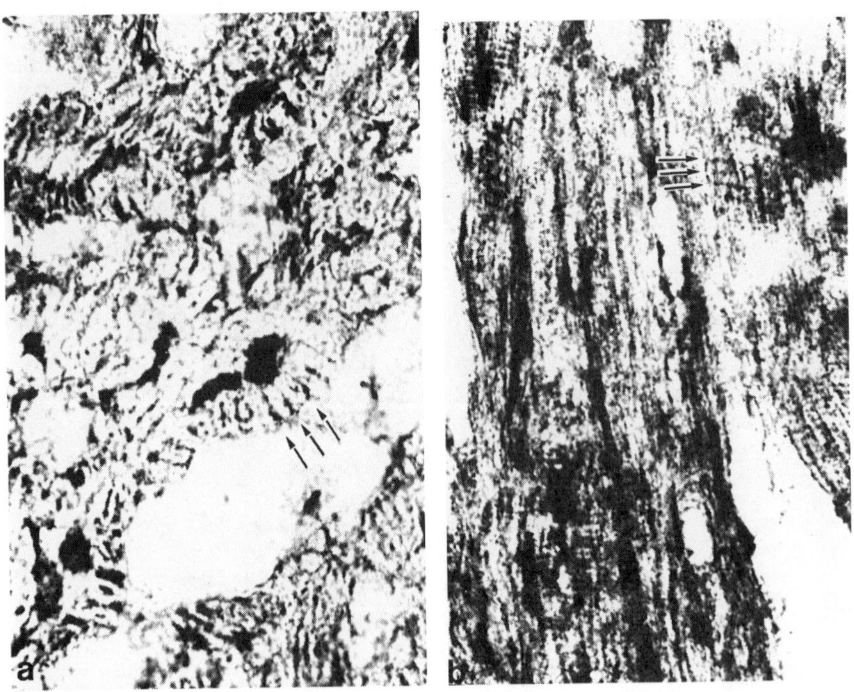

Fig 9. **In situ hybridization of myosin mRNA in adult rabbit ventricle.** Tissue hybridized to show the distribution of MHC mRNA in transversely (a) and longitudinally (b) sectioned cells. Arrows point to radial spokes in (a) and sarcomeric repeats in (b). Magnification X950.

In situ hybridization with non-isotopic biotin labelled riboprobe provides the ability to spatially locate mRNA species within the cell. The level of resolution attainable with enzymatic detection systems shows subcellular distributions and structural associations which merit further investigation. There is growing evidence for post-transcriptional regulation of gene expression in the cytoplasm and it is expected that mRNA distribution and interaction with other cellular components is important to these events. Myosin expression in cardiac myocytes provides an excellent model for these studies: myosin is highly expressed; rapid changes in isomyosins can be induced; and cardiac muscle has a highly organized cytoplasmic matrix in which mRNAs and their associated proteins exist.

SUMMARY

This chapter reviews a technique for *in situ* hybridization of myosin heavy chain mRNA in frozen sections of cardiac tissue. Production of biotin-labeled RNA probes (riboprobes) for *in situ* and filter hybridization is explained. Optimized protocols for fixation of frozen sections of muscle and hybridization of mRNAs are given. Detection of biotinylated riboprobes for light microscopy is done with streptavidin-alkaline phosphatase. The choice of appropriate controls for correct interpretation of endogenous mRNA are discussed. Results show the specific hybridization of myosin mRNA by a cRNA probe proven by the hybrids resistance to ribonuclease. A specific pattern of subcellular distribution of myosin mRNAs is observed in cardiac myocytes.

ACKNOWLEDGMENTS

This work was supported by grants from the American Heart Association and NIH HL-35728. DJD is supported by NIH training grant HL-07320.

REFERENCES

1. H.A. John, M.L. Birnstiel, and K.W. Jones. Nature 223, 582-587 (1969).
2. H.A. John, M. Patrinou-Georgoulas, and K.W. Jones. Cell 12, 501-508 (1977).
3. R.H. Singer and D.C. Ward. Proc. Natl. Acad. Sci., USA 79, 7331-7335 (1982).
4. J.B. Lawrence and R.H. Singer. Nucl. Acids Res., 13, 1777-1799 (1985).
5. J.B. Lawrence and R.H. Singer. Cell 45, 407-415 (1986).
6. R.H. Singer, J.B. Lawrence, and C. Villnave. BioTechniques 4, 230-250 (1986).
7. D.A. Melton, P.A. Krieg, M.R. Rebagliati, T. Maniatis, K. Zinn, and M.R. Green. Nucl. Acid Res. 12, 7035-7056 (1984).
8. P.R. Langer, A.A. Waldrop, and D.C. Ward. Proc. Natl. Acad. Sci., USA 78, 6633-6637 (1981).
9. K.H. Cox, D.V. DeLeon, L.M. Angerer, and R.C. Angerer. Develop. Biol. 101, 485-502 (1984).

10. D.A. Lynn, L.M. Angerer, A.M. Bruskin, W.H. Klein, and Angerer. Proc. Natl. Acad. Sci., USA 80, 2656-2660 (1983).
11. H. Hoefler, H. Childers, M.R. Montminy, R.M. Lechan, R.H. Goodman, and H.J. Wolfe. Histochem. J. 18, 597-604 (1986).
12. D.J. Dix and B.R. Eisenberg. J.Cell Biol. abstract (1987).
13. B.R. Eisenberg, D.J. Dix, and Z. Lin. Anat. Rec. 218, 39a-40a (1987).
14. A.M. Sinha, P.K. Umeda, C.J. Kavinsky, C. Rajamanickam, H.J. Hsu, S. Jakovcic, and M. Rabinowitz. Proc. Natl. Acad. Sci., USA 79, 5847-5851 (1982).
15. K. Struhl. BioTechniques 3, 452-453 (1985).
16. D. Hanahan in: DNA Cloning: A Practical Approach, D.M. Glover, ed. (IRL Press, Oxford 1985) pp. 109-135.
17. T. Maniatis, E.F. Fritsch, and J. Sambrook, Molecular Cloning: A Laboratory Manual (Cold Spring Harbor Laboratory, 1982).
18. L.M. Angerer and R.C. Angerer. Nucl. Acids Res. 9, 2819-2840 (1981).
19. H.C. Towle, C.N. Mariash, and J.H. Oppenheimer. Biochem. 19, 579-585 (1980).
20. P.S. Thomas. Proc. Natl. Acad. Sci., USA 77, 5201-5205 (1980).
21. M.A. Williams, Autoradiography and Immunocytochemistry (North-Holland Publ. Co., Amsterdam 1977).
22. R.M. Buckland. Nature 320, 557-558 (1986).
23. H.D. Webster, L. Lamperth, J.T. Favilla, G. Lemke, D. Tesin, and L. Manuelidis. Histochem. 86, 441-444 (1987).
24. D.J. Brigati, D. Myerson, J.J. Leary, B. Spalholz, S.Z. Travis, C.K.Y. Fong, G.D. Hsiung, and D.C. Ward. Virology 126, 32-50 (1983).
25. G.H. Smith, P.J. Douherty, R.B. Stead, C.M. Gorman, D.E. Graham, and B.H. Howard. Analyt. Biochem. 156, 17-24 (1986).
26. P. Liesi, J.P. Julien, P. Vilja, F. Grosveld, and L. Rechardt. J. Histochem. Cytochem. 34, 923-926 (1986).
27. G.V. Childs. Amer. J. Anat. 175, 125-289 (1986).

Analysis of Muscle Protein Expression with Monoclonal Antibodies and cDNA Probes.

Naoji Toyota, G. Raman, Arlene Sanchez, Joseph Bisaha, Steven Wylie, Rachel Rempel and David Bader

Department of Cell Biology and Anatomy
Cornell University Medical College
New York, New York 10021

INTRODUCTION

While it has long been known that atrial, ventricular and conduction system (CS) myocytes of the adult heart vary in their structure and function, little is known about the generation of these myocyte cell lineages during cardiac myogenesis. Recent studies from our laboratory [1,2,8,16] and from other groups [3,4] have shown that the diversification of these myocyte populations occurs early during heart development (stage 15 in the chick embryo). Our goal is to understand the cellular and molecular mechanisms by which cardiac myocyte determination and diversification are acheived. To examine these processes, we are presented with special problems. Among these are the small amount of material available for analysis due to the early emergence of specific myocyte types and the absence of cell lines with specific cardiogenic potential. To study the initial determination and diversification of cardiac myocytes, we have used the myosin heavy chain (MHC) as a marker of atrial, ventricular, and CS myocytes. The work of several groups has shown the tissue specific distribution of MHCs in myocytes of the adult heart [5-7]. We have isolated monoclonal antibodies (McAb) and cDNAs for the major MHCs in the heart as molecular markers of specific myocyte types. With these probes we have been able to follow specific cell lineages during cardiac myogenesis in vivo and in vitro, where complex cellular and developmental processes occur concurrently. Further, we have been attempting to clone atrial and ventricular specific transcripts in an effort to obtain new markers for these myocyte lineages.

In this review we describe the application of immunochemical techniques to the analysis of gene expression in the developing heart. Specifically, we will present our protocols for the analysis of MHC expression in cardiac myocytes and the screening of GT11 cDNA libraries with anti-myosin McAbs. In addition, we will present differential hybridization protocols which we are currently using to identify atrial and ventricular specific clones.

METHODS

Monoclonal antibodies used in this study. The cloning and characterization of the McAbs used here has been published elsewhere [1,2,9,10]. Their specific cross-reactivities in the heart are presented in TABLE I.

Biology of Isolated Adult Cardiac Myocytes
William A. Clark, Robert S. Decker, and Thomas K. Borg, Editors

TABLE I

	Atrial MHC	Ventricular MHC	CS MHC
MF20	+	+	+
B1	+	-	-
A19	-	+	-
ALD58	-	-	+

McAbs were affinity purified from conditioned cell culture media on columns of Sepharose 4B conjugated with specific myosins. Affinity columns were produced using the manufacturer's instructions (Pharmacia Fine Chemicals, Piscataway, N.J.) at 10mgs protein/ml of beads. After application of the supernatants to the columns, unbound proteins were washed from the beads with TBS (10mM Tris, pH 7.4, 150mM NaCl) and the affinity bound antibodies were eluted with 0.2M glycine (pH 2.2) into equal volumns of 0.2M Tris (pH 8.0). Fractions containing protein were dialyzed against TBS at 4°C and later stored at -20°C. When direct labelling of McAbs was desired, antibodies still bound to the myosin column (1ml of beads) were equilibrated with 150mM Na_2HPO_4 (pH 8.0). One ml of 10mg/ml TRITC or FITC (Molecular Probes, Junction City, OR) in 150mM Na_2HPO_4 (pH 8.0) was run into the column, the flow was stopped and the entire column placed on a rotator for 16 hours at 4°C in the dark. The column was then washed with TBS until no fluorochrome was found in the effluent. The affinity purified, directly labelled McAbs were eluted as noted above and the protein and fluorochrome to protein ratios determined according to [11]. Fluorochrome to protein ratios of 3-8:1 are preferable.

We have used these antibodies to study the initial expression of MHC in developing cardiac myocytes in vivo and in vitro using immunofluorescence microscopy, immunoblotting, and radioimmunoassay and to screen GT11 libraries. Each McAb we have used exhibits its own peculiarities in these assays. The general starting point for analysis of all anti-MHC antibodies employed in our laboratory is presented below. All procedures were performed at room temperature unless otherwise noted.

<u>Immunofluorescence Microsopy</u>

Cultured myocytes grown on collagen coated glass or plastic [2,10] were washed in ice cold TBS for 1 to 2 minutes with several changes and then fixed in ice cold 70% methanol for 1 to 2 minutes. The cells were again washed in TBS (2 to 3 washes; 2 minutes each) with a final wash with TBS containing 1% bovine serum albumin (BSA) for 10 minutes. The cultures were drained of liquid and reacted with fluorescently labelled McAb. We have found that noncompeting antibodies can be reacted with cells simultaneously. Affinity purified antibodies [1,2], labelled with TRITC or FITC were reacted at concentrations of 25-75ug/ml for 1 hour. The cells were then washed with TBS (3 to 5 washes; 2 minutes each) followed by distilled H2O (1 minute), and fixed in 4% formalin (5 minutes). We have found that such preparations are stable for approximately one month thereafter, increasing autofluorescence is detected on the FITC channel.

Immunoblotting

Standard gel electrophoresis followed by electrophoretic transfer (60 mA, 16 hours) to nitrocellulose paper according to Towbin et al [12] efficiently transfers 50-75% of MHC (10ug load of DEAE purified myosin) in 5-7.5% acrylamide gels. This is judged by Coomassie blue staining of gels after transfer. Three factors which affect MHC transfer and later reactivity of MHC with McAbs are: 1) 0.1% SDS in the transfer buffer is essential for efficient transfer; 2) acrylamide concentrations $>7.5\%$ in the gels decreases transfer of MHC and; 3) blots stored for more than one month may lose antigenicity with certain McAbs. After transfer, nitrocellulose papers were dried and rehydrated in TBS. Non-specific protein binding was blocked by washing papers with 1%BSA in TBS for 30 minutes with constant shaking. The nitrocellulose paper was then reacted with McAb at 25-75ug/ml for 15-30 minutes followed by immediate washing with TBS (5 washes; 5 minutes/wash). ^{125}I labelled goat-anti-mouse IgG (Cappel Laboratories, Cochranville, PA; prepared as [13]) was applied in a minimal volume at 10^6cpm/ml for 15 minutes. Immediate and extensive washing in TBS is essential to reduce background. Washes should be monitored for radioactivity until no counts remain in the washes. During the procedure, papers should never be allowed to dry. Nitrocellulose papers were finally dried and used to expose X-ray films with or without enhancing screens. Many McAbs which react with MHC in RIA, immunofluorescence microscopy and/or immunoprecipitation do not react with MHC after gel electrophoresis and transfer.

Solid phase radioimmunoassay

A description of myosin preparations from cultured cardiac myocytes is given. For myosin preparations from intact tissues, references are cited below. Seven day embryonic atrial and ventricular cultures plated at an initial density of 2.5×10^2 cells/mm^2 and grown for 7 days yield approximately 100ugs of partially purified myosin using the following protocol. (Note: This preparation is carried out in a cold room with ice cold solutions.) Cultures were washed in 3 changes of TBS and scraped in 10ml of TBS with 0.5% Triton X-100. The 10ml of cells/TBS/0.5% Triton was carried through all dishes. Dishes were then washed with an additional 10ml of TBS/0.5% Triton and after pooling the washes, the extract was centrifuged at 10,000rpm in a Sorvall SS34 rotor for 10 minutes at 4ºC. The pellet was washed in 10ml TBS and recentrifuged. This cycle was repeated once. The resulting pellet was extracted in 500ul of 0.5M NaCl, 10mM Na_2HPO_4, 10mM NaH_2PO_4, pH 8.0 for 30 minutes. Extraction was terminated by centrifugation in a microfuge for 5 minutes and the supernatant dialyzed against dH20 overnight. The crude myosin was collected by centrifugation (microfuge; 5 minutes) and redissolved in 0.6M NaCl. For most of our purposes, this impure preparation is adequate. When purer samples are desired, the myosin solution is made 5mM ATP and 5mM $MgCl_2$ and spun in a Beckman Airfuge for 15 minutes at 30psi. The resulting supernatant was dialyzed overnight against dH'0, centrifuged in a microfuge for 5 minutes and redissolved in 0.6M NaCl. Preparation of DEAE purified myosin from adult atrial and ventricular tissues was carried out as described in Zhang et al [16]. All these myosin preparations can be stored at -20°C in 50% glycerol. In our standard RIA (e.g. screening new antibodies), 1ug of protein in 25ul of 0.6M NaCl or 25 ul of each DEAE column fraction were applied to polyvinylchloride wells and air dried. Wells were washed with TBS (5 washes) with a final wash of TBS with 1%BSA. Forty ul of antibody solution was applied to the wells for 30 minutes after which the wells were subjected to 5 washes of TBS. Forty ul of ^{125}I labelled goat-anti-mouse antibody (10^6cpm/ml, prepared according to 13) were reacted with the preparation for 30 minutes followed by washing as stated above. Wells were cut out and counted in a gamma counter.

Screening GT11 cDNA Libraries with anti-MHC Monoclonal Antibodies

With the availability of cDNA expression vectors [14], it is possible to screen cDNA libraries with immunochemical probes. The following procedure has proved successful in the isolation of cDNA clones containing portions of transcripts or full length transcripts for troponin I, T and C [Toyota and Bader, manuscript in preparation] and ventricular MHC [Data presented here]. Ventricular and atrial GT10 and GT11 libraries were produced and characterized following standard procedures (Amersham, Arlington Heights, IL). Bacteria Y1088 and/or Y1090 were infected with GT11 for 30 minutes at 37°C, plated in LB top agarose containing 10mM $MgCl_2$ and grown at 37°C until plaques were first detected. 50mM isopropylthiogalactoside (IPTG) saturated and dried nitrocellulose filters were then applied to the plates for an additional 4 hours. Filters and the subjacent GT11 infected bacterial lawn were marked with asymmetric pinholes, removed, and washed with TBS with 0.5% Tween 20 (TBST; 10ml/100mm filter, 10 minutes/wash, 3 washes). TBST with 1% BSA (30 minutes) was used to block non-specific protein binding. Spent supernatants from hybridomas secreting anti-MHC antibodies (approximately 50ug/ml for McAb A19) were reacted with the filters for 16 hours at 4°C or 2 hours at room temperature, both with constant shaking.

The filters were then washed with TBST (3 washes; 10ml/wash) and reacted with HRP-labelled goat-anti-mouse (1:5000 dilution, Cappel Laboratories) for 1 hour at room temperature. After 3 washes with TBS (10ml/wash), the filters were reacted with diaminobenzidine (5mg/10ml) in 50mM Tris, pH 8.0 with fresh H_2O_2 (10ul/10ml of 30% stock). Positive plaques were identified as small brown circles (visible in 5 minutes) which match the periphery of the plaque. Interesting plaques were rescreened twice, phage DNA prepared [15] and the insert isolated after EcoR1 digestion.

Differential Hybridization of cDNA Libraries

Single strand atrial (At) and ventricular (Vt) cDNA were synthesized according to Natzle et al [20]. Reaction mixture contained: 50mM Tris-Cl (pH 8.3); 8mM MgCl; 30mM KCl; 0.5mM DTT; 2mM each dATP, dGTP, dTTP, 1.0ul human placental ribonuclease inhibitor (18U; Amersham), 40ug/ml oligo-dT (Collaborative Research, Lexington, Mass.), 5.0ul alpha-^{32}P-dCTP (3000 Ci/mmol, NEN), 8ug/ml polyA+ At or Vt RNA, 1.0ul Reverse Transcriptase (18U; Amersham) and adjusted to 20ul final volume with dH_2O. After incubation for 1.5 hours at 37°C 5ul of heat denatured salmon sperm DNA was added along with 12ul 7.5 M NH_4 HOAc (pH 7.5) and 90ul 100% ethanol and precipitated at -70°C for 30 min. cDNA was spun down, washed with 70% ethanol and redissolved in 97ul TE. mRNA was removed by adding 3ul 10N NaOH (0.3N final concentration) and incubated for 30 minutes at 37°C. The reaction was neutralized with 1.7ul glacial acetic acid (0.3M final concentration). The average length of cDNA was 1-2 Kb.

High frequency lysogeny (HFL) bacteria were infected with GT10 and plated in LB top agarose to yield a density of approximately 1000 plaques/150mm dish using standard techniques [15]. Transfer of DNA to GeneScreen Plus (NEN), prehybridization, hybridization and washing were done according to manufacturer's instructions. Two plaque lifts were taken from each plate (atrial or ventricular libraries) and probed with single strand cDNA from atrial and ventricular mRNA. Membranes were exposed to Kodak XAR film. Positive clones were identified by comparison between differentially probed membranes.

Interesting clones were isolated and rescreened twice. Large scale preparations of phage DNA were prepared and inserts subcloned into pUC 8 according to standard protocols [15].

Data are presented to show the characterization of one clone. Dot blot analysis was used to determine the tissue distribution of hybridizable message. 20ug of cardiac, fast skeletal and brain RNA were spotted onto GeneSreen (NEN). The 2.0Kb insert of one clone was gel purified for use as a probe on RNA dot blots. The probe was oligolabelled with ^{32}P dCTP according to the method of Feinberg and Vogelstein [21]. Prehybridization, hybridization, washing and autoradiography were done as per manufacturers instructions for GeneScreen (NEN).

Results and Discussion

Immunofluorescence microscopy. Double direct immunolabelling provides the easiest protocol for analysis of two different McAbs and, in addition, produces far less background than the indirect method. Problems arise when McAbs are insufficiently labelled or over labelled with fluorochrome. Fluorochrome to protein ratios lower than 3:1 are too low to provide adequate signal using standard epifluorescence microscopy. Ratios greater than 8:1 result in increased background presumably due to the denaturation of the IgG and its nonspecific interaction with the preparation. Increased time of reaction did not increase the signal and often increased the background. Finally, the length of time, concentration and nature of initial fixative can greatly alter the affinity of individual McAbs for their antigen. Figure 1 shows a typical atrial culture from a 7 day embryo after 7 days in culture. Three cells are seen in phase microscopy, two of which are cardiac myocytes. McAb MF20 recognizes all sarcomeric MHC, but not nonmuscle MHC, and thus serves as a positive indicator of muscle. The atrial specific antibody B1 reacts with only one of the two myocytes. Using this technique, we have been able to monitor fluctuations in MHC expression during cardiac myogenesis in vitro [2,8].

Figure 1

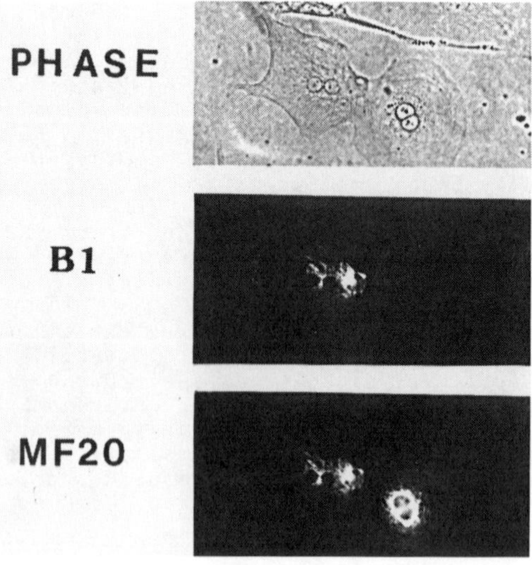

Immunoblotting. The reaction of anti-MHC McAbs with myosin after gel electrophoresis and transfer to nitrocellulose is highly variable. Many of our McAbs which are highly reactive with MHC in radioimmunoassay or in permeabilized cells do not react with immunoblots. Other McAbs non-reactive with blotted MHC show great affinity for transfered chymotryptic rod [data not shown]. In addition, McAbs known to react with two different MHC isoforms sometimes bind one MHC in immunoblots and not the other heavy chain. In other words, each anti-MHC McAb used in immunoblots must be characterized with reference to other immunochemical analyses. Our protocol uses incubation times much shorter than others presented in the literature. The time course of first and second antibody binding shows that greater than 50% of antibody binding occurs during the first 15 minutes of incubation under our experimental conditions. Thus, we have chosen short incubation times to limit background. Figure 2a shows the reaction of A19 with atrial and ventricular myosin. This antibody is highly reactive with ventricular MHC and shows only slight binding with atrial MHC on long film exposures. We have found that McAbs and polyclonal antibodies highly reactive in immunoblots provide the best probes for screening GT11 libraries.

Figure 2

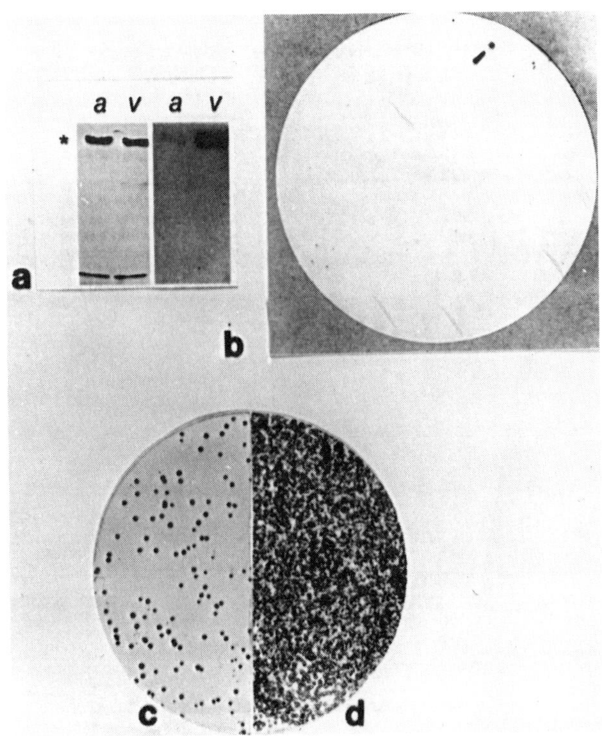

Solid Phase Radioimmunoassay. We have used RIA analysis to characterize MHC expression in various experimental systems. The binding of McAb to antigen appears to be independent of contaminating proteins as addition of non-reactive myofibrils to the first antibody reaction does not alter the affinity of the four McAbs for their antigens. Figure 3 shows the reaction of atrial MHC specific B1, ventricular MHC specific A19 and an anti C protein antibody MF1 with proteins from a ventricular myosin preparation separated by DEAE ion exchange chromatography. In this preparation, contaminating myofibrillar proteins are not retained by the column and are present in the void volume while myosin is eluted by the linear KCl gradient [17]. RIA analysis shows that MF1 reacts only with proteins in the void volume while A19 only binds fractions containing myosin. B1 binding is not detected in this ventricular myosin preparation. McAbs which do not react in immunoblots can be assayed for their specificity to myosin in this way. Further characterization of such anti-MHC antibodies requires the separation of light and heavy chains [18] and their reaction in RIA with the purified myosin subunits.

Figure 3

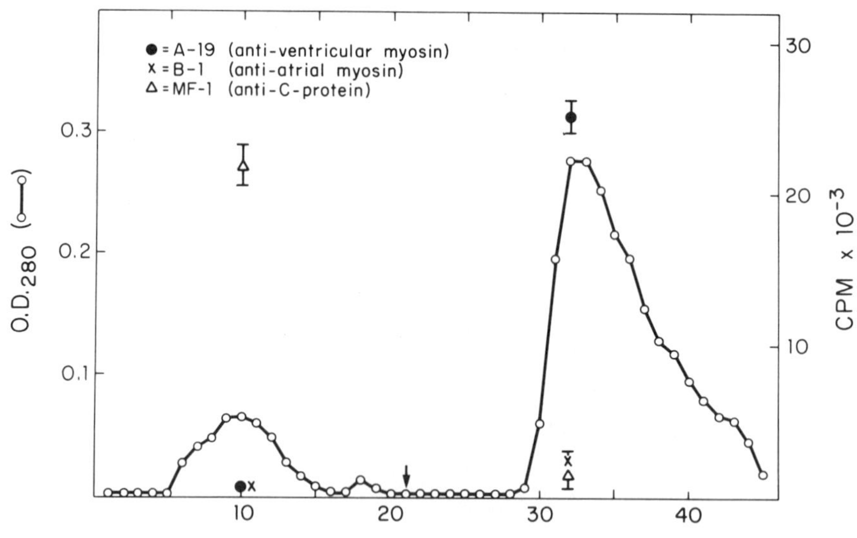

Screening GT11 cDNA Libraries with anti-MHC Monoclonal Antibodies. We have successfully screened expression vector libraries with mono- and poly- clonal antibodies. In screening MHC clones with McAbs, we have found it important that the McAb react with essentially denatured proteins on nitrocellulose paper and that the epitope on the MHC reside near the carboxyl terminus (The latter criterion is of course due to the priming of reverse transcription from the 3' end of the message.). Since the rod portion of the MHC is not thought to be extensively modified after translation, the binding of anti-rod antibodies is not likely to be dependent on post-translational modifications of the peptide. Thus, unmodified fusion peptides produced in bacterial hosts pose no problem to antibody binding. Figure 2 shows the isolation of a ventricular MHC cDNA using A19 as the probe. Approximately 104 plaques were screened in figure 3b and the fusion peptide of one clone was shown to react strongly (arrow). The plaque was identified, recloned twice (Fig. 2c and d), and a 2.0 Kb insert encoding MHC isolated using standard technology. The characterization of this MHC clone (GT/VMHC4.2) will be presented elsewhere. MF20 does not react with the fusion peptide of GT/VMHC4.2 even though this McAb binds ventricular MHC. An electron micrograph depicting the site of MF20 binding on the myosin molecule is presented in figure 4. This epitope is approximately 92nm from the end of the rod which, considering the three dimensional structure of the molecule [19], is approximately 629 amino acids from the carboxyl terminus. With the addition of 100-150 base pairs as an average length of the MHC nontranslated region and 25-50 bases for the poly A tail, this epitope is anticipated to encoded by sequences 5' to a 2.0 Kb cDNA. Thus, one should not expect MF20 to react with the fusion peptide of GT/VMHC4.2. For this reason, while MF20 has proven to be the McAb with the strongest reactivity in immunoblots, its usefulness in obtaining MHC clones from expression vector libraries has been somewhat limited.

Figure 4

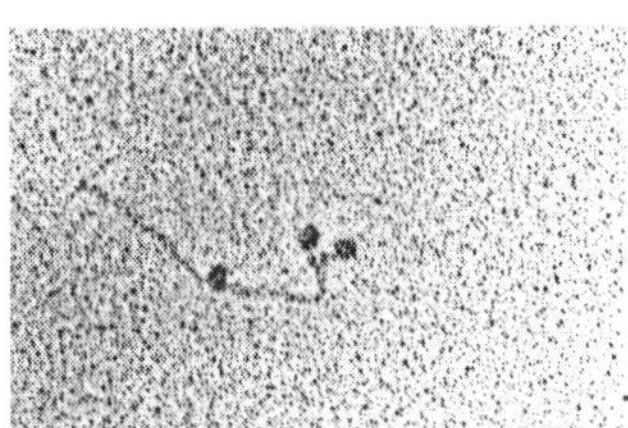

MF20 is seen as density at the mid-portion of the rod.

Differential screening of cDNA Libraries. Tissue specific transcripts in atrial and ventricular cDNA libraries were probed for by a differential hybridization technique. GT10 cDNA libraries were screened with cDNA produced from atrial and ventricular poly A+ RNA, positive clones were analyzed and compared. Approximately 90% of the positive plaques in the ventricular library were common to filters probed with At and Vt cDNA, therefore approximately 10% of the positive plaques screened were potentially unique under these experimental conditions. Four clones with potential specificity to the ventricle have been obtained. One of these clones has been shown by RNA dot blots to be muscle specific while not being truly ventricular specific (Figure 5). Sequence analysis of the 3' end of this cDNA has shown this polyadenylated transcript to be unlike any muscle specific gene product yet isolated (data not shown). Thus, this clone is of potential use in studying both cardiac and skeletal muscle lineage determination as it may represent a new muscle specific marker.

Using this approach, we hope to generate new non-myofibrillar markers for atrial and ventricular myocytes in order to study the determination and diversification of cardiac myocytes during embryogenesis.

Figure 5

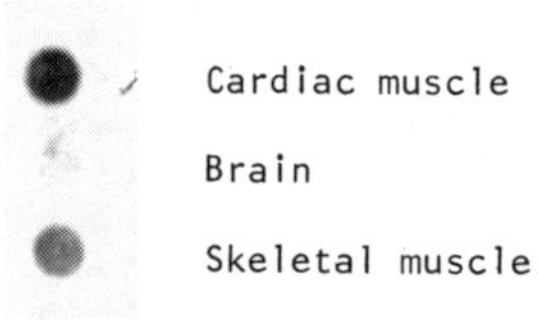

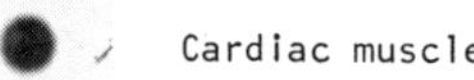

Summary

We have presented our basic protocols for the immunochemical analysis of muscle protein expression and the screening of expression vector libraries with anti-MHC McAbs. In addition, our techniques for differential screening of cDNA libraries were summarized. This was done in the hopes that other investigators may use them to their advantage and improve upon them.

Acknowledgements

We would like to thank Jim Dennis and Donald Fischman for the immunoelectron microscopic localization of the MF20 epitope. This work was supported by grants from the NIH (HL35776 and 37675) and the New York Heart Association to D.B. Dr. Bader was an Andrew W. Mellon Teacher-Scientist during time of this work. Dr. Raman is a recipient of a Norman and Rosita Winston Foundation Fellowship in Biomedical Research.

References

1. Gonzalez-Sanchez, A. and Bader, D. Develop. Biol. 103:151-158. 1984.
2. Gonzalez-Sanchez, A. and Bader, D. J. Cell Biol. 100:270-275. 1985
3. Sweeney, L., Manasek, F., and Zak, R. Circ. Res. 61:287-294. 1987.
4. Kulakowsky, R.R. Biophys. J. 47:311(abstract). 1985.
5. Sartore, S., Pierobon-Bormiolli, S. and Schiaffino, S. Nature 274:82-83. 1978.
6. Hoh, J.F.Y., McGrath, P.A., Hale, P.T. J. Cell. Molec. Cardiol. 10:1053-1076. 1978.
7. Chizzonite, R.A., Everett, A.W., Clark, W.A., Jakovcic, S. Rubinowitz, M. and Zak, R. J. Biol. Chem. 257:2056-2067. 1982.
8. Zadeh, B.J., Gonzalez-Sanchez, A., Fischman, D.A., and Bader, D.M. Develop. Biol. 115:204-214. 1986.
9. Bader, D., Masaki, T., and Fischman, D.A. J. Cell Biol. 95:763-770. 1982
10. Shafiq, S.A., Shimizu, T., and Fischman, D.A. Muscle and Nerve 7:380-387. 1984
11. Weir, D.M. Handbook of Experimental Immunology. Blackwell, Oxford. 1978.
12. Towbin,H., Stahelin, T., Gordon, J. PNAS. 76:4350-4353. 1979.
13. Reinach, F.C. and Fischman, D.A. J. Molec. Biol. 181:411-422. 1985.
14. Young, R.A. and Davis, R.W. PNAS. 80:1194-1198. 1983.
15. Maniatis, T, Fritsch, E.F., and Sambrook, J. Molecular Cloning. Cold Spring Harbor Laboratory, Cold Spring Harbor. NY
16. Zhang, Y., Shafiq, S.A., and Bader, D. J.Cell Biol. 102:1480-1484. 1986.
17. Richards, E.G., Chung, G.S., Menzel, D.B., and Olcott, H.S. Biochem.6:528-540. 1967.
18. Wagner, P.D. J. Biol. Chem. 256:2493-2498.
19. McLachlan, A.D. Ann. Rev. Biophys. Bioeng. 13:167-189. 1984.
20. Natzle, J.E., Hammonds, A.S., Fristrom, J.W. J. Biol. Chem. 261:5575-5583. 1986.
21. Feinberg, A. and Vogelstein, B. Anal. Biochem. 132:6-13. 1983.

MEASUREMENT AND INTERPRETATION OF CONTRACTION IN ISOLATED CARDIAC CELLS

JOHN W. KRUEGER
The Albert Einstein College of Medicine
1300 Morris Park Avenue
Bronx, N.Y. 10461

TABLE OF CONTENTS:

INTRODUCTION

The isolation of single cardiac cells with physiologic properties provides an opportunity to view the fundamental basis of cardiac function with unusual clarity. Since the myocytes are electrically coupled in the ventricle, each cell necessarily participates in the control of the heart beat. Inasmuch as each cell constitutes a physiologically complete unit, their uniform contraction reveals information about the nature of the pathways by which the cell's membranes influence contraction, the contractile behavior of the sarcomere, and a means by which extracellular factors could influence the function of the cell. Uniform shortening in the isolated cell frees the investigator from the uncertainties of heterogeneity which exist in intact tissue, but their nonuniform behavior also reveals important information. Contraction reflects the control of calcium ion around the sarcomere. Thus localized shortening within the cell reveals intracellular calcium movements, as well as situations when fluctuations of this ion may promote irregular activity of the heart. The nonuniform motions between sarcomeres may also reveal information about the mechanical nature of their interconnections. Thus properties of the cytoskeleton and its contribution to cardiac function can be examined.

This chapter focuses on the measurement of contraction in single myocytes which are isolated by enzymes and whose electrical membranes are intact. Consideration is limited to mammalian heart cells, as others have reviewed studies of contraction in amphibian myocytes [1]. The nature of shortening will be emphasized because only a few studies have characterized contractile tension in the electrically excitable cell [2,3]. A second emphasis here is on the relationship of contractile behavior in the isolated cell to that observed in intact muscle, both of which are stimulated electrically. As the experimental conditions are similar, this comparison presumably serves as a means of evaluating i) the status of the isolated cells and ii) other factors which physically influence cardiac function. Indeed, since contraction is the final step in a complex pathway it provides a most sensitive index of the state of the cell.

Biology of Isolated Adult Cardiac Myocytes
William A. Clark, Robert S. Decker, and Thomas K. Borg, Editors

However, this 'blessing' is a challenge in disguise!

MEASUREMENT OF CONTRACTILE SHORTENING IN UNATTACHED CELLS

The simplest method for detection of contraction of isolated cells relies on changes in the intensity of light transmitted through the cell during shortening [4]. The related techniques such as monitoring changes in cellular light scattering/optical density [5] or transparency by photodiodes [6,7] are awkward to quantify in terms of actual shortening. Virtually all of these methods rely ultimately on changes in the cell's optical properties which are due to its thickening rather than its force of contraction. Some of the difficulties are well recognized and have been alluded to in the past reports [8]; the chief being the absence of any simple physical relationship between shortening and optical scattering so that the system must be calibrated for each cell.

These approaches suffice for many applications where the precise details of sarcomere shortening are not required. However, photometric methods assume that light scattering depends only on cell length, irrespective of time in the contractile cycle. Moreover, the accuracy of photometric techniques will depend on the distribution of light in the specimen, and this is a function of its shape, its edge, and the particular type of microscopy used. Similar considerations apply to approaches in which the displacement of the edge of the cell is treated like the movement of an optical shutter.

Measurement of the dynamics of the sarcomere requires precise and rapid detection of the cell's structure. I review three independent methods which are based upon the self-scanned, linear array of photodidodes. The added advantage of direct measurement is that quantitative details of contraction in the isolated cell can be related more easily to studies in intact cardiac muscle.

Measurement of Sarcomere Length by Diffraction

As the smallest unit in the heart in which the pathways of activation and control are present, the isolated myocyte constitutes an ideal model by which to assess the microscopic nature of myofilament sliding. Ideally, we would like to measure the motions between the myofilaments, but individual thin and thick filaments can not be resolved with the light microscope. Fortunately, by virtue of their uniform lengths and their lateral alignment, the repeating arrays of myofilaments give to the cardiac cell its characteristic striated appearance. Since striations impart to the cell the properties of a diffraction grating, the separation of light in its diffraction pattern can be related to the predominant sarcomere length in the isolated cell. In practice, the light diffracted by the cell is collected by a high aperture microscope lens, in which case the colored diffraction pattern is easily seen by removing the eyepiece. If the cell is illuminated by a precise wavelength which is produced by a low power laser, its striations cause the diffracted light to interfere at precise angles, as shown in Figure 1.

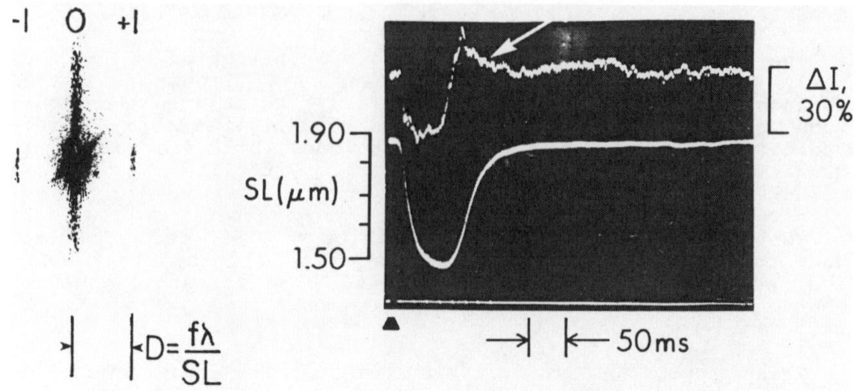

FIG. 1 (Left) Light diffraction pattern from a single cell. The separation between each order, D, is inversely proportional to sarcomere length, SL, and directly proportional to the wavelength of the laser, , and the focal length, f, of the lens system. (Right) Contractile changes in sarcomere length and first order intensity in the diffraction pattern. Rat myocyte.

Direct measurement of sarcomere length with precision and high speed requires a suitable way of detecting the position of the diffracted light. Usually the pattern of light occurring at the lens' rear focal plane is projected onto one of two types of sensors, either a barrier (i.e., 'lateral effect') photodiode or a linear array of photodiodes. Since the position of the diffracted light can be detected electronically, analogue circuits can be employed which rapidly compute sarcomere length during contraction [9]. With the single barrier photodiode, a photocurrent is generated where the light strikes the device; because its resistance is distributed, the relative amounts of current measured at the opposite sides of the barrier diode reveals the location of light. Thus, the position of the diffracted light can be determined instantaneously with relatively straightforward and inexpensive electronic circuits [9]. One advantage is that the intensity of the diffracted light is also available as the sum of the two photocurrents.

Detection of diffracted light position with the self-scanned linear array of photodiodes is considerably more involved, but it has one significant advantage in that the appearance of the diffracted light is immediately available. In the simplest terms, the video signal representing the profile of the first order diffracted light is integrated with each scan of the array. The total intensity of the integrated video signal is sampled and held for comparison to the next scan. The position on the array where the integrated intensity is equivalent to one half the value of the previous scan corresponds to the median position of the light [9]. In principle sarcomere length can be determined very rapidly, for the array can be scanned 2000 to 4000s. The speed at which the array can be scanned is enhanced by maximizing the amount of light striking its individual elements. So little light is available from the small amount of diffracting material in the single cardiac cell that some attention to the selection of the both the array and the cell proves worthwhile. The intensity in the diffraction pattern is proportional to its projected area: By enabling the scale of diffraction pattern to be reduced, arrays in which contiguous elements are sampled are the most practical. Cells which are wider have more diffracting elements and give the brightest diffraction patterns.

The unique advantage of the isolated cardiac cell is that it constitutes a discrete, easily defined population of sarcomeres. The cardiac cell is smaller than the area illuminated by the laser beam. Thus the population of sarcomeres sampled by diffraction remains constant with shortening so that the microscopic nature of myofilament sliding can be assessed [10]. For example, it has been suggested that striated muscle shortens by a series of small steps, possibly related to incremental changes in the lengths of some structural component of the sarcomere [11]. However, diffraction shows convincingly that the sarcomere shortens and relengthens smoothly in the unattached heart cell. This shows also that the structural elements which resist shortening and relengthen the heart cell constitute a mechanical continuum.

The use of the lens to collect and focus the light diffracted by the cell provides the Fraunhofer diffraction pattern. Conceptually, the pattern of light provides <u>some</u> of the information contained in the two-dimensional Fourier transform of the striated pattern of the cell. This provides some mathematical convenience to be applied to the diffraction analysis of cell structure. For example, one puzzling feature of cardiac sarcomere shortening is revealed by diffraction at very short sarcomere lengths. If the cell were a simple grating, then we would expect the intensity of the light to be uniquely related to sarcomere length. Yet the intensity of the diffracted light is always higher during relaxation phase, and it does not decrease as much as predicted when the cardiac sarcomere shortens to the known length of the thick filament [10]. However, the Fourier optical approach does not address the process by which sarcomeres are sampled by the diffraction method, since after all, the cell represents a grating in three dimensions rather than two. Fourier optics permit Illumination of the cell by a cone of light. This enhances sampling by diffraction, since the dependence upon a unique angle of incident light in volume diffraction [12] can then minimized. The contribution to the diffraction pattern is greatest from sarcomeres which are well ordered. While very small changes in the position of diffracted light can be detected, i.e., values typically equivalent to 0.25% the length of the sarcomere, these other factors will mitigate the certainty to which greater precision can be applied to the details of sarcomere motion.

The diffraction method I've described is designed to follow contraction rapidly in a single cell. Consequently it's elaborate insofar as the requirement for a suitable sensor with the requisite electronics and, for convenience, a microscope to visualize the cell. However, diffraction methods need not be complicated. Sarcomere length can be surveyed in large populations of heart cells using only a laser, a simple lens, and a ruler as shown in Figure 2. The cells settle to lie parallel to the bottom of the experimental chamber so that their long axes orient in two dimensions. Thus, the diffracted light occurs as a ring rather than discrete lines. The lens collects and focuses the light diffracted by the sample, so that the width of the incident beam no longer impairs the sharpness of the diffracted light.

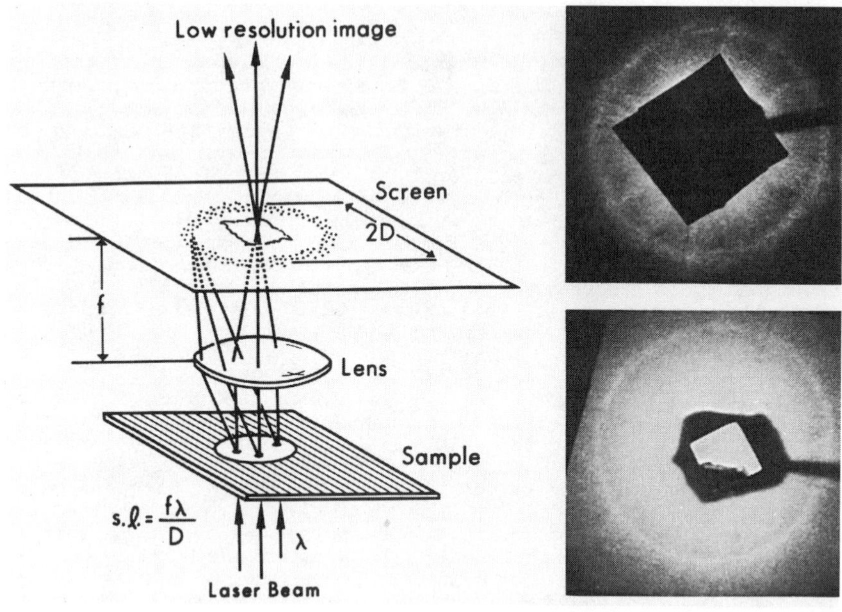

Fig. 2. (Left) A simple system for using diffraction to survey sarcomere length in populations of isolated heart cells. The mathematical symbols are the same as in figure 1. (Right) The annular diffraction patterns obtained from samples of (Top) prefixed myocardial fragments from the canine right ventricular free wall epicardium (SL = 2.24 um) and (Bottom) living, intact cells enzymatically isolated from rat myocardium (SL = 1.97 um). A barrier blocks the nondiffracted light to facilitate photography.

This inexpensive diffraction method can be used to circumvent the tedious process of microscopic measurement of many cells to obtain an average value for sarcomere length. The method constitutes a very simple way to study those factors which might influence sarcomere length in the various regions of the heart or in the isolated cell population. Self scanned photodiode arrays are made which have circular geometries so that synchronized contractions could be characterised in large samples with the circuit methods that I've already described.

Diffraction permits rapid measurement of sarcomere length with great precision in uniformly shortening intact cells, and it enables comparison of sarcomere behavior in muscle and in cells. Diffraction is not suitable for directly activated, permealized heart cells, because the pattern of the striations reverses at short lengths as predicted from the sliding filament mechanism [13]. Consequently the intensity of first order diffracted light becomes very weak. (For some reason, this does not occur in intact cells [10]!) Light scattering from micropipets or microtools make application of the diffraction technique difficult with electrophysiological studies. Moreover, it is inconvenient (and sometimes unpleasant!) to directly observe cells which are illuminated by laser light.

Measurement of Cell Length

A principle motivation for measuring the length of the cell occurs in electrophysiological studies where it is often inconvenient to visualize the sarcomeres. Here the photodiode array is aptly suited to monitor edge displacement [14,15] or the length of the isolated cell [16]. There are at least two schemes for extracting the edge displacement from the array's output. In the first scheme, the array gives a signal representing the sum of the total intensity projected onto all of the photodiodes [14]. In this case it is assumed that the cell behaves like a shutter and so, because of the array's geometry, the array's signal is proportional to the length of the projected shadow of cell. With the second approach, the array simply provides a videoscan of the cell's image, while a separate analogue circuit computes edge displacement at a preset level of the video signal [15].

Figure 3 illustrates the principles of measuring the position of an edge from the video-output of a self-scanned photodiode array. The inputs of the circuit consist of the respective timing pulses and the video output of the array. The array's timing pulse triggers a 'window' whose position and width are selected to overly the features of interest. (In Figure 3 this is restricted to the right end of the cell.) Consequently, the features from unwanted objects elsewhere in the image (i.e., micropipets, debris, et c.) do not interfere with the computation of displacement of the edge of the cell. The selected video signal then initiates a ramp which last as long as the video signal exceeds an adjustable threshold. The value of the ramp is sampled and held until the next scan is completed. Consequently, the amplitude of this signal is directly proportional to the absolute displacement of the video feature selected at the threshold level. The sampled length is refreshed with each scan of the array, so that edge displacements can be measured 1000/s. The relationship of these signals throughout a contraction in an isolated cell from Guinea Pig is shown in Figure 3.

The intensity variations in the cell renders unsuitable any approach based solely on the measurement of net intensity changes for the precise details of shortening. The general effect of measuring intensity alone is that velocity of shortening is underestimated since the contribution to the signal from the edge <u>increases</u> as the cell thickens.

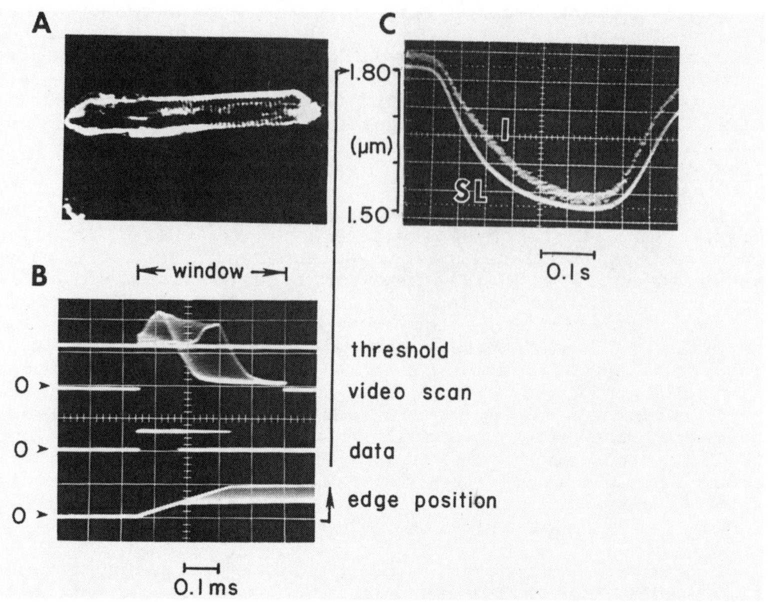

FIG. 3. Illustration of the method for measuring edge displacements in an isolated cardiac cell. A large and complex variation in the intensity distribution in the phase contrast image occurs at the edge of the cells (B). Thus, a threshold method is required to detect precisely the displacement of the edge of the cell, as shown in C.

The edge detector is ideal for studying the contractile properties of cells which are attached to suction pipets in electrophysiological measurements [15]. The virtue of the approach described here is the ease of use provided by the direct display of the video signal: The relevant feature of the cell is selected electronically so that unwanted information can be eliminated by visual inspection. Thus, pipets or other objects which must be be near the cell need not create difficulty. One inconvenience is that the point of attachment and the sarcomere length must be predetermined in each cell. As long as other techniques are used to confirm that sarcomere shortening is uniform, the precision can be very good (<0.01um/sarcomere), and it is limited only by the length of the free edge of the cell [15]. A similar scheme can be used to measure the absolute length of the cell [16]. The length of the cell can be also measured by counting the elements of the array representing the image of the cell, but then the excursions of the cell must encompass a suitable number of elements in order to insure an adequate measurement precision. Otherwise, the shortening of the cell will appear stepwise and the precision of obtaining the velocity of sarcomere motions will be compromised.

Direct Measurement of Sarcomere Length by FM Detection

Use of the self-scanned photodiode array provides a way to measure sarcomere length directly which is more convenient than either diffraction or edge detection. Since the elements in the array are scanned at a constant velocity, the spatial pattern representing the image of the striations is converted to a video signal whose frequency is inversely related to sarcomere length. The instantaneous frequency of the video signal can be converted to a voltage via the use of a special electronic circuit element known as the phase-locked loop, and sarcomere length can then be related to the detected voltage. This novel method, first devised by V.A. Claes, permitted sarcomere length to be measured directly from television images of isolated cells [17]. With their sensitivity to low-light levels, video systems permit precise visualization of sarcomeres by phase, polarization, or interference microscopy; however sampling is constrained by the slower field rates (5Ø-6ØHz) and the resolution is limited by the inherent nonlinearity and image retention of many videocameras. The photodiode array provides excellent linearity, and the amount of light available in bright field microscopy permits very high speed sampling of sarcomere length [18]. But in this case the striated image is formed by diffraction processes, and so the unique relation between the intensity in any striation and the precise components of the sarcomere is lost [19].

Figure 4 illustrates a method based on that described by Myers et al. [18] which is particularly suited for studying the motions <u>between</u> sarcomeres in various regions of the isolated heart cell. The sarcomeres are visualized with Hoffman-modulation contrast microscopy, a form of interference microscopy in which the intensity in the image is directly related to the gradients of refractive index in the specimen. Here the available light still permits sampling rates of 5ØØhz. The circuit computes the average sarcomere length which occurs within a selected portion, or 'window', of the video signal. Two windows enable simultaneous detection of the sarcomere motions which occur in two different parts of the cell.

Some features of nonuniform motion of the sarcomeres occur which can be applied to the mechanics of the cell. Figure 4B illustrates the behavior of two fields in a cell which is beating spontaneously and asynchronously. Each area was selected to encompass 4 sarcomeres and was separated from the other by approximately 22 microns. As sarcomeres in the first region shorten, they can stretch the sarcomeres in the distant region prior to the arrival of the propagated wave of contraction. The fact that lengthening in the inactive region coincides with shortening provokes questions about the mechanical nature and the distribution of the connections between the sarcomeres in the single cell. Since the unattached cell is assumed to be only minimally influenced by the substrate, the force which prelengthens the sarcomeres must arise within the cell. In this cell, the apex of stretch in the second region fortuitously occurs when the velocity of shortening is near zero in the first region. Since the two regions are in mechanical equilibrium we can estimate the amount of force exerted by the shortened sarcomeres. Specifically, the extensibility of inactive heart cells is generally known [2Ø,21], and so the force exerted by the shortening focus can be guaged by the strain imposed on the prestretched region. The shortened sarcomeres are also in equilibrium with the internal force which opposes shortening. Thus a direct method exists for calculating the internal load which resists shortening in the intact cell.

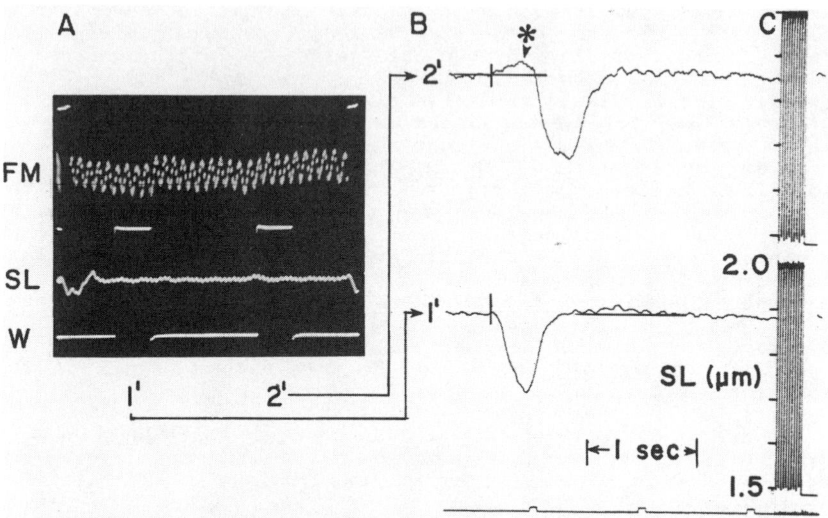

FIG. 4. (A) Principles of FM detection of striation spacing. Shown are the frequency modulated video signal representing the striations in a 2.Ø um grating, FM; the demodulated FM signal representing sarcomere length at respective location on the array, SL; and adjustable fields (1',2') where sarcomere length is computed, W. (B) Spontaneous changes in sarcomere length which occur at the respective locations indicated in A. Shortening at 1' simultaneously lengthens the sarcomeres at 2' (*) and vice versa. The amount of tension generated by the shortening focus can be estimated from the resistance to stretch in the unstimulated cell. (C) Calibration signal which spans the normal range of sarcomere shortening in the cardiac cell, 2.Ø > SL > 1.5 um.

The sarcomeres might prelengthen in the unattached cell for at least two reasons. First, the sarcomeres might be under slight compression by longitudinally arranged cytoskeletal elements in parallel to the sarcomere. Thus, net shortening in the length of the cell reduces tension in these elements elsewhere, an event which decompresses the sarcomeres. Alternatively, the sarcomeres could be under an extensile force, possibly created by internal hydrostatic pressure within the cell. Evidence could be cited for or against both possibilties, but either way the relations between sarcomere motions in the asynchronously beating cell ought to shed insights about the functional nature of the cytoskeleton and the origin of the restoring force in the unattached heart cell. The methods reveal also sarcomere shortening is less than maximal and that contractile activity need not propagate in the spontaneously beating cell. (The latter point is not shown here.)

EVALUATION OF ISOLATED CELLS BY THEIR CONTRACTILE BEHAVIOR

An overriding desire to establish the physiological status of isolated cells has prompted functional comparisons with the behavior of intact muscle. Yet analysis of contraction in isolated cells falls beyond many of the prior conventions established in muscle physiology, where interpretations are made relative to conditions in which force is defined or measured. Consequently, extrapolation between contraction in muscle and cells, however measured, requires some attention. This is especially true since few if any studies have systematically compared the respective preparations under truly similar conditions.

Terminology: Confusion often arises since the many terms used to describe cardiac cell contraction represent a legacy inherited from studies in muscle cell culture, biochemistry, and physiology. I will adopt the convention in which 'contraction' refers to synchronous contractile activation of the whole cell which follows an active depolarization of the cell membrane. Early studies also revealed that the unstimulated isolated cardiac cells can also 'beat' spontaneously in an asynchronous fashion. This spontaneous activity is characterised by a small focus of shortening and relengthening within the cell, the locus of which propagates longitudinally. This behavior can also be observed directly in intact muscle where such sarcomeric 'dithering' predominates at regions of damage [22] or when the stimulus interval is prolonged [23]. In other cases, the sarcomeres in the isolated cardiac cell may contract synchronously but spontaneously without external electrical stimulation. Finally, under some defined conditions, the sarcomeres in a small part of the isolated cell may contract synchronously in response to the localized depolarization of the cell membrane, but the locus of contraction does not spread to other parts of the cell [24].

Clarity is no less important when using terms such as 'nonbeating', 'quiescent', and 'resting', et.c. to describe the unstimulated cell. For example, some inactive cells may not contract at all if stimulated electrically. Here, 'quiescent' will refer to the general absence of visible spontaneous contractile activity between the interval of regular stimulation. Other cells may be electrically excitable, but have abnormal contractile function.

Sensitivity of contraction to calcium, and vice versa: Contractile shortening requires little development of tension and, presumably, minimal numbers of attached cross-bridges in the unattached cell. The presence of cross-bridges is thought to cooperatively enhance the sensitivity of the myofibril to calcium. (A corollary is that the extent and the velocity of shortening may be less sensitive to changes in intracellular calcium than are changes in force.) One consequence is that the fall of the intracellular calcium transient might be slowed in the unattached cell if the binding of calcium ion to the myofilaments is reduced at low tension, as is known to occur in intact heart muscle [25]. The small increment in cytosolic calcium produced by shortening can also prolong depolarization [26] and inhibit the electrogenic extrusion of calcium. The cell's content of calcium represents a complex balance between calcium binding to the myofilaments, other intracellular sites, and several transport processes within the sarcolemma. These facts suggest that dynamics of shortening will more closely mirror the transient rise and fall of calcium ion, uncomplicated by cooperative effects of cross-bridge formation. However, if less calcium is bound to the myofilaments it will be free to be transported out of the cell. Thus the consequence of shortening is that the cell's content of calcium ion may be reduced over a longer term by subtle shifts its calcium ion transport equilibria. The unloaded nature of contraction in cells may well alter their contractile and electrophysiological behavior when it is compared to intact muscle.

Cell Contraction versus Muscle Function

Contractile response to stimulation: Determining whether the contractile behavior observed in the isolated cell is representative of intact muscle amplifies the difficulties involved in extrapolating between the effects of contractile force and shortening. Ideally cells ought to be evaluated according to functional criteria. For example, it has been found that cells isolated from the rat heart which are quiesecent show little increase in the degree of shortening at higher stimulus frequencies, whereas cells which beat spontaneously show the negative effect on contractility that is usually associated with more rapid stimulation in rat heart muscle [27]. Yet, it should not be preassumed that a similar pattern of contractile response to stimulation in isolated cells and muscle preparations verifies their normal physiology, for it is likely that many isolated muscle preparations may be 'unrepresentative'. The negative force-frequency relation has been attributed to lack of adequate metabolic support rather than any special attribute of the excitation-contraction coupling pathway in rat heart muscle [28]. In this view, the force-frequency relation will reflect the dimensions of an isolated muscle specimen and will vary depending on the metabolic requirements of each species. In fact, a positive force-frequency relation has been observed in the isolated perfused rat heart [29], and a negative staircase is absent in isolated rat heart muscles which are thinner than 0.2 mm [30]. Comparisons between intact muscle and isolated cells must be made with caution, for even thin muscles may be too thick!

The contractile adjustment to the onset of regular stimulation emphasizes the unstimulated state of the cell, but this response appears to be too variable in quiescent cells [27] to be a definitive test of the cell's status. One possibility is that not all quiescent cells are alike. Gap junctions involute with time after the isolation of the cell [31], and so conditions other than the state of the cell's pathways for excitation-contraction coupling may contribute to their contractile response to stimulation.

Sarcomere shortening: The function of the heart cell is to contract, and so it be helpful to consider the ability of the isolated cell to withstand regular stimulation. Within this context, it may be important that cells which beat spontaneously do not appear to tolerate sustained stimulation at physiological rates [27]. If the content of calcium within the isolated cell is reduced, we might expect that less calcium was available for contraction. Yet the isolated cells can be found [10] in which the range of sarcomere shortening is in good agreement with that seen in intact muscles [32,33]. Extrapolation between the contractile behavior of muscle and cells requires that methods of measuring contraction be used which permit quantitative comparisons. For example, only a portion of the isolated muscle preparation shortens due to damage at the points of attachment [22]. In general, this means that the degree and velocity of shortening measured at the ends of a muscle preparation will be only 50 to 70% of the true values of the sarcomeres. Unless internal shortening was measured directly, the values of muscle shortening will have to be proportionally increased to enable firm comparison with the behavior of the isolated cell. Thus, the shortening measured in any cell which is said to be physiologic ought not to be less than that which occurs in the intact muscle preparation when comparable conditions of study are met, for it is difficult to imagine how the shortening of the muscle could exceed its components.

Shortening depends upon the difference between the initial and the final sarcomere lengths. Moreover, the maximum velocity of shortening is steeply dependent upon length at short sarcomere lengths in cardiac muscle [32]. Thus, cellular contractility may appear artificially reduced when the initial length of the sarcomere is shorter than its value *in situ*. Too often the extent and velocity of isolated cell shortening are expressed as only the absolute values for displacement (i.e., 'microns' and 'microns/sec'.). Such changes in shortening can not be easily related to absolute changes in contractility in the isolated cell unless sarcomere length is known.

Velocity of shortening and the internal resistance to sarcomere motion: Inotropic interventions which enhance sarcomere shortening also speed the velocity of shortening in the unattached heart cell, and latter is universally associated with an increase in the concentration of myoplasmic calcium in intact muscle. The precise mechanism by which calcium might increase the turnover of the cardiac cross-bridge remains elusive. It is well known that the velocity of muscle shortening is very sensitive to small increments in tension at the low force which characterises contraction in the unattached cell. If more sites for cross-bridge formation are exposed by calcium, then the alterations of the velocity of shortening reflect simply the ability to overcome a small but finite internal force which resist shortening in the unattached cell. But it is not clear whether the cell's resistance to shortening resides external or internal to the myofibril or, perhaps, even in an effect of calcium on the cross-bridge cycle itself. For example, marked slowing in the initial velocity of sarcomere shortening characterizes onset of contractile motions when stimulus rate is slowed in the isolated Guinea Pig heart cell (Refer to Figure 7B [15]). Presumbably, the pronounced slowing of early shortening can be associated with the reduced rate of delivery of calcium to the sarcomere. This interpretation, however, in turn requires that a finite resistance to shortening preexists in the unactivated sarcomere, since the little shortening which occurs at the slowed onset of contraction would be insufficient to increment a restoring force which is necessary to explain the effects by increased cross-bridge formation. Initial shortening may be slowed if active sarcomeres near the surface of the cell must overcome a resistance to shortening from their inactivated neighbors. Despite of their small size, it may inaccurate to assume that the distribution of activation within the cardiac cell is necessarily uniform [10]. If true, it is reasonable to suppose further that the microscopic appearance of the heart cell should reveal whether stimulus conditions alter the cell's reliance on selected intracellular pools of calcium for contractile activation.

Relengthening in cells and muscle: The peak velocity of relengthening is generally equal to the maximum speed of shortening in the unattached heart cell. In intact muscle, the peak velocity of relengthening also increases with shortening. In the latter case it must be remembered that shortening is always increased by lowering the external force on the isolated muscle preparation. The speeding of relengthening in muscle is presumed to be due to the presence of extracellular connections which are elastically distorted by shortening and thus serve to rapidly restore the sarcomere to its initial length. Unfortunately, few studies in isolated muscle observe contraction at the very low force which resists shortening in the unattached heart cell. Moreover, the deactivating effect of lower numbers of cross-bridges means that any external force, no matter how small, ought to relengthen the sarcomere more rapidly in muscle. In fact, when external forces are reduced to very low levels, relengthening slows dramatically in muscle even though its extent of shortening is increased [34]. Whereas unloaded muscle relengthens slowly, isolated cells appear to relengthen vigorously. This implies that the cell is the origin of the force which restores cardiac muscle to its rest length, for the mechanisms which govern relengthening the cell can only be slowed in intact muscle.

SUMMARY

The small internal force which resists sarcomere shortening in the isolated cell (Figure 4) appears to be of the same order as the 1-2% level of force which is estimated to relengthen the sarcomere in isolated muscle [35]. Although the isolated, unattached cell might appear at first to be an artificial representation of cardiac function, in fact the relengthening of the fibers of the heart during its filling occur at comparably low forces. This means that the mechanisms which control sarcomere shortening and relengthening in the isolated cell will be essential to a complete understanding of a fundamental basis of cardiac function.

The measurement of contraction is often synonymous with measurement of shortening or force. This encourages evaluation of isolated cells in terms of muscle function, although such comparison should be made with caution. The emphasis on measuring contraction should not detract with the possibilities inherent in the application of other techniques to observe the distribution of contraction. Holography of the cardiac cell [36] and the digital processing of its microscopic image [37] may reveal even more about the biophysics of cardiac cell structure. Observation of localized contractile phenomena can provide more specific information about the intracellular source and fate of calcium ion than is possible to resolve with measurement of whole cell currents or intracellular calcium indicators. The chief virtue of measuring the dynamics of the sarcomere is that the forces displacing the sarcomere can be established under defined conditions of myofilament overlap, and velocity which conform to prior convention in muscle physiology.

Acknowledgements: Supported, In part, by HL21325 (NIH), an Established Fellowship from the New York Heart Association, T32 GM 7288 (NIGMS), and the Martin Fund. I thank Barry London, Robert Smith, Adam Denton, Gerard Siciliano, Nadine Stram, and Hong Zhao for assistance.

REFERENCES

1. M. Tarr, Adv. Exp. Med & Biol. 161, 199-216 (1983).
2. A. Fabiato, J. Gen. Physiol. 78, 457-497 (1981).
3. A.J. Brady, G. Tan and N. V. Richiutti, Nature 282, 728-729 (1979).
4. O.M. Bucher, Exp. Cell Res. 13, 109-115 (1957).
5. G.B. Boder, J. Harley and I.S. Johnson, Nature 231, 531-532 (1971).
6. M.R. Mitchell, T. Powell, D.A. Terrar and V.W. Twist, Br.J. Pharm. 81, 543-550 (1984).
7. B. Koidl, G.Zernig and H.A. Tritthart, Bas. Res. Cardiol. Suppl.1, 111-116 (1985).
8. W.T. Clusin, J. Physiol. (Lond) 320, 149-174 (1981).
9. T. Iwazumi and G.H. Pollack, I.E.E.E. Trans. Biomed. Eng 26, 86-93 (1979).
10. J.W. Krueger, D. Forletti, and B. Wittenberg, J. Gen. Physiol. 76, 587-607 (1980).
11. G.H. Pollack, Circ. Res. 59, 1-8 (1986).
12. R. Rudel and F. Zite-Ferenczi, J. Physiol. (Lond) 290, 317-330 (1979).
13. J.W. Krueger and B. London, 119-134 in "Contractile Mechanisms in Muscle", G.H. Pollack and H. Sugi (eds), Plenum (1984).
14. G. Isenberg, Z. Naturforsch. 37c, 502-512 (1982).
15. B. London and J.W. Krueger, J. Gen. Physiol. 88, 475-505 (1986).
16. C.M. Phillips, V. Dutinh and S.R. Houser, I.E.E.E. Trans. BioMed. Eng. 33, 929-934 (1986).
17. N.M. deClerck, V.A. Claes, and D.L. Brutsaert, J. Mol. Cell Cardiol. 16, 735-745 (1984).
18. J. Myers, R. Tirosh, R.C. Jacobson and G.H. Pollack, I.E.E.E. Trans. BioMed Eng. 29, 463-466 (1982).
19. A.F. Huxley and R. Niedergerke, J. Physiol. (Lond) 144, 403-441 (1958).
20. A.J. Brady, J. Biomech. Eng. 106, 25-30 (1984).
21. D. Fish, J. Orenstein and S. Bloom, Circ. Res. 54, 267-276 (1984).
22 J.W. Krueger and G.H. Pollack, J. Physiol. (Lond) 251, 627-643 (1975).
23. J.W. Krueger and J.E. Strobeck, Eur. J. Cardiol. 7 (Suppl.), 79-96 (1978).
24. B. London, Biophys. J. 41, 180a (1983).
25. P.K. Housmans, N.K. Lee and J.R. Blinks, Science 221, 159-161 (1983).

26. M.J. Lab, D.C. Allen and C.H. Orchard, Circ. Res. 55, 825-829 (1984).
27. M. Capogrossi, A.C. Kort, H.A. Spurgeon and E.G. Lakatta, J. Gen. Physiol. 88: 589-613 (1986).
28. P.D. Henry, Am. J. Physiol. 228, 360-364 (1975).
29. F.J Meijler, Am. J. Physiol. 202, 636-640 (1962).
30. V.J.A. Schouten and H.E.D.J. ter Keurs, Pflügers Arch. 407, 14-17 (1986).
31. F. Mazet, B.A Wittenberg and D.C. Spray, Circ. Res. 56, 195-204 (1985).
32. G.H. Pollack and J.W. Krueger, Eur. J. Cardiol. 4(Suppl), 53-65 (1976).
33. H. Ter Keurs, W.H. Rijnsburger, R. van Heuningen and M.J. Nagelsmit, Circ. Res. 46, 703-714 (1980).
34. B.E. Strauer, Am. J. Physiol. 224, 431-434 (1973).
35. H. Ter Keurs, W.H. Rijnsburger and R. van Heuningen Eur. Heart J. 1 (Suppl A), 67-80 (1980).
36. R.S. Danziger, H.A. Spurgeon and M. Sharnoff, Biophys. J. 51, 110a (1987).
37. K. Roos, Biophys. J. 52, 317-327 (1987).

A TECHNIQUE FOR MEASURING CYTOSOLIC FREE Ca^{2+} WITH INDO-1 IN FELINE MYOCYTES.

William H. duBell, Charles Philips and Steven R. Houser*, Department of Physiology, Temple University School of Medicine, 3420 N. Broad St., Philadelphia, PA 19140.

Introduction

Cytosolic free calcium concentration, $[Ca^{2+}]_i$, fluctuates dramatically during the normal cardiac cycle. These changes in $[Ca^{2+}]_i$ are known to influence a host of physiological and biochemical processes in cardiac muscle. Of major importance in this regard is the fact that the transient elevation in $[Ca^{2+}]_i$ during systole, the so-called systolic "Ca^{2+} transient", triggers contraction in myocardial cells. The cellular processes which control both systolic and diastolic $[Ca^{2+}]_i$ in cardiac muscle are not easily studied in bulk muscle preparations or whole hearts because experimental conditions are difficult to control in these preparations. Two recent technical advances, however, now make it feasible to study important cellular processes involved in regulation of $[Ca^{2+}]_i$ in cardiac muscle cells. The first advance was the development of techniques for disaggregation of single myocytes from intact myocardium [1]. These techniques are summarized in a separate chapter of this book. Importantly, myocytes isolated with these techniques are able to withstand normal levels of extracellular Ca^{2+}, i.e. they are "Ca^{2+} tolerant" and recent studies [2] have shown that they retain the physiological properties of intact myocardium following isolation. In experiments using single myocytes and "patch type" suction micropipettes both the intracellular and extracellular environments can be independently controlled. The second technical advance has been the development of the fluorescent Ca^{2+}-indicators Fura-2 and Indo-1 [3] to measure $[Ca^{2+}]_i$ in single cells. These indicators offer significant advantages over other techniques for measuring $[Ca^{2+}]_i$ in cardiac muscle such as ion selective electrodes, metallochromic dyes and aequorin. A full discussion of the strengths and weaknesses of each of these techniques is beyond the scope of this chapter and can be found elsewhere [4]. The present chapter describes a technique which uses Indo-1 to measure $[Ca^{2+}]_i$ in single feline ventricular myocytes [5]. The reasons for choosing Indo-1 rather than Fura-2 will be discussed and the changes in the system that would be required to make it suitable for use with Fura-2 will be presented. It is important to point out that the system to be described can be used in conjunction with recently developed electrophysical [6] and contractile [7] techniques. In this fashion membrane currents, cell contraction and $[Ca^{2+}]_i$ can be measured simultaneously in the same myocyte. These powerful experimental approaches should provide new insight into basic processes involved in the regulation of $[Ca^{2+}]_i$ and excitation-contraction coupling in adult mammalian cardiac myocytes with intact sarcolemmae.

Properties of Indo-1

In order to study the Ca^{2+} transient in isolated single cardiac muscle cells, a probe is required that 1) can be incorporated into the cytosol, 2) is sensitive to Ca^{2+} over the range encountered from diastole (pCa approx. 7) through systole (pCa approx. 5), 3) has kinetics which are fast enough to follow the Ca^{2+} transient, 4) will not be subject to interference by competing ions, 5) produces a readily measurable signal and 6) will not overly influence cellular function [4].

Biology of Isolated Adult Cardiac Myocytes
William A. Clark, Robert S. Decker, and Thomas K. Borg, Editors

An increasingly popular strategy for measuring $[Ca^{2+}]_i$ in isolated cardiac myocytes has been to use the Ca^{2+}-sensitive fluorescent dyes developed in the laboratory of Roger Tsien [3,8]. Fluorescence is a property of certain molecules whereby a paired electron that has been excited into a high energy state by a photon of light decays back to the ground state and emits a photon, generally of lower energy than that which caused excitation [9]. Fluorescent molecules exhibit characteristic excitation and emission patterns. In the case of Ca^{2+}-sensitive fluorescent dyes, the binding of Ca^{2+} alters some quantifiable aspect of the excitation or emission characteristics of the molecule.

Until recently, the most commonly used of these fluorescent indicators was Quin-2 [8]. Quin-2 is an EGTA analogue which binds Ca^{2+} with 1-1 stoichiometry. When excited with light at 340 nm, this molecule emits light at 500 nm, the emission of which increases in a graded fashion, up to a saturating level, with the addition of Ca^{2+}. Quin-2 has been used extensively in suspensions of isolated myocytes to record steady and slowly changing Ca^{2+} levels [10,11,12,13] and even to record Ca^{2+} transients [14] but its usefulness is limited because the amount of intracellular Quin-2 required to produce an acceptable signal can buffer Ca^{2+} transients [3].

Fortunately, the more recently developed Indo-1 and Fura-2 [3] are more suitable for use in single isolated myocytes. As with Quin-2, both bind Ca^{2+} in 1-1 stoichiometry. However, they have emission intensities 30 times greater than Quin-2 and are more selective for Ca^{2+} over Mg^{2+} [3]. There are numerous reports of Indo-1 and Fura-2 being used to record Ca^{2+} transients in single, isolated cardiac myocytes [15,16,17].

The Ca^{2+} dependence of Fura-2 and Indo-1 fluorescence is different than that of Quin-2 in that there is a wavelength shift upon Ca^{2+} binding [3]. The Fura-2 shift is on the excitation side. When emission is monitored at 510 nm, peak emission in 0 Ca^{2+} occurs with an exciting wavelength of 380 nm and in saturating Ca^{2+} peak emission occurs with excitation at 340 nm. Indo-1, about which the bulk of this chapter is concerned, exhibits a wavelength shift on the emission side. When excited with light at 355 nm, the peak emission in 0 Ca^{2+} occurs at approximately 480 nm and shifts to near 410 nm in saturating Ca^{2+}. The wavelength shift exhibited by these two dyes is useful in that it can make calibration independent of the dye concentration. As will be discussed later, the ratio of emission at the two wavelengths can be used to calculate $[Ca^{2+}]_i$ and should allow, in principle, the use of standard calibrations, thus eliminating the need to calibrate the signal in each cell studied.

The rest of this section will concern the properties of Indo-1 as they apply to measuring $[Ca^{2+}]_i$ in single, isolated cardiac myocytes. Like the other Ca^{2+} sensitive fluorescent dyes Indo-1 can be incorporated into the cytosol either by direct injection of the Ca^{2+}-sensitive free acid (Indo-1 FA) by micropipette or by incubating a suspension of myocytes with the lipophilic acetoxymethyl ester of Indo-1 (Indo-1 AM). Once Indo-1 AM crosses the sarcolemma, the ester groups are cleaved by cytosolic esterases, leaving Indo-1 FA diffusion trapped within the cytosol. Figure 1 shows a series of emission scans of commercially available Indo-1 FA (Molecular Probes, Inc.) in approximate $[Ca^{2+}]$ of 0, 100 nM, 250 nM, 1000 nM and 1 mM (saturating). Excitation was at 352 nm (5 nm BW) and emission was scanned from 350 to 550 nm (10 nm BW). These scans show that emission at 410 nm increases and emission at 480 nm decreases in a graded fashion as Ca^{2+} is increased from 0 to 1 mM. [Based on this it would be expected that during a twitch, an Indo-1 loaded myocyte would show an increase in emission at 410 nm and a decrease in emission at 480 nm, both

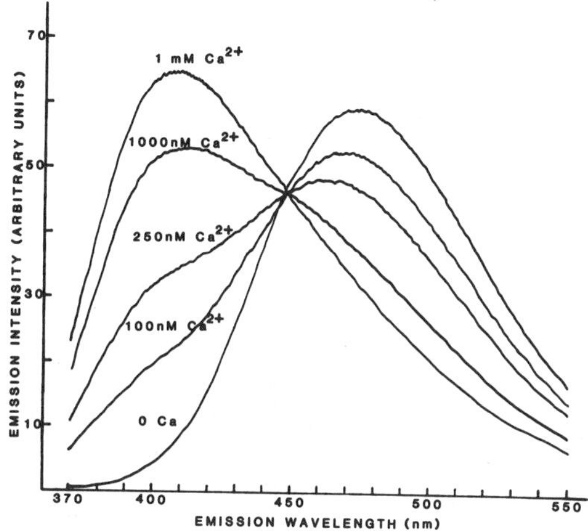

Fig. 1. Emission scans from solutions of Indo-1 FA (10 uM) in approximate $[Ca^{2+}]$ of 0, 100 nM, 250 nM, 1000 nM and 1.0 mM (saturating). The abscissa is the emission wavelength and the ordinate is fluorescence emission (arbitary units). Solutions contained 150 mM KCl, 5 mM Hepes, 4 mM EGTA; pH was set to 7.0 with KOH. The approximate Ca^{2+} values were calculated using an EGTA-Ca^{2+} dissociation constant at 2.45 x 10^{-6} M^{-1} [18] and verified using a Ca^{2+} electrode.

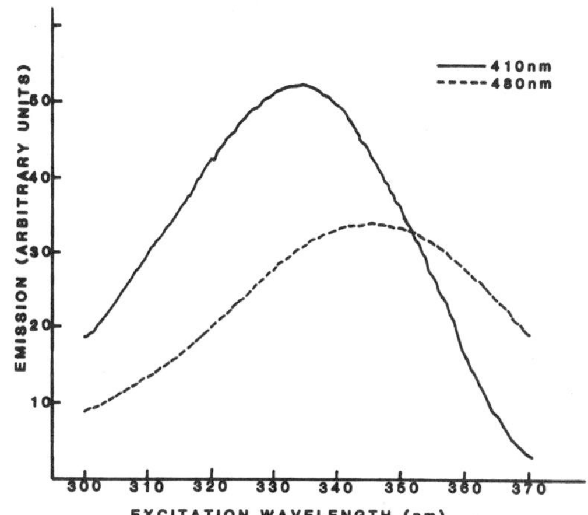

Fig. 2. Excitation scans of Indo-1 FA (1 uM) in 0 and 1 mM (saturating) Ca^{2+}. The abscissa is the excitation wavelength and the ordinate is emission intensity (arbitrary units). In 1 mM Ca^{2+} (solid line) emission was monitored at 410 nm (10 nm BW) and in 0 Ca^{2+} (dashed line) emission was monitored at 480 nm (10 nm BW). In both, excitation was scanned from 300 nm to 370 nm (5 nm BW). Gain settings were arbitrary, relative magnitudes of the peaks have no meaning. Solutions prepared as in Fig. 1.

of which would return to baseline as the cell relaxed.] Note that with an approximate [Ca^{2+}] of 250 nM, the concentration at which half of the Indo-1 should be bound to Ca^{2+} [3], the emission at each wavelength is approximately midway between the extremes. Although not shown here, emission scans of Indo-1 in 0 and 1 mM Ca^{2+} reveal superimposable scans with a peak at 450 nm. Awareness of this peak is important, as will be discussed later, because it can be helpful in detecting the presence of unhydrolyzed Indo-1 AM in myocytes loaded by this technique. Figure 2 shows excitation scans of Ca^{2+} saturated Indo-1 FA (solid line, emission monitored at 410 nm) and Indo-1 FA in 0 Ca^{2+} (dashed line, emission monitored at 480 nm). These show that both Indo-1 FA and the Indo-1 FA - Ca^{2+} complex show significant emission with excitation at 350 nm, the wavelength we have chosen for excitation.

The other factors relevant to the use of Indo-1 in recording Ca^{2+} in isolated myocytes are the association and dissociation kinetics of the Indo-1-Ca^{2+} reaction. A recent report by Jackson et al. [19] indicates that in stopped-flow spectrofluorimetric studies the association rate constant is $> 10^8$ M^{-1} sec^{-1} while the dissociation rate constant is 130 sec^{-1}. While these studies were not done in vivo they indicate that the kinetics of the Indo-1-Ca^{2+} reaction are fast enough to accurately track the Ca^{2+} transient.

Microfluorimeter for Indo-1

Optics

The instrument to be described was designed to use Indo-1 to quantify the rapid changes in free cytosolic calcium concentration that are thought to produce contraction in single cardiac myocytes. The basic requirements for such a system are the illumination of the Indo-1 loaded cell with 350 nm ultraviolet light, and the simultaneous measurement of the resulting fluorescence at 410 nm and 480 nm. The system we describe meets those requirements and is compact and modest in cost.

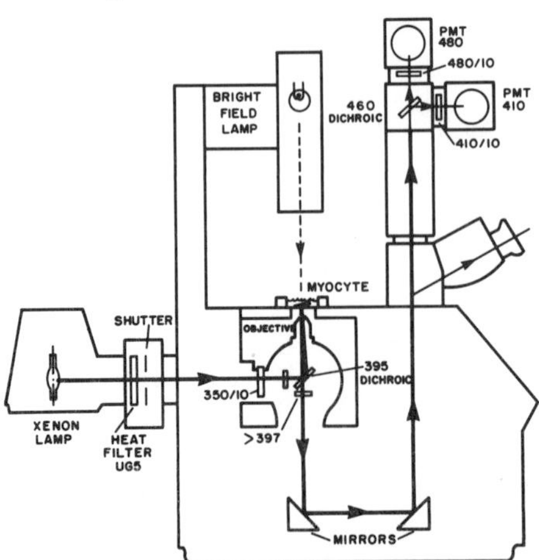

Fig. 3. Simplified schematic of optical system. See text for explanation.

Figure 3 is a simplified schematic of the fluorescence measurement system. All the optics are mounted in an inverted microscope (Zeiss IM). Excitation is via a 75W Xenon lamp (Hamamatsu L2174) because it provides wide band illumination including UV. Illumination with a mercury lamp was not as suitable as the Xenon lamp for reasons to be discussed later. The excitation wavelength is selected by a 350 nm (10 nm BW) interference filter (Corion P10-350-F-G833). A heat filter (Twardy Inc. UG5) protects the 350 nm filter as prolonged exposure to high temperatures will change the transmission characteristics of the excitation filter. An electromechanical shutter (Ilex Optical Co.) is placed in the excitation path so the myocyte is not illuminated unless fluorescence recordings are being made. This minimizes bleaching of the dye. The excitation light is directed upward by a 395 nm dichroic mirror (reflects UV light below 395 nm and passes light above 395 nm) and focused on the cell by the objective (Zeiss 40X Plan-Neofluar immersion lens). The resultant emission passes back through the objective and is transmitted by the 395 nm dichroic and a 397 nm barrier filter (which further rejects UV light from the recording system). Mirrors direct the fluorescent cell image to a trinocular which allows binocular viewing or measurement of the emission light intensity by the photomultiplier tubes (PMTs). The two PMTs are connected to a Zeiss filter cube which is mounted on a tower at the video port of the microscope. When the microscope is configured for light measurement, the emission beam is directed through the tower. A 460 nm dichroic beam splitter reflects the light with a wavelength below 460 nm to one PMT and passes light with a wavelength above 460 nm to the other. Wavelengths to be measured by the PMTs are selected with 410 nm (10 nm BW) (Oriel 53805) and 480 nm (10 nm BW) (Oriel 53850) interference filters. Shutters are placed in front of the PMTs to protect them when fluorescence recordings are not being made. The microscope is housed in an open front aluminum box 3' x 2' x 3' (HWD) lined with black felt. The Xenon lamp housing and shutter project out the back of the box through a close fitting hole to eliminate stray light from this source. All experiments described here were conducted in a darkened room.

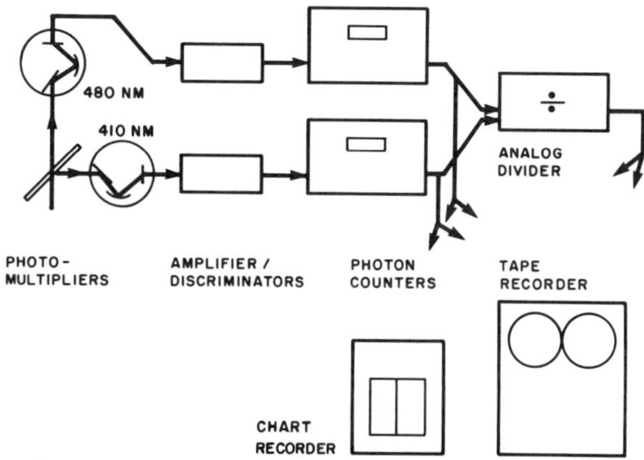

Fig. 4. Block diagram of electronics associated with fluorescence measurement system. The photon counting is done by two 2426 photometer systems, each comprised of 3150 SRF PMT housing, AD 126 amplifier/discriminator and 126 photometer (Pacific Instruments). The analog divider, built in our laboratory, uses an Analog Devices AD 534 multiplier.

Electronics

Figure 4 shows a block diagram of the electronics associated with the fluorescence measurement system. Output from each PMT (Hamamatsu R1527)is sent through an amplifier/discriminator to a photometer. Output from the photometer is sent to an analog divider which instantaneously computes I_{410}/I_{480}. The divider has a provision for removal of background signal from both wavelengths. The output from the divider, as well as the individual wavelength outputs can be recorded on a strip chart recorder (Gould) or FM tape (Vetters, Model D), for later analysis.

The photon counting method was used in all experiments conducted to date because it allows the experiment to be conducted at light levels 10 to 100 times lower than those required for recording in the PMT anode current mode.

The photon counting method operates as follows. For each photon converted to an electron at the photosensitive PMT cathode, a short pulse (< 10 ns) appears at the anode. A high speed voltage amplifier (x 100) boosts the level to the discriminator which separates photo-electron pulses from thermal electron pulses on the basis of pulse height.

The photon counters have both digital and analog outputs. In the experiments shown in this chapter the analog outputs were used. These outputs have user operated filters with time constants of 10 ms, 30 ms, 100 ms ... 100 sec. The setting can be changed depending on experimental needs. Specifically, if slow changes in $[Ca^{2+}]_i$ are to be recorded, a longer time constant setting would be used to reduce noise in the recording system.

Loading Indo-1

Because of its properties as a Ca^{2+} chelator, Indo-1, if present in high enough concentrations, could buffer the Ca^{2+} transients it is being used to study. Consequently, one goal of the loading procedure should be to have the lowest intracellular dye concentration possible. This will help to minimize Ca^{2+} buffering and other possible effects on myocyte physiology.

There are two basic techniques for loading myocytes with Indo-1 in particular and fluorescent dyes in general. The first, which we have chosen as our primary method, is to incubate a suspension of myocytes with the AM form of the dye. As this diffuses across cell membranes, cytosolic esterases cleave the ester groups, leaving the Ca^{2+}-sensitive FA diffusion trapped within the cytosol [20]. While, as will be discussed, there are potential problems with this technique that must be addressed, it is very convenient because it gives a large pool of myocytes with which to work. The second technique is to include FA as an ingredient of a micropipette filling solution and inject it directly into the cytosol of an impaled myocyte. For our purposes this is impractical because not all experiments require microelectrode impalements. However, this technique can be very useful for comparing the properties of myocyte generated Indo-1 FA to those of the commercially available compound.

In our early work with Indo-1 [15,21,22] we loaded the myocytes by a technique identical to that which we had used for Quin-2 loading [12], with the exception that the dye concentration was decreased from 25 uM to 10 uM. After isolation, myocytes were allowed to stabilize for 1 hour in

Krebs Henseleit buffer [(KHB), 133 mM NaCl, 5.4 mM KCl, 1.2 mM $MgSO_4$, 1.2 mM NaH_2PO_4, 25 mM $NaHCO_3$, 12.5 mM dextrose, 1 mM lactic acid and 3 mM Na-pyruvate] with 2.0 mM Ca^{2+} and 1% albumin at 37°C. The myocytes were then diluted to approximately 1 x 10^5 rod shaped cells/ml and loaded with Indo-1 AM (10 uM, from 1 mM stock in DMSO) for 30 minutes at 37°C. Myocytes were then washed twice in KHB to remove extracellular dye. As will be discussed later, this technique had significant effects on myocyte physiology.

Recently, Poenie et.al. [23] reported that loading newly fertilized egg cells with high concentrations of Fura-2 AM at physiological temperatures resulted in non-uniform loading within the population of cells and the gradual compartmentalization of dye away from the cytosol. To address this, a modified loading procedure was developed which involved premixing 5 uL of 10 mM Fura-2 AM (in DMSO) with 75 uL of fetal calf serum and 2.5 uL of 25% (w/w) solution of Pluronic F-127 (BASF Wyandotte Corp) in DMSO. Pluronic F-127 is a non-ionic emulsifier which helps to solubilize hydrophobic molecules in aqueous solutions. This mixture was added to 3 mls of cells (final dye concentration of 16 uM) and loading proceeded for 1 hour. It was noted that this procedure increased the uniformity of loading and decreased the compartmentalization of dye in these cells.

Our current loading procedure is derived from this approach and is very similar to a procedure recently described by Barcenas-Ruiz and Wier for loading Fura-2 AM into guinea pig myocytes [17]. 75 uL of fetal calf serum, 2.5 uL of 25% (w/w) Pluronic F-127 (in DMSO) and 10 uL of 1 mM Indo-1 AM (in DMSO) are premixed. (In practice, we generally make 10 ml of this solution, sonicate it for 30 minutes and freeze it in small aliquots for later use. Sonication ensures uniform solution of the Indo-1 AM and Pluronic F-127). The premixed solution of Indo-1 is added to 2 ml of myocytes (in KHB w/1% albumin and 2 mM Ca^{2+}, final dye concentration of 4.8 uM). Loading proceeds at room temperature for 2.5 minutes. A small aliquot of these myocytes is placed in the chamber on the microscope stage and allowed to settle for approximately 1 minute. They are then superfused with normal Tyrode solution (150 mM NaCl, 5.4 mM KCl, 1.2 mM $MgCl_2$, 10 mM dextrose, 2.5 mM Na-Pyruvate, 5 mM Hepes, pH = 7.4) with 2.0 mM Ca^{2+} for at least 10 minutes before study.

We have found that dye loading is much more uniform within the myocyte population since we started using this technique. This is probably because the loading solution is much more homogeneous with respect to Indo-1 AM. As will be discussed later, it also seems to diminish compartmentalization of Indo-1 within the myocytes. We have also noticed that detectable signals can be obtained from myocytes loaded for as little as 1 min although the signal to noise ratio is much better after 2.5 minutes and myocyte physiology seems to be only slightly affected.

As mentioned previously, loading with Indo-1 AM is our preferred technique. However, it is also possible to directly add Indo-1 FA to a cell by including it as an ingredient in a micropipette filling solution and either pressure injecting it into the myocyte or allowing it to diffuse from the pipette tip. Some experiments of this type can be important for comparing the responses of the Indo-1 FA produced by the myocyte and that which is commercially available. Although we have no direct experience with this technique, Barcenas-Ruiz and Wier have used it to load guinea pig myocytes with Fura-2 [17]. Microelectrodes contained .050 or .070 mM Fura-2 FA. Following impalement, myocytes were loaded by diffusion for 5-10 minutes. These experiments showed that Ca^{2+} transients measured with Fura-2 AM loaded myocytes and Fura-2 FA injected myocytes were not different. It should be noted that for a system such as the one described in this chapter, in which the entire myocyte is projected onto the PMTs, the Indo-1 FA in the micropipette would add significant background. This would have to be subtracted unless some way were devised to mask the microelectrode.

Typical Response of an Indo-1 Loaded Myocyte

Figure 5 shows Ca^{2+} transients recorded from an Indo-1 AM loaded myocyte. The myocyte was field stimulated from rest at approximately 0.2 Hz at 24°C. The individual wavelength recordings show the expected behavior, with I_{410} increasing and I_{480} decreasing following stimulation. The I_{410}/I_{480} (ratio) recording reveals that the Ca^{2+} transient recorded with Indo-1 rises very rapidly following stimulation. Also, importantly, the Ca^{2+} transient shows the expected physiology with the first transient being small and prolonged with respect to the steady state and subsequent Ca^{2+} transients increasing in magnitude and decreasing in duration until the steady state is reached (Beat 6). This is expected based on the well known contractile staircase shown by these myocytes when stimulated from rest. Although not shown here, previous work from this lab has demonstrated that the upstroke of the Ca^{2+} transient recorded from Indo-1 AM loaded feline ventricular myocytes leads the development of shortening [21]. More recent work (not shown) has demonstrated that the timing of the Ca^{2+} transient with respect to cell shortening may be very similar to the timing of the aequorin recorded Ca^{2+} transient and developed tension in cat papillary muscle [24].

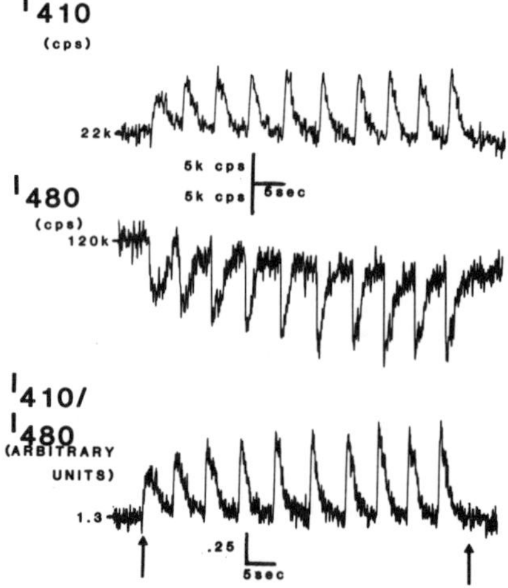

Fig. 5. Ca^{2+} transients from an Indo-1 AM loaded feline ventricular myocyte. Top record is I_{410} (minus system background) and middle record is I_{480} (minus system background), both in photon counts/second (cps). Myocyte autofluorescence is not subtracted. Bottom record is I_{410}/I_{480} (with system background subtracted from each wavelength). This record is calibrated in volts and includes several gain constants. The individual wavelengths were filtered with a photometer time constant of 30 msec, recorder filtering was 16 Hz. Stimulation was initiated at first arrow and terminated at second arrow.

Calibration

In order for Indo-1 to be useful as anything other than a qualitative indicator of the Ca^{2+} transient, it is necessary to calibrate the fluorescence emission in terms of Ca^{2+}. One potential advantage of Indo-1 (and Fura-2) is that there is a wavelength shift upon Ca^{2+} binding. This means that unlike that of Quin-2, the calibration of Indo-1 should be independent of dye concentration [3].

In the case of Quin-2, the magnitude of emission at 500 nm increases in a graded manner with Ca^{2+}. Thus $[Ca^{2+}]$ can be determined using the following equation [3]:

$$[Ca^{2+}] = K_D \frac{F-F_{min}}{F_{max}-F}$$

where K_D is the Quin-2-Ca^{2+} dissociation constant, F is the emission above background of the Quin-2 loaded preparation and F_{min} and F_{max} are the emissions in 0 and saturating Ca^{2+}, respectively. F only has quantitative meaning in the context of F_{min} and F_{max}. Thus, F_{max} and F_{min} must be determined for each preparation by using digitonin or a Ca^{2+} ionophore to expose the cytosolic Quin-2 to saturating Ca^{2+} (F_{max}) and then chelating the Ca^{2+} with EGTA or quenching all Ca^{2+} sensitive emission with Mn^{2+} (F_{min}) [3].

In the case of Indo-1, however, the shift in the emission peak upon binding to Ca^{2+} can obviate the need to determine a minimum and maximum fluorescence for each preparation. The following equation is used to determine $[Ca^{2+}]$ [3]:

$$[Ca^{2+}] = K_D \frac{R-R_{min}}{R_{max}-R} \beta$$

In a system such as the one described here, R is the ratio of fluorescence at 410 nm (I_{410}) to that at 480 nm (I_{480}), Rmin is I_{410}/I_{480} in 0 Ca^{2+}, Rmax is I_{410}/I_{480} in saturating Ca^{2+} and β is the ratio of I_{480} in 0 Ca^{2+} to I_{480} in saturating Ca^{2+}. The β term is a consequence of the derivation of the calibration equation as explained by Grynkiewicz et al. [3]. These ratios can be determined experimentally and then, potentially, regarded as constants. The major part of this section will discuss techniques for determining these values. A small portion at the end will be devoted to other possible strategies for calibrating this dye.

In solutions, Rmin, Rmax and β are easily determined. To determine R_{min} and R_{max}, solutions of 5 uM Indo-1 FA are prepared in 0 and saturating (>0.1 mM [3]) Ca^{2+} and I_{410} and I_{480} recorded. Background is measured by using identical solutions without dye. After background subtraction R_{min} and R_{max} can be calculated. β is merely the ratio, after background subtraction, of I_{480} in 0 Ca^{2+} to I_{480} in saturating Ca^{2+}. It is essential to the accuracy of the calibration, however, that when determining β, the concentration of Indo-1 in the two solutions be identical.

In myocytes loaded with Indo-1 AM, however, a calibration of this type is not a simple matter. It is necessary to alternately deplete the cell of Ca^{2+}, exposing Indo-1 to 0 Ca^{2+} (R_{min}) and then saturate the cytosolic dye with Ca^{2+} (R_{max}) without causing the loss of dye from the cytosol. This can be done by exposing an Indo-1 AM loaded myocyte to a Ca^{2+} ionophore, such as ionomycin. In the presence of 0 extracellular Ca^{2+}, intracellular Ca^{2+} will leave the cell, reduce cytosolic Ca^{2+} to 0 and establish R_{min}. Upon changing the external solution to 2 mM Ca^{2+}, Ca^{2+} will enter the cell, cause hypercontraction, saturate the dye and establish R_{max}. Assuming no loss of dye from the cell, β can be calculated from I_{480} in 0 and saturating Ca^{2+}. (An alternate approach to determining β is to use thin solutions of Indo-1 FA in 0 and saturating Ca^{2+}. Again, it is essential that the dye concentration be identical and that the thickness of the solutions be the same). Figure 6 shows an experiment in which the emission of an Indo-1 AM loaded myocyte is calibrated by this technique.

There are potential problems with this approach. Ionomycin does not bind appreciable amounts of Ca^{2+} at pH < 7.0. Therefore, it is essential that the pH inside and outside the cell be appreciably above this. An alternate Ca^{2+} ionophore, Bromo-A23187, can be used. This molecule has Ca^{2+} binding properties similar to the commonly used A23187 but is not fluorescent [25]. However, this molecule does not seem to insert well in 0 Ca^{2+} so it may be necessary to add it in the presence of some low concentration of Ca^{2+} (100 nM or 250 nM) before changing to 0 Ca^{2+} for determining R_{min}.

A recent report by Li, Autschuld and Stokes has mentioned another consideration [26]. They state that myocytes that have hypercontracted can still have some ATP dependent Ca^{2+} sequestration and extrusion capability that, even in the presence of the ionophore, can prevent the establishment of a true R_{max}. They suggest superfusing the myocyte with glucose free solution and adding the mitochondrial inhibitor CCCP and the NADH dehydrogenase inhibitor amytal to deenergize the myocyte before adding the ionophore.

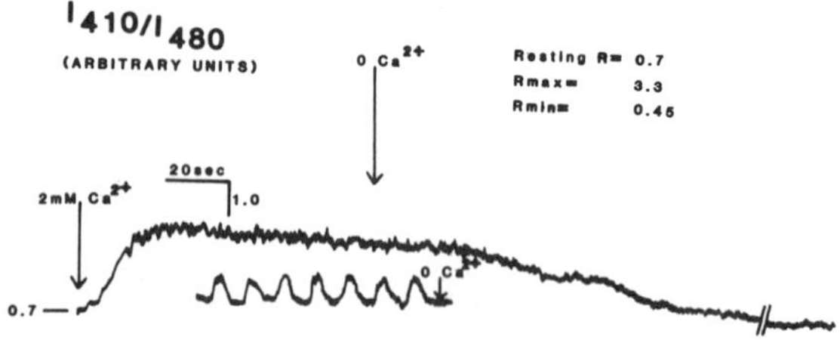

Fig. 6. Calibration experiment done as described in text. Tracing represents I_{410}/I_{480}. Inset portion is a series of stimulated twitches (0.2 Hz, 24°C). Arrow on inset indicates where twitches stopped when superfusing solution was changed to 0 Ca^{2+} Tyrode solution (4 mM EGTA). After cell was stabilized in 0 Ca^{2+}, flow was stopped. 100 uM ionomycin (in Tyrode solution with 0 Ca^{2+}) was added (not shown). After 2 minutes, flow was resumed with 0 Ca^{2+} Tyrode solution. At arrow, solution was changed to Tyrode solution with 2 mM Ca^{2+}. R_{max} was 3.3. At second arrow, solution was changed to Tyrode solution with 0 Ca^{2+}. Time elapsed during gap in record was 90 sec. R_{min} was 0.45. β, (calculated from I_{480} record, not shown) was 1.53. Calculated resting $[Ca^{2+}]_i$ was 40 nM, calculated peak $[Ca^{2+}]_i$ was 600 nM. All solutions used in calibration were set to a pH of 8.0. Individual wavelengths were filtered with a photometer time constant of 100 msec, recorder filtering was at 15 Hz.

As will be discussed later, before a calibration can be done which will have meaning in other myocytes loaded by the AM technique, it is necessary to be able to subtract the background fluorescence contributed by the myocyte and be confident that all the Indo-1 FA is sequestered in the cytosol. However, once these concerns have been addressed the R_{min}, R_{max} and β values should be usable in all myocytes studied as long as the fluorescence measurement system remains unchanged.

Other potential strategies for calibrating Indo-1 do exist. One is to use either of the two wavelengths at which Indo-1 emits and calibrate as with Quin-2. Another is to permeabilize the myocyte membrane with ionomycin or bromo-A23187 and then superfuse with solutions of known Ca^{2+} (0, 100 nM, 250 nM, 1000 nM, 2 mM). As cytosolic Ca^{2+} equilibrates with each solution, a ratio is determined which would correspond to this Ca^{2+}. By plotting R vs Ca^{2+}, one could estimate $[Ca^{2+}]_i$ in the preparation. Both of these techniques, however, require that calibration be done in every cell from which quantitative data are required. Because of the fragile nature of single isolated myocytes, these techniques would be expected to have a low probability of success.

Technical Considerations

In this section we describe the philosophy behind our system design. These design choices stem primarily from our desire to simultaneously record the Ca^{2+} transient, electrophysiological events and contraction in single isolated cardiac myocytes. We will also discuss potential pitfalls and how they can be avoided or mitigated.

The first consideration was whether to use Indo-1 or Fura-2. Indo-1 was chosen because the wavelength shift upon Ca^{2+} binding occurs on the emission side. This means that wavelength separation can be effected by a simple beam splitter placed upstream from two filtered PMTs. This allows for rapid time response because both wavelengths can be monitored simultaneously. This would not be the case with a Fura-2 system because some sort of provision, such as a high speed chopper, would have to be made for alternating between the two excitation wavelengths. An aditional consideration was that the Indo-1 system is inherently vibration free, an advantage when microelectrodes are used to record electrophysiological parameters.

The system we describe gives the desired rapid response, is vibration free, compact in size and moderate in cost. The optical system is mounted on a standard vibration table and the electronics are rack mounted. We have chosen to use filters rather than monochromators for wavelength selection because of their large area, small size, moderate cost, high efficiency and compatibility with the microscope technology.

The proper choice of certain components is necessary for good performance. These will be detailed, beginning with the UV source. A Xenon lamp with excitation below 360 nm is necessary for a good 410 nm response. Figure 2 shows that emission at 410 nm is critically dependent on excitation wavelength. In this regard, we have found that use of a mercury lamp with its sharp 365 nm line results in a very poor signal to noise ratio (or no response) at 410 nm. The Xenon lamp should be stable with a guaranteed noise spec.

It is well known that many glasses begin to attenuate light below 350 nm and information on the response of optical parts such as objective lenses, condenser lenses, and internal relay lenses is not easily obtained.

While quartz lenses pass UV easily, they are very expensive. We have, therefore, tested numerous microscope objectives for their ability to pass 350 nm excitation light. This is a critical issue because excitation light must be below 360 nm in order for the dual emission properties of Indo-1 to be optimally utilized. The Zeiss 40X Plan-Neofluar immersion objective lens is the best non-quartz lens we have tested to date. The standard condenser and relay lenses with the Zeiss microscope have been adequate.

Presently we are collecting light from the entire 40X field. This results in a significant background fluorescence since the myocyte covers only a portion of the field. This background is electronically subtracted before the ratio is computed. However, the background also contributes noise to the system and the signal to noise ratio could possibly be improved by masking the surrounding area. We have attempted to eliminate the background by using a pinhole to project only a portion of the myocyte image to the PMTs. However, we have found that this induces a significant motion artifact into our recordings. We have also considered the use of a slit between the myocyte and the PMTs to allow the entire myocyte to be projected while restricting the amount of surround which is projected. However, this would require either the ability to change the alignment of the slit or the selection of only those myocytes with the proper orientation. Thus, for our purposes, the simplest approach is to illuminate the whole field, collect from the whole field and subtract the background.

Because the entire field is imaged, care must be taken to ensure that the entire field projects to the active area of the PMTs. In this regard, a 125 mm focal length lens (Edmund Scientific) was used in the base of the tower to reduce the diameter of the image seen by the PMTs from 16 mm to about 8 mm, since the PMT active area is 10 mm at its minimum. In a related consideration, it is important that the entire field be uniformly illuminated with excitation light. This can be tested by moving an Indo-1 AM loaded myocyte around the field. Uniform illumination exists if I_{410} and I_{480} do not vary with the position of the myocyte.

The PMTs used in our system are a compact, high performance, low cost type (Hamamatsu R 1527HA). The associated electronics (two Pacific Instruments 2426 systems) provide both photon counting and anode current measurement. This system seems to have the temporal response characteristics needed to follow Ca^{2+} transients in cardiac myocytes. Along these lines, the time response of the analog output was checked by an optical step test and found to be within the resolution of the test, about 10 ms.

Although this system was designed for use with Indo-1, it can readily be used as a microfluorimeter for any dye with a single excitation and one or two emissions simply by changing filters. Conversion to use with Fura-2 while maintaining fairly rapid response characteristics and simultaneous ratio recording would be more difficult. The system would require a chopper to alternate excitation between 340 and 380 nm. It could use a single Xenon lamp, possibly in a square housing, without mirrors, with outputs on two adjacent faces. The two beams could be separately filtered, chopped with a fairly large (5"-6" dia.) half circular wheel at a 30 Hz frequency, phase locked to the power line and recombined with a 360 nm dichoric mirror. This would allow use with TV. In addition, the output of the single photomultiplier, after passing through its amplifier/discriminator would be gated into two separate counters. Commercially available systems (e.g. Photon Technology International) tend to emphasize monochromators but possibly their chopper could be adapted to a more compact, lower cost, filter system. It should be kept in mind, however, that the short 340 nm excitation light needed for Fura-2 puts additional demands on all optical components and quartz optics might be necessary in some or all portions of the excitation light path.

In addition to technical considerations regarding the fluorescence measurement system, there are also concerns about dye loaded myocytes which must be addressed. Chief among these are the potential for 1) overloading myocytes with Indo-1, 2) cellular compartmentalization of Indo-1 as well as incomplete hydrolysis of the AM compound and 3) motion artifact. Dye overloading is a concern because excess Ca^{2+} buffering will both diminish and slow the Ca^{2+} transient. Dye compartmentalization and motion artifact are perhaps of more concern because both can cause inaccurate fluorescence ratios and thus result in a fluorescence transient which is not a true indicator of the Ca^{2+} transient.

Because Indo-1 FA is a Ca^{2+} chelator, it can act as a Ca^{2+} buffer. In light of this, part of the strategy for using this indicator should be to load only as much as necessary to obtain an acceptable signal. In the accompanying table, contractile parameters of non-loaded myocytes are compared with those of myocytes loaded for 2.5, 10 or 30 minutes by the technique described previously. As loading time is increased, peak shortening decreases and the time to peak is prolonged. Figure 7 shows steady state shortening from a non-loaded myocyte and one loaded for 30 minutes. The changes in twitch parameters as loading time is increased are most likely caused by an increase in cytosolic Ca^{2+} buffering capacity. In our system, acceptable signals can be obtained with a loading time as short as 2.5 minutes, with only minimal effects on contractile parameters. An additional reason for keeping loading to a minimum is that for each ester group cleaved, 2 H^+ ions and 1 molecule of formaldehyde are released [20]. These can have deleterious effects on myocyte function.

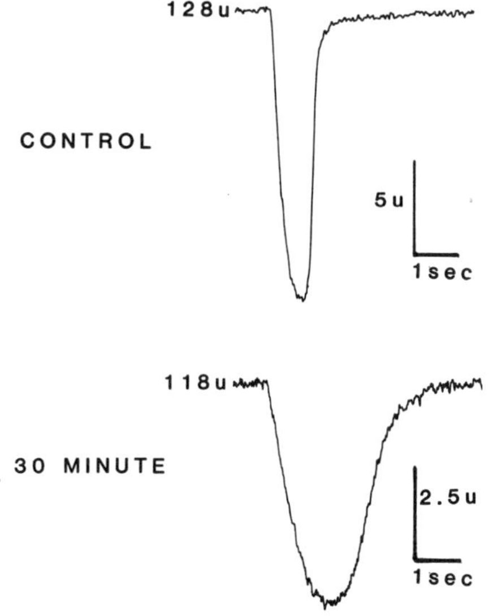

Fig. 7. Comparison of steady state shortening from a myocyte loaded with Indo-1 AM (by procedure described in text) for 30 min. and a non-loaded myocyte. Myocytes were field stimulated at 0.2 Hz, temperature was 24°C.

TABLE: Contractile parameters of myocytes loaded with Indo-1 AM

Loading Time (min)	Shortening (% resting length)	Time to Peak Shortening (msec)
Control	12.2	750
2.5	10.6	817
10	9.4	942
30	9.3	1616

Two of the key assumptions on which the ratio technique of calibrating Indo-1 is based are 1) that there is complete conversion of the Indo-1 AM to Indo-1 FA and 2) that all the Indo-1 FA so produced is trapped in the cytosol. The presence of non-Ca^{2+} sensitive fluorescence (beyond that contributed by the myocyte, which can be quantified and corrected for) in the cytosol or of Ca^{2+}-sensitive fluorescence in compartments other than the cytosol can lead to errors in computation of the ratio, invalidate the calibration constants and even result in inaccuracies in the Ca^{2+} transient waveform. Previous reports of non-hydrolyzed Indo-1 AM and compartmentalized dye in epithelial cells [27] and isolated cardiac myocytes [22] do exist. However, in both of these cases, loading was carried out at 37°C for long periods (30 minutes and longer). It was recently reported that in newly fertilized PtK1 [23] cells loaded with Fura-2, compartmentalization was eliminated by loading at room temperature in the presence of Pluronic F-127. In addition, Barcenas-Ruiz and Wier [17] report that in guinea pig myocytes loaded by a procedure similar to that used in our studies, there is very little bound or non-cytoplasmic Fura-2. In our Indo-1 loaded myocytes this also seems to be the case.

Addressing the possibility of non-cytoplasmic dye is fairly simple. Exposing the myocyte to digitonin will selectively permeabilize the sarcolemma leaving other membrane bound compartments intact. If fluorescence rapidly falls to background, it is a good indication that the dye was limited to the cytosol [17]. Detection of non-Ca^{2+} sensitive emission is a bit more difficult. One possible technique [22] is to load a suspension of myocytes, wash thoroughly to remove extracellular dye and then permeabilize the sarcolemma with digitonin. This should release the cytosolic dye to the surrounding medium. After centrifugation, the supernatant can be scanned in a fluorescence spectrophotometer and the resulting scans compared with scans of Indo-1 FA.

The presence of some motion artifact is also possible in a system such as this and must be considered as a potential source of error. It is unlikely to be a significant factor in our system because the entire myocyte is illuminated and projected on to the PMTs. (We have been able to induce significant motion artifacts by either restricting the excitation light to illuminate only a portion of the myocyte or by illuminating the whole myocyte and monitoring emission from only a spot. This is probably because, in both cases, the myocyte changes in thickness during contraction and relaxation, resulting in changes in optical pathlength and the amount of dye in the optical pathway.) In addition, the fact that the upstroke of the Ca^{2+} transients recorded in our system leads the upstroke of the twitch [21] argues against the presence of a significant motion artifact.

Summary

We have described a microscope designed for use with the Ca^{2+}-sensitive fluorescent dye Indo-1. It can be easily adapted to allow simultaneous recording of $[Ca^{2+}]_i$, electrophysiological events and cell contraction, making it a very useful system for studying excitation-contraction coupling in isolated cardiac myocytes.

Acknowledgements

Supported by NIH Grants HL33921 and HL33648 and fellowships from Berlex Labs., Inc. and Southeastern Pa. Chapter of the AHA.

References

1. L.H. Silver, E.L. Hemwall, T.A. Marino and S.R. Houser, Am. J. Physiol. 245, H891-H896 (1983).
2. S.R. Houser, A. Bahinski and L.H. Silver, Am. J. Physiol. 248, H622-H630 (1985).
3. G. Grynkiewicz, M. Poenie and R.Y. Tsien, J. Biol. Chem. 280, 3440-3450 (1985).
4. J.R. Blinks, W.G. Wier, P. Hess and F.G. Prendergrast, Prog. Biophys. Molec. Biol. 40, 1-114 (1982).
5. C.M. Philips, W.H. duBell and S.R. Houser, Proc. 39th Ann. Conf. Eng. in Med. and Biol. 28, 65 (1986).
6. O.P. Hamill, A. Marty, E. Neher, B. Sakmann and F.J. Sigworth, Pflugers Arch. 391, 85-100 (1981).
7. C.M. Philips, V. Duthinh, S.R. Houser, IEEE Trans. Biomed. Eng. Vol. BME-33, 929-934 (1986).
8. R.Y. Tsien, Biochemistry 19, 2396-2404 (1980).
9. J.R. Lakowicz, Principles of Fluorescence Spectroscopy, Plenum Press, NY, NY (1983).
10. T.R. Powell, P.E.R. Tatham and V.W. Twist, Biochem. Biophys. Res. Comm. 122, 1012-1020 (1984).
11. S.S. Sheu, V.K. Sharma and S.P. Banerjee, Circ. Res. 55, 830-834 (1984).
12. W.H. duBell and S.R. Houser, Biophys. J. 49, 350a (1986).
13. W.H. duBell and S.R. Houser, Cell Calcium 8, 259-268 (1987).
14. A.P. Thomas, M. Selak and J.R. Williamson, J. Mol. Cell. Cardiol. 18, 541-545 (1986).
15. W.H. duBell, C.M. Philips and S.R. Houser, J. Gen. Physiol. 88, 20a (1986).
16. M.B. Cannell, J.R. Berlin and W.J. Lederer, Biophys. J. 49, 466a (1986).
17. L. Barcenas-Ruiz and W.G. Wier, Circ. Res. 61, 148-154 (1987).
18. D.M. Bers, Am. J. Physiol. 242, C404-C408 (1982).
19. A.P. Jackson, M.P. Timmerman, C.R. Bagshaw and C.C. Ashley, Febs Letters 216, 35-39 (1987).
20. R.Y. Tsien, Nature 290, 527-528 (1981).
21. W.H. duBell and S.R. Houser, Biophys J. 51, 110a (1987).
22. W.H. duBell and S.R. Houser, Fed. Proc. 46, 1095 (1987).
23. M. Poenie, J. Alderton, R. Steinhardt and R. Tsien, Science 233, 886-889 (1986).
24. J.P. Morgan and J.R. Blinks, Can. J. Physiol. Pharmacol. 60, 524-528 (1982).
25. C.M. Deber, J. Tom-Kun, E. Mack and S. Grinstein. Analytical Biochem., 146, 349-352 (1984).
26. Q. Li, R.A. Autschuld and B.T. Stokes, Biochem. Biophys. Res. Comm. 147, 120-126 (1987).
27. A. Luckhoff, Cell Calcium 7, 233-248 (1986).

WHOLE CELL VOLTAGE CLAMP TECHNIQUES AND THE MEASUREMENT OF CURRENTS IN THE ISOLATED HEART CELL PREPARATION

R. L. WHITE
Department of Neuroscience
Albert Einstein College of Medicine
Bronx, NY 10461

CHARACTERISTICS OF THREE APPROACHES FOR WHOLE CELL VOLTAGE-CLAMPING WITH PATCH ELECTRODES

The cardiac myocyte preparation allows the study of the electrophysiological characteristics of single cells isolated from the electrical influence of their neighbors through gap junctions. Also, these cells are free from uncontrolled neural, hormonal, and extracellular ion effects. Many studies, including several presented at this meeting, have characterized several passive and active electrical membrane properties of cardiac myocytes. The voltage clamp technique is used to systematically study electrical properties of membranes and can be employed in several ways: the whole cell recording technique using a continuous voltage clamp with a single patch electrode; the discontinuous voltage clamp using a single patch electrode or a microelectrode; and conventional two electrode techniques. Each has technique has unique advantages and disadvantages for recording from isolated cardiac myocytes.

Whole cell recordings using a continuous voltage clamp circuit with a single electrode.

The whole cell recording technique was developed and popularized several years ago by Neher and his colleagues [1,2]. The unique advantage of this technique is that the cell membrane is minimally damaged in the process of establishing electrical continuity with the cytoplasm. Conventional microelectrodes are usually pulled for high resistance (small tips) to minimize membrane damage upon electrode penetration, but high resistance electrodes are noisy and have difficulty passing current, often rectifying. Patch type electrodes are low in electrical resistance and establishing a gigaseal insures minimal membrane damage and leakage of the extracellular solution into the cell. However, the large tip diameter of the patch pipette may allow significant dialysis of the cytoplasm with the patch electrode solution. This may or may not be an advantage depending on the goals of the experiment. When one wants to perturb a membrane process and record the resulting ionic concentration changes in the cytoplasm, dialysis by the patch electrode represents a chemical load which will dampen the physiological response of the cell. On the other hand, the soluble components of the cytoplasm may be effectively controlled once any intracellular buffer systems are overcome. This technique has to be approached cautiously, however, and the extent of any dialysis should be confirmed by independent measurements of the cytoplasmic constituent concentration changes. When this was done in snail neurons, a patch pipette with a tip one-third the diameter of the cell was able to achieve a 90% change in cytoplasmic K^+ concentration in 30-90 sec [3]. The situation was quite different when dialysis of cytoplasmic H^+ was attempted. The patch pipette was filled with 100 mM buffer at a pH near the pK of the buffer and had a tip diameter one-third the diameter of the cell, but adequate change of intracellular pH required 8-10 min. [3].

The principle disadvantage of the whole cell recording technique which uses a single recording electrode and a continuous voltage clamp circuit (such as the current to voltage converter circuit popularly used in a whole cell voltage clamp paradigm) is a large series resistance which can be only partially compensated. Since the patch electrode measures voltage and passes current at the same time in this voltage clamp paradigm, the measured intracellular potential is reduced by a factor (ΔP) equal to R_e*I_m; where R_e is the resistance of the patch electrode and Im is the measured membrane current. Series resistance compensation is accomplished by summing a potential equal to $-\Delta P$ with the command potential. Series resistance compensation circuits form a positive feedback loop within the voltage clamp circuit. The gain of this loop must be less than 1 at all frequencies or the

Biology of Isolated Adult Cardiac Myocytes
William A. Clark, Robert S. Decker, and Thomas K. Borg, Editors

voltage clamp circuit will oscillate. In practice, 80-90% of the series resistance artifact can be compensated if phase anomalies within the feedback loop caused by the patch electrode capacitance and stray capacitance at the input of the I-V converter are carefully neutralized. Series resistance compensation is set on the assumption that electrode resistance is neither time nor current dependent. This may not always be the case, especially when large currents are passed through the electrode. Electrodes may also change resistance over time due to current-induced polarization or partial sealing over, so periodic re-compensation of series resistance should be done over the course of an experiment. Another difficulty with series resistance is the magnitude of the uncompensable component and its effects on accurate measurement of membrane conductances. In order to maintain good voltage control of the sarcolemmal membrane in a single myocyte, the impedance of the voltage clamp should be no more than one-tenth that of the peak conductance of the sarcolemma. In the voltage clamp experiment illustrated in Figure 1, a patch electrode was sealed on to a single myocyte and continuity was established with the cytoplasm by rupturing the membrane patch. The uncompensated series resistance was about 4 Mohms (0.25 uS). We were able to reduce the effective series resistance to about 0.7 Mohms (1.4 uS) with series resistance compensation. Under these conditions, peak sarcolemmel membrane conductance should not have exceeded 0.14 uS or good control[1] of the membrane voltage would have been lost in a graded manner as conductance increased from 0.14 uS. The voltage clamp record (Fig. 1) shows a family of slow inward currents elicited by a voltage steps (-35 mV to -5 mV) from the holding potential of -45 mV. The cell input conductance was about 1 nS at the holding potential and increased to about 14 nS (transient membrane conductance plus leak conductance) during the peak inward current shown. In this case, the largest membrane conductance was 1% of the voltage clamp conductance and good voltage control of the membrane was maintained. While

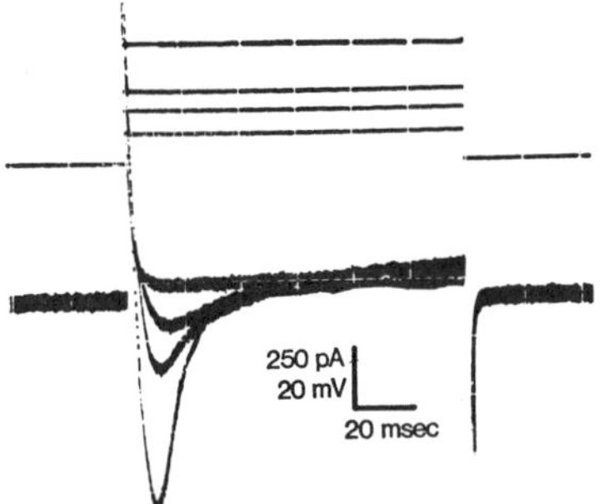

Figure 1. Oscillograph of slow inward currents elicited from a single, voltage clamped ventricular myocyte. The whole cell voltage clamp technique with a single electrode was used. The cell was held at -45 mV to inactivate the fast inward current then stepped to increasingly positive potentials. The voltage (top traces) and current (bottom traces) were successive sweeps which were superimposed. Membrane leakage currents were very low and not subtracted from these traces. Calibrations: top trace, 20 mV; bottom trace, 250 pA; time scale 20 msec.

this DC analysis is simplistic and voltage clamp admittance should be assessed, it gives the investigator an easily calculated place to start from. It is important to point out that the investigator will not be aware of voltage clamp escape by examining the voltage trace because the voltage record from this whole cell recording technique is the command potential and not the measured cell membrane potential. This situation is made even more acute with the double whole cell recording technique which uses two independent voltage clamp circuits to measure junctional conductance between a pair of cardiac myocytes [4]. In this case, two

---

[1] We arbitrarily define "good voltage clamp control" as achieving a transmembrane potential within ±10% of the command potential over the entire range of membrane conductances encountered during an experiment.

patch electrodes are used and the residual series resistance component is the sum of the uncompensated series resistance in each electrode (see [5] for a discussion of current pathways in pairs of isolated myocytes). Using the compensated electrode resistances cited in the experiment in Figure 1, peak junctional conductance should not exceed 0.07 uS for good membrane voltage control, and the maximum conductance one would measure in a hypothetical experiment with both electrodes at zero separation in a single cell is 0.7 uS.

Voltage-clamping using discontinuous single electrode and two electrode continuous voltage clamp circuits with patch electrodes.

The two electrode continuous voltage clamp uses separate voltage recording and current passing electrodes. Since no current is passed through the voltage recording electrode, the resistance of the current electrode and a variable portion of the cell cytoplasm (depending on electrode separation) are included within the feedback loop of the voltage clamp circuit. Series resistance ceases to be a significant problem in either the discontinuous single electrode or the two electrode continuous voltage clamp paradigms since electrical resistance (R_S) to the cell cytoplasm through the current electrode is:

$$R_S = \frac{Re}{1 + A*(R_i/(R_i + R_e))}$$

where A is the open loop gain of the voltage clamp circuit, R_e is the resistance of the current passing electrode, and R_i is the cell input resistance.

The discontinuous voltage clamp technique alternately measures voltage and passes current through a single electrode[2]. The measured membrane voltage is compared with the command voltage to produce an error voltage and the clamp circuit applies a voltage to the electrode, based on the magnitude and polarity of the error voltage, which corrects the membrane voltage. The minimum rate at which this process must occur for good membrane voltage control is determined by: 1) the time constant of the cell; 2) the rate and magnitude of membrane conductance changes; and 3) the rate of change of the command potential.

For a cell held at a constant potential, the minimum switching rate (in units of time) should be at least one-tenth the cell time constant. The steady-state membrane potential of a typical cardiac myocyte with a time constant of 12 msec can be controlled with a cycle of measuring voltage and passing current which is completed in 1.2 msec. The discontinuous nature of voltage sample, however, puts another constraint on the minimum switching rate. Sampling theory shows that accurate representation of time varying signals which were sampled as discrete points in time is only possible when the sampling rate (frequency) is at least twice that of the fastest Fourier components comprising the signal. Sampling rates less than the "Nyquist sampling criterion" produce aliasing errors (spurious low frequency waveforms and "beating" of the original signal with the sample frequency). Accurate membrane voltage control requires a sampling frequency which is at least twice that of the significant[3] high frequency Fourier components comprising the command voltage waveform (see [6] for a formal discussion). A similar sampling rate criterion exists when eliciting membrane conductance changes. The slow inward calcium current, for example, peaks in less than 10 msec and has significant Fourier components extending to about 2 kHz. The minimum sample rate should be 4 kHz, but unless the command voltage step is slowed and

---

[2] Note that the apparent open loop gain of a discontinuous voltage clamp circuit is 0.5 times the gain of the circuit when switching is inhibited due to the 50% duty cycle.

[3] If the command voltage waveform is a square pulse, then odd order harmonic components extend quite far up in the frequency spectrum. We feel that when amplitudes of these components are less than 1% of the amplitude of the fundamental, they can be ignored. Incidentally, the faster the rise time of the step, the greater and more numerous are the high frequency components. Rounding the leading and trailing edges of the step is very useful.

rounded the sample rate must be much higher to achieve good membrane control during the capacitive transient.

The maximum sampling rate is set by the electrode time constant. The application of voltage to the electrode results in charging of the electrode capacitance. This charge must be dissipated before an accurate sample of membrane voltage can be taken. The usual route for electrode capacitive charge dissipation, in view of the 1 x 10^{12} ohm input resistance of the electrometer[4], is across the tip resistance. An example using a conventional microelectrode of about 50 Mohms resistance and 1 pf of un-neutralized electrode capacitance gives an electrode time constant of 50 usec and a maximum switching rate of perhaps 4-5 kHz. This rate is just fast enough for the slow inward current if the electrode remains stable at 50 Mohms. One can improve this situation dramatically by using the discontinuous voltage clamp circuit with patch electrodes in the whole cell recording configuration and fabricating the patch electrodes for minimum electrode capacitance with Sylgard (see below). The time constant of this system can be as low as 0.6 usec, allowing switching rates approaching 100 kHz (limited now by internal circuit considerations rather than the electrode). Gigaseal formation on cell membranes with patch electrodes can be readily monitored with conventional electrometers by passing small test currents through the electrode. At the moment gentle suction on the pipette forms the gigaseal, the voltage deflection in response to the current pulse becomes very large (often saturating the electrometer). Rupturing the membrane patch with stronger suction (or brief overcompensation of capacitance) results in recording the resting potential of the cell.

Patch electrodes can also be used with a conventional two electrode voltage clamp circuit. In this case, the advantage is minimal sarcolemmal damage and the opportunity to dialyze the cell cytoplasm especially if patch electrodes are used for both voltage and current. If only one electrode is a patch electrode, low noise considerations and freedom from iontophoretically induced accumulation of charged molecules dictate that it should be the voltage electrode. The large open loop gain of a properly designed and implemented two electrode voltage clamp circuit will reduce the resistance of the current microelectrode by a factor of almost 10^5.

FABRICATION OF PATCH ELECTRODES

We routinely make electrodes for "gigaseal" recordings by pulling 1.2 mm glass capillary tubing with a Kopf (Tujunga, CA) model 720 puller. We use A-M Systems (Everett, WA) #6020 filament glass, however WPI (Hamden, CT) and others market similar if not the same glass, all of which seem to come from Glass Company of America in Bargaintown, New Jersey. The tubing is drawn from Corning 7740 ("Pyrex") glass and the pulling characteristics seem to vary some from one batch of glass to the next, possibly reflecting variation in Corning's formulation of 7740. Electrodes are pulled in two stages. The initial pull thins the electrode down to about 20% of its initial diameter and the final pull separates and forms the electrode. Kopf sells an attachment for pulling patch electrodes in two stages, but we find that we can fashion a temporary stop from a 35 mm film can cut such that it fits around the sliding vertical shaft of the lower electrode clamp and this works as well as the attachment.

We polish the electrodes on the stage of a microscope at about 500x with the aid of a 100 um diameter platinum-iridium filament bent into a "hairpin" shape. A dissecting microscope illuminator supply provides the low (4-7 VAC) voltage necessary to heat the filament to a red-orange color. We cannot resolve the tip of the electrode well enough to see its actual shape so we approach the filament with the electrode, apply heat and look for a change in the diffraction pattern at the tip. Electrode tip size is gauged by the well known bubble test. We use a Touhy-Borst adapter (#3097; Becton, Dickinson and Co., Rutherford, NJ) and a 10 cc syringe. The electrode is mounted directly in the Touhy-Borst adapter and the tip is immersed in methanol. Starting at the 10 cc volume mark, the syringe plunger is depressed. The volume mark where bubbles are first seen is noted as the bubble test number. We routinely use electrodes testing at 3.0 to 3.5 on the bubble test. These

---

[4] One could design a shorting electrometer, but it wouldn't be easy!

electrodes will have a resistance of about 3-8 Mohms when filled with the patch solution described below.

Electrode capacitance is reduced in several ways. We generally follow the recommendations of Corey and Stevens [2] and have coated electrode tips with Sylgard (Dow Corning Corp., Midland, MI). While this is a singularly effective means of reducing tip capacitance, it is time consuming and effective application requires winding a wisp of catalyzed but uncured resin to within 50 uM of the tip without clogging the tip. This method of electrode capacitance reduction can also be applied to conventional microelectrodes and is most useful when using a discontinuous (switching) voltage clamp. However we recommend using patch electrodes with this circuit (see Section I). We speed the curing of Sylgard by either passing the electrode through the heated coil of the electrode puller or by baking in a vacuum oven at $150^{o}C$ for a few minutes.

ELECTRODE HOLDERS AND FILLING SOLUTIONS

We mount the electrodes in electrode holders with side ports and silver wires (#PC-S3; E.W. Wright, Guilford, CT). The outside surface of these holders were coated with conductive paint (Ladd Research Industries, Inc. Burlington VT). The side port facilitates the application of suction or pressure, while the silver paint serves to reduce capacitance to ground. We have machined electrode holders from Teflon (TFE) similar to the E.W. Wright design for critical low noise recordings on excised patches. These holders are shielded with copper foil (which is available from music stores specializing in electric guitars). The connection of the electrode shield is always to the output of the negative capacitance circuit in our recording apparatus, since this facilitates current injection through the capacitor formed by the shielding and the core conductor (silver wire and electrode filling solution). Our TFE electrode holders have the advantage in this application of providing a uniform dielectric material since the insulator of the BNC connector into which the electrode holder fits is also TFE. The filling solution for patch recording has changed some over the years in our lab, but the current composition (in mM) is: K-aspartate (110); KCl (13); NaCl (7); EGTA (5); HEPES (10); glucose (5.4); pH=7.1. We don't routinely use ATP as a constituent of our patch solution and we think that a cautionary statement about this compound is necessary. The use of ATP in patch recordings arose because large "ATP-depletion" currents are induced under some recording conditions. These conditions may arise because either intracellular high energy phosphates and substrates necessary to maintain these metabolites are dialyzed below some critical level by the patch electrode. Obviously, this condition is exacerbated by large, low resistance patch electrodes and/or a cell preparation which is metabolically compromised. The reason for caution in using ATP in the pipette occurs due to ATP's role as a putative neurotransmitter. Recent reports [7] including one presented at this meeting indicate that ATP (and ADP) act through a membrane receptor to increase Ca^{++} conductance in the sarcolemmal membrane. The diffusion of patch solution (with ATP) from the pipette could activate ATP receptors and lead to an increase in intracellular Ca^{++}. This situation is most acute as the pipette is being brought close to the cell prior to forming a gigaseal and some investigators have noticed sarcomere shortening and contractions symptomatic of calcium overload when ATP was added to the pipette filling solution (A. Talo, personal communication). Any accumulation of ATP in a small recording dish (see [8]) from multiple gigaseals (or attempts) would be eliminated if the dish were perfused continuously with fresh solution.

CIRCUITRY

Voltage clamp circuits for whole cell recording

A single electrode continuous design

The design principles of the circuitry used to voltage clamp cells using the whole cell technique with a single electrode are well described in the literature [2]. Figure 2 is a schematic diagram of the single electrode circuit we use to patch clamp myocytes. Device A1 and resistor r1 comprise the headstage which is a current to voltage (I-V) converter (perhaps more familiarly known to electrophysiologists in its form as a virtual ground circuit). The + input of A1 is driven by the command voltage via the output of amplifier A4. The - input is connected to the patch pipette and is forced to the command potential by feedback through r1. We will refer to the voltage appearing at the inputs of A1 as the applied pipette potential. The value selected for r1 determines the current to voltage conversion ratio (in amps/volt). Since the most suitable operational amplifiers for the headstage of a patch clamp have a maximum output voltage near ±10 V, r1 also determines the maximum clamp current (I_{max}) which the circuit is capable of passing ($\pm I_{max} = \pm 10/r1$). I_{max} during a voltage clamp experiment is most likely to peak during steps to new potentials when capacitive currents dominate. In a typical voltage clamp experiment designed to investigate cellular properties

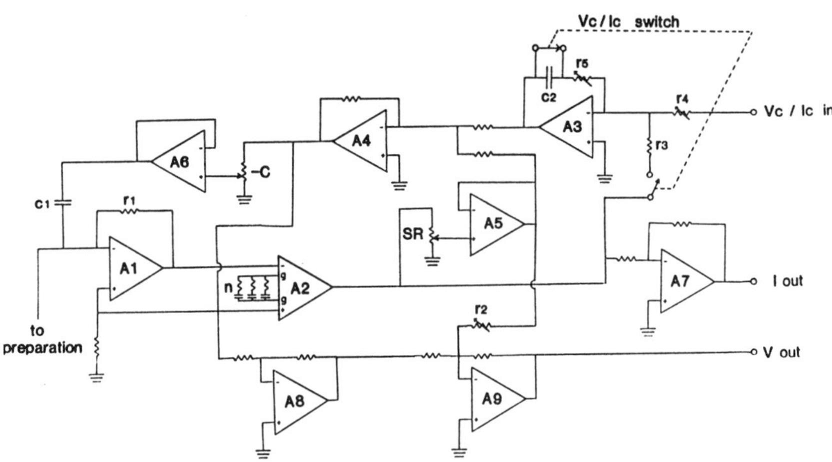

Figure 2. A schematic diagram of the single electrode continuous voltage clamp circuit. A1 (OPA 104) is the headstage amplifier. A2 (INA 101) is an instrumentation amp with an external gain network (n). A3 and A4 are the V_c amplifiers. A5 is the series resistance compensation amp. A6 is the capacitive transient cancellation amp. A7 inverts the current signal before output. A7 and A9 amplify the pipette potential and subtract series resistance compensation before output. All devices except those noted are Burr-Brown OPA 102's. SR and -C are 20 kohm 10 turn pots. All resistors are 10 kohm 1% except r2 (see text), and r3 - r5 which are 100 kohm trimmers. Capacitor c1 is formed by the input BNC, while c2 is hand selected for stability in the I_c mode.

associated with the slow inward current, the cell might be held at -50 mV and stepped to +10 mV to elicit the maximum inward Ca^{++} current. The command potential can change at the rate of 2 V/usec in even modest circuit designs[5] and a typical 110 x 25 x 5 um ventricular myocyte has an input capacitance (C_i) of about 100 pf [4]. Capacitive current (I_c) is Ci*dV/dt or 200 uA. If this current is to be supplied by the I-V converter, the sum of r1 and series resistance must be 50 kohms, a value far lower than can be achieved with this circuit. One solution to this problem is to slow the rate of change of the command potential so that the step from -50 mV to +10 mV occurs in 100 usec. In this case, I_c is 60 nA and a value of 100 Mohms for r1 (I_{max} = 100 nA) is feasible. Another solution is to use a circuit external to the I-V converter to supply the capacitive membrane current during a step voltage command. This circuit (not a part of the voltage clamp circuit in Figure 1) duplicates the circuit (Fig. 1; A6 with -C) used to supply current to charge the capacitance of the patch electrode except that the command voltage is AC coupled and filtered before

---

5 We assume for the purposes of this discussion that the leading edge of command voltage step is a ramp, an approximation (see the published oscillograph for the large signal pulse response in the specification sheets for an LF 356 op amp) which makes dV/dt a constant.

being applied to the amplifier input. The output from this circuit would be summed with the output from A6 to supply both cell membrane and electrode capacitive current via c1. For this scheme to work properly, series resistance compensation must be applied to the command signal *after* feeding the capacitive transient cancellation circuits.

Clamp current is the difference signal between output of the I-V converter and the command potential. A2 is an instrumentation amplifier which is a device, with an internally closed feedback loop, whose primary function is to accurately amplify low level difference signals in the presence of a larger ground referred signal. The network (n) connected to the "g" (gain) terminals alters the frequency response of A2 to compensate for the decrease in the frequency response of the I-V converter caused by r1 and stray capacitance (see [2] for a formal discussion of I-V high frequency roll-off). The values for the capacitors and resistors in n are selected by cut and try with the criteria being the minimum rise time in current steps injected into the input of the voltage clamp circuit. Current steps are injected by bringing a 4 cm length of wire connected to the output of a low distortion triangle wave generator in proximity to the input thus forming an air gap capacitor. The output of A2 is the inverted clamp current which is re-inverted by A7 to become I_{out} which gives inward currents through the cell membrane a negative polarity, the usual electrophysiological convention. The inversion of the clamp current at A2 simplifies adding series resistance compensation (Fig. 1; A5 and SR) and current clamp circuitry (Fig. 1; c2, r3, r5, and switch) by minimizing the number of inverting stages. Minimizing the number of stages comprising loops within the total circuit minimizes phase lags and anomalies as well as minimizing the parts count.

Devices A3 and A4 with their associated resistors amplify the command voltage signal input (V_c). Series resistance is summed with the command voltage at A4 to form the applied pipette potential. Resistor r2 subtracts the series resistance compensation signal from the inverted applied pipette potential at A9. A9 re-inverts the signal so that V_{out} is the command potential minus series resistance compensation. In the current clamp mode when the command current signal I_c is zero, V_{out} is the cell membrane resting potential. The V_c/I_c switch applies the inverted clamp current to the input of A3 in the current clamp position via r3. Capacitor c2 increases the gain of A3 at low frequencies, while r5 limits the gain reduction at high frequencies.

A two electrode continuous design

The design principles of the circuitry used to voltage clamp cells using two electrodes are well known and differ from the one electrode continuous design in one key point mentioned previously, the current passing electrode and the cell form the feedback network of an operational amplifier (the voltage clamp circuit). The overall design objective is to make the gain and the bandwidth of the individual stages in the voltage clamp circuit as high as possible to achieve a large gain bandwidth product for the overall circuit. Since feedback and thus the gain of the voltage clamp circuit will change as a function of the input resistance of the cell, this insures an ample feedback signal to control the voltage across the membrane of the cell even under conditions where the current electrode is high in resistance and the cell membrane is very conductive. The large gain bandwidth product of this circuit also allows us to dispense with most inter-electrode shielding as long as the included angle between the electrodes is at least 120°. Figure 3 is a schematic diagram of the two electrode circuit we use to voltage clamp myocytes. Device A1 and resistor r1 comprise the current headstage which is an I-V converter previously described above. The pipette command voltage is the output of A7, a 10X gain high voltage amplifier. A2 is an optically coupled isolation amplifier and is analogous to the instrumentation amplifier (A2 in Fig. 2) discussed in the previous section. An optically coupled isolation amplifier is used rather than an instrumentation amplifier in this design because: 1) the high voltage output of A7 precludes the use of commercially available committed differential amplifiers without employing some form of isolation; 2) the minimum common mode rejection ratio (CMRR) necessary to amplify a 1 mV (equal to 1 nA) signal in the presence of a 150 V ground referred (common mode) signal is 103.5 db, a performance difficult to obtain in a differential amplifier design, but easy in an isolated amplifier design; and 3) isolation of the headstage I-V converter allows the use of a fast, high performance, low voltage op amp with low input noise (Burr-Brown OPA 101). The choice of optical rather than transformer coupling was made on the basis of the superior frequency response and low noise of the optically coupled design. Linearity and temperature stability are achieved by coupling light from an LED driven by the output of A1' back to the input of A1' as well as forward to A2' (Fig. 3). A3 is the voltage headstage and is a simple follower with a gain of 1. A4 and its feedback network (gain is 10X), c1, and -C is the negative capacitance circuit. DC is a simple DC command circuit.

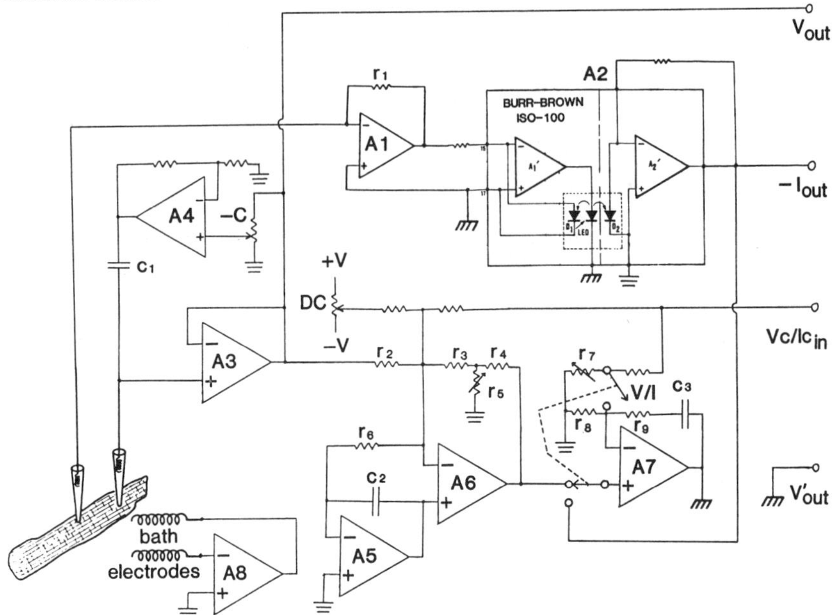

Figure 3. A simplified schematic diagram of a two electrode continuous voltage clamp circuit. A1, A3-A5, and A8 are Burr-Brown OPA 101 BM's. A1 and A1' are operated from an isolated $^{+}$15 V power supply (B.B. 722). A2 is an optically coupled isolation amplifier (B.B. ISO 100 CP) and A7 is a high voltage op amp (B.B. 3583) operated at $^{+}$150 V. A6 is a very high speed op amp (Analog Devices HOS 050A). Not shown are power supply connec-tions, some DC off-set circuits, the TTL connections for the V/I switch, and the inverter circuit for I_{out}. V/I, represented schematically as a DPDT switch, is made from two CMOS dual channel analog switches (DG-300; Siliconix, Inc.). ⏚ is an isolated ground plane driven by the output of A7.

The main clamp amplifier consists of A5-A7. Most of the gain is developed by A6 (Analog Devices HOS 050A; gain bandwidth product = 1 GHz), a very high speed, low noise op amp developed for video applications. The principle disadvantage of the HOS 050A is its huge initial input offset potential of 35 mV and a concomitant high temperature coefficient of offset drift. This disadvantage was solved by using a low drift amplifier (Fig. 3, A5, c2, and r6; A5 = B.B. OPA 104) to sense input offset voltage at the - input of A6 and correct it by driving the + input [9]. Capacitor c2 feeds the high frequency part of the signal around A5 (feedfoward design), so the very high gain bandwidth product of A6 is preserved along with the very low (250 uV) initial input offset voltage and drift of A5. The gain (A_V) of the A5-A6 combination is set by the local feedback network[6] consisting of r2-r5:

$$A_V = rf/r2$$

[6] We call this network <u>local</u> because the cell and the current electrode form an external feedback network for the entire clamp circuit.

Resistor network r3-r5 forms a "T" attenuation network whose effective resistance (rf) is:

$$rf = r3 + r4 + \frac{r3*r4}{r5}$$

When r5 is set to zero, rf becomes infinite and A_V becomes the open loop gain of A5-A6. This is the setting at which we operate the voltage clamp circuit after instabilities from switching to the voltage clamp mode have settled. The gain of the voltage clamp circuit is further enhanced at low frequencies by capacitor c3 in the feedback loop of A7.

The current clamp mode is analogous to that discussed previously for the single electrode clamp and is done by disconnecting the main clamp amplifier from A7 and connecting the output of the current measuring circuit to A7. Since we connected the output of A1 to the - terminal of A2, the output of the current monitor is inverted, so no additional inverter stage is necessary. The other section of the V/I switch is closed to connect I_c as well as r7 to the summing junction of A7. Current commands are fed via I_c and r7 is placed in parallel with r8 to increase the gain of A7.

SUMMARY

Three protocols for voltage-clamping isolated myocytes along with the advantages and disadvantages of each technique were discussed. Single electrode voltage clamp circuits using current-to-voltage converters as the first stage have a significant series resistance problem when used to voltage clamp myocytes. This disadvantage is overcome by employing discontinuous single electrode or continuous two electrode voltage clamp circuits. The electrode time constant, however, becomes a limiting factor in the performance of the discontinuous voltage clamp. Patch electrodes, by reducing the access resistance to the cytoplasm of the cell, offer significant advantages over microelectrodes when used with single or double electrode voltage clamp circuits. We presented two circuits for voltage or current clamping: 1) a single electrode circuit using an I-V converter as the headstage; and 2) a two electrode circuit which uses an I-V converter and optically coupled isolation amplifier to measure current, a very fast op amp, and a high voltage output stage.

REFERENCES

1. Hamill, O.P., A. Marty, E. Neher, B. Sakmann, and F.J. Sigworth. Pfluegers Archiv. 391, 85-100 (1981).
2. Sakmann, B. and E. Neher. Single-channnel Recording (Plenum Press, New York 1983).
3. Beyerly, L. and W.J. Moody. J. Physiol. 376, 477-491 (1986).
4. White, R.L., D.C. Spray, A.C.C. de Carvalho, B.A. Wittenberg, and M.V.L. Bennett. Am. J. Physiol. 249(Cell Physiol. 18), C447-C455 (1985).
5. Wittenberg, B.A., R.L. White, R.D. Ginsberg, and D.C. Spray. Circ. Res. 59(2), 143-150 (1986).
6. Brigham, E.O. The Fast Fourier Transform (Prentice-Hall, Inc., Englewood Cliffs NJ 1974).
7. Benham, C.B. and R.W. Tsien. Nature 328, 275-278 (1987).
8. Wittenberg, B.A., J. Doeller, R. Gupta, and R.L. White in: The Biology of Isolated Myocytes. T. Borg, W. Clark, and R. Decker eds. (Elsevier Amsterdam 1988).
9. Graeme, J.G. Designing with Operational Amplifiers: Applications Alternatives (McGraw-Hill New York 1977).

ACKNOWLEDGMENTS: I wish to thank my friends and colleagues in the Depts. of Neuroscience and Physiology and Biophysics for many helpful discussions in these matters. Supported by NIH HL-33655 and NS 07512.

BIOCHEMISTRY OF ISOLATED MYOCYTES

Beatrice A. Wittenberg, Albert Einstein College of Medicine, Bronx, N.Y. and Robert A. Haworth, University of Wisconsin, Madison.

OVERVIEW

The broad scope of the biochemistry section testified to the range of opportunity which isolated adult heart cells offer for biochemical investigation.

In his opening remarks Dr. Howard Morgan addressed the question of the usefulness of the isolated adult cardiac myocyte model for the elucidation of biochemistry observed in the whole heart. He pointed out that each model for experimental investigation of the heart has its strengths and its weaknesses. The choice of model should be determined by the question being asked, and by the limits which the experimental investigation of the question imposes. Papers presented in the Biochemistry Section exploited several specific advantages of the isolated cell model in physiological and pathological states.

1. Short defined diffusion distances permit definition of the extracellular medium and simultaneous monitoring of the intracellular milieu. Reports described the spectroscopic monitoring of intracellular myoglobin (Wittenberg and Wittenberg); fluorescence measurements of intracellular calcium (Hansford and Moreno-Sanchez); and Ca^{2+} uptake (Kaminishi and Kako) in intact cells.

2. Isolated cells allow solution biochemistry while preserving intracellular structure, compartmentation and functional intracellular interactions. Many reports exploited this advantage. Reports described the functional interactions of sarcoplasmic myoglobin with mitochondrial oxidative phosphorylation (Wittenberg and Wittenberg); sarcoplasmic free calcium with mitochondrial pyruvate dehydrogenase, mitochondrial $NADH/NAD^+$, and oxidative phosphorylation (Hansford and Moreno-Sanchez); extracellular oxidants with intracellular calcium homeostasis (Kaminishi and Kako) and with sarcoplasmic and mitochondrial adenine nucleotides (Andersson, Sundberg and Rajs). Effects of extracellular hypoxia, substrate deprivation and deenergization on the intracellular adenine nucleotide pool were described by Altschuld, Gamelin, Kelley, Lambert, Mackall and Brierley; and also by Pinson, Venturi and De Jong. Effects of extracellular hormones on: intracellular glucose oxidation (Chen and Downing); sarcolemmal receptor binding, and intermediates involved in signal transduction to the sarcoplasm (Eckel and Reinauer; Shanahan and Edwards; Buxton; Lundgren, Terracio, Allen and Borg; Jones, McDonaugh and Brown) were reported.

3. A preparation of isolated myocytes permits the study of myocyte biochemistry with minimized contribution from non-myocyte heart cells. Reports in which this was important were in the study of adenine nucleotide catabolism (Altschuld et al, Pinson et al), lipoprotein lipase activity (Severson), and the study of alpha, adrenergic effects (Buxton; Jones et al).

Biology of Isolated Adult Cardiac Myocytes
William A. Clark, Robert S. Decker, and Thomas K. Borg, Editors

SUMMARY OF FINDINGS

The control of respiratory rate

Wittenberg and Wittenberg presented data which showed that a fraction (30%) of the basal respiratory rate of cells in suspension was proportional to the fraction of oxymyoglobin, under conditions where sufficient oxygen was present to fully saturate cytochrome oxidase. These conditions were achieved by carbon monoxide competitive blockade at partial pressure ratio of carbon monoxide to oxygen of 1:1, insufficient to inhibit cytochrome oxidase directly but high enough to bind to myoglobin. The authors conclude that oxymyoglobin delivers a flow of oxygen to intracellular cardiac mitochondria.

Hansford and Moreno-Sanchez showed that a rough correlation exists between respiration rate and the logarithm of intracellular Ca concentration , when cells are loaded with Ca^{++} by veratridine treatment or K^{+} depolarization. Pyruvate dehydrogenase was activated, but mitochondrial $NADH/NAD^{+}$ ratios decreased, indicating that the stimulation of respiration exceeded that of the dehydrogenases.

Oxidant-induced damage

Kaminishi and Kako showed that H_2O_2 acted like ouabain in causing a stimulation of Ca uptake, resulting in a decline in cell viability. They concluded that H_2O_2 inhibited the NaK ATPase by an iron-catalyzed Haber-Weiss reaction.

Andersson et al showed that the lipophilic oxidant, tert-butyl hydroperoxide, caused a loss in cell viability and a decline in ATP. They find that the mitochondrial adenine and pyridine nucleotides persisted longer than the cytosolic pools. They suggest that mitochondrial nucleotides played a functional role in toxic cell injury.

Regional creatine kinase distribution

Smith et al found evidence for a moderate but significant difference in creatine kinase activity between different regions of the heart. When expressed as activity per cell, instead of activity per mg protein, the activity in the right ventricular free wall was less than that in the left ventricle and septum. This suggests a greater activity per cell in cells which sustain a greater load. They also observed that in hearts made hypertrophic by renal hypertension the activity per mg protein decreases, but the activity per cell remains the same. This also suggests that the activity is determined by load and not by cell size, if it is assumed that the hypertrophy was sufficient to normalize wall stress.

Adenine nucleotide metabolism in anoxia and ischemia

Altschuld et al showed that ATP regenerated by reoxygenation after a period of anoxia originated from IMP rather than from adenosine. They also found that the conditions at the time of ATP depletion determined whether AMP was degraded to IMP or to adenosine: if glycolysis was inactive, IMP was formed; if glycolysis was active, adenosine was formed.

Pinson et al presented a model for ischemia using cultured (Neonatal) heart cells. Extracellular volume was made small so that excreted metabolites were accumulated at high concentration. Effects of glucose deprivation and anoxia were reported. Glucose was found to protect strongly against depletion of ATP and phosphocreatine. Release of a portion of cytosolic enzymes was observed before the onset of irreversible cell damage and was arrested on reoxygenation, whereas lysosomal enzyme release occurred later and was not reversible.

Glucose transport and oxidation in diabetes, and the mechanism of action insulin

Chen and Downing presented data showing that cells from strepto-zotocin-diabetic rats oxidized glucose at impaired rates which could be restored only partially to normal by insulin addition. T_3, T_4 and norepinephrine had little further effect. Insulin given (i.v.) to the rats 30 min. before sacrifice, on the other hand, resulted in complete restoration of glucose oxidation in cells subsequently isolated.

Using measurements of 3-0-methylglucose uptake rate, Eckel and Reinauer found an unaltered sensitivity of Zucker (obese) rat heart cells to insulin. The maximal effect of insulin was decreased in cells from Zucker rats, while cells from diabetic BB rats showed a reduced sensitivity but an unaltered maximal effect.

To elucidate the role of receptor internalization in insulin action, Eckel and Reinauer blocked internalization with phenylarsine oxide, and found the onset of insulin action was delayed. They concluded that receptor internalization promotes insulin action.

Shanahan and Edwards investigated the role of cGMP analogues and stimulation of glucose transport. They found that cGMP analogues and stimulators of guanylate cyclase stimulated glucose transport, inhibitors of guanylate cyclase blocked the response to insulin, and inhibitors of phosphodiesterase with some selectivity for cGMP stimulated glucose transport at low concentrations. They propose an involvement of cGMP as an inducer of glucose transport in mammalian heart cells, and its involvement in the stimulation of glucose transport by insulin.

Adrenergic and cholinergic receptors function

Buxton has found that alpha stimulation promotes cAMP degradation in myocytes, and that the alpha receptor action apparently is mediated by a GTP-dependent transducer. He has now investigated how this action might be mediated. He showed that alpha stimulation results in transient IP_3 formation, as has been found in other cell types. Both alpha-stimulated IP_3 formation and cAMP degradation were inhibited by phorbol ester. He concluded that the activation of cAMP degradation may be mediated by IP_3, perhaps as a consequence of IP_3-induced Ca release.

Lundgren et al showed that the number of beta receptors on adult rat heart cells was maintained for ten days in culture, although the cAMP response to beta stimulation tended to increase.

Jones et al, like Buxton, reported increased IP_3 formation in permeable cells in response to GTP S, suggesting a role for a G protein in regulation of PI hydrolysis, as in other cell types. They also found an increased release of arachidonic acid after norepinephrine or carbachol treatment, and investigated the mechanism of this. No increase in intracellular Ca resulted from hormone treatment, even though IP_3 was formed; on the other hand phorbol ester increased arachidonic acid release. This supported a mechanism mediated through protein kinase C activation, rather than through Ca activation of phospholipase A_2, though several interpretations were possible.

Severson reported that isoproterenol had no effect on lipoprotein lipase activity in cardiac myocytes, even though an increase in the activity ratio for phosphorylase was detected. Heparin released lipoprotein lipase into the medium without any detectable reduction in myocyte lipoprotein lipase activity.

SUMMARY DISCUSSION SESSION, FRIDAY, MORNING

The biochemistry discussion section addressed the question of myocyte preparation: For biochemical measurements it is important to maximize the yields of calcium tolerant cells both in order to minimize selection of specific cells and to have enough material for assay.

There was general agreement that the low calcium, collagenase perfusion is crucial for good yield although a variety of conditions are equally effective, as long as there is good perfusion. Many successful perfusions use balanced salt solution supplemented with amino acids with pH buffering either by HEPES or bicarbonate. Bicarbonate buffering requires control of CO_2 in the gas equilibration. Many investigators use perfusion at 37°C. At different temperatures it is important to optimize O_2 of the gas equilibration.

Dr. Altschuld reported that the method of killing the rat affected some properties of the myocytes subsequently isolated. In experiments where the rate of Ca entry into ATP-depleted cells was measured, she found that the rate was much lower when rats were anesthetized with pentobarbital (i.p.) before excision of the heart than when cells were isolated from rats killed by guillotine. It was speculated that the difference could be caused by the large and rapid release of catecholamines that occurs on decapitation. Dr. Claycomb noted that a good preparation was obtained even if 20-30 minutes elapsed between decapitation and the mounting of the heart for perfusion. Some investigators noted that they carefully massaged the heart during perfusion (without bruising) to achieve washout of visible blood. Some investigators used heparin, but others found it unnecessary if hearts were excised and cannulated sufficiently rapidly to avoid clotting. Dr. Claycomb used adenosine to dilate blood vessels during perfusion. Recirculating perfusion is used by many investigators, who also use 7-10 ml/min perfusion rates. Some investigators maintain a constant pressure head, while others maintain a constant flow rate during perfusion. For 350 to 450g rats 20-30 minute collagenase perfusions were reported. Calcium is diminished to low levels of about 10-50 uM for the initial portion of the collagenase perfusion. Dr. Haworth reported that concentrated amino acid solutions in glass bottles (100 x MEM amino acids, Flow Labs) contain 2 to 3 mM Ca. If this is added to the Ca free perfusate this Ca must be removed, since the resulting Ca concentration is too high, and the hearts become patchy, resulting in a low yield. He also reported that 1 mM Ca could be reintroduced into the perfusate after 20 min of collagenase perfusion without damge to the cells, resulting in a improvement in % rod-shaped cells in the final preparation. Dr. Altschuld commented that she now also follows this procedure. Others increase the calcium to this level after removing the heart from the cannula or after cell isolation.

At any rate 1 mM calcium should be introduced before final use of the cells both to get rid of calcium intolerant cells and to improve the long term viability of calcium tolerant cells. In addition to the importance of the length of time of Ca deprivation, it is also possible that the length of time after restoration of Ca to the cells is a significant variable in determining their measured biochemical properties. Considerable variability is reported in relation to the basal rate of glucose transport, from essentially zero to values similar to the insulin-stimulated rate. Dr. Eckel commented that bovine serum albumin raised the basal rate of glucose transport, to a degree variable between lots. Dr. Altschuld noted that it is also important to analyze lots of bovine serum albumin (BSA) for efficacy in maintaining viability. Dr. Wittenberg uses extensive dialysis of BSA first against 2 changes in EDTA to remove some of the heavy metal contaminants and then four changes in balanced isotonic buffered salt solution. Taurine addition to the MEM, was reported by Dr. Wittenberg to diminish myoglobin leakage from cells. Optimal collagenase preparations are difficult to define because identical analyses provided by the manufacturer may give variable yields. Collagenase, trypsin and clostripain with variable proteases are part of collagenase Type II supplied by Worthington which is used effectively by several investigators. Collagenase preparations should be tested for optimal properties for the particular purpose of the heart cell preparation. Maximum yield, high ATP and phosphocreatine levels, optimum contractile and electrophysiological properties, are among the most sensitive assays.

A NEW FUNCTION OF MYOGLOBIN REVEALED IN CARDIAC MYOCYTES

Beatrice A. Wittenberg and Jonathan B. Wittenberg, Albert Einstein College of Medicine, 1300 Morris Park Avenue, Bronx, N.Y. 10461

Classic hypotheses for the role of myoglobin in aiding respiratory oxygen uptake by the heart are: short-term oxygen storage and facilitation of oxygen diffusion [1,2]. Beat-to-beat fluctuation in stores of myoglobin-bound oxygen observed in the saline-perfused heart [3,4,5], may be damped by reserves of hemoglobin-bound oxygen held in the capillaries of the blood perfused normal heart.

The need for myoglobin has been established by studies of blood perfused skeletal muscle _in situ_ [6] and by studies of saline-perfused heart [7,8]. Inactivation of myoglobin in blood-perfused muscle sharply reduces work output and oxygen utilization [6]. Inactivation of myoglobin in the arrested, saline-perfused heart leads to rapid depletion of intracellular ATP and phosphocreatine [8].

A preparation of fiber bundles teased from pigeon breast muscle is favorable to demonstrate myoglobin-enhanced oxygen transport [9]. The diffusion path from outside to the innermost mitochondria of the bundle is very long. In experiments using fiber bundles, inactivation of myoglobin roughly halved respiratory oxygen uptake at oxygen pressures where oxygen supply was limiting oxygen uptake.

Myoglobin-facilitated oxygen diffusion is a consequence of the reversible binding of oxygen to myoglobin. The molecular mechanism has been established by experiments in model systems [10,11]. Myoglobin molecules, wandering in solution in a random walk, constantly combine with and dissociate diatomic oxygen. During the time that a myoglobin molecule carries a bound oxygen molecule, it may undergo translational displacement through the solution. In the presence of a gradient of oxygen pressure, provided that the oxygen pressure on the downhill side is low enough to at least partially desaturate the myoglobin, there will also be a gradient of myoglobin fractional saturation with oxygen. The consequence is a net flux of oxymyoglobin molecules carrying bound oxygen molecules (and an equal and opposite flux of deoxymyoglobin molecules). The flux of myoglobin-bound oxygen is the facilitated flux and is additive with the simple diffusive flux of dissolved oxygen.

The diffusive flux is proportional to the oxygen pressure gradient, while facilitated flux is proportional to the concentration of myoglobin and the steepness of the gradient of myoglobin oxygenation. Total flux is the sum of the two. Calculation suggests that each flux will contribute about half of the oxygen influx into normally working muscle [12,13].

A suspension of isolated heart cells offers the experimental advantage that the steady state extracellular oxygen pressure may be set to any desired value. Previously we have studied heart cells at low extracellular oxygen pressure to learn the steepness of intracellular oxygen pressure gradients. Oxygen uptake by these isolated heart cells does not become oxygen limited until intracellular myoglobin is largely deoxygenated and extracellular oxygen pressure is less than 1.0 torr. We find that oxygen pressure differences within the respiring myocyte are small and that the largest part of the oxygen pressure difference, 20 torr, from the capillary

Biology of Isolated Adult Cardiac Myocytes
William A. Clark, Robert S. Decker, and Thomas K. Borg, Editors

lumen to mitochondria of the working heart must be extracellular [14].

If the extracellular oxygen pressure is made large (greater than 40 torr) intracellular myoglobin of a suspension of cardiac myocytes will be almost fully saturated with oxygen and the gradient of myoglobin oxygenation, on which facilitated diffusion depends, will vanish. The gradient of oxygen pressure to the mitochondrion will be large, and the maximum diffusive oxygen flux will exceed mitochondrial oxygen consumption. When these experiments are carried out in steady states [14], the storage function of myoglobin also vanishes. Cytochrome oxidase is not oxygen-limited and experiences oxygen pressures 20-200-fold that required to maintain the normal, largely oxidized, state seen in resting myocytes. Carbon monoxide now blocks oxygenation of sarcoplasmic myoglobin selectively without perturbing the optical spectrum of intracellular cytochrome oxidase.

Carbon monoxide competes with oxygen for binding to intracellular myoglobin. At constant P_{O2} and increasing P_{CO}, an increasing fraction of myoglobin is ligated to carbon monoxide (at the oxygen pressures used, the balance is oxymyoglobin). Myoglobin is almost entirely converted to the carbon monoxide form when the ratio P_{CO}/P_{O2} approaches 1:1. At this ratio, and indeed up to a ratio of 20:1, optical spectra indicate no ligation of carbon monoxide to intracellular cytochrome oxidase, which remains in its normal, largely oxidized state. Carbon monoxide blockade of myoglobin oxygenation abolishes about one third of the total respiration of resting cardiac myocytes [15]. This may be called the myoglobin-dependent respiration. This myoglobin-dependent oxygen uptake is inversely proportional to the fractional saturation of sarcoplasmic myoglobin with carbon monoxide and is proportional to the fraction of sarcoplasmic oxymyoglobin. Half inhibition was achieved at different P_{CO} in experiments at different P_{O2}, but always when myoglobin was half saturated with carbon monoxide. This indicates that the effect of carbon monoxide is exerted on myoglobin and cannot be ascribed to inhibition of other cellular functions.

We conclude that cardiac mitochondria accept two additive, simultaneous flows of oxygen: the well-known flow of dissolved oxygen to cytochrome oxidase (about two thirds of the total respiration in these experiments) and a flow of myoglobin-bound oxygen to a mitochondrial terminus (the myoglobin-dependent respiration) [15]. The myoglobin-mediated oxygen flow supports ATP generation in the physiological range of oxygen pressure.

These experiments were possible because suspensions of isolated cardiac myocytes lend themselves to: 1) precise control of extracellular gas pressures; 2) accurate measurement of steady state oxygen uptake; 3) optical spectroscopy with well defined intracellular path length. Ligation of intracellular myoglobin and oxidation/reduction state of components of the intracellular, mitochondrial electron transport chain are learned from the optical spectra.

METHODS

Preparation of Isolated Heart Cells

This preparation is described in a chapter in this volume (16).

Measurement of Steady State Respiration and Optical Spectra

The observation chamber and method have been described [14,15].

Analytical Measurements

ATP and phosphocreatine are measured using ion exchange HPLC, with a modification of the method of Harmsen et al [17]. We use ammonium salts instead of potassium salts in our eluting buffers. We use a Perkin Elmer Series 400 liquid chromatograph with LC-85B variable wavelength detector and LCI-100 integrator. A sample of heart cells (1 ml; 10^6 cells per ml) is added to 0.4 ml of ice cold 3M perchloric acid and immediately frozen in liquid nitrogen. The sample is cautiously returned to ice temperature, centrifuged to remove precipated protein, neutralized with KOH and again centrifuged to remove potassium perchlorate. This procedure minizimes loss of phosphocreatine. An aliquot (100 ul sample loop) is fractionated on a Partisil SAX 10 anion exchange column fitted with a guard column. The column is eluted first with 0.005 M H_3PO_4 adjusted to pH 2.85 with ammonium hydroxide for 10 min at 1 ml/min. Ten minutes after injection a gradient is started with .75 M ammonium phosphate replacing the original buffer at 4% per minute at a flow rate of 2 ml/min.

Protein is determined by the method of Lowry et al [18].

ACKNOWLEDGEMENTS

This work was supported in part by NIH HL 19299 and HL33655 (to B.A.W.) and by Research Grants DMB 84-16001 and PCM 84-16016 (to J.B.W.) from the United States National Science Founcation. J.B.W. is a Research Career Program Awardee 1-K6-733 of the United States Public Health Service, National Heart, Lung, and Blood Institute.

REFERENCES

1. J.B. Wittenberg, Physiol. Rev. 50, 559-636 (1970).

2. J.B. Wittenberg and B.A. Wittenberg in: Oxygen and Living Processes, D.L. Gilbert, ed. (Springer Verlag, New York 1981) pp. 177-199.

3. M. Tamura, N. Oshino, B. Chance and I.A. Sibver, Arch. Biochem 191, 8-22 (1978).

4. I.E. Hassinen, J.K. Hiltunen, and T.E.S. Takala, Cardiovasc. Res. 15, 86-91 (1981).

5. L. Caspary, J. Hoffmann, H.R. Ahmad, and D.W. Lubbers, Adv. Exptl. Med. Biol. 191, 263-270 (1985).

6. R.P. Cole, Resp. Physiol. 53, 1-14 (1983).

7. J.R. Bailey and W.R. Driedzic, Am. J. Physiol. 251, R1144-R1150 (1986).

8. D.J. Taylor, P.M. Matthews and G.K. Radda, Resp. Physiol. 63, 275-287 (1986).

9. B.A. Wittenberg, J.B. Wittenberg and P.R.B. Caldwell, J. Biol. Chem. 250, 9038-9043 (1976).

10. J.B. Wittenberg, Biol. Bull. 117, 402 (1959).

11. P.F. Scholander, Science 131, 585-590 (1960).

12. J. Wyman, J. Biol. Chem. 241, 115-121 (1966).

13. J.D. Murray, Lectures on Nonlinear-differential equation models in Biol. (Clarendon Press, Oxford 1977).

14. B.A. Wittenberg and J.B. Wittenberg, J. Biol. Chem. 260, 6548-6554 (1985).

15. B.A. Wittenberg and J.B. Wittenberg, Proc. Natl. Acad. Sci. in press Nov. 1987.

16. B. A. Wittenberg, J.E. Doeller, R.K. Gupta and R.L. White in: Biology of Isolated Adult Cardiac Myocytes (1988).

17. E. Harmsen, P.Ph. DeTombe, and J.W. DeJong, J. Chromat. 230, 131-136 (1982).

18. O.H. Lowry, N.J. Rosebrough, A.L. Farr, and R.J. Randall, J. Biol. Chem. 193, 265-275 (1951).

MECHANISM OF H_2O_2-INDUCED ACCELERATION OF CALCIUM INFLUX INTO ISOLATED RAT HEART MYOCYTES.

T.Kaminishi and K.J.Kako*
Department of Physiology, University of Ottawa, Ottawa, Ontario, K1H 8M5

A number of reports have appeared in recent years indicating that generation of oxygen free radicals is involved in some disease states including ischemia-reperfusion injury (1 for review). The most likely source of free radicals appears to be activated polymorphonuclear leucocytes which produce H_2O_2, superoxide radicals and secondarily-generated hypochlorite (2). Another possible source is xanthine oxidase which may be produced under hypoxic conditions.

However, the mode of action of reactive oxygen intermediates in causing cellular injury remains largely unknown. We investigated in our previous studies the effect of H_2O_2 on isolated Na^+K^+ATPase preparations. Our results indicated that H_2O_2 suppressed the enzyme activity, ouabain binding and sulfhydryl content, suggesting that enzyme protein was modified by the action of free radicals (3,4). However, whether or not such a mechanism of free radical action may be operative in a more integrated biological system is not known. Therefore, we have investigated effects of several oxidants on Ca^{2+} influx of heart myocytes. A number of advantages to using isolated, calcium-tolerant, adult rat heart cell preparations have been recognized (5,6). Ca^{2+} influx was chosen as an indicator for changes in intracellular calcium homeostasis, since the latter is difficult to quantify.

Adult rat heart myocytes were isolated by perfusion and incubation in medium containing collagenase (Fig.1). Viabilities, as judged by trypan blue exclusion and rod cell morphology (5), were changed little over 3 h in

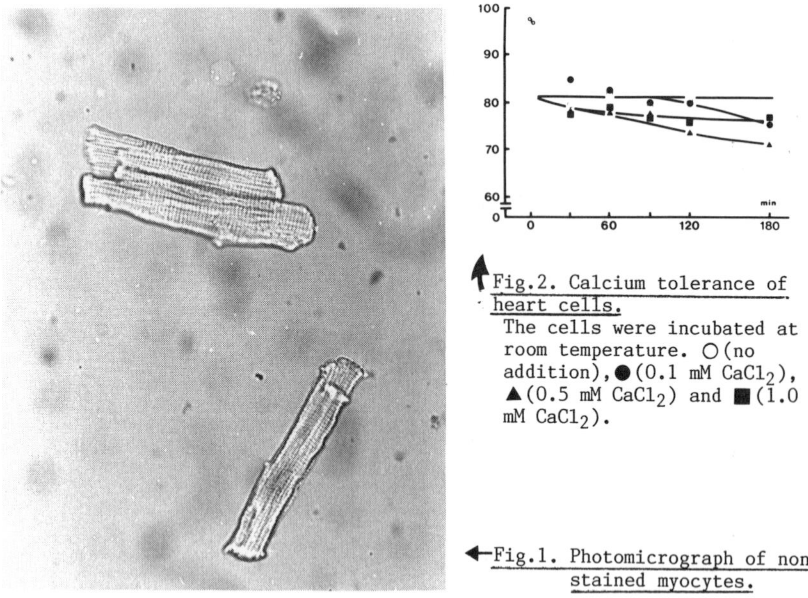

Fig.2. Calcium tolerance of heart cells.
The cells were incubated at room temperature. ○(no addition), ●(0.1 mM $CaCl_2$), ▲(0.5 mM $CaCl_2$) and ■(1.0 mM $CaCl_2$).

Fig.1. Photomicrograph of non-stained myocytes.

* address for correspondence.

Biology of Isolated Adult Cardiac Myocytes
William A. Clark, Robert S. Decker, and Thomas K. Borg, Editors

the presence of 1 mM $CaCl_2$ (Fig.2). Several oxidants, viz. H_2O_2, hypochlorite, ammonium persulfate, t-butyl hydroperoxide, etc., accelerated the advance of contracture of myocytes in a concentration- and time-dependent manner (Figs.3 & 4)(MS submitted for publication). The rate of Ca^{2+} influx into the cell was examined with $[^{45}Ca]Cl_2$. Following various times of incubation, cell suspensions were filtered by suction through a Millipore filter. The myocytes took up $[^{45}Ca]^{2+}$ rapidly during the first few min upon addition of radioactive $CaCl_2$. The amount of Ca^{2+} uptake reached a plateau approximately in 10 min (Fig.5). Ca^{2+} uptake by myocytes, measured in this manner, increased very rapidly for the first 30 min following the addition of 2.5 mM H_2O_2 to the cell suspension. Uptake was essentially unchanged between 60 and 120 min after H_2O_2 addition, and therefore, influx of $[^{45}Ca]^{2+}$ into cardiomyocytes was determined 60 min following addition of the oxidant. The influx was found to be increased by 2.5 mM H_2O_2 twofold (Fig.5). Ca^{2+} influx stimulated by H_2O_2 was suppressed by increasing $[Na^+]o$ to 194 mM. The increased medium Na^+ concentration by itself did not influence the Ca^{2+} uptake. By contrast, lowering of $[Na^+]o$ to 15 mM increased Ca^{2+} uptake (Fig.6). Ouabain (1 mM) similarly increased Ca^{2+} uptake (6), but a further addition of H_2O_2 to the incubation mixture containing ouabain did not increase the Ca^{2+} uptake (Fig.7). Increasing the Na^+ concentration of the medium containing ouabain to 194 mM inhibited the increase in Ca^{2+} uptake. These maneuvers, i.e., raising or reducing the medium Na^+ concentration, or addition of ouabain, did not significantly alter cell viabilities. These observations suggest that H_2O_2-induced acceleration in cell contracture was independent of the increase in Ca^{2+} influx. Thus, our results support those obtained by Altschuld et al. (7) and Starke et al. (8), who demonstrated that not intracellular calcium homeostasis per se, but some other factors, for example, an interrelationship between decrease in cytosolic ATP level and increase in free calcium concentration, are associated with the progress of hypercontracture of isolated myocytes.

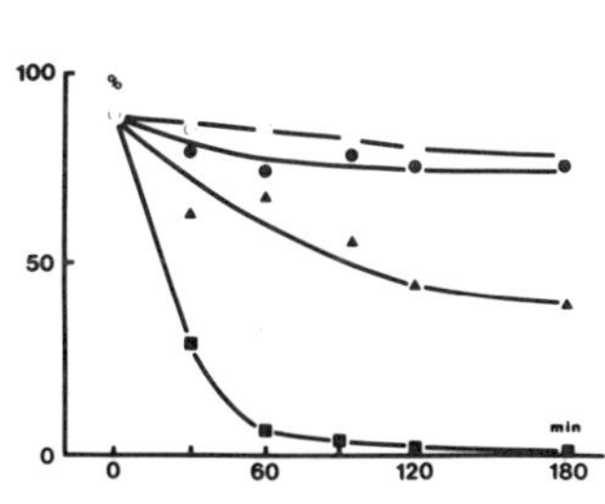

Fig.3. Effects of H_2O_2 on viabilities of myocytes. ○(no addition),●(1 mM), ▲(2.5 mM) and ■(5 mM).

Fig.4. Photomicrograph of contractured cells.

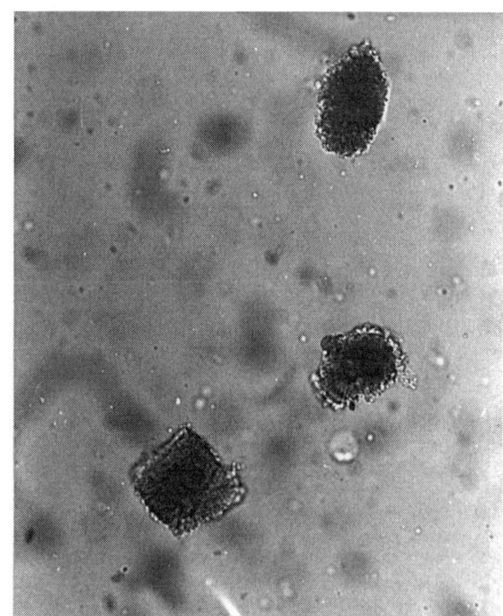

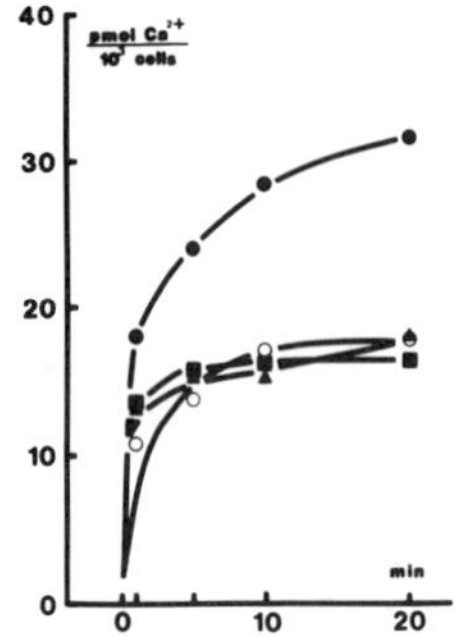

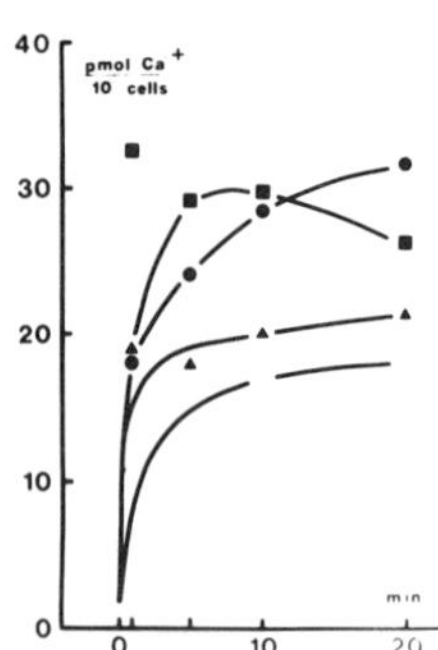

Fig.5. (left) Effects of H_2O_2 and high $[Na^+]o$ on Ca^{2+} uptake by myocytes. ○ (no addition), ● (2.5 mM H_2O_2, 120 mM Na^+), ■ (2.5 mM H_2O_2, 194 mM Na^+) and ▲ (194 mM Na^+).

Fig.6. (right) Effects of H_2O_2 and low $[Na^+]o$ on Ca uptake by myocytes. ○ (no addition), ● (2.5 mM H_2O_2, 120 mM Na^+), ■ (2.5 mM H_2O_2, 15 mM Na^+) and ▲ (15 mM Na^+).

Involvement of sarcolemmal Na^+/Ca^{2+} exchange is further indicated by the experiment in which medium pH was decreased from 7.3 to 6.5. H_2O_2-induced acceleration in Ca^{2+} uptake was suppressed to nearly the control level at pH 6.5 (9). These results suggest that the action of H_2O_2 is mediated by the enhancement of Ca^{2+} influx via sarcolemmal Na^+/Ca^{2+} exchange activity. The Bmax of ouabain binding to myocytes was 3.69 ± 0.13 amol/cell (n = 8), which was reduced by 2.5 mM H_2O_2 to 1.01 amol/cell, and by 5 mM to 0.64 amol/cell, supporting the view that H_2O_2 or H_2O_2-derived free radicals inhibited Na^+K^+ ATPase activity.

The possibility that Ca^{2+} influx was accelerated by enhanced intracellular Ca^{2+} uptake or opening of Ca^{2+} channels was examined next. Reduction in the intracellular ATP level by an uncoupler, CCCP (6), decreased Ca^{2+} influx and accelerated advance of contracture. The results suggest that mitochondria released Ca^{2+} and their Ca^{2+} uptake decreased, as consequences of reduction of proton gradients of the inner membrane. Administration of hypochlorite reduced also Ca^{2+} influx, probably through the inhibition of intracellular Ca^{2+} uptake. The H_2O_2-induced increase in Ca^{2+} uptake was not significantly changed by the addition of diltiazem, verapamil or amiloride, suggesting that Ca^{2+} channels did not play a major role in H_2O_2-stimulation of Ca^{2+} influx. 3-aminobenzamide has been used as an inhibitor of poly(ADP-ribose) polymerase, which is activated upon addition of H_2O_2 to tumour cells, P388D1, and human lymphocytes. Inhibition of the enzyme was found by other investigators to prevent injury caused by H_2O_2 (10). However, the decrease in viability and the increase in Ca^{2+} influx, induced by H_2O_2in isolated rat heart cells, were both uninfluenced by 3-aminobenzamide.

Deferoxamine suppressed significantly the H_2O_2-stimulated Ca^{2+} uptake (Fig.8) and ameliorated the oxidant-induced membrane damage, as indicated by trypan blue permeability. These results suggest that the effect of H_2O_2 is mediated through the transition metal ion-catalyzed free radical reaction.

Our results presented here suggest that although the progress of hypercontracture of cardiomyocytes was accelerated by exposure to H_2O_2,

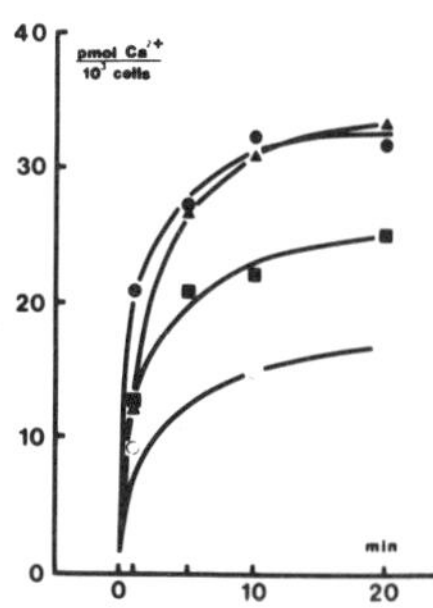

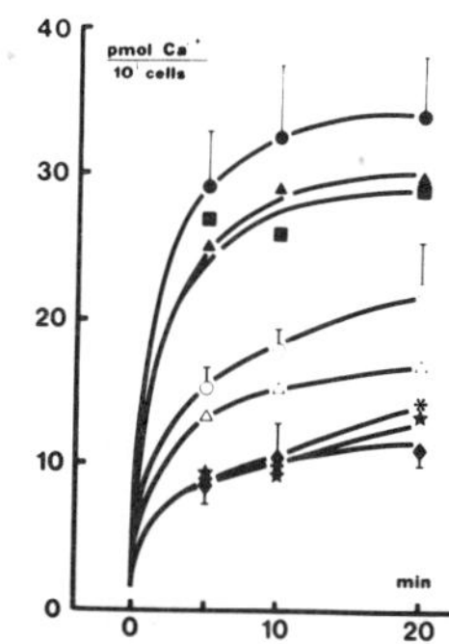

Fig.7. (left) Effects of ouabain on Ca^{2+} uptake of cardiomyocytes. ○ (no addition), ▲ (1 mM ouabain), ● (1 mM ouabain + 2.5 mM H_2O_2) and ■ (1 mM ouabain + 194 mM Na^+).

Fig.8. (right) Effects of deferoxamine on Ca^{2+} uptake by cardiomyocytes. Deferoxamine, 20 mM, was added to myocyte suspension 1 h before addition of H_2O_2. ● (60'), ■ (90') and ▲ (120') with H_2O_2 alone; ◆ (60'), * (90') and ✳ (120') with H_2O_2 and deferoxamine; ○ (60') and △ (120') with deferoxamine alone.

hypercontracture per se was not the principal cause of increased Ca^{2+} influx. The dose-response relationship between H_2O_2 and Ca^{2+} influx indicated that the highest Ca^{2+} influx was found at around 2.5 mM, and Ca^{2+} influx began to decrease at higher doses of H_2O_2, despite the fact that the advance of hypercontracture was directly proportional to the dose of H_2O_2. Furthermore, other oxidants caused hypercontracture of myocytes without augmenting Ca^{2+} influx.

In conclusion, the results of our experiments indicated that 1) 2.5 mM H_2O_2 significantly accelerated Ca^{2+} uptake by isolated adult rat heart cells, 2) this stimulation was caused by the inhibition of Na^+K^+ ATPase and the resultant enhancement of Na^+/Ca^{2+} exchange activity, 3) the effect of H_2O_2 was mediated by the iron-catalyzed free radical reaction, and 4) the effect was not primarily associated with increased flux through slow channels, decreased ATP levels or hypercontracture.

REFERENCES

1. K.J.Kako, Jikeikai Med.J. 32, 609-639 (1985)
2. S.J.Weiss & A.F.LoBuglio, Lab.Invest. 47, 5-18 (1982)
3. K.J.Kako, J.Mol.Cell.Cardiol. 19, 209-211 (1987)
4. K.J.Kako, M.Kato, T.Matsuoka & A.Mustapha, Am.J.Physiol. 253 (in press)
5. B.B.Farmer, M.Mancina, E.S.Williams & A.M.Watanabe, Life Sci. 33, 1-18 (1983)
6. R.A.Haworth, A.B.Goknur, D.R.Hunter, J.O.Hegge & H.A.Berkoff, Circ.Res. 60, 586-594 (1987)
7. R.A.Altschuld, W.C.Wenger, K.G.Lamka, O.R.Kindig, C.C.Capen, V.Mizuhira, R.S.Vander Heide & G.P.Brierley, J.Biol.Chem. 260, 14325-14334 (1985)
8. P.E.Starke, J.B.Hoek & J.L.Farber, J.Biol.Chem. 261, 3006-3012 (1986)
9. J.E.Ponce-Hornos, G.A.Langer & L.M.Nudd, J.Mol.Cell.Cardiol. 14, 41-51 (1982)
10. I.U.Schraufstatter, P.A.Hyslop, D.B.Hinshaw, R.G.Spragg, L.A.Sklar & C.G.Cochrane, Proc.Natl.Acad.Sci.US 83, 4908-4912 (1986)

OXIDATIVE STRESS IN THE MYOCARDIUM. A STUDY ON THE MECHANISM(S) FOR CYTOTOXICITY

B.S. ANDERSSON,* M. SUNDBERG,** AND J. RAJS**
Departments of *Toxicology and **Forensic Medicine, Karolinska Institutet, Box 60400, 104 01 Stockholm, Sweden

INTRODUCTION

Isolated cardiac myocytes have become a useful model system for the study of myocardial function. Incubation of these cells in a synthetic medium, and under different concentrations of oxygen, allows an evaluation of cellular responses to pharmacological and physiological variables. Furthermore, isolated myocytes are also used in studies of ischemia- and chemical-induced cell injury to the myocardium [1,2]. Several molecular mechanisms have been proposed to explain the critical event(s) which result in cardiotoxicity. These include the binding of a compound or its metabolite to cellular macromolecules [3] or the depletion of high-energy phosphates [4]. However, the structural and metabolic abberations which characterize chemical-induced cell injury to the myocardium remain incompletely understood.

"Oxidative stress" in biological systems is defined as an imbalance in the pro-oxidant/anti-oxidant ratio, which results in accumulation of reactive oxygen species within the system [5]. This stimulates a variety of biochemical alterations to occur such as oxidation of soluble and protein thiol groups, as well as peroxidation of polyunsaturated fatty acids. For instance, the cardiotoxicity induced by antineoplastic anthracyclines has been suggested to involve oxidative stress [6].

The aim of the present study was to induce the state of oxidative stress in isolated myocytes using menadione and tert-butyl hydroperoxide (tBH) as model compounds. This may provide an evaluation of the morphological and biochemical changes associated with oxidative damage to the myocardium.

METHODS

Cardiac myocytes were isolated from Sprague-Dawley rats (200-300 g) by retrograde perfusion, followed by incubation in collagenase containing medium as described by Andersson et al. [7]. Cell viability, morphology and cell count were evaluated in a hemocytometer in the presence of 0.2% trypan blue. The yield of myocytes was 5-8 x 10^6/heart, about 80% were viable by trypan blue exclusion, and 60-75% showed rod-shaped configuration. Digitonin fractionation of myocytes was carried out by treating the cells with digitonin (0.1 mg/10^6 myocytes) in Eppendorf tubes (1.5 ml), and centrifuging treated cells through a silicone oil-mineral oil layer (ratio 6:1) into 40% glycerol [7]. This procedure released more than 90% of the sarcoplasmic marker enzyme lactate dehydrogenase (LDH) without affecting mitochondrial integrity, as assayed by measuring release of the mitochondrial marker enzyme glutamate dehydrogenase (GDH). Ninety percent of GDH but only 5% of LDH were retained in the particulate fraction after digitonin treatment of the myocytes.

Incubations (0.25 x 10^6 myocytes/ml) were performed in rotating round-bottom flasks at 37°C in Krebs-Henseleit buffer (pH 7.2), containing $CaCl_2$ (50 µM), HEPES (11 mM), BSA (1% W/V), glucose (10 mM), taurine (30 mM), creatine (20 mM) and rat plasma levels of 20 amino acids under an

Biology of Isolated Adult Cardiac Myocytes
William A. Clark, Robert S. Decker, and Thomas K. Borg, Editors

atmosphere of carbogen.

Determination of adenine and pyridine nucleotides in the sarcoplasmic and nonsarcoplasmic compartments was carried out by digitonin fractionation, except that 0.25 ml 1M perchloric acid substituted for the glycerol as the bottom layer in the centrifuge tubes. The perchloric acid extracts were neutralized with $NaHCO_3$, and the supernatants were analyzed for ATP, ADP, AMP, NADP and NAD contents by high-performance liquid chromatography using a Waters radial compression Z-module with a Radial-PAK 5 μ Bondapack C_{18} column cartridge [8]. Data represent the average of at least 3 different myocyte preparations.

RESULTS AND DISCUSSION

Effects of menadione and tBH on cell morphology

Freshly isolated myocytes, incubated as described in METHODS, maintained both their rod-shaped structure and viability for up to 3 hours. However, incubation in the presence of menadione (100 μM) resulted in a 70% loss of rod-shaped myocytes (Fig. 1) and a 55% decrease in viability after 60 minutes. By 90 minutes incubation, 16% of the total myocytes still maintained their rod-shaped structure, while almost 30% of the cells were viable. At this timepoint, virtually all myocytes exposed to tBH (100 μM) were in the round hypercontracted configuration. Of these round cells, about 25% excluded trypan blue. In contrast to menadione, which induced trypan blue uptake into rod-shaped myocytes, tBH caused an initial blebbing of the myocyte plasma membrane, which was apparent within 15 minutes. Further incubation produced a conversion of myocytes to the round hypercontracted configuration, and finally uptake of trypan blue. Although both compounds produce oxidative stress in cells, they appear to cause morphological changes by different mechanisms.

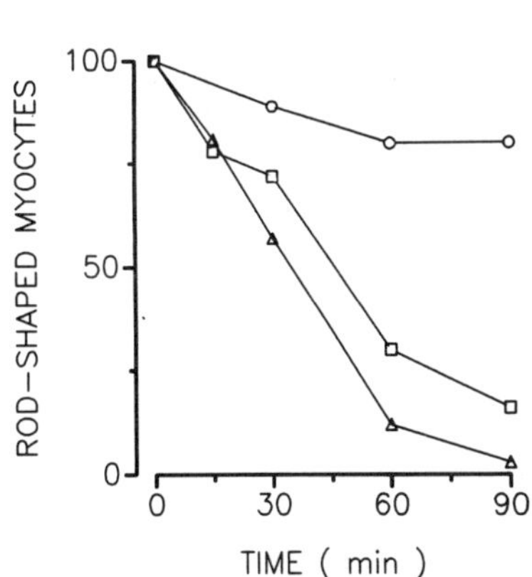

FIG. 1. EFFECT OF tBH AND MENADIONE ON CELL SHAPE OF ISOLATED MYOCYTES. Percent of cells at time 0. Control (o), tBH (Δ), Menadione (□)

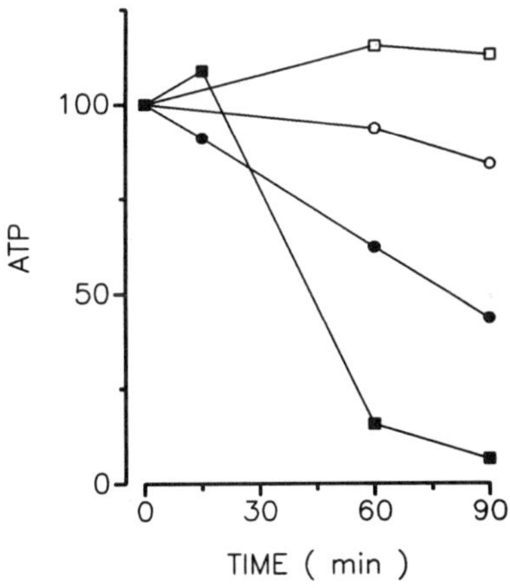

FIG. 2. EFFECT OF tBH ON ATP LEVELS IN ISOLATED MYOCYTES. Percent of ATP level at time 0. Control-sarcoplasmic (□), Control-nonsarcoplasmic (o), tBH-sarcoplasmic (■), tBH-nonsarcoplasmic (●)

Effect of tBH on the adenine nucleotide pool

Isolated myocytes incubated under anaerobic conditions in the absence of glucose lose most of their ATP, even though cell viability remains high [9]. However, in the present study, where myocytes were incubated aerobically with glucose in the presence of tBH (100 μM), there was a marked effect on cell shape and viability as well as adenine nucleotide content. Fig. 2 shows the effect of tBH on the cellular ATP levels. In the sarcoplasmic compartment, ATP was rapidly lost following 15 minutes incubation, resulting in a 95% depletion of this nucleotide at 90 minutes. A slower continous decline was observed in the nonsarcoplasmic fraction, which contained 44% of the initial ATP at this point. Also the myocyte content of ADP was affected by exposure to tBH. A progressive loss occurred in the sarcoplasm (87%), whereas the nonsarcoplasmic pool only decreased by 20% after 90 minutes (data not shown). In contrast to these two nucleotides, AMP was detected only in the nonsarcoplasmic compartment, presumably the mitochondria, an observation previously reported by Geisbuhler et al. [9]. Treatment of myocytes with tBH for 90 minutes decreased the mitochondrial AMP content by 35% (not shown).

These results show that tBH causes an alteration in the myocardial energy metabolism. The extensive loss of ATP from the sarcoplasm indicates an imbalance between the production of ATP and its utilization. Since the mitochondria are the primary site for ATP generation under aerobic conditions [10], it seems possible that tBH exerts its effect on these organelles. Furthermore, we observed a slightly higher concentration of ATP in the nonsarcoplasmic compartment compared to the sarcoplasm (4.5 vs. 4.0 n mol/10^6 cells, respectively, after 90 minutes incubation with tBH), suggesting that the translocation of ATP out of the mitochondria may also be inhibited.

Effect of tBH on pyridine nucleotides

Tert-butyl hydroperoxide caused an elevation (40%) of NADP in the sarcoplasmic compartment after 15 minutes incubation (Table I). This initial increase was followed by a rapid decline of the nucleotide, and 40% remained in the sarcoplasm by 90 minutes exposure to tBH. In contrast, the nonsarcoplasmic compartment showed a slower, continous decrease of NADP, which resulted in a 35% depletion. Using the isolated perfused heart model, Ishikawa and Sies [11] showed that perfusion with 100 μM tBH resulted in a rapid oxidation of myocardial glutathione, which was maximal already within 5 minutes. The initial increase in NADP level observed in the present study may therefore be a consequence of the glutathione reductase mediated reduction of GSSG formed in the glutathione peroxidase catalyzed metabolism of tBH. It is interesting to speculate on an enhanced activity of the mitochondrial nicotinamide nucleotide transhydrogenase for generation of NADPH, resulting in an increased consumption of the elctrochemical proton gradient (Δp), which is the driving force for the synthesis of ATP. This may be one of the mechanisms for reducing the ATP level during the metabolism of organic hydroperoxides by myocytes, and which is currently under investigation in our laboratory.

The sarcoplasmic level of NAD did not appear to increase to the same extent as NADP, whereas there was a more pronounced depletion of the nucleotide upon prolonged exposure to tBH (Table I). Also in the nonsarcoplasmic pool, the loss of NAD was greater than for NADP. Since most of the NAD is found in the nonsarcoplasmic compartment, i.e. mitochondria [7,9], these results further support the hypothesis that tBH affects mitochondrial function. One possible site of action for this compound may be a component of the mitochondrial electron transport chain, resulting in a decreased capacity of the mitochondria to oxidize NADH. This would then affect the generation of Δp, and subsequently reduce the mitochondrial capacity to synthesize ATP.

TABLE I. Effect of tBH on oxidized pyridine nucleotides in isolated myocytes.

Incubation Time (min.)	NADP Sarco-plasmic	NADP Nonsarco-plasmic	NAD Sarco-plasmic	NAD Nonsarco-plasmic
15	140	94	108	94
90	40	65	15	43

Data represent percent of nucleotide level at time 0.

SUMMARY

The results presented in this study show that generation of oxidative stress in isolated cardiac myocytes produces marked alterations in the morphology of these cells. The loss of rod-shaped configuration is associated with an extensive decrease in the cellular ATP level, and further by an increased uptake of trypan blue into the cells. These results suggest that changes in mitochondrial function, which result in a decreased capacity to synthesize ATP, may be an underlying mechanism for cardiotoxicity induced by substances whose metabolism produces oxidative stress.

ACKNOWLEDGEMENTS

This study was supported by a grant from Karolinska Institutet. We thank Dr. D. Thompson for his helpful comments during manuscript preparation.

REFERENCES

1. G.P. Brierley, C. Hohl, and R.A. Altschuld, Adv. Exp. Med. Biol. 161, 231-248 (1983).
2. C. Paul, A. Tomingas, J. Rajs, I. Anundi, J. Högberg, and C. Peterson, Acta Pharmacol. et Toxicol. 51, 292-299 (1982).
3. B.K. Sinha in: Cardiovascular Toxicology, E.W. Van Stee, ed. (Raven Press, New York 1982) pp. 181-197.
4. R.B. Jennings, H.K. Hawkins, J.E. Lowe, M.L. Hill, S. Klotman, and K.A. Reimer, Am. J. Pathol. 92, 187-214 (1978).
5. H. Sies in: Oxidative Stress, H. Sies, ed. (Academic Press, London 1985) pp. 1-8.
6. J. Doroshow, and P. Hochstein in: Pathology of Oxygen, A.P. Autor, ed. (Academic Press, New York 1982) pp. 245-275.
7. B.S. Andersson, M. Sundberg, and J. Rajs, Manuscript submitted for publication.
8. B.S. Andersson, and S. Uhlig, Manuscript submitted for publication.
9. T. Geisbuhler, R.A. Altschuld, R.W. Trewyn, A.Z. Ansel, K. Lamka, and G.P. Brierley, Circ. Res. 54, 536-546 (1984).
10. L.M. Mela-Riker, and R.D. Bukoski, Ann. Rev. Physiol. 47, 645-663 (1985).
11. T. Ishikawa, and H. Sies, J. Biol. Chem. 259, 3838-3843 (1984).

USE OF ISOLATED ADULT CARDIAC MYOCYTE TECHNIQUE TO CALCULATE PER CELL ACTIVITY OF CREATINE KINASE IN NORMAL AND HYPERTROPHIED MYOCARDIUM

Shirley H. Smith*, Martha F. Kramer**, Ilana Reis**,
Sanford P. Bishop*, Joanne S. Ingwall**
*Department of Pathology, University of Alabama at Birmingham,
VAMC Birmingham; **Department of Medicine, Harvard Medical School,
Brigham and Women's Hospital, Boston, Massachusetts

ABSTRACT

Creatine kinase (CK) activity quantified on the basis of tissue concentration (IU/mg protein) showed decreased activity in hypertrophied myocardium. Using the isolated myocyte technique to measure cell volume, we calculated the cell content (μIU/cell) of CK. A difference in cell size was demonstrated, but there was no difference ($p<0.05$) in cell content of CK in hypertrophied cells. Thus, the apparent decrease in enzyme activity in hypertrophied myocardium was due to dilution of the enzyme within the cell.

INTRODUCTION

Isolated adult cardiac myocytes have been used for morphometric analysis in various types of hypertrophy [1,2]. This procedure allows analysis of size and shape of myocytes and of variations of these properties within the myocardium [1,3]. We have employed the isolated myocyte technique to estimate the creatine kinase enzyme activity of left ventricular free wall cells in normal and two-kidney, one clip renal hypertensive rats. By analyzing the activity of creatine kinase per cell in normal and hypertrophied myocardium, we were able to assess whether or not changes in activity kept pace with the enlargement of the cell.

MATERIALS AND METHODS

Two-Kidney, One Clip (2K1C) Renal Hypertension:

Weanling male Sprague-Dawley rats (50-75 g) from Charles River Laboratories were placed in two study groups: 2K1C and nonoperated control. In 2K1C rats, the left renal artery was clipped (0.20 mm ID clip) under ketamine anesthesia (100 mg/Kg IP). The rats grew for 6 weeks. Weekly tailcuff pressures were measured using a Narco Biosystems PE-300 electrosphygmomanometer.

Criteria for Selection of Animals Accepted for Study:

Due to the variable response of each rat to the clipping procedure, not all rats are expected to develop hypertension. The procedure optimally results in compensatory hypertrophy of the right kidney and slight atrophy of the left kidney, consistently associated with high blood pressure [4]. Only 2K1C rats with 0.4-0.9 left/right kidney weight ratios were accepted for study.

Myocyte Isolation:

Eight 2K1C and 12 control rats were killed by decapitation, the hearts removed, and weighed. The hearts were cannulated by the aorta and

Biology of Isolated Adult Cardiac Myocytes
William A. Clark, Robert S. Decker, and Thomas K. Borg, Editors

perfused for 2 min. with calcium-free Joklik medium (GIBCO Labs) containing EGTA (0.5 mM) followed by a 15 min. collagenase (Sigma Chemical, 0.5 g/l) digestion on a modified Langendorff apparatus at pH 7.4 and 37°C [5,6]. The left ventricular free wall was minced and passed through a sieve (250 μ nylon mesh), and the isolated cells were fixed by addition of an equal volume of phosphate-buffered 2% glutaraldehyde (300 mOsM) to the media containing the cells. Glass slide smears from each group were examined microscopically to insure that each preparation consisted of at least 80% cylindrical myocytes. Each sample was prepared for cell volume studies by centrifugation (1000 rpm) through 5 ml of a 6% ficoll gradient to remove debris. The supernatant was discarded and the pellet resuspended in glutaraldehyde. The collagenase-softened myocardial tissue remaining in the nylon mesh was immediately frozen in liquid nitrogen and stored at -70°C for biochemical studies.

Cell Volume Measurement:

An aliquot of isolated fixed myocytes from the left ventricular free wall of each heart was suspended in Isoton II (Coulter Electronics). Cell volume was measured by a Model ZH Coulter Counter interfaced to a microprocessor. The cells (20,000 to 40,000 per sample) passed through a 140 μm aperture. The lower window threshold was set to exclude objects less than 5000 fl. A shape factor adjustment of 1.08 was used, as myocytes are roughly rod-shaped and pass lengthwise through the electric field [7,8]. Mean cell volume from each sample was used for statistical analysis.

Creatine Kinase (CK) Activity:

Frozen samples were weighed (10-20 mg) and homogenized for 10 sec. at 4°C in 0.1 M KPO_4 buffer containing 1 mM EGTA and 1 mM β-mercaptoethanol, pH 7.4 (1 ml buffer/5 mg tissue). Aliquots were removed for protein analysis [9]. Triton X was added to the homogenate to a final concentration of 0.1% for enzyme assays.

Total CK activity was measured using a Calbiochem CK-NAC Reagent Kit (Behring Diagnostics), which employs the hexokinase reaction to measure the amount of ATP produced from creatine phosphate. Duplicate assays were measured spectrophotometrically using a Gilford Stastar III Spectrophotometer interfaced to a Gilford System 5 Automatic Enzyme Analyzer [10,11]. Enzyme activities were expressed as International Units per mg protein (IU/mgP).

Per Cell Content of Enzyme Activity:

Cell content (μIU/cell) of CK was calculated from tissue concentration (IU/mgP) and cell volume (where 1 mg wet weight = 1 μl) using the following formula:

μIU/cell = (IU/mgP)x(mgP/mg wet weight)x(femtoliters/cell)/1000.

Statistical Analysis:

Biochemical and morphologic parameters were compared by the unpaired Student's t-test. Values were reported as mean $\pm$ SEM. A p value <0.05 was considered statistically significant.

RESULTS

Heart Weight and Blood Pressure Measurement:

Blood pressure was elevated in 2K1C rats (196 mmHg ± 9 SEM) above control (135 ± 3). Total heart weight was 41% higher in the 2K1C group (1.79 g ± 0.08) compared to the control group (1.27 ± 0.03). Body weight was not different.

Myocyte Volume:

In 2K1C hypertension, mean myocyte volume was significantly higher than in control animals (p=0.000014) (Table I).

Creatine Kinase (CK) Activity:

Tissue Concentration (IU/mgP):

The tissue concentration of CK decreased by 24% in 2K1C rats (p=0.011) (Table I).

Cell Content (μIU/cell):

However, the activity of CK per cell showed no difference from control (p=0.387) (Table I). Thus, although the number of activity units per mg protein decreased, the larger cells in the hypertrophied myocardium contained the same number of enzyme activity units per cell.

TABLE I. Cell volume (fl), tissue concentration (IU/mgP) of creatine kinase (CK), and cell content (μIU/cell) of CK of left ventricular free wall myocytes in hypertensive (2K1C) and control rats. Values are reported as mean ± SEM. *=p<0.05 compared to control.

	CELL VOLUME (fl)	CK (IU/mgP)	CK (μIU/cell)
CONTROL	25392 ±1101	4.96 ±.35	19.4 ±1.7
2K1C	37391* ±2086	3.78* ±.25	20.3 ±2.9

DISCUSSION

These data indicate that apparent differences in enzyme activity which occur in cardiac hypertrophy when measured as tissue concentration (IU/mgP) may not reflect the content of the individual cell. Previous studies have shown that tissue concentration of CK decreases in hypertrophied myocardium [12,13]. In the present study, the 24% decrease in tissue concentration of CK disappeared when the enlarged volume of the cell was taken into account. Cell content (μIU/cell) did not change, even though myocyte size increased by 47%.

The contribution of non-myocyte material to CK activities measured in this study using collagenase-digested tissue is small, since non-myocytes contain very low CK activity relative to cardiac myocytes. The use of only a few isolated myocytes to measure enzyme activity might serve to demonstrate even greater differences between tissue concentration and cell content. Due to the possible contribution of extracellular water to the wet weight of the frozen sample used for enzyme assay, the presumption that 1 mg wet weight is equal to 1 μl of volume may underestimate the absolute cell content of enzyme.

Although this study demonstrated no change in total CK/cell, other studies have suggested that the isoenzyme composition of CK shifts in hypertrophied hearts [12,14]. Future studies should include an in depth analysis of CK isozymes.

REFERENCES

1. S.H. Smith and S.P. Bishop, J. Mol. Cell. Cardiol. 17, 1005 (1985).
2. A.M. Gerdes, J. Kriseman and S.P. Bishop, Lab. Invest. 48(5), 598 (1983).
3. S.H. Smith, M. McCaslin, C. Sreenan and S.P. Bishop, J. Mol. Cell. Cardiol. (in press).
4. S.H. Smith and S.P. Bishop, Hypertension 8(8), 700 (1986).
5. J.W. Dow, N.G.L. Harding and T. Powell, Cardiovasc. Res. 15, 483 (1981).
6. T. Powell and V.W. Twist, Biochem. Biophys. Res. Comm. 72, 327 (1976).
7. G.B. Nash, P.E.R. Tatham, T. Powell, V.W. Twist, R.D. Speller and L.T. Loverlock, Biochim. Biophys. Acta. 587, 99 (1979).
8. J. Hurley, Biophys. J. 10, 74 (1970).
9. O.H. Lowry, N.J. Rosebrough, A.L. Farr and R.J. Randall, J. Biol. Chem. 193, 265 (1951).
10. S.F. Rosalki, J. Lab. Clin. Med. 69, 696 (1967).
11. G. Szasz, J. Waldenstrom and W. Gruber, Clin. Chem. 25, 446 (1979).
12. J.S. Ingwall, M.F. Kramer, M.A. Fifer, B.H. Lorell, R. Shemin, W. Grossman, P.D. Allen, New Eng. J. Med. 313, 1050 (1985).
13. J.S. Ingwall, F.R. Badke, R.S. Pavelec, J.W. Covell, Circulation 54(4)(Suppl II), II-59 (1976).
14. J.S. Ingwall, Eur Heart J. 5(Suppl F), 129 (1984).

DEGRADATION AND RESYNTHESIS OF ADENINE NUCLEOTIDES IN ADULT RAT HEART MYOCYTES: ROLE OF THE PURINE NUCLEOTIDE CYCLE

RUTH A. ALTSCHULD, LILI M. GAMELIN, ROBERT E. KELLEY, DOROTHY K. WIMSATT, LYNN E. APEL, and GERALD P. BRIERLEY
Departments of Physiological Chemistry and Pathology and Division of Cardiology, Department of Internal Medicine, The Ohio State University Medical Center, Columbus, Ohio 43210

INTRODUCTION

During myocardial ischemia or hypoxia, when energy use exceeds ATP production, the cytosolic energy charge declines and AMP increases. The subsequent degradation of AMP by 5' nucleotidase and release of adenosine (ADO) by the myocytes produces vasodilation. Slight transient imbalances between ATP production and consumption are thus corrected by an increase in coronary blood flow. In global ischemia, however, ADO production does not increase the delivery of oxygen and metabolic substrates; AMP accumulates to high concentrations and is slowly degraded to ADO, inosine (INO), and the purine bases [1]. AMP can also be degraded by the purine nucleotide cycle enzyme, AMP deaminase, but only small amounts of IMP are detected in globally ischemic rat hearts [2,3]. By contrast, there is substantial production of IMP by high-flow Langendorff hearts deenergized by perfusion with hypoxic, glucose-free buffers [2]. Isolated myocytes incubated under similar conditions also accumulate large amounts of IMP, and during reaeration IMP declines and the size of the adenine nucleotide pool increases [3].

The present studies were undertaken to characterize the pathways for adenine nucleotide degradation more precisely using a preparation of calcium-tolerant adult rat heart myocytes. Rapidly deenergized myocytes show a clear progression of adenine nucleotide degradation from AMP to intracellular ADO and IMP, followed by exit of ADO from the cell and conversion to INO. The relative amounts of ADO and IMP produced by rapidly and synchronously deenergized myocytes can be altered by prior metabolic activity, epinephrine, and the ADO deaminase inhibitor, coformycin.

METHODS

Myocytes were isolated as previously described [4] and suspended in a HEPES-buffered Krebs-Henseleit medium supplemented with vitamins, amino acids and 2% bovine serum albumin. However, for more recent experiments, the rats were anesthetized with pentobarbital to comply with newly-issued guidelines on the care and use of laboratory animals. In all previous work from this laboratory, the rats were sacrificed by decapitation. Cells were incubated at 37°C, pH 7.4 in the above buffer and sedimented through bromododecane into perchloric acid for measurement of nucleotides and nucleosides by HPLC [4]. All data are presented as means ± S.E.M.

RESULTS AND DISCUSSION

A recent study from this laboratory [4] established that when myocytes are incubated anaerobically without added glucose, ATP declines from 27 to less than 1.0 and adenine nucleotides from 34 to 8 nmoles/200,000 cells in 45 min at 37°C (200,000 myocytes ≈ 0.9 mg "Lowry" protein). The decline in adenine nucleotides is accounted for

Biology of Isolated Adult Cardiac Myocytes
William A. Clark, Robert S. Decker, and Thomas K. Borg, Editors

by increases in extracellular ADO and INO and by a 5-7 nmole/mg increase in intracellular IMP. Reaeration for 15 min increases the size of the adenine nucleotide pool to 12-15 nmoles per mg and there is an equivalent decline in IMP. In cells with purine nucleotides labeled by preincubation with ^{14}C-ADO, the specific activity of the resynthesized ATP, as measured by on-line liquid scintillation HPLC, approximates that of IMP and not extracellular ADO. These data indicate that IMP can be reaminated quite rapidly in isolated myocytes and the purine nucleotide cycle is fully functional in these cells.

The contribution of the purine nucleotide cycle to myocardial adenine nucleotide synthesis and degradation is somewhat controversial [5,6]. Takala et al [7] found that the activity of purine cycle enzymes was much higher than observed rates of NH_3 production in the perfused heart, suggesting perhaps that these enzymes are subject to as yet undefined controls. In our studies of deenergized myocytes [3,4], we found the rate and extent of AMP deaminiation to be variable and extremely sensitive to incubation conditions. As shown in TABLE I, IMP production during hypoxic incubations without added glucose can be affected both by the ADO deaminase inhibitor, coformycin, and seemingly, by the method used to sacrifice the donor rat.

TABLE I. Effects of coformycin on IMP production by deenergized myocytes

Coformycin		Anaesthesia	nmoles IMP/mg; 45 min anoxia	
1	0	none	5.6 ± 1.5	
2	5 μM	none	6.8 ± 0.7	1 vs 2, NS
3	0	pentobarbital	3.8 ± 0.5	
4	5 μM	pentobarbital	7.6 ± 0.8	3 vs 4, $p < 0.01$

With prolonged oxygen and glucose deprivation, metabolite data represent average values over a heterogenous population of myocytes [8]. To study AMP degradation under better-controlled conditions, we developed a procedure for converting nearly all of the cellular adenine nucleotides to AMP within less than a minute. Results of a typical experiment are shown in FIG. 1.

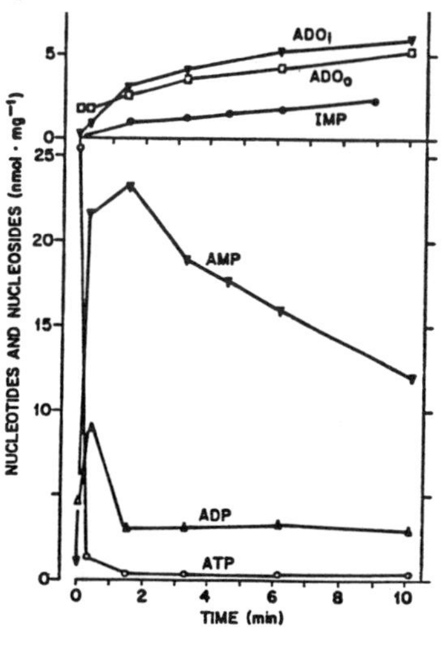

FIG. 1. Time course of changes in cellular ATP, ADP, AMP, IMP and ADO (ADO_i) and extracellular ADO (ADO_0) in rapidly deenergized myocytes. The cells were incubated 30 min with 11 mM glucose, 5 μM coformycin and 1 μg/ml rotenone. At time zero, 5 mM iodoacetate and 10 μM CCCP were added to inhibit glycolysis and activate mitochondrial ATPase activity. (Reproduced from ref. #4 with permission)

Under the conditions of FIG. 1, where myocytes are maintaining ATP stores solely through anaerobic glycolysis, sudden deenergization causes an appreciable buildup of intracellular ADO with gradual efflux to the suspending medium. The alternate pathway for AMP degradation, deamination to IMP, is relatively slow. However, as shown in TABLE II, if the period of anaerobic glycolysis is eliminated and iodoacetate, CCCP, and a respiratory inhibitor are added simultaneously after 30 min aerobic incubation, IMP production increases whereas degradation of AMP to ADO declines.

TABLE II. Effects of prior anaerobic glycolysis on IMP and ADO production by rapidly deenergized myocytes

Minutes	IMP (nmoles/mg)		ADO (nmoles/mg[a])	
	control	glycolyzing	control	glycolyzing
0	0.04 ± 0.01	0.2 ± 0.05	1.2 ± 0.1	2.1 ± 0.2
5	10.4 ± 0.2	2.7 ± 0.7	6.2 ± 0.7	9.7 ± 0.4
10	11.0 ± 1.1	4.2 ± 1.2	7.0 ± 0.9	11.7 ± 0.2

a) ADO = the sum of intracellular and extracellular ADO as determined by HPLC of the suspending medium and of extracts of the sedimented myocytes.

b) Rapid denergization was produced with 10 µM CCCP, 3 mM amytal, and 5 mM iodoacetate (IAA). The simultaneous addition of rotenone and IAA does not produce respiratory inhibition; thus amytal was used as an alternative inhibitor of NADH dehydrogenase.

As shown in FIG. 2, the inhibitory effect of anaerobic glycolysis on IMP production in subsequently deenergized myocytes can be overcome by inclusion of 1 µM epinephrine during the anaerobic incubation with rotenone. Epinephrine at this concentration had no discernable effect on ATP content after 30 min incubation with rotenone and 11 mM glucose (30 vs 29 nmoles/mg), but lactate production was increased slightly (481 ± 22 vs 406 ± 24 nmoles/mg/30 min, n=6).

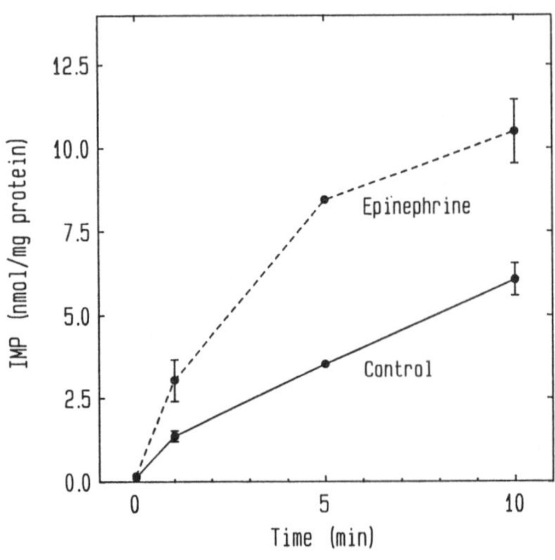

FIG. 2. Effects of epinephrine (1 µM) on IMP production by rapidly deenergized myocytes. Myocytes were incubated 30 min with 1 µg/ml rotenone, 11 mM glucose, and where indicated, 1 µM epinephrine. At time zero, 5 mM iodoacetate and 3 µM CCCP were added to inhibit glycolysis and stimulate mitochondrial ATPase activity. ATP fell to less than 1 nmole/mg by 1 min in both cases.

The results of the present study establish that myocardial AMP deaminase is under metabolic and hormonal control. The pronounced inhibitory effect of a period of anaerobic glycolysis on subsequent IMP production during rapid deenergization may explain the low levels of IMP found in globally ischemic hearts. Such an inhibitory effect could result from an accumulation of lactate, NADH, or H^+, but its reversal by epinephrine, which accelerates lactic acid production by respiration-inhibited myocytes, suggests a more complicated mechanism. The stimulation of IMP production by coformycin was an unwelcome finding. We had hoped to use the compound to inhibit AMP deaminase, but concentrations up to 500 μM have been ineffective. The stimulation shown in TABLE 1 may be secondary to inhibition of ADO deaminase. Finally, the effects of anaesthesia vs decapitation for removal of donor rat hearts require comment. Since changing to pentobarbital anaesthesia, we have noted several subtle changes in the properties of our myocytes. In addition to apparent effects on AMP deaminase, we note a decrease in the rate of ATP depletion during oxygen and glucose deprivation and a decrease in the rate of increase in free Ca^{2+} after ATP exhaustion in individual cells as reported by single cell fura-2 fluorscence microscopy [9]. Some such changes are reversed, at least in part, by 1 μM epinephrine.

ACKNOWLEDGEMENTS

These studies were supported, in part, by a grant-in-aid from the Central Ohio Heart Chapter, Inc. and United States Public Health Services Grant HL 36240.

REFERENCES

1. R.B. Jennings and C. Steenbergen, Jr. Ann. Rev. Physiol. 47, 727 (1985).
2. S.M. Humphrey, D.G. Hollis and R.N. Seelye, J. Mol. Cell. Cardiol. 16, 1127 (1984).
3. T. Geisbuhler, R.A. Altschuld, R.W. Trewyn, A.Z. Ansel, K. Lamka, and G.P. Brierley, Circ. Res. 54, 536 (1984).
4. R.A. Altschuld, L.M. Gamelin, R.E. Kelley, M.R. Lambert, L.E. Apel, and G.P. Brierley, J. Biol. Chem., in press (1987).
5. E. Zoref-Shani, G. Kessler-Icekson, L. Wasserman, and O. Sperling, Biochim. Biophys. Acta 804, 161 (1984).
6. H. Taegteyer, J. Mol. Cell. Cardiol. 17, 1013 (1985).
7. T. Takala, J.K. Hiltunen, and I.E. Hassinen, Biochem. J. 192, 285 (1980).
8. R.A. Haworth, D.R. Hunter, and H.A. Berkoff, Circ. Res. 49, 1119 (1981).
9. Q. Li, R.A. Altschuld, and B.T. Stokes, This Volume (1988).

THE EFFECTS OF OXYGEN DEPRIVATION AND VOLUME RESTRICTION ON THE METABOLISM OF CULTURED HEART CELLS

ARIE PINSON,* RAMESH VEMURI,* MARCEL MERSEL,** AND J.W. DE JONG***

*Laboratory for Myocardial Research, The Hebrew University-Hadassah Medical School, Jerusalem, Israel; **Centre de Neurochimie, Strasbourg, France; ***Thorax Center, Erasmus University, Rotterdam, The Netherlands

INTRODUCTION

The heart is essentially an oxidative organ, which depends predominantly upon oxidative phosphorylation [1,2]. Within seconds of oxygen deprivation, it switches to anaerobic glycolysis in order to maintain the cellular energy charge [3,4]. However, cellular high energy phosphates (HEP) rapidly decline and purine and oxypurine production increases [5,6]. Heart cells in culture have been used as a model system for studying oxygen deprivation [7-9], although enzyme release, a marker of cell damage, could only be detected after long periods under anoxic conditions; and uncouplers and/or metabolic inhibitors were employed in some of these experiments [10].

Recently, we have shown that reduction of the volume of extracellular fluid to a minimum so that the height of the liquid above the cells approximates in size to a single cultured cell, simulating a true "non-circulating microenvironment" [11]. Under anoxic conditions, cellular damage, as reflected in enzyme release, was inversely proportional to the volume of the medium [11], presumably attributable to the effects of catabolic products (i.e., lactic acid) that remain in the vicinity of the cells. Reduction of the extracellular volume *per se* did not have any deleterious effects. Larger volumes (1-2 ml/35 mm diameter Petri dish) gave rise to less cellular damage under anoxia, apparently owing to the "washout" of catabolic products into the extracellular space.

In this report, the term anoxia refers to cell cultures incubated with 2 ml oxygen-deprived medium per Petri dish, and "ischemia" to plates with either 0.2 or 0.4 ml medium.

The overall aim is to present a bird's-eye view of some of the key metabolic events occurring under conditions of oxygen deprivation.

MATERIALS AND METHODS

Preparation of heart cell cultures [12,13] and the conditions simulating anoxia and "ischemia" have been described extensively [11,14,15].

RESULTS AND DISCUSSION

Table I shows LDH release during glucose and oxygen deprivation. After 2 h under anoxic and "ischemic" conditions, 11% and 30% of the cellular LDH were released, respectively; lactate production was higher, by 77% in "ischemia" as compared to anoxia; and glycogen content fell by 27% and by 51%, in anoxia and "ischemia", respectively. Other cytoplasmic enzymes, CPK and GOT, displayed similar release patterns.

Biology of Isolated Adult Cardiac Myocytes
William A. Clark, Robert S. Decker, and Thomas K. Borg, Editors

TABLE I. LDH and lactate release, and cellular glycogen utilization during anoxia and "ischemia"

Incubation time (min)	Normoxia	Anoxia	"Ischemia"
	LDH (mIU/plate)		
30	5±0.57	10±1.01	20±1.5
60	7±0.52	27±2.3	90±9.3
120	10±2.6	85±9.5	240±10
180	15±1.4	145±10	460±21
240	19±1.5	400±23	765±35
	Lactate (mmol/plate)		
30	0.13±0.02	0.41±0.12	0.42±0.13
60	0.19±0.13	0.78±0.18	0.99±0.22
120	0.21±0.15	0.98±0.78	1.74±0.46
180	0.29±0.10	1.71±0.61	2.09±0.24
240	0.32±0.08	1.94±0.52	2.66±0.35
	Glycogen (μg/plate)		
30	218±2.1	209±8.1	207±4.3
60	216±3.1	191±3.8	180±6.5
120	203±7.6	185±4.8	123±8.3
180	198±5.4	144±6.4	84±10.1
240	191±6.1	68±9.21	26±13.5

Initial values (100%); LDH --> 800±18mIU/plate; glycogen --> 255±30 μg/plate.

Heart cells contain high levels of glycogen - a substrate utilized during oxygen deprivation, which is more efficient than glucose as an anaerobic source of ATP since it provides an additional mole [16]. The catabolic products of ATP activate phosphorylase (from the a to b form), further increasing the rate of glycogen breakdown. However, presence of both glucose and glycogen enhanced cell resistance during oxygen deprivation, manifested in delayed degradative phenomena and enzyme release [14].

The release pattern of hexosaminidase, a lysosomal marker, is presented in Table II; and data for other lysosomal enzymes (e.g., β-galactosidase) follow similar trends. Marked release of these enzymes, beginning 2 h after anoxic injury, lagged behind that of the cytoplasmic ones - clearly indicating a well defined sequence of events under these conditions.

TABLE II. Release of hexosaminidase during normoxia, anoxia, and "ischemia"

Incubation time (min)	Normoxia	Anoxia	"Ischemia"
30	-	1.5	1.8
60	1.5	2.0	2.5
120	2.5	3.2	4.5
180	3.0	13.5	21.8
240	3.8	23.0	36.5

Results are expressed as % of total activity.

Protein degradation was calculated from the ^{14}C-phenylalanine release from prelabelled proteins [17] (see Table III). There is good correlation between the rate of lysosomal release and other manifestations of cellular injury. Protein degradation during normoxia may be taken as the normal controlled rate of protein turnover [17], whereas even the small amounts of lysosomal enzymes released during the first 120 min presumably account for the uncontrolled protein degradation, which is accelerated concomitantly on further release of these enzymes with the progress of anoxia.

TABLE III. ^{14}C-phenylalanine release into the extracellular medium

Incubation time (min)	Normoxia	Anoxia	"Ischemia"
30	1.0	1.3	2.5
60	1.4	2.5	3.75
120	2.25	3.75	6.5
180	2.75	6.5	11.8
240	4.0	13.0	20.75

Results are expressed as % of total radioactivity [17].

Preincubation with 100μM chloroquine, which is rapidly taken up by lysosomes [18] with a stabilizing effect [19,20], delayed lysosomal enzyme release and decreased protein degradation [15].

High energy phosphate was more rapidly degraded during "ischemia" than in anoxia. Cellular ATP levels decreased, after the first hour, by 33.7% during anoxia and by 57.85% during "ischemia", and by 49.4% and 87%, respectively, after another hour under these conditions, and were also reflected in further degradation to purines [15]. Creatine phosphate (CP) levels fell even more rapidly. It should be noted that large-scale lysosomal enzyme release began when the cellular energy charge (EC) was almost completely exhausted. Although the presence of glucose delayed cellular EC depletion, it did not have a similar effect on HEP content during normoxia. In anoxia, the cells were capable of synthesizing ATP from glycogen and from other nucleotide catabolites (ADP and AMP) and via the salvage pathway. During "ischemia", however, ATP synthesis was presumably inhibited by catabolites that remained in the vicinity of the cells.

Sarcolemmal transformations were manifested in both functional impairment and structural modifications; cellular Na^+ and Ca^{2+} were increased and K^+ released.

Increasing amounts malonyldialdehyde (MDA), a product of lipid peroxidation, were formed, and cholesterol loss from the sarcolemma - exarcerbated by the marked decline in HEP and lysosomal enzyme release - took place. The sarcolemma underwent profound structural modifications, which were reflected in the degree of accessibility of surface phospholipids (PL) to lactoperoxidase-glucose oxidase radioiodination [21]. Thus, the PE/PC labelling ratio increased from about 1.0 in normoxia to 2.4 in "ischemia". The data indicated that this was not due to PL loss, but rather to redistribution of the various PL classes between the two sarcolemmal leaflets [15].

CONCLUSIONS

Oxygen deprivation coupled with extracellular volume restriction in heart cell cultures has proved to be a valuable model for anoxia and "ischemia" at the cellular level. Events take place in a well defined sequence. In a reversible phase shortly after the onset of "ischemia", cytoplasmic enzymes are released, probably indicating sarcolemmal reorganization accompanied by partial HEP depletion. During the subsequent irreversible stage, CP and ATP are almost completely exhausted, concomitantly with lysosomal enzyme release. Further studies along these lines should furnish data concerning reoxygenational and reperfusional repair, and, in the long term, may have clinical implications.

ACKNOWLEDGMENTS

This work was partially supported by grants from the Chief Scientist of the Israel Ministry of Health; the Ministry of Education and Science of the state of Niedersachen, FRG; the Mr. and Mrs. D. Vidal-Madjar Foundation for Heart Research, Paris, France; Mrs. F. Berk, Brussels, Belguim, in memory of her daughter Mrs. Iva Mis; and Visiting Fellowships from INSERM, France, The Dutch Heart Foundation, and ZWO, The Netherlands.

REFERENCES

1. D.J. Hearse, J. Mol. Cell. Cardiol. 9, 605-616 (1984).
2. A.J. Doorey and W.H. Barry, Circ. Res. 53, 192-201 (1983).
3. S.H. Taylor, Br. Heart J. 33, 329-333 (1971).
4. W. Haider, F. Eckersberger, and E. Wolner, Anesthesiology 60, 422-429 (1984).
5. D.K. Reibel and M.J. Rovetto, Am. J. Physiol. 237, H247-H252 (1979).
6. B. Schoutsen, J.W. de Jong, E. Harmsen, P.P. De Tombe, and P.W. Achterberg, Biochim. Biophys. Acta 762, 519-524 (1983).
7. D. Acosta, M. Puckett, and R. McMillin, In Vitro 14, 728-732 (1978).
8. A. Van der Laarse, A. Hollaar, L.J.M. Van der Valk, and S.A.G.J. Witteveen, J. Mol. Med. 3 123-131 (1978).
9. T.J.C. Higgins, D. Allsopp, and P.J. Bailey, J. Mol. Cell. Cardiol. 12, 909-927 (1980).
10. T.J.C. Higgins, D. Allsopp, P.J. Bailey, and E.D.A. D'Souza, J. Mol. Cell. Cardiol. 13, 599-615 (1981).
11. R. Vemuri, S. Yagev, M. Heller, and A. Pinson, In Vitro 21, 521-525 (1985).
12. S. Yagev, M. Heller, and A. Pinson, In Vitro 20, 893-898 (1984).
13. A. Pinson in: The Heart Cell in Culture (Vol. I), A Pinson, ed. (CRC Press Inc., Boca Raton 1987, in press).
14. R. Vemuri, M. Heller, and A. Pinson, Bas. Res. Cardiol. 80(suppl. 2), 165-169 (1985).
15. R. Vemuri, Ph.D. thesis, Hebrew University-Hadassah Medical School, 1986.
16. J.R. Neely, M.J. Rovetto, and J.F. Oram, Prog. Cardiovasc. Dis. 15, 289-329 (1972).
17. K.N. Mayorek, A. Pinson, and M. Mayer, J. Cell Physiol. 98, 587-595 (1979).
18. F.Z. Meerson, V.E. Kagan, Y.P. Koslov, L. M. Belkind, and Y.V. Arkipenko, Bas. Res. Cardiol. 10, 465-485 (1982).
19. R.M. Rodout, R.S. Decker, and K. Wildenthal, J. Mol. Cell. Cardiol. 10, 175-183 (1978).
20. M. Vibo and B. Poole, J. Cell Biol. 63, 430-440 (1974).
21. A. Benenson, M. Mersel, M. Heller, and A. Pinson, in: Studying Cardiac Membranes (Vol.II), N.S. Dhalla, ed. (CRC Press Inc., Boca Raton 1984) pp. 59-81.

HORMONAL ACTION ON GLUCOSE OXIDATION BY FRESHLY ISOLATED CARDIAC MYOCYTES FROM ACUTELY DIABETIC RATS

Victor Chen, and S. Evans Downing
Department of Pathology, Yale University School of Medicine, 310 Cedar Street, New Haven, CT 06510

ABSTRACT

The effects of different hormones on glucose utilization by freshly isolated Ca^{2+}-tolerant cardiac cells from 48-60 hr streptozotocin-diabetic rats were examined. Both the yield and viability of isolated myocytes from diabetic rats were comparable to those of normal animals. The rate of glucose (5 mM) oxidation was significantly decreased (-50%) in myocytes of diabetic rats. Inclusion of insulin (5 mU/ml) in the incubation medium partially reversed the diminished rate of glucose oxidation, but not to normal. Incubating diabetic cells with T_3 (5 ng/ml), T_4 (200 ng/ml) or norepinephrine (2 ng/ml) also partially restored the level of glucose oxidation. The changes with each of these hormones were substantially less than that with insulin, however. The insulin effect on glucose oxidation remained unaltered by the addition of thyroid hormones or norepinephrine individually, but was slightly augmented in the presence of all three hormones. Regardless, the oxidation rate remained 25-40% below normal. Impairment in glucose oxidation by isolated myocytes from diabetic rats was corrected only when the animals were given insulin in vivo. These findings indicate a spectrum of hormonal trophic effects on glucose oxidation in diabetic myocytes, with insulin exerting the greatest influence. Differences in response to in vivo and in vitro insulin treatment suggest that additional factors may be responsible for the depressed glucose oxidation.

INTRODUCTION

In experimental diabetes, glucose oxidation by the myocardium is greatly reduced as a result of diminished glucose transport and phosphorylation, and substrate inhibition of regulatory enzyme in the oxidative pathway [1-4]. The impairment is generally considered to be a result of insulin deficiency because it is corrected by insulin treatment as in reduced cardiac function [5,6]. However, depressed heart function in diabetic rats is also restored in these animals by giving thyroid hormones [5]. The purpose of this study was to examine the individual and combined effects of insulin, thyroid hormones and norepinephrine on altered glucose utilization in freshly isolated myocytes from acutely diabetic rats.

MATERIALS AND METHODS

Diabetes was induced in male Sprague-Dawley rats (225-250g) by a single intravenous injection of streptozotocin in citrate buffer at a dose of 65 mg/kg body weight. Control rats were injected with citrate buffer. They were used 48-60 hr after injection. Blood samples were taken and assayed for plasma glucose (Glucostat, Worthington Diagnostics). Hearts were excised,

Biology of Isolated Adult Cardiac Myocytes
William A. Clark, Robert S. Decker, and Thomas K. Borg, Editors

rinsed and used for the isolation of myocytes as previously described [7], except that initial perfusion of isolated hearts with collagenase was maintained by a Langendorff column of 70-80 cm H_2O pressure. Cells from 2-4 hearts were pooled and resuspended in Joklik buffer containing 1% fatty-acid free bovine serum albumin (BSA), 1 mM $MgSO_4$, 1.5 mM $CaCl_2$, 1 mM L-carnitine and 5 mM non-labelled glucose. They were used immediately in the following experiments.

A dose response curve of insulin on glucose oxidation in diabetic myocytes was obtained. The reaction was initiated by adding U-^{14}C -glucose to alliquots of cell suspensions preincubated without or with insulin at different concentrations for 15 min. The production of $^{14}CO_2$ from labeled glucose during 40 min. incubation was determined [7]. Similarly, the effects of T_3 (5 ng/ml), T_4 (200 ng/ml) and norepinephrine (2 ng/ml) on glucose oxidation was evaluated. To determine in vivo insulin effects, diabetic rats were given regular insulin intravenously (1U, bolus) or NPH-insulin subcutaneously (5U/kg) 1 and 2 hr, respectively, before use.

RESULTS

Plasma glucose levels of control and diabetic rats were 7.1$\pm$0.8 (N=6) and 23.1$\pm$0.5 (N=47) mM, respectively. The yield of isolated myocytes from diabetic rats was comparable to that of the controls (averaging 1.13 and 1.02 x 10^7/heart). Viability of cells before (78.5$\pm$0.8 and 77.3$\pm$1.5) and after (72.2$\pm$0.8 and 70.0$\pm$1.8) 40 min incubation, was similar between the two groups.

The dose-response relationship between insulin and glucose oxidation in diabetic cells is shown in Fig. 1. The insulin effect was evident at 2.5 mU/ml. Maximum stimulation was achieved at 5 mU/(2.2x10^{-8}M). Therefore, the myocytes were incubated with insulin at 5 mU/ml in the subsequent experiments.

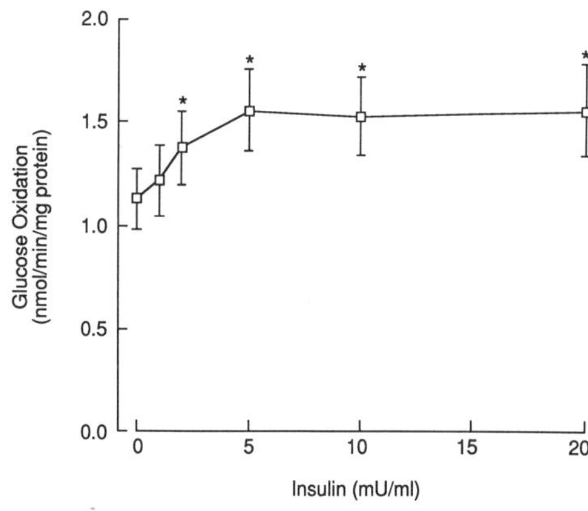

FIG. 1. Dose-response curve relating insulin concentrations to glucose oxidation by isolated myocytes from diabetic rats. Values are means $\pm$ SE of 5 experiments. *$P < 0.05$ compared with cells incubated without insulin.

Glucose utilization by isolated myocytes from diabetic rats was markedly reduced (Fig. 2). The decrease was partially alleviated ($P < 0.05$) by insulin. Adding T_3, T_4 and norepinephrine also partially restored glucose oxidation ($P < 0.05$). The change with each hormone was less, however, than with insulin. The insulin effect on diminished glucose oxidation was not altered by the thyroid hormones or norepinephrine individually, but was slightly enhanced in the presence of all three hormones. Nevertheless, the oxidation rate remained below normal. The inability of insulin to completely restore glucose utilization was not due to substrate limitation because a similar insulin effect was demonstrated when diabetic myocytes were incubated with 25 mM glucose (data not shown). The diminished glucose oxidation was fully restored to normal in cells from diabetic rats receiving in vivo insulin treatment, regardless of the route of administration (Fig. 3).

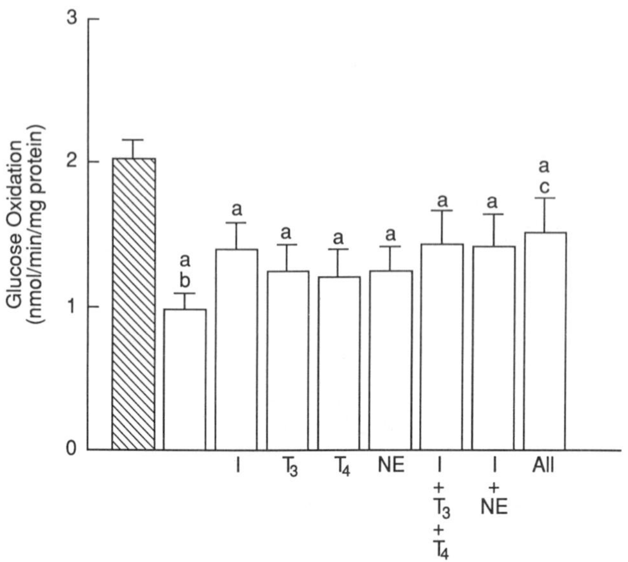

FIG. 2. Glucose oxidation by isolated myocytes from control (hatched bar) and diabetic rats (open bars) in the absence and presence of insulin (I), thyroid hormones (T_3, T_4) and norepinephrine (NE). Values are means $\pm$ SE of 6 experiments. a, $P < 0.01$ from controls. b, $P < 0.05$ from hormone treated diabetics. c, $P < 0.05$ from diabetics treated with insulin only.

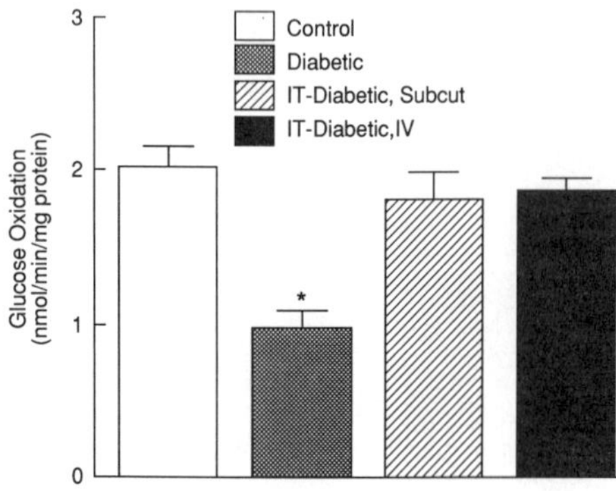

FIG. 3. Glucose oxidation by isolated myocytes from control (open bar), untreated diabetic (dotted bar) and diabetic rats administered insulin subcutaneously (5U/hr, hatched bar) or intravenously (1U bolus, solid bar). Values are means $\pm$ SE of 4-6 experiments. *$P \leq 0.001$ from controls.

DISCUSSION

The present findings demonstrate significant trophic effects by several hormones on glucose oxidation by isolated myocytes from acutely diabetic rats. Insulin was found to exert the greatest influence. Irrespective of the hormone tested, whether singly or in combination, the reduced oxidation rate was only partially corrected. Although the insulin effect was most profound, it became fully manifested only when it was given in vivo. This suggests that additional factors may be responsible for the altered glucose oxidation.

The inability of insulin to completely reverse impaired glucose oxidation may be related to a feedback mechanism involving the endogenous fatty acids. Fatty acid uptake by myocytes is elevated due to accelerated lipolysis of adipose tissue (unpublished observation). Since glucose oxidation is reduced in the presence of fatty acids [4], accumulation in the diabetic myocytes may have inhibited glucose oxidation, even when insulin was present. This inhibitory action by fatty acids may also explain why, in contrast to the diabetic myocytes, glucose oxidation by isolated perfused hearts from diabetic rats is restored to normal by in vitro insulin treatment [8]. Presumably the endogenous fatty acids are rapidly metabolized by diabetic hearts as a result of the greater energy demands, and therefore do not interfere with the insulin action. It should also be recognized that findings from quiescent myocytes reflect basal metabolic requirements of the cells, whereas those obtained from isolated hearts depend on contractile activity.

ACKNOWLEDGEMENTS

We thank Veronika Walton and Abolfath Aminiafshar for their expert technical assistance.

These studies were supported by a grant from the National Institutes of Health (HL-33646)

REFERENCES

1. H.E. Morgan, E. Cadenas, D.M. Regen, and C.R. Park, J. Biol. Chem. 236, 262-268 (1961).
2. P.J. Randle, E.A. Newsholms, and P.B. Garland, Biochem. J. 93, 973-976 (1964).
3. D.M. Regen, W.W. Davis, H.E. Morgan, and C.R. Park, J. Biol. Chem. 239, 43-49 (1964).
4. V. Chen, C.D. Ianuzzo, B.C. Fong, and J.J. Spitzer, Diabetes 33, 1078-1084 (1984).
5. D.W. Garber, A.W. Everett, and J.R. Neely, Am. J. Physiol. 244, H592-H598 (1983).
6. A.G. Tahiliani and J.H. McNeil, Can. J. Physiol. Pharmacol. 64, 188-192 (1986).
7. V. Chen, G.J. Bagby, and J.J. Spitzer. Am. J. Physiol. 245, C46-C51 (1983).
8. L.H. Opie, K.R.L. Mansford, and P. Owen, Biochem. J. 124, 475-490 (1971).

INSULIN RECEPTORS AND GLUCOSE TRANSPORT IN ISOLATED ADULT CARDIAC MYOCYTES: SIGNALING PATHWAYS AND DIABETES INDUCED ALTERATIONS

JÜRGEN ECKEL AND HANS REINAUER
Diabetes Research Institute, Auf'm Hennekamp 65,
D-4000 Düsseldorf 1, Federal Republic of Germany

INTRODUCTION

Stimulation of glucose transport has been recognized to represent one of the most prominent actions of insulin on target tissues [1] and the mechanisms of transmembrane signaling have been the focus of extensive investigations during recent years [for review, see 2]. Insulin action on cardiac glucose uptake has been studied using the isolated perfused rat heart [3,4], however, until recently cellular events could not be ruled out due to the complexity of that model system resulting in an incomplete understanding of the molecular basis of cardiac insulin action.

Our laboratory has approached these problems by using freshly isolated and primary cultured adult rat heart cells. This resulted in a detailed description of cardiac insulin receptors [5-10] and provided some insights into the mechanisms of insulin action under normal [11-14] and pathological [15-16] conditions. In the present paper we report on the existence of multiple pathways of insulin action, which may undergo diabetes induced alterations.

METHODS

Calcium-tolerant myocytes from adult rat were isolated by perfusion of the heart with collagenase followed by additional trypsin treatment, as detailed previously [11]. Culturing of these cells was performed as outlined recently [9]. Measurements of insulin binding and 3-O-methylglucose transport were conducted in Hepes buffer at 37°C using the oil centrifugation technique [5]. Insulin internalization was monitored using a recently developed dissociation procedure [14]. Isolation and characterization of cardiac myocytes from diabetic animals have been described in detail before [15,16].

RESULTS AND DISCUSSION

Characteristics of cardiac insulin receptors

Binding of ^{125}I-labelled insulin to cardiac myocytes was found to be saturable, highly specific, partially reversible, and pH-, time- and temperature-dependent, in agreement with recent findings in other target tissues [for review, see 17]. Scatchard analysis of binding data suggested the presence of both high- and low-affinity insulin receptors. At physiological temperatures about 100,000 high-affinity sites per myocyte could be detected with a K_d of 0.3 nmol/l. These high-affinity sites appear to be strictly dependent on the ionic environment, since removal of calcium and/or magnesium resulted in a total loss of these sites [13].

It may be argued that the number of cell surface receptors is affected by the isolation procedure. This was evaluated by monitoring insulin binding to cardiocytes immediately after isolation and during different stages of the culture period. As presented in Fig. 1, after removal of serum, which may act by inhibition of protein degradation [18], cultured cells exhibited the same level of insulin binding as freshly isolated cells. Moreover, an identical receptor number and affinity were observed in freshly isolated and

Biology of Isolated Adult Cardiac Myocytes
William A. Clark, Robert S. Decker, and Thomas K. Borg, Editors

primary cultured cardiac myocytes [9].

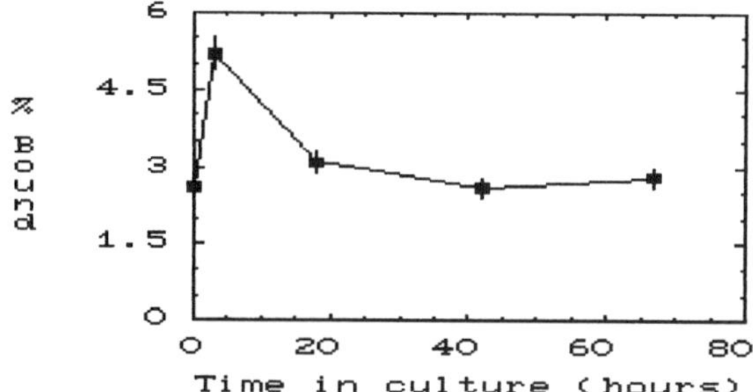

Fig. 1. Insulin binding to cardiac myocytes as a function of culture period. Determinations of specific insulin binding were performed in monolayer as detailed in [9] after keeping cells in culture medium for indicated times. Insulin binding at zero time was measured immediately after isolating the cells. Data are mean ± SEM of 3 separate experiments.

Coupling of insulin receptors to the glucose transport system

Two lines of evidence argue in favour of a highly efficient coupling between insulin receptors and the cardiac glucose transporter. First, half-maximal action occured at an insulin concentration of 0.3 nmol/l corresponding to the high-affinity constant of the insulin receptor, second, the onset of insulin action was very rapid with a lag-phase of only 20 seconds. These observations suggest generation of an intracellular signal as a consequence of the initial insulin-receptor interaction. Autophosphorylation of the receptor may represent such an early event [17]. Consistently, we succeeded in demonstrating autophosphorylation of the β-subunit of insulin receptors purified from cardiac myocytes [19]. Furthermore, this phosphorylation step fits well to our earlier [20] observations on the involvement of ATP and magnesium in the stimulatory action of insulin in the isolated cardiac cell.

Extensive investigations on the fate of receptor-bound insulin have now ruled out a complex chain of events subsequent to the initial binding step, involving receptor-mediated endocytosis, lysosomal degradation of insulin and perhaps of the receptor, and recycling of internalized receptors back to the cell surface [21,22]. Our laboratory has reported comparable findings using freshly isolated [7] and cultured cardiac myocytes [10]. The physiological implications of insulin internalization, however, remain obscure. In order to rule out a possible relationship between this process and the stimulation of glucose transport, the kinetics of insulin internalization have been determined and correlated to the onset of insulin action. As shown in Fig. 2, insulin internalization increased linearly up to 10 min followed by a slower phase up to 60 min. It is noteworthy that under these conditions insulin binding already reaches a plateau by at least 5 min. As can be seen from the data, the kinetics of insulin internalization were comparable to the time course of the onset of insulin action on glucose transport. A rapid phase up to 8 min resulted in a transport stimulation of about 80%. After that time point a much slower phase was observed, but the stimulatory action of insulin still significantly increased by 57% reaching a maximal transport stimulation of about 130% after 30 - 60 min of incubation. A proportionate increase in insulin internalization between 10 and 60 min paralleled the slower phase of glucose transport stimulation. This striking kinetic similarity points to a possible functional relationship between the two reactions.

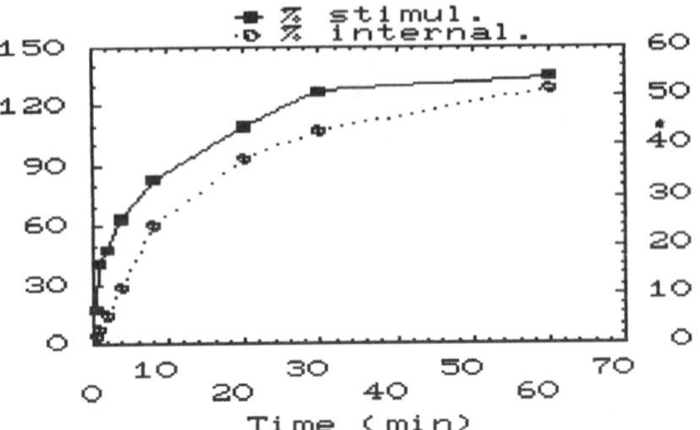

Fig. 2. Time course of insulin internalization (········) and onset of insulin action (——) on 3-O-methylglucose transport. For details, see [14].

In order to substantiate the relationship between insulin processing and insulin action, attempts have been made to selectively block internalization of the hormone. This was achieved by treatment of cells with phenylarsine oxide, a drug which has been reported to inhibit endocytosis in isolated cells [23]. Under these conditions initial insulin action was totally abolished. It should be noted that viability, ATP-content and β-receptor-mediated effects remained unaltered after treatment of cells with phenylarsine oxide [14]. The lysosomal inhibitor chloroquine, which does not affect insulin internalization, was without effect on the initial stimulatory action of insulin. However, steady-state (60 min) action was reduced by 60%, a finding which completely disagrees with earlier reports using isolated adipocytes [24]. The precise mechanism of the lysosomal pathway is not known. Thus, not insulin degradation but a degradative step in general may be involved in mediating steady-state insulin action. Taken together, very early processing of insulin receptor complexes and subsequent degradative steps appear both to be involved in mediating the stimulatory action of insulin on the glucose transport system of the isolated cardiac cell.

Effects of diabetes

Besides functional changes multiple biochemical alterations have been observed in the diabetic myocardium [25] from both type I- and type II-diabetic subjects. However, it is not clear if defects in the signaling pathways outlined above may be responsible for myocardial insulin resistance. Cardiac myocytes isolated from genetically obese (fa/fa) Zucker rats and spontaneously diabetic BB rats have been used to study these relationships. Myocytes from Zucker rats exhibited a decreased number of low-affinity insulin receptors (50%) and a largely (70%) decreased internalization of the bound hormone. This may represent an important defect in the signaling pathway, since hormonal processing was found to be related to its action (see above). Consistently, the responsiveness of the glucose carrier towards stimulation by insulin was significantly decreased. Moreover, basal activity of the transporter was reduced, representing an additional defective site.

In contrast to the Zucker rat, insulin binding and internalization, basal glucose transport and insulin responsiveness remained unaltered in cells isolated from diabetic BB rats. However, the sensitivity of the carrier was markedly reduced with an increase in the coupling time by 400% from 5 to 20 min in cells from control and diabetic animals, respectively. These data suggest that multiple alterations of transmembrane signalling at the receptor and the postreceptor level may be associated with the diabetic syndrome.

ACKNOWLEDGMENTS

This work was supported by the Ministerium für Wissenschaft und Forschung des Landes Nordrhein-Westfalen, the Bundesministerium für Jugend, Familie und Gesundheit, and the Deutsche Forschungsgemeinschaft (SFB 113).

REFERENCES

1. Czech, M.P., Diabetes 29, 399-409 (1980).
2. Houslay, M.D. and Heyworth, C.M., Trends Biochem. Sci. 8, 449-452 (1983).
3. Morgan, H.E., Randle, P.J. and Regen, D.M., Biochem. J. 73, 573-579 (1959).
4. Fischer, U., Acta Biol. Med. Germ. 26, 87-99 (1971).
5. Eckel, J. and Reinauer, H., Biochim. Biophys. Acta 629, 510-521 (1980).
6. Eckel, J. and Reinauer, H., Biochem. Biophys. Res. Commun. 92, 1403-1408 (1980).
7. Eckel, J. and Reinauer, H., Biochem. J. 206, 655-662 (1982).
8. Eckel, J., Offermann, A. and Reinauer, H., Basic Res. Cardiol. 77, 323-332 (1982).
9. Eckel, J., van Echten, G. and Reinauer, H., Am. J. Physiol. 249, H212-H221 (1985).
10. Van Echten, G., Eckel, J. and Reinauer, H., Biochim. Biophys. Acta 886, 468-473 (1986).
11. Eckel, J., Pandalis, G. and Reinauer, H., Biochem. J. 212, 385-392 (1983).
12. Eckel, J. and Reinauer, H., Biochim. Biophys. Acta 736, 119-124 (1983).
13. Eckel, J. and Reinauer, H., Diabetes 33, 214-218 (1984).
14. Eckel, J. and Reinauer, H., Biochem. J., in press.
15. Eckel, J., Wirdeier, A., Herberg. L. and Reinauer, H., Endocrinology 116, 1529-1534 (1985).
16. Eckel, J., Röhn, G., Kiesel, U. and Reinauer, H., Diabetes Res. 4, 79-83 (1987).
17. Czech, M.P., Ann. Rev. Physiol. 47, 357-381 (1985).
18. Frelin, C., J. Biol. Chem. 255, 11149-11155 (1980).
19. Häring, H.U., Machicao, F., Kirsch, D., Rinninger, F., Hölzl, J., Eckel, J. and Bachmann, W., FEBS Lett. 176, 229-234 (1984).
20. Eckel, J. and Reinauer, H., Basic Res. Cardiol 80, Suppl. 2, 103-106 (1985).
21. Carpentier, J.L., Gorden, P., Freychet, P., Le Cam, A. and Orci, L., J. Clin. Invest. 63, 1249-1261 (1979).
22. Marshall, S., J. Biol. Chem. 260, 13517-13523 (1985).
23. Wiley, H. S. and Cunningham, D.D., J. Biol. Chem. 257, 4222-4229 (1982).
24. Häring, H,U., Biermann, E. and Kemmler, W., Am. J. Physiol. 240, E556-E565 (1981).
25. Opie, L.H., Tansey, M.J. and Kennely, B.M., S. Afr. Med. J. 56, 207-211 (1979).

$Alpha_1$-Adrenergic Receptor Signal Transduction in the Adult Rat Cardiac Myocyte

IAIN L. O. BUXTON and KURT O. DOGGWILER Department of Pharmacology, University of Nevada School of Medicine, Reno, Nevada 89557-0046

INTRODUCTION

We have previously demonstrated that the ventricular myocyte of rat heart possesses a large compliment of alpha-adrenergic receptors of the $alpha_1$ subtype [1]. Radioligand binding studies employing purified myocyte membranes have shown that norepinephrine (NE) competition of [^{3}H]prazosin binding is regulated by added GTP, suggesting that the $alpha_1$ receptor is coupled to an effector via a GTP binding protein. Our studies of the coupling of the $alpha_1$ receptor to response in the myocyte reveal that the occupation of receptor by agonist leads to both the acceleration of cyclic AMP (cAMP) degradation [2] and an increase in the hydrolysis of phosphatidylinositol [3]. In order to explain the role of the $alpha_1$ receptor in the regulation of both cAMP and inositol phosphate second messenger generation, we have studied cAMP-phosphodiesterase (cAMP-PDE) activity and inositol trisphosphate (IP_3) formation in the myocyte.

METHODS

Ventricular myocytes were prepared from enzyme perfused rat hearts as previously described [4]. Briefly, hearts were excised from phenobarbital anesthetized Sprague Dawley rats and mounted via the aorta in a warmed (32°), oxygenated perfusion chamber of our own design that is capable of perfusing 12 hearts simultaneously. Following 30min of collagenase (1mg/ml; Cooper T-II) perfusion in a recirculating fashion, the right and left ventricles were removed and teased apart. Myocytes were purified by successive unit gravity sedimentation in Krebs buffer with BSA (0.01%) and calcium (0.2mM). Following purification the calcium concentration was increased to 1.0mM. The preparation is visably homogenious and contains 75-85% rod-shaped cells excluding trypan blue. Myocytes are used 30-60min following their preparation.

Cardiac myocyte cAMP-PDE was measured in both homogenates and cell fractions by the method of Thompson et al [5] and in the intact myocyte by labeling cells with [^{3}H]adenine after the method of Shimizu et al [6]. For in vivo assay of cAMP-PDE, the cells were labeled at 35° for 60-90min with [^{3}H]adenine (10uCi/ml) in Krebs buffer containing 1mM calcium. Washed myocytes were then stimulated as a concentrated cell suspension (2-4 x 10^6 cells/ml) with 1uM isoproterenol (INE) for 3min to generate [^{3}H]cyclic AMP within the cell. Following this stimulation, cells were rapidly diluted with Krebs buffer containing a final concentration of either 1uM propranolol (PROP), for control degradation, or PROP plus 10uM NE as net $alpha_1$ stimulation (alpha + beta stimulation + beta antagonist). Samples were removed at various times, acidified with trichloroacetic acid (5% final) and the [^{3}H]cAMP remaining determined by separation over Dowex-50 and alumia columns as described by Salomon et al [7].

Biology of Isolated Adult Cardiac Myocytes
William A. Clark, Robert S. Decker, and Thomas K. Borg, Editors

Inositol phosphates were measured essentially as described by Abdel-Latif [8]. Cells were labeled with [^{3}H]myo-inositol (15uCi/ml x 90min at 35°), washed three times and added to washed testtubes. TCA was added following the desired treatment, (5% final) and the sample extracted with ether, lypholized, resuspended in 10mM TRIS buffer (pH 7) and loaded on a Dowex-1 column. The inositol phosphates were specifically eluted with increasing concentrations of ammonium formate. Columns were calibrated with [^{3}H] standards of IP_1, IP_2 and IP_3. Recovery of IP_3 was 78%.

RESULTS AND DISCUSSION

In order to determine if alpha$_1$ receptor activation couples to the activation of a cAMP-PDE in the myocyte, we measured PDE activity in vitro either by adding NE and GTP or other modifiers to the assay, or by first stimulating the tissue with alpha agonist and then quick freezing the tissue in liquid N_2 and then assaying the "fossil" activation in homogenates and fractions. Neither approach to the study of alpha$_1$ regulation of cAMP-PDE activity in the myocyte was successful. In contrast, it was possible to demonstrate the alpha$_1$ effect in the intact cell as shown in figure 1.

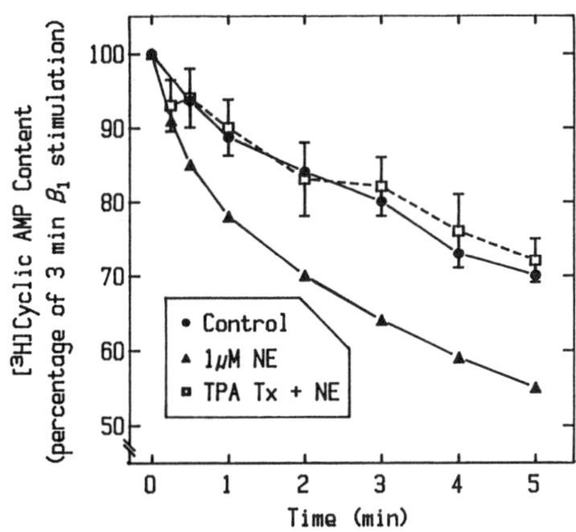

Figure 1. Myocytes were labeled with [^{3}H]adenosine as described above. At time 0, cells had already been stimulated for 3min with INE (1uM) then diluted in the presence of PROP (1uM). Data are the mean +/- SEM, n=3.

When myocytes were pretreated for 20min with the C-kinase agonist, phorbol,12-myristate,13-acetate (TPA), the ability of NE to accelerate degradation of beta receptor stimulated cAMP accumulation was abolished. Thinking that this effect of TPA might be due to alteration of the inositol phosphate pathway, as suggested by Orellana [9], and thus was a decrease in the availability of $[Ca^{2+}]_i$ for activation of a Ca^{2+} sensitive cAMP-PDE, we measured the formation of inositol phosphates in the myocyte before and after TPA treatment (Figure 2). Norepinephrine stimulation of the cardiac myocyte leads to a

185% increase in IP_3 generation at 3min. Control experiments revealed that this effect was due to $alpha_1$ receptor activation (blocked by prazosin but not yohimbine) and not beta receptor stimulation (not ellicited by isoproterenol). When cells are pretreated with TPA however, this effect of NE to stimulate formation of IP_3 is abolished.

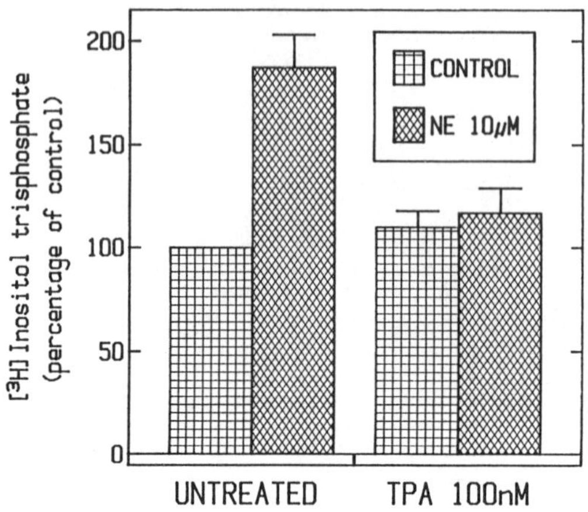

Figure 2. Myocytes prelabeled with [^{3}H]inositol were pretreated either with or without TPA (100nM) for 20min prior to stimulation with NE (10uM). IP_3 was separated as described in METHODS. The average signal measured in the untreated control was 285dpm. Data are mean +/- SEM, n=3.

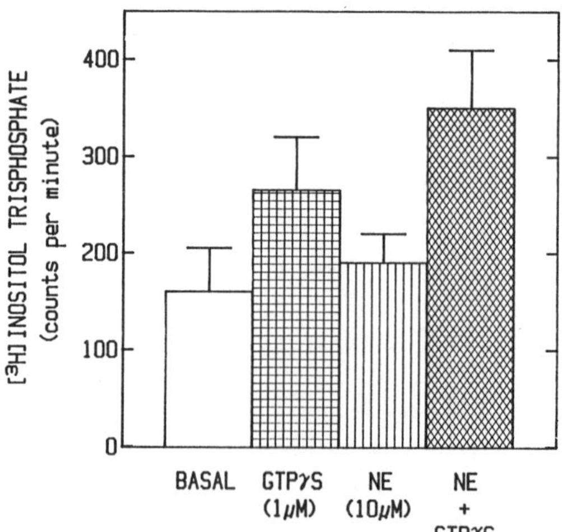

Figure 3. [^{3}H]inositol labeled myocytes were incubated in normal Krebs buffer with 3mM octyl-B-D-glucopyranoside for 5min prior to addition of agonists. Data are mean +/- range in two experiments performed in triplicate.

Our inability to assay the $alpha_1$ receptor activation of cardiac myocyte cAMP-PDE in the in vitro assay, while not conclusive evidence that the receptor does not couple directly to a cAMP-PDE, does suggest that this effect is subordinate to the action of another receptor coupled event. The fact that TPA pretreatment can both abolish the $alpha_1$ stimulation of phospholipase C (PLC), and eliminate the acceleration of cAMP degradation is strong, albeit indirect, evidence that the $alpha_1$ effect on myocyte cAMP is due to some consequence of the formation of IP_3. The most likely, but by no means the only event that would explain cAMP-PDE activation, would be that IP_3 releases Ca^{2+} that then activates a cAMP-PDE. In order to accumulate further evidence that the $alpha_1$ receptor couples directly to the activation of PLC, we investigated the role of GTP in receptor activation of IP_3 formation. As shown in Figure 3, addition of NE to permeabilized cells did not lead to IP_3 formation (presumably due to the vast dilution of cellular GTP) while addition of the hydrolysis resistant GTP analogue GTPgamma-S (1uM) did. Indeed when both agonist and GTPgamma-S were added a very large increase in IP_3 was measured. These data argue strongly that the results we have previously obtained (ie. GTP alters receptor affinity for agonist in radioligand binding experiments) are due to the presence of a GTP binding regulatory protein coupling the $alpha_1$ receptor to PLC activation.

TABLE I. Effects of Cholera and Pertussis toxin on $Alpha_1$ receptor mediated IP_3 formation in the adult cardiac myocyte.

TREATMENT	IP_1	IP_2	IP_3	cAMP	
	(percentage of O-time)			(%INE+CAR)	(%CONT)
Untreated	163/12	130/8	155/18	65/9	-
Pertussis	158/9	143/12	150/13	104/10	-
Cholera	146/10	125/11	142/12	-	632/98

For IP measurements, rat myocytes were incubated with pertussis toxin (100ng/ml), cholera toxin (30ug/ml) or nothing for 30min prior to NE (10uM) stimulation for 3min. Cyclic AMP accumulation following muscarinic stimulation (100uM carbachol=CAR) in the presence of 3uM INE (3min), or that following cholera toxin treatment was used as a positive control for pertussis effects on G_i and cholera effects on G_s respectively. Data are the mean/SEM, n=3.

The data above, in table I, clearly demonstrate that the effects of both pertussis toxin on G_i and cholera toxin on G_s can be measured in the myocyte. Because treatment of myocytes with either toxin does not alter the $alpha_1$ effect on IP_3 formation (Table I), we do not believe that the GTP regulatory protein responsible for coupling the $alpha_1$ receptor to PLC is either G_i or G_s. It is likely then, that another GTP binding protein exists in the myocyte and couples the $alpha_1$ receptor to response. This protein might conveniently termed $G_s{}^p$ as we believe it will be shown to be homologous with such proteins in other tissues that couple a variety of receptors to activation of PLC.

SUMMARY

We have studied the transduction of signal following $alpha_1$ receptor activation in the ventricular myocyte purified from adult rat heart. These cells are readily produced in large numbers, (12 hearts from 300g rats yeilds 8-10 x 10^7 myocytes that are 75-85% rod shaped cells). These are highly responsive cells that share the expected biochemical homology with the intact heart. Our data show that the acceleration of cAMP degradation that is measured following $alpha_1$ receptor stimulation in these cells is not the result of direct coupling of receptor to a cAMP-PDE, but rather, occurs as a consequence of $alpha_1$ receptor coupling to PLC. Our data suggest that regulation of both the secondary alpha-adrenergic effects on cAMP as well as direct stimulation of IP_3 formation (ie. inhibition by TPA) is the result of activation of myocyte C-kinase. We believe it is likely that this activation of protein kinase C may occur normally when diacylglycerol and Ca^{2+} become more available following $alpha_1$ receptor stimulation and might explain receptor desensitization in the cell. Furthermore, we explain the effects of GTP on $alpha_1$ receptor affinity for agonist in radioligand binding assays as the result of a GTP binding protein that couples the $alpha_1$ receptor to its effector. We do not find that this protein is either G_i or G_s, the GTP regulatory proteins known to regulate adenylate cyclase in the myocyte, but must be a distinct protein as has been suggested in heart by Masters et al [10].

ACKNOWLEDGMENTS

This work was supported by NIH grant HL 35416 to ILOB and a grant from the Nevada affiliate of the American Heart Association.

REFERENCES

1. Buxton, I.L. and Brunton, L.L., Am. J. Physiol. 251: H307 (1986).
2. Buxton, I.L. and Brunton, L.L., J. Biol. Chem. 260: 6733 (1985).
3. Brown, J., Buxton, I.L. and Brunton, L.L., Circ. Res. 57: 532 (1985).
4. Buxton, I.L. and Brunton, L.L., J. Biol. Chem. 258: 10233 (1983).
5. Thompson, W.J., Brooker, G. and Appleman, M.M. in: Methods in Enzymology (Academic Press, Fl.) 38: 205 (1974).
6. Shimizu, H., Daley, J.N. and Creveling, C.R., J. Neurochem 16: 1606 (1969).
7. Salomon, Y., Londos, C. and Rodbell, M., Anal. Biochem. 58: 541 (1974).
8. Abdel-Latif, A.A. in: Pharmacological Reviews 38: 227 (1986).
9. Orellana, S.A., Solski, P.A., and Brown, J.H., J. Biol. Chem. 260: 5236 (1985).
10. Masters, S., Martin, M., Harden, T. and Brown, J.H., Biochem. J. 227: 933 (1985).

BETA-RECEPTOR DENSITY AND FUNCTION ARE MAINTAINED BY ADULT CARDIAC MYOCYTES AS THEY PROGRESS INTO CULTURE

Evy Lundgren*, Louis Terracio**, Donald O. Allen** and Thomas K. Borg**.
*Department of Medical and Physiological Chemistry, Box 575, S-751 23 Uppsala, Sweden.
**Departments of Anatomy, Pharmacology and Pathology, University of South Carolina, Columbia, SC 29208.

INTRODUCTION

It is well established that catecholamines, by acting through α- and β-receptors (1,2) modulate a variety of physiological responses in the heart including increased rate and force of cardiac contraction (3,4). By stimulation of the β-adrenergic receptors the membrane bound enzyme adenylate cyclase is activated and adenosine 3',5'-monophosphate (cAMP) is accumulated and induces an array of mechanisms that regulate cardiac contraction.

Recent technical advances have made cultures of adult cardiac myocytes available as potential models in the study of cardiac function (5,6,7). In order to establish optimal culture conditions allowing for biochemical and pharmacological investigations, we have studied the attachment of isolated adult myocytes to extracellular matrix components. We have shown that adult myocytes adhere to the basement membrane components collagen type IV (C IV) and laminin (LN) and these substrates are necessary for establishment of high density cultures (6).

When maintained in culture, adult myocytes undergo major morphological changes (6). The freshly isolated rod-shaped myocyte spreads out into a flattened cell in culture. However, we have shown that the cells have reorganized actin-filaments and that they contract spontaneously. Other investigators have shown that adult myocytes _in vitro_ have normal resting potentials (8), adult metabolic patterns (5) and distinctive T-tubules (9) supporting the fact that the cultured adult myocyte is not dedifferentiated but has adapted its morphology to culture conditions.

To further investigate the function and retention of adult characteristics by cultured myocytes, the density of β-receptors and the response to β-receptor stimulation after different times in culture was studied.

MATERIALS AND METHODS

Adult rat cardiac myocytes were isolated as previously described (10) and suspended in F12K culture medium supplemented with 20 % fetal bovine serum (FBS) and antibiotics. Culture dishes (35 mm; Corning) were coated with 20 µg/ml of LN as earlier described (6) and the myocytes were plated at a density of 1×10^5 cells per dish. The cells were fed with fresh medium every other day and to inhibit growth of fibroblasts 10 µg/ml of cytosine arabinoside (ARA-C; Sigma) was added to the medium.

Iodocyanopindolol (^{125}I-CYP) obtained from New England Nuclear was used to identify β-receptor sites on the cultured cells. The cell cultures were washed and the radioligand was added at various concentrations in F12K containing 50 µg/ml of phentolamine (Ciba Geigy AG). The cells were then incubated in the presence or absence of 10 µg/ml of propranolol (Sigma) for specific and nonspecific binding, respectively. After an incubation

Biology of Isolated Adult Cardiac Myocytes
William A. Clark, Robert S. Decker, and Thomas K. Borg, Editors

of 60 minutes at 37°C, the cells were washed three times (5 minutes each) at 37°C and the cells were digested in 0.5 M NaOH. Radioactivity was determined from duplicated dishes with a gamma counter and protein was analyzed in separate dishes according to Lowry et al. (11). Specific binding was defined as total binding minus nonspecific binding. The number of binding sites was analyzed according to Scatchard (12).

The response to β-receptor stimulation was examined by incubating cultured myocytes with 1 μM of (-)-isoproterenol (Sigma) in F12K medium for 2 minutes at 37°C. The incubation was stopped by aspirating the medium and adding 1 ml of 5 % TCA and cAMP was analyzed by the method of Harper et al. (13). Protein was determined as described above.

RESULTS AND DISCUSSION

The specific binding of ^{125}I-CYP to adult myocytes was saturable with increasing concentration of the ligand and after 60 minutes of incubation at 37°C. Figure 1a show specific and nonspecific binding of ^{125}I-CYP to freshly isolated myocytes and maximal specific binding was achieved at 60 pM. Scathchard analysis of the specific binding is shown in figure 1b. The number of binding sites in this experiment was 42 fmoles/mg protein.

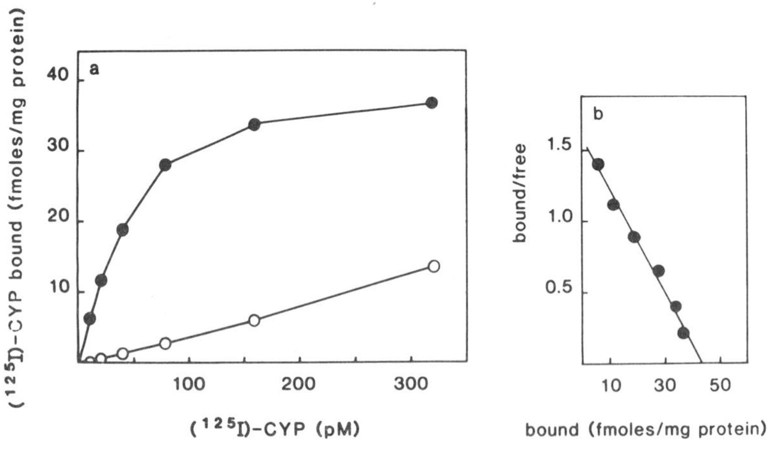

Figure 1. a. Specific (●) and nonspecific (○) binding of ^{125}I-CYP to freshly attached adult myocyte; b. Scatchard analysis of the specific binding data presented in fig. 1a.

Saturable binding and low nonspecific binding indicated that ^{125}I-CYP was applicable for β-receptor binding studies on intact cells. These advantages of ^{125}I-CYP compared to other radiolabelled β-receptor ligands have been discussed by others (14,15,16). The binding of ^{125}I-CYP to cultured adult myocyte was furthermore displaced by isomeres of propranolol and isoproterenol both in a pharmacological and stereospecific way.

Binding of ^{125}I-CYP to adult myocytes was studied after 1 hour, 2 days, 5 days, and 10 days in culture and showed that the β-receptor density calculated per mg protein was similar during the 10 day culture period at a density of approximately 50 fmoles/mg cell protein (table I), indicating that the myocytes maintain their β-receptors in culture. In freshly isolated myocytes this is equivalent to 60,000 binding sites/myocyte.

TABLE I. Number of β-receptors on adult myocytes after different times in culture.

	time in culture			
	1 hour	2 days	5 days	10 days
number of β-receptors fmoles / mg protein n=4±SEM	50±9.9	44±11.0	34±6.1	54±6.3

In parallel with the β-receptor experiments, the concentration of cAMP in cultures of myocytes was determined as well as the ability of the myocytes to respond to β-receptor stimulation after different times in culture (Table II). There was at least a two fold increase in cellular content of cAMP after β-receptor stimulation with isoproterenol at all times studied indicating that adult myocytes preserved their β-receptor function in culture.

TABLE II. Cellular concentration of cAMP in adult myocytes after different times in culture. cAMP was determined before (nonstimulated myocytes) or after (stimulated myocytes) incubation with isoproterenol.

concentration of cAMP pmoles / mg protein n=9±SEM	time in culture			
	1 hour	2 days	5 days	10 days
nonstimulated myocytes	6.4±0.3	8.9±0.6	9.3±0.9	15.8±0.9
stimulated myocytes	17.2±0.8	23.9±1.1	23.4±1.7	60.0±3.8

SUMMARY

Adult myocytes maintained a density of β-receptors in culture that was similar to freshly isolated myocytes and increased the cellular concentration of cAMP after β-receptor stimulation. These results indicate that cultured adult myocytes retain functional β-receptors and should be useful in studies of cardiac function at the cellular level.

ACKNOWLEDGEMENTS

This research was supported from grants from NIH HL-33656, HL-24935, HL-37669 and Swedish Medical Research Council 07466.

REFERENCES

1. R.P. Ahlquist, Am. J. Physiol. 153, 586-600 (1948).
2. B.B. Hoffman and R.J. Lefkowitz, Ann. Rev. Physiol. 44, 475-484 (1982).
3. A.M. Katz, Adv. Cyclic Nucl. Rec. 11, 303-343 (1979).
4. G.L. Stiles, M.G. Caron and R.J. Lefkowitz, Am. J. Physiol. 64, 661-743 (1984).
5. W.C. Claycomb, A.H. Burns and E.D. Shepherd, FEBS Lett. 169, 261-266 (1984).
6. E. Lundgren, L. Terracio, S. Mårdh and T.K. Borg, Exp. Cell Res. 158, 371-381 (1985).
7. S.L. Jacobson and H.M. Piper, J. Mol. Cell. Cardiol. 18, 661-678 (1986).
8. C.F. Meier Jr, G.M. Briggs and W.C. Claycomb, Am. J. Physiol. 250, H731-H735 (1986).
9. R.L. Moses and W.C. Claycomb, Am. J. Anat. 164, 113-131 (1982).
10. E. Lundgren, T.K. Borg and S. Mårdh, J. Mol. Cell. Cardiol. 16, 355-362 (1984).
11. O.H. Lowry, N.J. Rosebrough, A.L. Farr and R.J. Randall, J. Biol. Chem. 193, 265-275 (1982).
12. G. Scatchard, Ann. NY Acad. Sci. 51, 660-672 (1949).
13. J.F. Harper and G. Brooker, J. Cyclic Nucl. Res. 1, 207-218 (1975).
14. G. Engel, D. Hoyer, R. Berthold and H. Wagner, Naunyn-Schmiedeberg's Arch. Pharmacol. 317, 277-285 (1981).
15. H. Porzig, C. Becker and H. Reuter, Naunyn-Schmiedeberg's Arch. Pharmacol. 321, 89-99 (1982).
16. M. Schonberg, S.A. Morris, A. Krichevsky and J.P. Bilezikian, Cell Diff. 12, 321-327 (1983).

GUANINE NUCLEOTIDE-REGULATED INOSITOL POLYPHOSPHATE PRODUCTION IN ADULT RAT CARDIOMYOCYTES

Linda G. Jones and Joan Heller Brown
Department of Pharmacology, M-036, School of Medicine, University of California at San Diego, La Jolla, CA 92093

INTRODUCTION

The stimulation of both α_1-adrenergic and muscarinic cholinergic receptors has been shown to promote phosphoinositide (PI) hydrolysis in the heart [Reviewed in Ref. 1]. This may seem puzzling since these receptors are generally thought to provoke opposing functions in the heart, the α_1-adrenergic stimulation serving an excitatory role and muscarinic stimulation an inhibitory role in modulating contractility and rate.

It is now well-established that $InsP_3$ serves a role in the mobilization of calcium in a number of systems [2,3]. It is of interest to determine whether both α_1-adrenergic and muscarinic stimulation lead to the production of $InsP_3$ in the heart. In addition, evidence for the existence of a guanine nucleotide-binding protein that regulates phospholipase C activity continues to increase although the nature of this G-protein has not yet been established [4]. The studies shown here provide further evidence for the production of the inositol polyphosphates subsequent to both α_1-adrenergic and muscarinic stimulation and for the regulation of these responses by guanine nucleotides.

METHODS

Cardiomyocyte preparation.

Ventricular cardiomyocytes were prepared from adult male Sprague-Dawley rats (300-350 g, Charles River Laboratories, St. Louis, MO) by a procedure modified from that previously described [5]. In brief, excised hearts were mounted by the aorta in a perfusion apparatus which maintained the temperature (32° C) and flow rate of the calcium-free, bicarbonate-buffered medium (continually gassed with 95% O_2/ 5% CO_2). The hearts were perfused with this medium containing collagenase (1.2 mg/ml) for 45-55 minutes. Following this perfusion, the hearts were teased apart and treated with the enzyme buffer for an additional 10 minutes. The dissociated tissue suspension was filtered, and the cells gently pelleted through a 1% BSA solution. Four settling steps with the reintroduction of 1 mM calcium in the final 2 washes were performed before the cells were resuspended in the labeling medium. Approximately 8 x 10^6 cells per heart were routinely isolated of which 51-68% were rod-shaped and excluded trypan blue.

Phosphoinositide assay.

Purified cardiomyocytes were resuspended in the purification buffer containing 1 mM CaCl2, 1-5% fetal calf serum, 1% fungibact and 3-20 μCi/ml [^{3}H]inositol. Following 8-18 hours of labeling, cells were washed and resuspended in the same buffer at a density of 0.3-0.5 x 10^6 cells per ml. Cells to be permeabilized were resuspended in an intracellular buffer which contained an ATP-regenerating system, 150 nM free calcium and 50 μg/ml saponin for 2 minutes and then gently washed and pelleted before resuspension in the intracellular buffer without saponin. Assays were initiated by the addition of 1 ml of the cell suspension (permeabilized or nonpermeabilized) to a 10x concentration of the appropriate drugs. All assays were carried out in the presence of 100 μM ascorbate and 10 mM LiCl

Biology of Isolated Adult Cardiac Myocytes
William A. Clark, Robert S. Decker, and Thomas K. Borg, Editors

of TCA (10% final) to the reaction mixture, and the cell supernatant ether-extracted. Assays using permeabilized cells were stopped by the rapid centrifugation of the cell suspension and the separation of the reaction medium (into which the inositol phosphates had been released) from the cell pellet. The [^{3}H]inositol phosphates were separated by anion exchange column chromatography following a modification of the procedures described by Berridge et al. [6] and by Batty et al. [7]. Radioactivity in all the eluted fractions was quantified by liquid scintillation counting. Identification of the inositol phosphates in the elution fractions was verified by the elution profiles of tritiated standards.

Data were analyzed using the unpaired Student's t-test [8]. The p values were obtained using a one-tail test. Data are means ± S.E.

RESULTS

As previously shown [9] stimulation of both the α_1-adrenergic and the muscarinic cholinergic receptors promote phosphatidylinositol (PI) hydrolysis in radiolabeled ventricular cardiomyocytes purified from adult rats. Alpha$_1$-adrenergic stimulation promotes a 5-8x increase in the accumulation of the total inositol phosphates in the intact cardiac cell preparation while the response to muscarinic stimulation is always less with a 1.5-2x increase in the breakdown products. Also, the two responses are additive suggesting independent mechanisms. In this report, we demonstrate the accumulation of inositol bis- and tris-phosphates ($InsP_2$ and $InsP_3$) within one minute of exposure to norepinephrine (Table 1). The accumulation of $InsP_3$ and $InsP_2$ suggests that a polyphosphatidylinositol-specific phospholipase C (PPI-PLC) is activated. Hormone does not induce a significant increase in the accumulation of InsP until after one minute suggesting that the formation of InsP is subsequent to the metabolism of the inositol polyphosphates.

TABLE 1. Stimulation of inositol phosphate accumulation at one minute by 30 μM norepinephrine in intact adult rat cardiomyocytes.

	InsP	$InsP_2$	$InsP_3$
Control	3656 ±117	800 ±14	122 ±4
Norepi	4043 ±292	969 ±42 p=0.002	152 ±10 p=0.01

A permeabilized cell preparation was used to determine whether a guanine nucleotide-binding protein transduces receptor stimulation to PI turnover. The activation of a PPI-PLC appears to be regulated by guanine nucleotides as GTP and its analogs, GTPγS and GppNHp, promote significant increases in the accumulation of the inositol phosphates while AppNHp does not (Figure 1). This figure also shows that the response to hormone is at least additive, if not synergistic with GTPγS. Furthermore, the nonhydrolyzable GDP analog, GDPβS, inhibits GTPγS stimulation of $InsP_{1-4}$ accumulation by more than 50% providing further evidence for a specific guanine nucleotide effect.

Pertussis toxin has been shown to ADP-ribosylate the α subunit of several guanine nucleotide-binding proteins, and this is associated with an inhibition of the coupled response [10]. To determine whether a pertussis toxin-sensitive substrate was involved in the transduction of PI hydrolysis in the rat cardiomyocyte, we measured the accumulation of the inositol phosphates following overnight incubation with increasing concentrations of pertussis toxin. We found that pretreatment for 18 hours with pertussis toxin fails to diminish the accumulation of the inositol phosphates stimulated for 30 minutes with norepinephrine (Table 2).

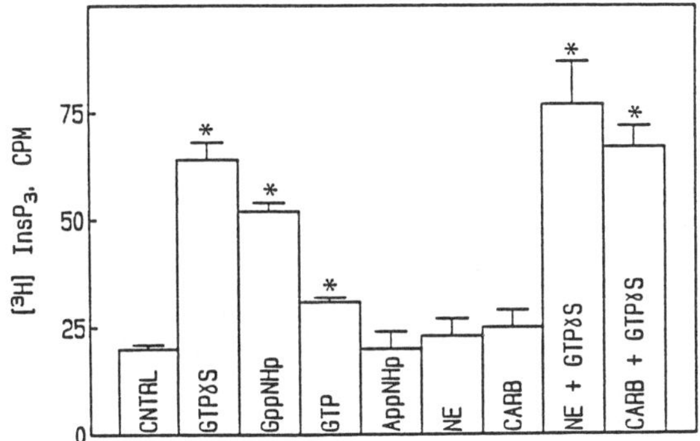

Figure 1. $InsP_3$ released over 30 minutes into medium of permeabilized rat cardiomyocytes in response to 30 μM guanine nucleotides, AppNHp, norepinephrine (NE), and 1 mM carbachol, (* denotes $p \leq 0.0005$). Similar results were obtained for $InsP_2$ and InsP in this experiment.

TABLE 2. Accumulation of the inositol phosphates following overnight pretreatment with pertussis toxin (PT).

	CONTROL				NOREPINEPHRINE (30 μM)			
PT,μg/ml:	0	30	100	300	0	30	100	300
InsP	2854	2702	3060	3124	8085	8561	10504	10608
$InsP_2$	402	378	389	425	804	806	882	880
$InsP_3$	41	41	46	52	76	97	101	116

DISCUSSION

The second messenger role of $InsP_3$ in the release of calcium from intracellular stores has been well-established in numerous systems [2,3]. More recently, a role for $InsP_4$ in regulation of calcium at the plasma membrane has been described [11]. It has thus become important to determine whether these inositol polyphosphates are formed in the heart following stimulation by agonists known to induce phosphatidylinositol hydrolysis and, if formed, whether they serve a similar function.

Our current data demonstrate the production of $InsP_3$ in adult rat heart cells in response to norepinephrine and carbachol. Poggioli et al. [12] have also recently demonstrated the production of $InsP_3$, $InsP_2$ and InsP in rat ventricle in response to α_1-adrenergic, muscarinic and electrical stimulation. We have shown in the embryonic chick heart cell that Ins 1,4,5-P_3, Ins 1,3,4-P_3 and $InsP_4$ are formed in response to muscarinic cholinergic stimulation as well as to guanine nucleotides in the permeabilized cell preparation [13]. While we have not employed HPLC to separate the isomers of $InsP_3$ in the rat heart cells, Renard and Poggioli [14] have shown in rat heart slices the formation of both the 1,4,5- and 1,3,4- isomers of $InsP_3$. They also demonstrated $InsP_3$ kinase activity in an <u>in vitro</u> assay. We have found that stimulation by GTPγS in the permeabilized rat heart cell promotes a significant ($p<0.003$) increase in the $InsP_4$ fraction (data not shown). These data with those describing $InsP_3$ kinase activity suggest that the phosphorylation of InsP3 to InsP4 occurs in the rat heart cell though whether it is consequent to hormone stimulation remains to be determined.

We now show also that the accumulation of the inositol phosphates in the adult rat cardiomyocyte is regulated by guanine nucleotides since the addition of GTP, GTPγs or GppNHp significantly increases the accumulation of the inositol polyphosphates in the permeabilized cell while AppNHp does not. The failure of pertussis toxin to block PI hydrolysis in rat cardiomyocytes as in the chick heart cell [15] suggests that the putative G-protein involved in the regulation of phospholipase C in the heart is not G_i or G_o; both of these have been shown in heart tissue to be ribosylated by pertussis toxin [16]. It has recently been demonstrated that pertussis toxin does not affect the positive inotropic response to α_1-adrenergic stimulation in rat left auricles [17]. In addition, there is a positive inotropic response to muscarinic stimulation that also is not affected by pertussis toxin [18].

Whether the formation of $InsP_3$ serves to mobilize calcium in the heart remains to be determined. To date, we have not observed a calcium-induced increase in fura-2 fluorescence following agonist exposure in either the embryonic chick or adult rat heart cell although marked increases are observed in response to the calcium ionophore ionomycin and the sodium channel activator veratridine (PM McDonough, personal communication). As we have previously discussed in more detail [1], it may be that the other branch of the PI pathway, the activation of protein kinase C, is responsible for the cellular effects observed in the heart upon stimulation of PI hydrolysis.

ACKNOWLEDGEMENTS

This work was supported by NIH Grants HL28143 and HL17682 to JHB. LGJ is a postdoctoral fellow previously supported by PHSHL-07444 6-404814-24106 and currently by the California Heart Association.

REFERENCES

1. JH Brown and LG Jones in: Phosphoinositides and Receptor Mechanisms, JW Putney, Jr, ed (Alan Liss, Inc, New York 1986) pp 245-270.
2. MJ Berridge and RF Irvine, Nature 312, 315-321 (1984).
3. JW Putney, Jr, Am J Physiol 252 (Gastrointest Liver Physiol 15), G149-G157 (1987).
4. S Cockcroft, Trends Biochem Sci 12, 75-78 (1987).
5. ILO Buxton and LL Brunton, J Biol Chem 258, 10233-10239 (1983).
6. MJ Berridge, CP Downes, and MR Hanley, Biochem J 206, 587-595 (1982).
7. IR Batty, SR Nahorski, and RF Irvine, Biochem J 232, 211-215 (1985).
8. SA Glantz in: Primer of Biostatistics (McGraw-Hill Book Company, New York 1981) pp 63-93.
9. JH Brown, IL Buxton, and LL Brunton, Circ Res 57, 532-537 (1985).
10. AG Gilman, Ann Rev Biochem 56, 615-649 (1987).
11. RF Irvine and RM Moor, Biochem J 240, 917-920 (1986).
12. J Poggioli, JC Sulpice, and G Vassort, FEBS Lett 206, 292-298 (1986).
13. LG Jones, D Goldstein, and JH Brown, Circ Res, in press 1988.
14. D Renard and J Poggioli, FEBS Lett 217, 117-123 (1987).
15. SB Masters, MW Martin, TK Harden, and JH Brown, Biochem J 227, 933-937 (1985).
16. JM Martin, DD Hunter, and NM Nathanson, Biochemistry 24, 7521-7525 (1985).
17. M Bohm, W Schmitz, and H Scholz, Naunyn-Schmiedeberg's Arch Pharmacol 335, 476-479 (1987).
18. T Tajima, Y Tsuji, JH Brown, and AJ Pappano, Circ Res in press 1987.

ISOPROTERENOL HAS NO EFFECT ON HEPARIN-RELEASABLE LIPOPROTEIN LIPASE ACTIVITY IN CARDIAC MYOCYTES FROM ADULT RATS

DAVID L. SEVERSON, ROGAYAH CARROLL, AND MARK LEE
Department of Pharmacology, Faculty of Medicine, The University of Calgary, Calgary, Alberta T2N 4N1 Canada

ABSTRACT

Heparin induced the rapid release of lipoprotein lipase (LPL) into the incubation medium of cardiac myocytes. Incubation of myocytes with 10 μM isoproterenol for 30 min. did not influence this heparin-releasable LPL activity. Preincubation of the post-heparin medium with ATP, $MgCl_2$ and the catalytic subunit of cyclic AMP-dependent protein kinase had no effect on LPL activity.

INTRODUCTION

The degradation of triacylglycerol-rich lipoproteins occurs at the luminal surface of the vascular endothelium in the heart, as a result of the presence of LPL at the surface of endothelial cells [1,2]. LPL is not synthesized by endothelial tissue cells. Instead, the enzyme is synthesized in other cardiac tissue cells and then is transported to the capillary endothelium. The identity of the cell(s) that provide the precursor of the functional LPL at the endothelial cell surface is controversial. In cell cultures from newborn rat heart, LPL activity associated with mesenchymal cells was much greater than activity in cardiac muscle cells [3,4]. However, LPL activity has been detected in myocyte preparations from adult rat hearts [5-7], and all the activity in whole heart preparations from fed rats was recovered in cardiac myocytes [8], indicating that myocytes are the major, if not exclusive, cellular site for LPL synthesis in adult hearts.

The secretion of LPL from neonatal heart mesenchymal cells [4] and from cardiac myocytes isolated from adult rats [9-11] can be induced by the addition of heparin to the culture or incubation medium. Friedman et al [12] have recently reported that incubation of mesenchymal heart cells with isoproterenol for 30 min. produced a 3-fold increase in heparin-releasable LPL activity. Our objective, therefore, was to determine if isoproterenol treatment of cardiac myocytes from adult rat hearts would produce a similar increase in the activity of heparin-releasable LPL.

METHODS

Calcium-tolerant myocytes were isolated from the hearts of adult male rats (200-280 g) and were suspended in Joklik minimum essential medium containing 1.5 mM $CaCl_2$ and 1% (w/v) defatted albumin [13]. Myocytes (approx. 4×10^5 cells/ml) were incubated at 37°C under an atmosphere of 95% O_2 5% CO_2 in the absence and in the presence of 10 μM isoproterenol. After 30 min. of incubation, heparin was added to a final concentration of 5 U/ml, and the incubation was continued for another 5-20 min. At various time intervals, aliquots (1 ml) of the incubation were removed and centrifuged for 10 sec at 15,000 x g in an Eppendorf microcentrifuge. The medium was decanted into tubes and frozen until assayed for LPL activity.

LPL activity in the medium was assayed with a ^{3}H-triolein emulsion as described previously [7,11]. In some experiments, the post-heparin medium collected after centrifugation was preincubated for 10 min. with 1 mM $MgCl_2$,

Biology of Isolated Adult Cardiac Myocytes
William A. Clark, Robert S. Decker, and Thomas K. Borg, Editors

1 mM ATP and 10 μg catalytic (C) subunit of cyclic AMP-dependent protein kinase (kinase A; generously provided by Dr. M.P. Walsh, University of Calgary) prior to the addition of the substrate emulsion for the determination of LPL activity.

RESULTS

Incubation of cardiac myocytes for 30 min. resulted in the release of a small amount of LPL into the medium (Fig. 1,A). The addition of heparin, however, produced a rapid secretion of LPL into the incubation medium. The activity of LPL in the post-heparin medium was 6-fold greater than the pre-heparin medium activity (Fig. 1,B). Heparin probably can displace LPL from binding sites that are at or near the cell surface of cardiac myocytes, as proposed for mesenchymal cells [12] and adipocytes [14].

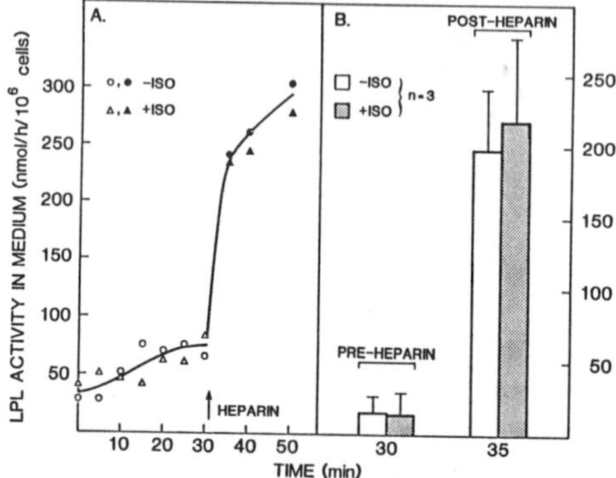

Fig. 1. Effect of isoproterenol on the heparin-induced release of LPL into the incubation medium of cardiac myocytes. In panel B, results are presented as the mean ± S.E.M.

The presence of 10 μM isoproterenol in the incubation medium had no effect on heparin-releasable LPL activity (Fig. 1, A and B). Isolation of cardiac myocytes did not damage the β-adrenergic receptor since isoproterenol did increase cyclic AMP levels [13] and the phosphorylase a activity ratio (results not shown).

Oscai et al [15] have reported that preincubation of a post-heparin fraction from perfused hearts with ATP, $MgCl_2$ and the catalytic subunit of protein kinase A produced a two-fold increase in LPL activity. This result could not be reproduced when post-heparin medium from cardiac myocytes was preincubated under similar experimental conditions (Table I).

The catalytic subunit was able to catalyze the phosphorylation of histone and the activation of adipose tissue hormone-sensitive lipase (results not shown).

DISCUSSION

The incubation of cardiac myocytes with isoproterenol for 30 min. did not influence the heparin-induced release of LPL into the medium. It is clear, therefore, that myocytes from adult rat hearts are different from neonatal heart mesenchymal cells where incubation with isoproterenol for 30 min, resulted in a substantial increase in heparin-releasable LPL activity [12].

TABLE I. Effect of preincubating post-heparin medium from cardiac myocytes with ATP, $MgCl_2$ and the catalytic subunit (C subunit) of protein kinase A on LPL activity.

Additions to Preincubation	LPL Activity[a) nmol/h/10^6 cells
None	537 ± 21
$MgCl_2$ (1 mM), ATP (1 mM) + C subunit (10 μg)	505 ± 48

a)Mean ± S.D. for 3 experiments with fresh post-heparin medium

Results from experiments to determine the effects of short-term perfusion of rat hearts with catecholamines on heparin-releasable LPL activity have been contradictory. Simpson [6] reported that isoproterenol increased LPL activity in post-heparin perfusates, but Stam and Hulsmann [17] found that perfusion of hearts with norepinephrine for 5 min. did not change post-heparin LPL activity. The results of Stam and Hulsmann [17] are consistent with our inability to produce any direct activation of LPL in the post-heparin medium of myocytes following a preincubation with ATP, $MgCl_2$ and the C subunit of kinase A. An explanation for the discrepancy between these results and the observations of Oscai et al [15] is not apparent. Although LPL in adipocytes can be inactivated by catecholamines [18], this result is not due to a direct covalent modification of the enzyme [19] but reflects an inhibition of LPL synthesis and stimulation of enzyme degradation [18].

On the other hand, experiments involving a more chronic exposure of hearts to agents that increase cyclic AMP content have provided more consistent evidence for an activation of heparin-releasable LPL. Perfusion of rat hearts for 2 and 4 hours with norepinephrine or glucagon resulted in an increase in heparin-releasable LPL activity with a corresponding fall in the heparin-nonreleasable or residual LPL activity in the heart homogenates [20], suggesting that these hormones can stimulate the translocation of LPL from a cardiac cell compartment to the vascular endothelium. Administration of cholera toxin to intact rats also increased heparin-releasable LPL activity from perfused hearts after 16-17 hours [21,22], but under these experimental conditions, the residual LPL activity in heart homogenates was also increased [21,23]. Clearly, cardiac myocytes will have to be exposed to isoproterenol for longer periods of time (4-24 hours) in order to determine if changes in heparin-releasable LPL activity can be observed. A 24-hour incubation of cultured mesenchymal cells with cholera toxin resulted in a 6-fold increase in heparin-releasable LPL activity [24]. LPL is synthesized as an inactive proenzyme that is activated by glycosylation [14,20,25]. Terminal processing in the Golgi may also be important for the secretion of active enzyme [25]. Therefore, further experiments with cardiac myocytes will have to assess the effect of catecholamines on LPL activity and the processing of the enzyme protein by glycosylation.

REFERENCES

1. A. Cryer, Int. J. Biochem. 13, 525-541 (1981)
2. M. Hamosh and P. Hamosh, Molec. Aspects Med. 6, 199-289 (1983).
3. T. Chajek, O. Stein and Y. Stein, Biochim. Biophys. Acta. 488, 140-144 (1977).
4. T. Chajek, O. Stein and Y. Stein, Biochim. Biophys. Acta. 528, 456-465 (1978).
5. G.J. Bagby, M.S. Liu, and J.A. Spitzer, Life Sci. 21, 467-474 (1977).
6. G.V. Vahouny, A. Tamboli, M. Vander Maten, H. Jansen, J.S. Twu and M.C. Schotz, Biochim. Biophys. Acta. 620, 63-69 (1980).

7. I. Ramirez, A.J. Kryski, O. Ben-Zeev, M.C. Schotz and D.L. Severson, Biochem. J. 232, 229-236 (1985).
8. P. Chohan and A. Cryer, Biochem. J. 174, 663-666 (1978).
9. P. Chohan and A. Cryer, Biochem. J. 186, 873-879 (1980).
10. A. Cryer, P. Chohan and J.M. Smith, Life Sci. 29, 923-929 (1981).
11. I. Ramirez and D.L. Severson, Biochem. J. 216, 233-238 (1986).
12. G. Friedman, T. Chajek-Saul, O. Stein and Y. Stein, Biochim. Biophys. Acta 877, 112-120 (1986).
13. A.J. Kryski, K.A. Kenno and D.L.Severson, Amer. J. Physiol. 248, H 208-216 (1985).
14. C. Vannier, E.Z. Amri, J. Etienne, R. Negrel and G. Ailhaud, J. Biol. Chem. 260, 4424-4431 (1985).
15. L.B. Oscai, R.A. Caruso and W.K. Palmer, Biochem. Biophys. Res. Commun. 135, 196-200 (1986).
16. J. Simpson, Biochem. J. 182, 253-255 (1979).
17. H. Stam and W.C. Hulsmann, Eur. Heart J. 6, 158-167 (1985).
18. K.L. Ball, B.K. Speake and D.S. Robinson, Biochim. Biophys. Acta 877, 399-405 (1986).
19. J.C. Khoo, D. Steinberg, J.J. Huang and P.R. Vagelos, J. Biol. Chem. 251, 2882-2890 (1976).
20. H. Stam and W.C. Hulsmann, Biochim. Biophys. Acta. 794, 72-82 (1984).
21. H. Knobler, T. Chajek-Saul, O. Stein, J. Etienne and Y. Stein, Biochim. Biophys. Acta 795, 363-371 (1984).
22. W.C. Hulsmann and M.L. Dubelaar, Biochim. Biophys. Acta 875, 69-75 (1986).
23. W.C. Miller, W.K. Palmer, D.A. Arnall and L.B. Oscai, Can. J. Physiol. Pharmacol. 65, 60-63 (1987).
24. G. Friedman, T. Chajek-Saul, O. Stein and Y. Stein, Biochim. Biophys. Acta 752, 106-117 (1983).
25. T. Chajek-Saul, G. Freidman, H. Knobler, O. Stein, J. Etienne and Y. Stein, Biochim. Biophys. Acta 837, 123-134 (1985).

CELL AND MOLECULAR BIOLOGY OF CULTURED ADULT CARDIAC MYOCYTES

Radovan Zak*, Robert S. Decker**, and William A. Clark***
*The University of Chicago, **Northwestern University Medical School, and
***Michael Reese Hospital, Chicago, IL.

INTRODUCTION

A number of studies in this volume illustrate that the isolated adult cardiac myocyte displays a variety of morphological, physiological and biochemical characteristics similar to its *in vivo* counterpart during the first few hours after isolation. Maintaining these cells for more prolonged periods permits the evaluation of cellular functions such as gene regulation and protein synthesis which cannot be determined during a few hours of observation. The papers presented in this section address the biology of cardiac myocytes maintained for days to weeks following isolation. While unique studies related to the ability to maintain and observe the cell in a totally defined environment are possible in this model, it is important to recognize that as the cell is maintained for more than a short period outside the heart, it may be undergoing a form of adaptation to a new environmental state where its activity is no longer representative of its activity in its native state. There are some differences of opinion, however, in distinguishing normal versus adaptive activity which are discussed in several papers presented in this section.

Establishing Long-Term Cultures of Adult Cardiac Myocytes

Major progress has been made in the preparation of calcium tolerant cells which survive in culture for a number of weeks and which continue to display characteristics of cardiac myocytes. The first requirement for long term maintenance of cylindrical myocytes appears to be attachment to a suitable adhesive substrate such as laminin or type IV collagen. All adult cardiac myocytes that have been cultured in serum supplemented media ultimately flatten and spread in culture. Simpson, Decker and Decker illustrated that as the myocytes spread, cytoskeletal and myofibrillar elements were remodeled extensively. Their observations suggested that changes in actin and tubulin were correlated with cell spreading while alterations in desmin and vinculin were closely associated with the reorganization of the contractile apparatus. That such changes might be initiated at the time of myocyte isolation was suggested by J.S. Frank who showed that calcium depletion stripped portions of the sarcolemmal glycocalyx and may have disrupted cytoskeletal components immediately subjacent to the cell surface. Similar relationships between contractile, cytoskeletal and membrane proteins were also elegantly demonstrated by Messina et al., using rapid freeze-deep etch techniques with immunogold. They then illustrated the distribution of alpha-actinin in the Z-line and spectrin in a Z-line-like structure and subjacent sarcolemmal regions.

One of the more disturbing facets about culturing adult myocytes is the precipitous decline in cell number that accompanies prolonged culture. Part of this decline may be by a process of rapid contracture and cell death. In this process, the myofibrils contract in uncontrolled way, the membrane is ruptured and the cellular component (such as soluble proteins, ribosomes and even mitochondria) become expelled from the cells interior. This event occurs very rapidly and is similar to some cases of cardiac injury (calcium paradox). What makes this of interest is that such a disruption of cells accompanied by disorganization of myofibrillar mass also accompanies cell death seen in ischemia. Thus, we have a model

Biology of Isolated Adult Cardiac Myocytes
William A. Clark, Robert S. Decker, and Thomas K. Borg, Editors

of cell death which potentially could be studied *in vitro* under defined conditions. Even in cells which survive initial attachment and plating in culture, there are further losses. Piper and Jacobson, as well as others, report that approximately 50% of the freshly attached myocytes fall off the culture plates by 2 weeks *in vitro*, regardless of which substrate adhesives were initially employed to attach the cells. Considerable controversy has ensued, with serum factors, extracellular substrates, and the ability of the myocytes to develop focal contacts representing central themes in the discussion on the maintenance of cell numbers. Since a consensus of opinion noted that successful attachment of freshly isolated myocytes would ensure their survival, the development of an "appropriate" extracellular substratum might increase the number of myocytes that survive long term culture.

Gene Regulation, Protein and DNA Synthesis in Cultured Myocytes

A significant reason for studying isolated cardiac myocytes in long term culture is to evaluate their response to factors which regulate their protein synthetic and growth activity. One of the more striking aspects of cultured cardiac myocytes is their resumption of DNA replication. Both Claycomb and Nag report that significant DNA synthesis is observed following maintenance of myocytes in culture for more than a week. Nag has also reported karyokinesis in myocytes, but complete mitosis has not been reported. The fact that the fully differentiated muscle cells resume DNA synthesis is of great interest since studies of intact hearts previously led to the conclusion that DNA synthesis is irreversibly lost during differentiation of heart muscle cells. That the cells become active with respect to DNA synthesis has drawn focus to this preparation for studies of cell transformation into lines. If this were accomplished, the tools of cardiovascular research would be expanded considerably.

Claycomb also reports that DNA synthesis can be stimulated by treatment of the cells with the phorbol ester TPA. He reports that this treatment stimulates the activation of proto-oncogenes, c-FOS and c-Myc, which are involved in the regulation of proliferation. However, treatment with TPA also appears to *inhibit* the expression of mRNA for differentiated muscle proteins, myosin HC and M-creatine kinase.

Protein synthesis was evaluated directly in cultured myocytes in four studies. Bugaisky et al. compared total protein synthesis in myocytes maintained for 2 or 13 days in culture. No differences were reported in the radioautographic labeling pattern of 1d SDS-PAGE separated, ^{35}S-labeled proteins, and thus, no qualitative differences were apparent in the types of proteins synthesized in myocytes maintained in culture over this period. However, both Bugaisky and Nag reported that changes were evident in myosin isoform expression from a predominance of type V1 to an increase in type V3 in myocytes maintained in serum for 2 weeks in culture. This shift in isoforms was delayed in the presence of T3. Terracio et al. showed by labeling and immunoprecipitation of labeled proteins from the culture medium that cultured myocytes also continued to synthesize and secrete type IV collagen and laminin during the period from 1 to 14 days in culture.

While these studies each indicated that typical proteins continued to be expressed by cultured adult myocytes, the study of Haddad et al. revealed that the rate of protein synthesis in general, and myosin heavy chain synthesis in particular, were dramatically reduced in cultured myocytes from the rates observed in the intact heart. Fractional protein synthesis rates for myosin heavy chain were as much as 10 times lower than comparable rates for this protein in the intact heart.

Ultimate understanding of how protein synthesis is regulated in the myocyte may come from exploration of factors which permit gene expression in the cytoplasm. In the study of Cribbs et al., promoter sequences of the cardiac alpha and beta myosin heavy chain gene were transfected into a number of cell types. Using a chloramphenicol acetyl-transferase (CAT) marker gene conjugated to the myosin promoter region, myosin gene regulation was studied in a number of cell types. This study showed that the alpha myosin heavy chain was constituently expressed in all cell types reported, whereas the beta myosin heavy chain gene was only expressed in differentiated muscle cultures. The cultured adult myocyte model may provide an excellent environment to examine regulatory factors involved in the expression of myosin isoform and other differentiated gene products by transfection.

Adaptation of Isolated Myocytes to Culture

Of considerable interest is the question whether the changes of cultured cardiac cells should be viewed as "dedifferentiation" or adaptation to culture conditions. This question is difficult to answer. The fact that cell specific proteins continue to be expressed and that no other phenotypes appear upon culture seems to indicate that the cells have retained their differentiated state, but have adapted to conditions of culture. On the other hand, the fact that the cells resumed DNA synthesis and have a much reduced rate of differentiated protein synthesis is consistent with the definition of non-differentiated cells. It is thus imperative to use descriptive terms such as "morphological dedifferentiation" so that no confusion will result from studies of the heart. One has to use clear-cut markers of cell phenotype or well defined properties in defining the state of differentiation. Moreover, it has to be recognized that even cells of living tissue do possess considerable plasticity which allow them to modify their phenotype in response to various environmental stimuli.

Previous observations from Moses and Claycomb have clearly illustrated that adult myocytes undergo profound structural reorganization during prolonged cell culture, regardless of whether they are cultured on native plastic or on an extracellular substratum such as fetal bovine serum or laminin. Following attachment, the cells flatten and send out stellate pseudopodia. The cells also temporarily loose their cross-striated appearance and resume DNA synthesis, which is followed by nuclear division. Although excellent arrangements of filaments with cross-striated patterns are later established, the cells remain stellate. The principal concern of most laboratories is whether these structural alterations reflect an "adaptation" of the adult cell to a two dimensional environment or overt "dedifferentation" of the myocyte to a more "primitive" state. Although we cannot presently distinguish between these alternatives, the observations presented at this workshop provide considerable new information on the behavior of adult myocytes in culture.

The observations and discussion presented here indicate that the cultured adult cardiac myocyte undergoes a remarkable subcellular reorganization when it is placed in culture. Several factors clearly affect its ability to spread *in vitro* and immunofluorescent and structural studies demonstrate that a dramatic remodeling of its myofibrillar apparatus and cytoskeleton attends this phenomena. These results suggest an enormous plasticity in response to an environmental change in the cultured adult myocyte. Further study will establish the value of this model as an experimental tool to directly study cardiac biochemistry, physiology, gene regulation, protein metabolism, mechanics and structure function relationships.

PROTEIN EXPRESSION IN CULTURED ADULT RAT CARDIAC MYOCYTES

L.B. Bugaisky, R.S. Hall, S.B. Thompson and R. Zak*.
The University of Alabama at Birmingham, Departments of Pathology; Cell Biology and Anatomy. *The University of Chicago, Departments of Medicine, Physiological and Pharmacological Sciences.

ABSTRACT

We have isolated and maintained adult rat cardiac myocytes in culture for several weeks. During this period of time the cells undergo a morphological transformation, yet, remain highly differentiated. Little change is observed in the overall pattern of protein synthesis and the *in vivo* myosin phenotype continues to be expressed for the first 7-10 days. These cells should provide a good system to study regulation of cardiac myocyte growth devoid of systemic influences.

INTRODUCTION

The long-term culture of adult cardiac myocytes provides a means to investigate those factors which act directly at the cellular and molecular level to produce growth, differentiation and adaptation to stress in the adult heart. Such a system is of major importance to the study of heart related problems including cardiac hypertrophy, ischemia and congenital heart disease since it will provide the opportunity to separate secondary and tertiary systemic effects on the heart from those which are a direct consequence of primary stimuli to the myocyte itself. While investigations have taken place over the last 20 years using embryonic or neonatal cells in culture, such studies may not be valid for extrapolation to the intact adult heart. Cells obtained from hearts of embryonic or newborn rats have different biochemical and physiological properties than the same cells obtained later in the life of the animal. For example, embryonic or neonatal cells in culture appear to retain the capacity for cell division, which adult cells do not. Thus, the response of cultured embryonic myocytes to hypoxia may not be valid for extrapolation to the *in vivo* adult heart. In order to obtain a better system to study growth regulation at the cellular and molecular level, we have maintained isolated adult rat cardiac myocytes in culture for several weeks. In this report we present a characterization of these cells both in terms of the general pattern of protein synthesis as well as myosin isoform expression. The latter represents a major marker of growth and differentiation in cardiac muscle.

METHODS

Isolated adult cardiac myocytes for cell culture were obtained from 175-225 gm female rats. Myocyte isolation was based on the procedures of Claycomb and Palazzo [1] and Borg et al. [2]. Hearts were retrogradely perfused through the ascending aorta with 1.0-1.2 mg/ml of collagenase (Worthington CLS or Sigma Type I) in Joklik's Minimal Essential Medium containing taurine and glutamic acid at 37°C. Following 30-45 minutes of perfusion, hearts were removed from the apparatus and isolated myocytes obtained from the softened pieces of tissue were placed in Joklik's medium containing 5% calf serum (Hyclone). Following washing and sedimentation at unit gravity, the cells were placed into Basal Eagles Medium plus 5% calf serum and allowed to attach to 6 cm dishes precoated with 15μgm of

Biology of Isolated Adult Cardiac Myocytes
William A. Clark, Robert S. Decker, and Thomas K. Borg, Editors

laminin (GIBCO). After 24 hours, cytosine arabinoside was added to a final concentration of 0.1 mM and left in the medium for 3-4 days to inhibit fibroblast proliferation. Thereafter, the media was changed every second day.

RESULTS AND DISCUSSION

Freshly isolated cells which attached to the laminin coated dishes were cylindrical, contained evident cross-striations and rarely demonstrated spontaneous contractility (Fig 1A). Over the next 7-10 days in culture the isolated myocytes underwent a dramatic morphological transformation from the initial cylindrical cell with evident cross-striations to one which was more pleiomorphic (Fig 1B). During the initial period of change the cross-striations were lost; however, with increasing time in culture they reappeared. Myocytes are non-beating during the first several days, by five days in culture ,however, at least 50% of the cells contract with an average rate of at least 170 beats per minute.

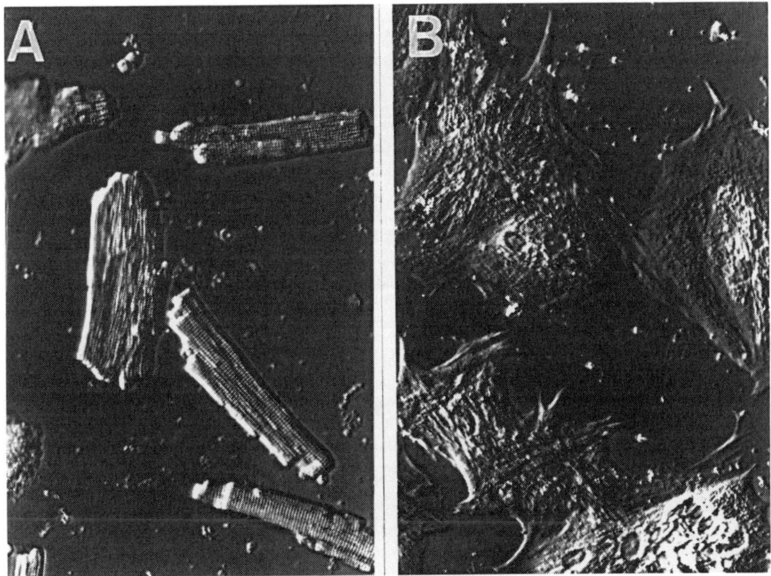

FIG. 1. Adult cardiac myocytes in culture for 3 hours (A) and 14 days (B).

Despite the morphological adaptation to culture, the isolated myocyte still maintains many characteristics of the adult myocyte phenotype. During the period of greatest morphological change we have labelled the myocytes with ^{35}S-methionine to observe the relative pattern of protein synthesis. Following cell labelling, proteins were extracted and analyzed by 1-dimensional gel electrophoresis. With the possible exception of actin (arrow), few if any qualitative differences occur in the pattern of protein expression between days 1 and 13 in culture (Fig 2). This is somewhat surprising when one considers the dramatic

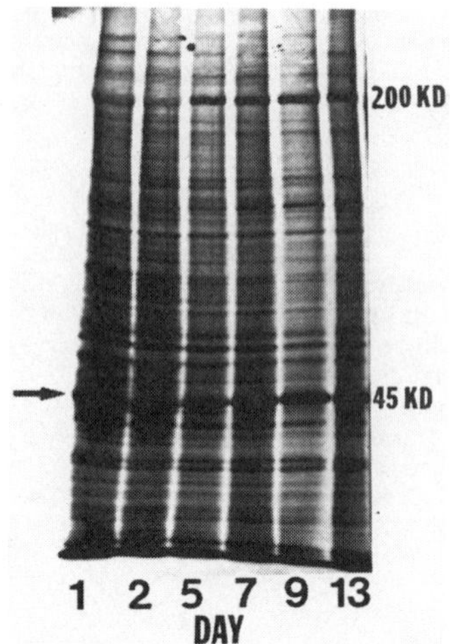

FIG. 2. Pattern of protein synthesis in cultures of adult myocytes during thirteen days in culture. Six cm. culture dishes were labelled for 2 hours with 25 Ci/ml of ^{35}S-methionine and then proteins extracted for gel analysis.

morphological changes these cells go through during the first week in culture. More subtle changes however, such isoform as variations in structural and functional protein may in fact be occurring. To investigate this possibility, we have also examined specific protein synthesis in terms of myosin isoform expression. Changes in the percentages of myosin isoforms in the rat heart have been shown to occur during development, as well as during physiological and pathological interventions. Using native gel electrophoresis we have observed only the V1 isoform during the early period in culture (Fig. 3). Expression of only this isoform continues during the first 7-10 days in culture. This is

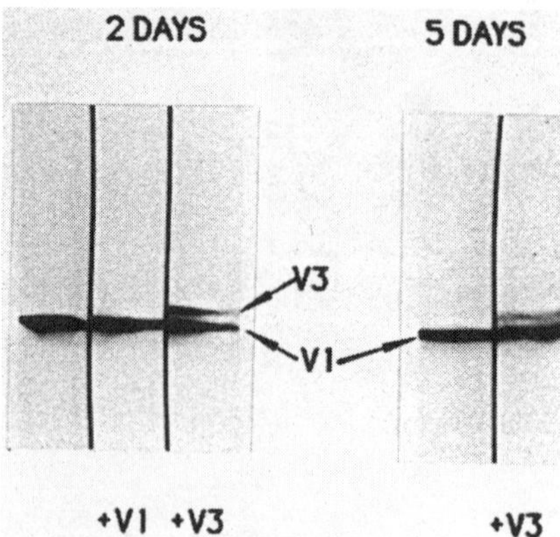

FIG. 3. Myosin isoform expression during the first five days in culture. A V1 and/or V3 standard was added to the cell extract to determine the identity of the single band.

similar to the pattern of expression found in the *in vivo* heart and is representative of the adult myocyte phenotype. It is possible to prolong the expression of the V1 myosin isoform even longer, if the cells are switched from medium with calf serum to serum-free medium. We have used PC-1 medium (Ventrex Corp.) for this purpose and have observed continued expression of V1 myosin for an additional 10 days [3]. This medium contains insulin, transferrin, fatty acids, T3 and proprietary proteins but does not contain such traditional growth factors as EGF, FGF or PDGF. The use of the serum-free medium provides a more carefully controlled environment for the examination of growth regulation and should be useful for future studies. Based on our characterization of cultured adult myocytes which demonstrate that a high degree of differentiation is maintained in culture, we feel that the isolated cardiac myocyte represents a good *in vitro* system for the future study of those factors which act *directly* on the adult cell to produce growth, differentiation and adaptation to stress in the intact heart. Furthermore, because these cells maintain many of thr *in vivo* characteristics of the adult myocyte they also represent a system for extrapolation of *in vitro* results to the intact heart.

This work was supported by grants from the N.I.H. and the American Heart Association.

REFERENCES

1. W.C. Claycomb and M.C. Palazzo. Dev. Biol. 80, 446-482 (1980).
2. T. Borg, K. Rubin, E. Lundgren, K. Borg, and B. OBrink, Dev. Biol. 104, 86-96 (1984)
3. L.B. Bugaisky and R. Zak. J. Cell Biol. 103, 119a (1986)

ISOLATION AND CULTURE OF HUMAN ADULT CARDIAC MYOCYTES

Lawrence B. Bugaisky
Department of Pathology; Cell Biology and Anatomy, The University of Alabama at Birmingham, Birmingham, Alabama

ABSTRACT

We have isolated and cultured adult human myocytes from cardiac tissue obtained during transplantation. Three out of four hearts contained approximately 65% binucleated cells while the fourth contained only 51.5%. Myocytes capable of being cultured were those which were cylindrical upon initial plating. They then underwent a morphological transformation similar to cultured rat myocytes, however, the human cells, never began to beat spontaneously. Based on our initial success, we feel that cultured human myocytes represent a useful system for the study of living human cardiac cells. Furthermore, with increased experience it should be possible to obtain sufficient numbers of these myocytes for biochemical studies of heart disease in man.

INTRODUCTION

During the last ten years the study of cultured adult cardiac myocytes has rapidly proceeded from descriptions of isolation procedures for obtaining a few selected viable cells to reports resulting from the utilization of reasonably large quantities of cells. Despite significant progress in the isolation and culturing of adult cells obtained from several mammalian species, however, with the exception of a single report [1], little has appeared concerning the use of isolated adult human cells. While the availability of tissue is admittedly limited, there are likely to be opportunities for the study of adult human myocytes in several institutions across the country. This is particularly true in those areas where cardiac transplantation occurs on a regular basis. The potential for insights into understanding myocyte adaptation or lack thereof to coronary artery disease is great. Successful cultures of large numbers of human cardiac myocytes should eventually produce significant advances in our understanding myocyte growth as it applies to the human heart. With this goal in mind we have begun to study the isolation and culture of myocytes isolated from normal and diseased human cardiac tissue. In this report, we will present our results as well as some of the problems we have encountered.

METHODS

Tissue Availability: Cardiac tissue was obtained from hearts of patients undergoing cardiac transplantation. In cases where tissue was obtained from the diseased hearts of transplant recipients, tissue was available shortly after extirpation into 4°C Krebs-Henseleit (usually 5-30 minutes). In other cases, tissue was obtained during valve procurement from normal hearts (usually 8-12 hours after extirpation). During the period following extirpation these hearts had been maintained in Krebs-Ringer Lactate at 4°C.

Cell Isolation and Culture: Cell isolation is based on the procedure of Jacobson et al. [1] and was performed using the "finger apparatus" which he described in an earlier report [2]. This consists of two

Biology of Isolated Adult Cardiac Myocytes
William A. Clark, Robert S. Decker, and Thomas K. Borg, Editors

interdigitating sets of thin teeth or fingers. Since the fingers are made of teflon, they have a high degree of flexibility and are presumably very gentle on the tissue during the dissociation procedure. The top part of the apparatus is attached to a motor capable of turning at 10-15 rpm. 750-1000 mg of tissue obtained from the free wall of the left ventricle is processed at one time. Following dissection, the tissue is placed in Calcium Magnesium Free solution and the fat removed. The tissue is then minced with a scissors and initially digested for 7 minutes in 0.25% trypsin in Joklik's Minimal essential medium containing glutamic acid and taurine [3]. Following this digestion as well as the next two series of digestions, the supernatant which presumably contains released cells is removed and added to Joklik's medium containing 5% calf serum.

After the trypsin digestion, the remaining tissue is treated three times for 15 minutes each with 0.1% collagenase and then three times with 0.05% collagenase. Liberated cells are allowed to sediment at unit gravity in the Joklik's medium plus 5% calf serum. Cells from all dissociations are combined in a 1:1 mixture of Joklik's and Basal Eagles Medium (BME) containing 5% calf serum and allowed to attach to laminin (15 µgm/dish) precoated dishes. After a minimum of 3-4 hours the medium is replaced with 100% BME + 5% calf serum. All medium contains 1% penicillin-streptomycin-neomycin and 1.5% kanamycin (GIBCO).

RESULTS AND DISCUSSION

The procedure described above results in a population of cylindrical myocytes with evident cross-striations that can be maintained in cell culture for up to 14 days. The greatest obstacle at the moment however, for the successful use of these cells as a system to study cardiac biochemistry is that the final percentage of calcium-tolerant cells is rather small. Therefore, in order to obtain as much useful information as possible from the isolation of these cells, we have fixed aliquots of cells early in the isolation procedure when greater numbers of cylindrical cells are present and obtained nuclei counts on hematoxylin-eosin stained slides. Both mono- and binucleated myocytes were easily found in hearts from individuals between 16 and 69 years of age of which two different types cells are shown Figure 1. In figure 1A the nuclei are located in close proximity to each other while in 1B they are a substantial distance apart. It is yet to be determined whether these different spatial arrangements of nuclei have any significance concerning the physiological or pathological state of the heart *in vivo*. While admittedly based on a very limited sample, there does not appear to be any difference in the percentage of mono- and binucleated cells in normal hearts over a 33 year time span, i.e. between 36 and 69 years of age (Table 1). Interestingly, a 20 year old female with a cardiomyopathy had the same percentage of binucleated cells as a normal 69 year old male, while a normal 16 year old male had about 25% fewer binucleated cells than the older male. While conclusions may be premature at this point, it might be suggested that in the heart of the 20 year old female, hypertrophy accompanying the cardiomyopathy is a sufficient growth stimulus to cause a premature decrease in the percentage of mononucleated cells. In this regard, Clubb et al. [4] have suggested that binucleation was accelerated in the neonatal spontaneously hypertensive rat due to the early onset of cardiac hypertrophy.

Our attempts to culture the isolated adult cells have met with mixed success. One constant in the several preparations has been that those cells which we can maintain in culture are the ones which are cylindrical and attach rapidly to the dish following upon plating. This is true regardless of the source (normal or diseased) or the length of time since extirpation of the heart. We have also had greater success in obtaining cells from tissue obtained from normal hearts than from the diseased

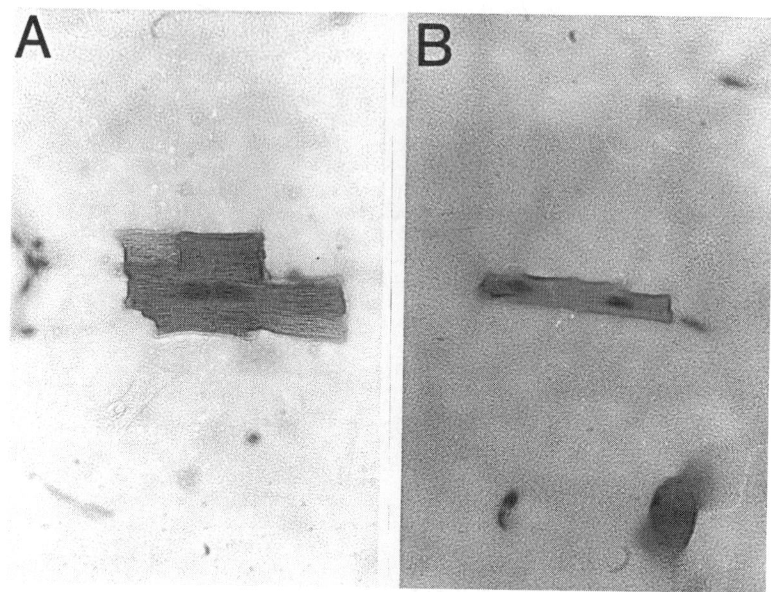

FIGURE 1. Human cardiac myocytes stained with hematoxylin-eosin. Figure 1A illustrates a cell containing two nuclei in close proximity to one another and was obtained from the heart of a 36 year old male while the cell in figure 1B was obtained from a 16 year old male.

TABLE I. Nuclei counts in adult human cardiac myocytes

	Mononucleated	Binucleated
16 YR OLD MALE	51.5%	49.5%
36 YR OLD MALE	34.4%	65.6%
69 YR OLD MALE	34.7%	65.3%
20 YR OLD FEMALE (Cardiomyopathy)	32.9%	67.1%

hearts. This is despite the fact that the normal hearts have usually been extirpated 10-12 hours prior to cell isolation.

Enzymatic treatment, by itself, does not appear to cause serious damage since we have observed large numbers of cylindrical cells in intact heart tissue which became soft during enzymatic treatment. This tissue was fixed prior to separation into single cells. The problem with cell damage most likely occurs during both the physical separation into isolated cells and the reintroduction of physiological levels of calcium. Those cells which survive the enzymatic treatment and cell isolation appear to behave somewhat similar to other types of mammalian adult myocytes which have been observed in culture. The cylindrical cells attach rapidly to the laminin coated dishes and as shown in Fig 2A are still cylindrical after three days in culture. The spreading out process appears to take longer and unlike rat cells, even after three days we have not observed significant sarcoplasmic extensions. With increasing time in culture, the myocytes begin to demonstrate a more spread out, pleiomorphic shape (Fig. 2B); however, they do not possess spontaneous contractility. Another major

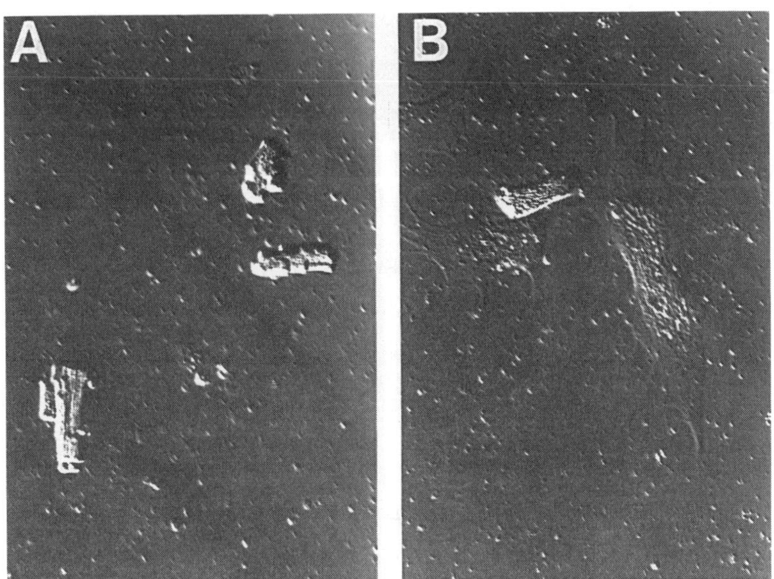

FIGURE 2. Adult human myocytes in culture. Figure 2A demonstrates cells which have been in culture for 3 days while those in figure 2B have been in culture for 10 days.

difference from the rat cells is that we have not observed the reappearance of cross striations in our cells and with increasing time in culture, the cells morphologically resemble fibroblasts. Based on our initial successes and an optimistic outlook, it is felt that with increasing improvements in isolation and culturing, adult human myocytes should prove to be a useful system for the study of cardiac muscle biology.

REFERENCES

1. S.L. Jacobson, M. Banfalvi and T.A. Schwarzfeld. Basic Res. Cardiol. 80, Suppl. 1, 79-82 (1985).
2. S.L. Jacobson. Cell Structure Funct. 2, 1-9 (1977).
3. W.C. Claycomb and M.C. Palazzo. Dev. Biol. 80, 446-482 (1980).
4. F.J. Clubb, D. Bell, J.D. Kriseman and S.P. Bishop. Lab. Invest. 56, 189-197 (1987).

INFLUENCE OF TISSUE CULTURE CONDITIONS ON CARDIOMYOCYTE DEVELOPMENT IN VITRO

STUART L JACOBSON,* H. MICHAEL PIPER,** AND PETER SCHWARTZ***
*Department of Biology, Carleton University, Ottawa, Ontario, Canada, K1S 5B6; **Physiologisches Institut I, Universität Düsseldorf, Moorenstr. 5, D-4000 Düsseldorf 1, FRG; ***Zentrum Anatomie, Universität Göttingen, Kreuzbergring 36, D-3400 Göttingen, FRG.

INTRODUCTION

Experience with cultured adult cardiomyocytes is still in a nascent state. Currently, three primary culture systems are in most frequent use (1): (i) a serum free culture of rapidly attached cells on serum precoated dishes, in which the cells maintain their in-vivo morphology, but do not survive for several weeks (2), (ii) a culture with high serum concentrations, in which the cells attach late, spread extensively, and can be maintained for months (1,3), and (iii) a culture of cells attached on a laminin substratum on which the cells can keep an elongated morphology even when spread, and can be cultured in presence of serum for several weeks (4,5). The aim of this study was a systematic investigation of the influence of the attachment mode and medium additions such as sera, extracellular matrix proteins and growth factors on survival and morphological development of adult cardiomyocytes in culture.

METHODS AND MATERIALS

Adult rat cardiomyocytes were isolated as previously described (2) and plated at a density of 4×10^3 /cm^2 on Falcon tissue culture plastic dishes coated with various substrates: (i) on dishes preincubated for 8 h with 4% fetal calf serum (FCS, from Gibco) according to (2)(**d-FCS**), (ii) on dishes coated with 1.25 and 12.5 µg laminin / cm^2 (1 X Laminin, 10 X Laminin; **d-1L**, **d-10L**) according to (4), (iii) on non-treated dishes (d-tcp), and (iv) on siliconized glas, to prevent attachment. For cultures of type (i) and (ii) cells were plated in M199 + 4 % FCS and M199, respectively. After 4 h the medium was changed for the maintenance medium, either M199 or M199 + 20% FCS. For cultures (iii) and (iv) cells were plated directly in one of the maintenance media, and the media were not changed until day 6. For the first 5 days in all cultures the maintenance media contained 10 µM cytosine-β-D-arabinofuranoside (ARA-C, from Sigma). At times indicated, cultures were washed twice with culture medium, and the attached cells were counted. In further experiments the influence of medium supplements other than 20 % FCS were investigated in cultures of the above types (i) and (ii): addition of 2 % FCS, 10 % autologous rat serum, laminin (50µg/ml), fibronectin (100 µg/ml), collagen IV (80 µg/ml), fibroblast growth factor (100 ng/ml), basic fibroblast growth factor (2 ng/ml), endothelial cell growth supplement (150 µg/ml),nerve growth factor (50 ng/ml), multiplication stimulating activity (250 ng/ml). Laminin was a generous gift from T. Borg, Columbia, SC, growth factors were obtained from Collaborative Research. Processing for electron microscopy has been described (2).

RESULTS

The use of ARA-C during the first 5 days ARA-C effectively prevents the growth of non-muscle cells. Cells on siliconized glas surfaces deteriorat during the first 3 days to round, blebbed cell remnants, with or without the presence of FCS. Already after 1 hour most of the floating rod-shaped cells form network-like cell clusters, particularly in the presence of 20% FCS, but these cell-cell contacts do apparently not sufficiently support cell survival. On d-tcp on which the large majority of cells do neither attach soon after plating, cells also deteriorate in the absence of FCS. But if the medium is supplemented with 20% serum, only half of the initially rod-shaped

Biology of Isolated Adult Cardiac Myocytes
William A. Clark, Robert S. Decker, and Thomas K. Borg, Editors

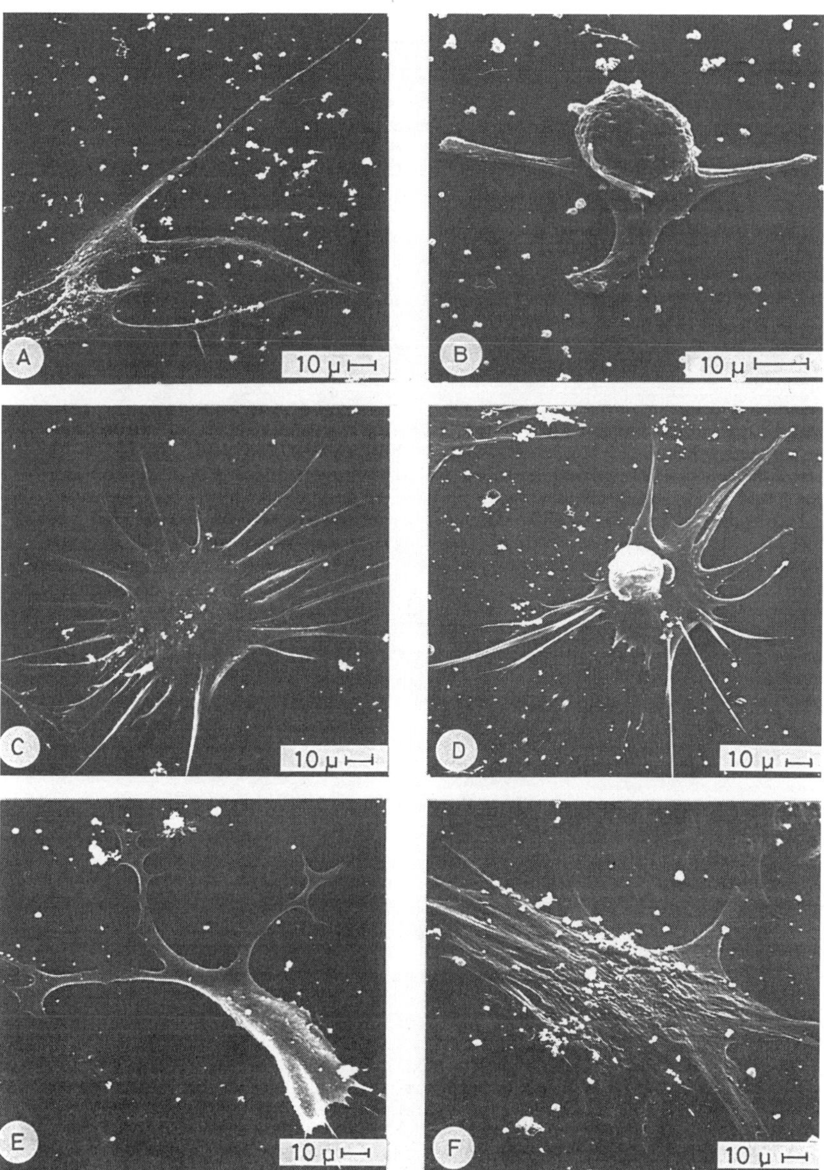

Plate 1: Typical phenotypes of cultured cardiomyocytes after 9 days in culture (scanning EM). **A.** d-FCS, no serum. Long extended, thin cell. **B.** d-tcp, 20 % FCS. Cell with blob and short, thick extension. **C.** d-FCS, 20% FCS. Flat spread cell with long thin extensions. No blob. **D.** d-FCS, 20% FCS. Flat spread cell with thin extensions, and with blob. **E.** d-1L, 20% FCS. Cell body voluminous and elongated, long thin extensions from the cell's ends, no blob. **F.** d-10L, 20% FCS. Flat, spread cells with thick extensions, no blob.

TABLE 1. Attached cells in cultures on 4 different substrates, with 20% or 0% FCS, from 4 h to 9 days after plating. Number of cells attached on serum precoated dishes set at 100 % (3 x 10^3 / cm^2). Mean values from 3 experiments. The predominant phenotype is indicated by abbreviations: rod, rod-shaped; rnd, round; sp,spreading; sp-l, spread,elongated; sp-b; spread,broad. Culture medium 199, with ARA-C during the first 5 days. On tissue culture plastic the majority of cells is not attached during the first 5 days. In this case the morphology of the majority of all cells is given in brackets.

dish	FCS		TC Plastic		10 X Laminin		1 X Laminin	
FCS	20%	0%	20%	0%	20%	0%	20%	0%
4h	100 rod	100 rod	11 (rod)	11 (rod)	92 rod	92 rod	88 rod	88 rod
d3	64 rnd,sp	48 rod	23 (rnd)	8 (rnd)	73 rod,sp	54 rod	61 rod,sp	42 rod
d6	53 sp-b	29 rod,sp	43 rnd,sp	3 rnd	67 sp-l	41 rod,sp	54 sp-l	30 rod,sp
d9	52 sp-b	14 sp-l	45 sp-b	1 sp-b	63 sp-b	35 sp-l	49 sp-b	21 sp-l

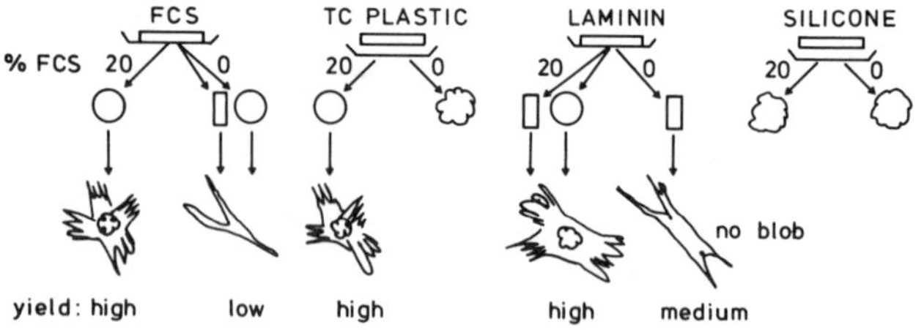

cells turn into blebbed cell remnants. The other half is transformed into smooth round cells (3) which attach in 3-5 days to the plastice surface and begin to spread (**Plate 1.B**).

Most of the cells that have attached rapidly to d-FCS (2), undergo the same sequence of morphological changes in presence of 20% FCS as on d-tcp, but in an accelerated manner and with a slightly higher number of cells surviving on day 9. After 9 days the cells are spread, most into a flat, broad form (**Plate 1.C,D**). Many of the cells carry round "blobs" on their cell body which eventually disappear. These blobs seem to contain the condensed remnants of the initially elongated cell. If FCS is omitted on d-FCS, rod-shaped cells preserve their elongated morphology for the first 6 days. Those that have lost this morphology will detach and can be removed by a medium change. This serum-free culture, however, is not usable beyond 1 week in culture, because then two thirds of the cell population have been lost. The few cells remaining attached after this time develop very thin, long extensions spreading from a still elongated, but atrophic cell body (**Plate 1.A**).

With 20% FCS present, after 9 days cells on d-1L or d-10L are extensively spread, but most of them do not pass through an intermediate round stage. On day 9 blobs are rare (**Plate 1.F**). In serum-free medium the pattern of cell spreading is different. As on d-FCS, the elongated cells spread at their ends (**Plate 1.E**), but already on day 2. And they do not become so atrophic. In the presence of serum, the number of cells surviving is larger, but also continuously decreasing.

The effect of fetal calf serum on 9 day survival proved to be dependent on the quality of the batch. Among 5 batches tested at a 20 % concentration (from Gibco and Boehringer) numbers of attached cells after 5 days varied between 38 and 52 % (% as for Table 1). Sera with fewer cells remaining in culture, also induced less broad spreading. Among the batches, the order of potency for cell survival was not identical with that for rapid attchment on d-FCS. On all substrates, long term survival with 2 % FCS was lower than with 20 % (e.g., on d-10L on day 9: 41% instead of 63%). Cell spreading was also less extensive than with 20% FCS. The effect of 10 % autologous rat serum resembled that of 2 % FCS in cell maintenance (on d-L10 on day 9: 46% instead of 63%) and cell spreading. On d-tcp, 10% rat serum failed completely to promote cell attachment and spreading and the cells deteriorated during the first 3 days. All extracellular matrix components and growth factors listed in Methods and Materials failed to change the results of the culture experiments, both with FCS present and without.

DISCUSSION

The results of this study demonstrate the predominant importance of fetal calf serum for long-term cultures of adult cardiomyocytes. Autologous rat serum cannot replace it in d-tcp cultures, since it seems to lack factors that promote the dedifferentiation/redifferentiation cycle in these cultures. Rat serum, however, has previously been shown to give good rapid attachment if it is used for the pretreatement of culture dishes (2,6). The right selection of a fetal calf serum batch is of crucial importance for promoting rapid cell attachment on d-FCS (2,6), as well as for maintaining cells for longer period in culture, irrespective of the initial mode of attachment. Sera with poor survival rates in culture also caused less cell spreading. This may indicate that cells with extensive spreading, and this means cells which have lost the typical in-vivo shape, are best adapted to the isolated state.

Added to the culture medium, laminin, which might be thought to interact with cell metabolism through laminin receptors (4), had no effect, neither did a selection of other extracellular matrix components and classical growth factors. In the presence of 20% FCS the number of cells established in culture after 9 days was similar for d-FCS, d-tcp, and on laminin. Laminin as a substratum, however, reduced the number of cells which transitorily become round during the first 5 days. After more extended periods in culture (30 days), however, all three cultures exhibited the same networks of synchronously beating, spread cells. In the absence of serum, laminin supports the maintenance of an elongated spread cell type for some longer time than d-FCS, but the non-spread, in-vivo morphology is retained for the first few days best on d-FCS.

Thus, for long-term cultures d-FCS, d-tcp, and d-1L or d10L can be used equally when 20 % FCS is added to the medium. If cardiomyocytes are to be maintained in culture for several hours up to a few days, d-FCS seems the model of choice.

REFERENCES

1. S.L. Jacobson, and Piper, H.M., J. Mol. Cell. Cardiol. 18, 61-678 (1986)
2. H.M. Piper, I. Probst, J.F. Hütter, and P.G. Spieckermann, J. Mol.Cell. Cardiol. 14, 397-412 (1982).
3. S.L. Jacobson, Cell Struct. Funct. 2, 1-9 (1977)
4. E. Lundgren, T. Borg, and S. Mardh, J. Mol. Cell. Cardiol. 16, 803-811 (1984)
5. G. Cooper, W.E. Mercer, J.K. Hooper, P.R. Gordon, R.L. Kent, I.K. Lauva, and T.A. Marino, Circ. Res. 58, 692-705 (1986).
6. H.M. Piper, R. Spahr, I. Probst, and P.G. Spieckermann, Basic Res. Cardiol. 80 (Suppl. 2), 175-180 (1985)

DIFFERENTIAL REGULATION OF CARDIAC MYOSIN HEAVY CHAIN GENE PROMOTERS

L. L. Cribbs*, N. Shimizu*, C. E. Yockey*, S. Jakovcic*, and P. K. Umeda*
*Department of Medicine, The University of Chicago,
950 E. 59th Street, Chicago, IL 60637

INTRODUCTION

Mammalian ventricular muscle contains two well-defined forms of myosin heavy chains (HC), α and β [1,2,3] that specify isomyosins having high and low ATPase activities, respectively [4]. The expression of the α and β isoforms follows a defined development pattern [5,6] that can be altered by hormonal state [7]. In addition, the expression of these HCs also depends on the metabolic status of the muscle [8] and the hemodynamic load [9]. Analyses at the molecular level show that these alterations in α and β expression are primarily controlled at the pretranslational level [5,10,11]. Thus, the response of cardiac myosin HC expression to such diverse physiological conditions suggests a complex mechanism for differentially regulating transcription of these genes, possibly involving several independent processes.

The genes specifying ventricular α and β myosin HCs have been isolated and their 5' coding and flanking regions characterized in detail [3,12,13]. We report here the use of DNA transfection experiments to further study transcriptional regulation of the rabbit α and β myosin HC genes. We show that whereas the α promoter is constitutively expressed in many cell backgrounds, the β promoter is selectively up-regulated during skeletal muscle differentiation. Furthermore, we have determined that DNA sequences mediating muscle-specific regulation reside within at least 300 bps upstream from the cap site. The results suggest that the tissue-specific expression of the cardiac β promoter is mediated through positive regulatory mechanisms, whereas that for the α promoter relies on suppression or other mechanisms.

METHODS

The cell lines used in these experiments were HeLa cells maintained in Dulbecco's modified Eagle's medium supplemented with 10% fetal calf serum, and a mouse myoblast cell line, 10T1/2aza23A2 [14], maintained in basal minimal Eagle's medium supplemented with 15% fetal calf serum. Primary skeletal muscle cultures were prepared from 12-day-old embryonic chicken pectoralis muscle essentially as described in [15].

DNA transfections were carried out using the calcium-phosphate procedure of Wigler et al. [16]. One to thirty μg of plasmid DNA containing the myosin HC promoter region linked to the gene for bacterial chloramphenicol acetyltransferase (CAT) was used to transfect either subconfluent cultures of cells (HeLa, 10T1/2 23A2) or primary cultures of chick myoblasts. The precipitate was added directly to cultures and incubated either 4 hours (10T1/2aza23A2 and primary cultures) or overnight (HeLa cells). The media was replaced with fresh media, and the cultures incubated for an additional 24 to 48 hours.

CAT activity in the cell extracts was assayed 48 to 72 hours following transfection according to the method of Gorman et al. [17]. The acetylation of ^{14}C-chloramphenicol was monitored by thin layer chromatography on silica gel plates and visualized by autoradiography. In some experiments, the plasmid pSV2-βgal, containing the *E. coli* β-galactosidase gene under the control of the SV40 early promoter, was cotransfected (2 μg per culture) with the CAT plasmids. Cell extracts were assayed for β-galactosidase according to Miller [18] using chlorophenyl red-β-D-galactopyranoside as the substrate.

Published 1988 by Elsevier Science Publishing Co., Inc.
Biology of Isolated Adult Cardiac Myocytes
William A. Clark, Robert S. Decker, and Thomas K. Borg, Editors

RESULTS

The structure of the 5' ends of the rabbit cardiac myosin HC α and β genes is shown schematically in FIG. 1. Just upstream from the first exon of each gene are sequences corresponding to the TATA and CCAAT eukaryotic promoter consensus elements. To examine transcription from these cardiac myosin HC promoters, restriction fragments (indicated by brackets) containing the putative promoter elements along with the first exon of each gene were subcloned immediately upstream from the bacterial CAT gene in $pA_{10}CAT_{3M}$ (pCAT3M) [19]. pMHC-α contains a 466 bp fragment including 418 bps upstream from the cap site, and pMHC-β has a 782 bp fragment with 682 bps of upstream sequences. These plasmids were then transfected into eukaryotic cells, and the function of the promoters was determined by the expression of CAT activity. Since CAT is not normally present in eukaryotic cells, the enzyme activity is a sensitive marker for gene expression.

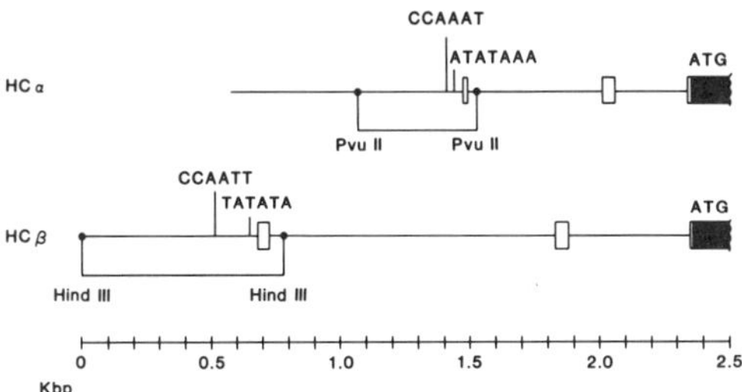

FIG. 1. 5' Flanking regions of the rabbit cardiac myosin HC genes.

The function of the α and β promoters in three different cell types is shown in FIG. 2. In each case pCAT3M, having no promoter, served as a background control while pSV2-CAT was used as a positive control for CAT expression. In HeLa cells (FIG. 2A), the α promoter was quite active as seen by the high CAT activity, whereas the β promoter showed no detectable signal. A comparable pattern of expression was seen for both the α and the β promoters in other heterologous cell systems tested, including human hepatoma (HepG2), rat pituitary (G/C), African green monkey kidney (CV-1) and mouse embryonal carcinoma (P19) (data not shown). The results indicate that the structurally identified α promoter is functional, but it is active in cells that apparently do not express the endogenous α gene.

Similar results were also observed in undifferentiated skeletal myoblasts. As shown in FIG. 2B, the α promoter is expressed in a myogenic cell line derived from the pluripotent mouse embryonic 10T1/2 cells prior to terminal differentiation, but the β promoter remains inactive.

The evaluation of promoter function following differentiation of the mouse myogenic cell line was difficult since the process extends over 8 to 10 days by which time the transient expression of CAT activity was very low. However, in primary chick skeletal muscle cultures (FIG. 2C and 3), where differentiation is completed over a 24-hour interval (between 48 and 72 hours in culture), expression of the β promoter is selectively induced following fusion while the activity of the α promoter increases approximately 2-fold. The specificity of the β promoter for the differentiated state is also demonstrated by blocking the differentiation of the cultured myoblasts with the thymidine analogue, bromodeoxyuridine (BUdR) [15]. As shown in FIG. 3, the exogenous β (but not the α) promoter ceases to function when muscle differentiation is blocked with BUdR. Thus, whereas the α promoter shows constitutive expression in many cell backgrounds, the β promoter region used in these experiments apparently directs both muscle- and stage-specific regulation in skeletal muscle.

To directly demonstrate the role of selective gene sequences in mediating the stage-specific regulation of the β gene, we have examined the

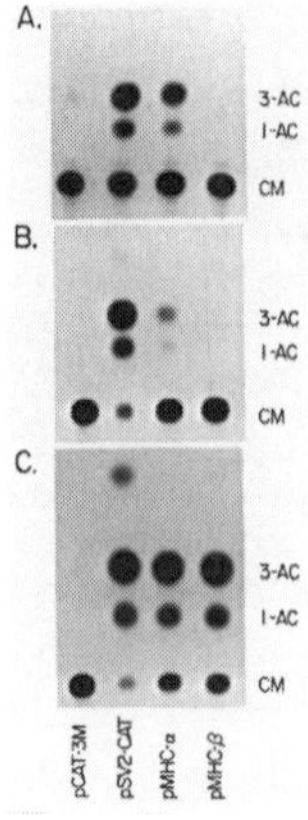

FIG. 2. CAT activity in cells transfected with the myosin HC-CAT plasmids.

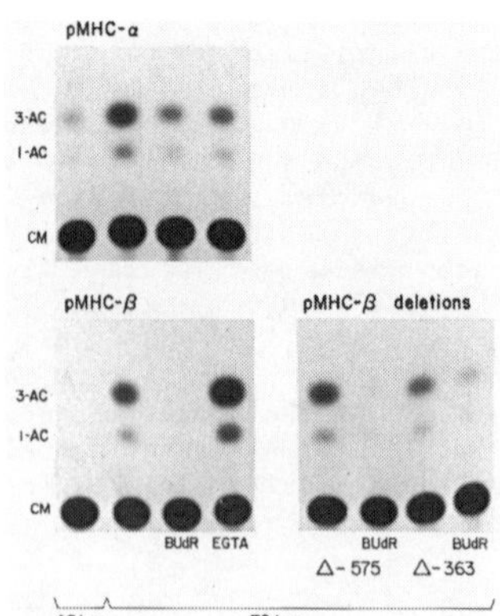

FIG. 3. CAT activity in primary skeletal muscle cultures.

function of a series of 5' deletion mutants of the β promoter. Two examples are shown in FIG. 3. The results reveal (data not shown) that both muscle- and stage-specific expression of pMHC-β are lost when sequences between -293 and -226 bps of the cap site are deleted. Since the later deletion does not alter the CAAT and TATA motifs, the data suggest that specific cis-acting elements mediate regulated expression of the β promoter.

DISCUSSION

We initiated the analysis of rabbit cardiac myosin HC gene expression at the transcriptional level using DNA mediated gene transfer experiments. By transfecting chimeric genes containing the α and β promoter sequences linked to bacterial CAT into cultured cells, we have shown that the 5' regions tested are capable of driving transcription from the cardiac myosin HC promoters. While the analysis has been limited to heterologous and skeletal muscle cells, the results reveal some basic differences in the way the two promoters may be regulated, consistent with their antithetical regulation in cardiac muscle.

In this study, expression of pMHC-β was specifically limited to differentiated skeletal muscle. The induction of the cardiac gene in skeletal muscle is not unexpected. In mammals, the β cardiac myosin HC is expressed in early embryonic and slow skeletal muscles. The deletion analysis indicates that activity is controlled by cis-acting sequences distinct from those necessary for a functional promoter, and the inhibition of function by BUdR shows the specificity for terminal differentiation. The results suggest that tissue-specific expression of the β gene (at least in skeletal muscle) is mediated through a positive regulatory element(s) requiring muscle specific signals or factors that are induced during differentiation.

By contrast, the expression of pMHC-α appears to be constitutive regardless of the cell background or state of differentiation. While some increase in promoter function occurs in differentiated skeletal muscle, the effect is only 2-fold at most (adjusting for differences in transfection efficiency between experimental cultures). The unusual activity does not appear to result from the juxtaposition of vector and selected flanking sequences of the α gene. RNase protection experiments indicate transcription from the correct cap site in the chimeric gene, and the function of the promoter remains largely unchanged in 5' deletions of pMHC-α and in constructs containing an additional 1.5 kbp of 5' upstream sequences. Thus, the difference in the activity of the transfected promoter sequences and the endogenous gene suggests that the former has escaped the normal mechanisms mediating tissue-specific expression. It is possible that expression of the endogenous gene in heterologous cells is repressed either by the chromatin conformation, or the state of methylation. Alternatively, pMHC-α may lack sequences that would act to repress the α gene in non-homologous cell types. Thus, in contrast to the β-promoter, activation of the α gene does not appear to depend solely on positive mechanisms.

Whether the same general patterns of regulation operate on the α and β myosin HC genes in cardiac muscle is unclear. These results, however, provide a basis for examining the transcriptional regulation of these genes in isolated cardiac myocytes by DNA-mediated gene transfer experiments.

ACKNOWLEDGEMENTS

This work was supported by United States Public Health Service Grants HL20592 and HL09172, and was done under the tenure of an Established Investigatorship of the American Heart Association with funds contributed in part by the Chicago Heart Association. L.L.C. is a Senior Research Fellow of the Chicago Heart Association.

REFERENCES

1. J.F.Y. Hoh, G.P.S. Yeoh, M.A.W. Thomas and L Higginbottom, FEBS Lett. 97, 330-334 (1979).
2. A.M. Sinha, P.K. Umeda, C.J. Kavinsky, C. Rajamanickam, H-J. Hsu, S. Jakovcic and M. Rabinowitz, Proc. Nat. Acad. Sci. 79, 5847-5851 (1982).
3. V. Mahdavi, A.P. Chambers and B. Nadal-Ginard, Proc. Nat. Acad. Sci. 81, 2626-2630 (1984).
4. B. Pope, J.F.Y. Hoh and A. Weeds, FEBS Lett. 118, 205-208 (1980).
5. A-M. Lompre, B. Nadal-Ginard and V. Mahdavi, J. Biol. Chem. 259, 6437-6446 (1984).
6. R.A. Chizzonite, A.W. Everett, W.A. Clark, S. Jakovcic, M. Rabinowitz and R. Zak, J. Biol. Chem. 257, 2056-2065 (1982).
7. I.L. Flink, J.R. Rader and E. Morkin, J. Biol. Chem. 254, 3105-3110 (1979).
8. W. Dillman, Molec. Cell. Endocrinol. 34, 169-181 (1984).
9. J-J. Mercadier, A-M. Lompre, C. Wisnewsky, J-L. Samuel, J. Bercovici, B. Swynghedauw and K. Schwartz, Circ. Res. 49, 525-532 (1981).
10. A.M. Sinha, A.W. Everett, P.K. Umeda, R. Zak, S. Jakovcic and M. Rabinowitz, Circ. Res. 66, II-259 (1982).
11. A.W. Everett, P.K. Umeda, A.M. Sinha, S. Jakovcic, M. Rabinowitz and R. Zak, Biochemistry 23, 1596-1599 (1984).
12. P.K. Umeda, J.E. Levin, A.M. Sinha, L.L. Cribbs, D.S. Darling, D.J. Ende, H-J. Hsu, E. Dizon and S. Jakovcic in Molecular Biology of Muscle Development, C. Emerson, D. Fischman, B. Nadal-Ginard and MAQ. Siddiqui, eds. (Alan R. Liss, Inc, NY 1986) pp. 363-371.
13. D.J. Friedman, P.K. Umeda, A.M. Sinha, H-J. Hsu, S. Jakovcic and M. Rabinowitz, Proc. Nat. Acad. Sci. 81, 3044-3048 (1983).
14. S.F. Konieczny and C.P. Emerson Jr, Cell 38, 791-800 (1984).
15. R. Bischoff and H. Holtzer, J. Cell Biol. 44, 134-150 (1970).
16. M. Wigler, R. Sweet, G.K. Sim, B. Wold, A. Pellicer, E. Lacy, T. Maniatas, S. Silverstein and R. Axel, Cell 16, 777-785 (1979).
17. C.M. Gorman, L.F. Moffat and B.H. Howard, Mol. Cell. Biol. 2, 1044-1051 (1982).
18. J.H. Miller, Experiments in Molecular Genetics,(Cold Spring Harbor, Cold Spring Harbor Laboratory).
19. L.A. Laimins, P. Gruss, R. Pozzatti and G. Khoury, J. Virol. 49, 183-189 (1984).

"DEDIFFERENTIATION" OF THE CULTURED ADULT CARDIAC MUSCLE CELL BY TPA

WILLIAM C. CLAYCOMB
Department of Biochemistry and Molecular Biology
LSU Medical Center, New Orleans, Louisiana 70112

INTRODUCTION

The terminally differentiated adult rat ventricular cardiac muscle cell when grown in culture has been shown to maintain most of the ultrastructural, biochemical and physiological properties of the *in situ* adult cardiac myocyte. These highly differentiated cells do not revert back to an undifferentiated or embryonic-like state when cultured and hence serve as a good model for *in vitro* studies of the adult heart muscle cell. One nonadult like feature of these cultured cells is that they incorporate radioactive thymidine into nuclear DNA [1-3]. We have shown previously that this [^{3}H] thymidine incorporation is into DNA that is replicating semiconservatively [1] and thus is not due to some type of DNA repair phenomenon. These cells also reacquire the activity of enzymes which are needed to replicate DNA [1]. Previously, DNA replication and cell division in ventricular cardiac muscle cells was believed to be permanently and irreversibly repressed during early neonatal development of the rat. Our laboratory has initiated studies to determine if the DNA synthetic activity in cultured adult rat ventricular cardiac myocytes could be stimulated and to explore the mechanisms involved with the reinitiation of DNA replication in these terminally differentiated cells.

TPA STIMULATES CARDIAC MYOCYTE DNA SYNTHESIS

A variety of growth factors, hormones, and chemicals were tested for their effect on DNA synthesis in cultured adult cardiac myocytes. By far the greatest stimulation has been observed with the phorbol ester tumor promoter TPA (12-0-tetradecanoyl-phorbol-13-acetate). TPA produced a consistent 3-fold stimulation in DNA synthesis and further autoradiographic experiments established that this stimulated DNA synthesis was due to cells not previously synthesizing DNA being induced to enter the S phase of the cell cycle. In order to understand the mechanism involved with the reactivation and stimulation of DNA synthesis in cultured myocytes the effect of TPA on the ultrastructure and on expression of several genes in these cells was examined.

Adult rat ventricular cardiac muscle cells were isolated and cultured by our standard procedures [4,5]. Cytosine arabinoside was added for the first seven days of culture to eliminate fibroblast and other nonmuscle cell contamination [4,5]. The cells were then cultured for various periods of time in the presence and absence of 50 ng/ml of TPA (preliminary studies had shown that this was the optimal concentration). Total cellular RNA was isolated by the guanidinium isothiocynate/CsCl procedure. RNA was size fractionated on 1.2% agarose - 2.2 M formaldehyde gels and transfered to Zeta-Probe nylon membranes. The membranes were then hybridized with the indicated ^{32}P-labeled DNA probe. Autoradiography was performed using Kodak X-Omat RP film and Dupont lighting-plus intensifying screens at -70°C.

TPA INHIBITS MUSCLE SPECIFIC GENES AND ACTIVATES SEVERAL PROTO-ONCOGENES

Figure 1 shows the effect of TPA on the expression of myosin heavy chain and M-creatine kinase genes. This phorbol ester essentially turns off the expression of these differentiation-specific muscle genes.

Biology of Isolated Adult Cardiac Myocytes
William A. Clark, Robert S. Decker, and Thomas K. Borg, Editors

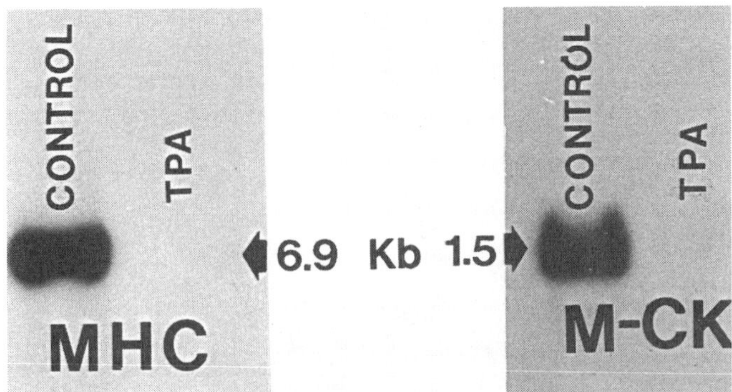

FIG. 1. Northern blot analysis of the effect of TPA (50 ng/ml) on the expression of myosin heavy chain (MHC) and M-creatine kinase (M-CK) genes in cultured adult rat ventricular cardiac muscle cells. Myocytes were treated with TPA for 5 days (day 7 of culture to day 12), total RNA was isolated and electrophoresed (15 µg/lane), transfered to nylon membrane and hybridized to the indicated radioactive DNA probe. The estimated size of the transcripts being expressed is given in Kb.

We have previously examined the expression of 13 proto-oncogenes in proliferating and terminally differentiated rat cardiac muscle cells [6] and have found that several of these genes are actively expressed only in the less differentiated neonatal cells. The effect of TPA on the expression of several of these proto-oncogenes was tested and the results are shown in Figs. 2 and 3. TPA rapidly and transiently induces the expression of c-fos with the maximum activity being seen 60 minutes after its addition to the cultured myocytes. c-myc expression was first seen in TPA-treated cultures at 4 hours and persisted for at least 12 hours thereafter (Fig. 2).

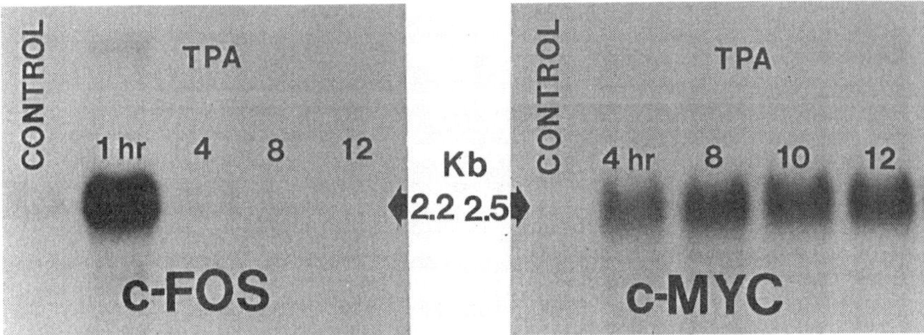

FIG. 2. Northern blot analysis of the effect of TPA (50 ng/ml) on the expression of c-fos and c-myc in cultured adult rat ventricular cardiac muscle cells. Cells were treated for the indicated time periods.

The expression of proto-oncogenes coding for proteins with tyrosine kinase activity (c-abl and c-src) were also observed to be induced by TPA (Fig. 3).

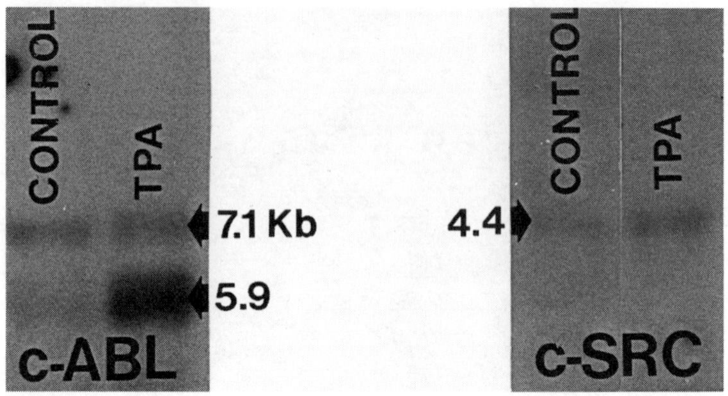

FIG. 3. Northern blot analysis of the effect of TPA (50 ng/ml) on the expression of c-abl and c-src in cultured adult rat ventricular cardiac muscle cells. Cells were treated with TPA for 48 hours.

CONCLUSION

These studies suggest that TPA is stimulating DNA synthesis in these cells by activating genes involved with cell proliferation and DNA replication and inactivating genes involved with terminal differentiation. Our morphological studies have shown that TPA treated myocytes are embryonic-like in appearance in that they lose their highly ordered myofibrillar ultrastructure. Most of the effects of TPA are known to be mediated by a serine-threonine-specific calcium/phospholipid-dependent protein kinase (protein kinase C) [7,8]. The normal cellular effector of this enzyme is diacylglycerol (DAG) [7,8]. We have observed that several different DAGs would mimic all of the effects of TPA on these cultured adult cells which indicates that TPA is indeed acting through activation of protein kinase C.

The cellular homologues of acutely transforming retroviral oncogenes termed proto-oncogenes are thought to play an important role in the regulation of normal cellular proliferation and cellular differentiation. The studies reported here show that TPA is able to induce in these cultured adult myocytes several proto-oncogenes whose expression is observed only in actively proliferating neonatal rat cardiac muscle cells [6]. This may mean that these proto-oncogenes function in some manner in the regulation of cardiac muscle DNA replication and cell proliferation. This TPA system may provide a means to determine how these genes are involved with these processes in the cardiac myocyte.

In summary, these TPA studies demonstrate a structure-function relationship between the degree of morphological differentiation of the ventricular cardiac muscle cell, gene expression and DNA synthetic activity. These cells appear to be very plastic in that they readily adapt to standard culture conditions and their genetic program can be easily manipulated by growth factors, hormones and chemicals. This TPA induced "dedifferentiation" of the cultured adult cardiac muscle cell may provide a system which can be used to study myocyte differentiation and how DNA synthesis and cell proliferation are permanently repressed *in vivo* during the early development of the mammalian heart.

This work was supported by NIH Grants HL 25873 and HL 35632.

REFERENCES

1. W.C. Claycomb and H.D. Bradshaw, Jr., Develop. Biol. 90, 331-337 (1983).
2. W.C. Claycomb and R.L. Moses, Exp. Cell Res. 161, 95-100 (1985).
3. A.C. Nag and M. Cheng, Tiss. Cell 18, 491-497 (1986).
4. W.C. Claycomb and M.C. Palazzo, Develop. Biol. 80, 446-482 (1980).
5. W.C. Claycomb and N.A. Lanson, Jr., In Vitro 20, 647-651 (1984).
6. W.C. Claycomb and N.A. Lanson, Jr., Biochem. J. IN PRESS (1987).
7. Y. Nishizuka, Nature 308, 693-698 (1984).
8. Y. Nishizuka, Science 225, 1365-1370 (1984).

STRUCTURAL ORGANIZATION, DNA SYNTHESIS AND EXPRESSION OF MYOSIN ISOFORMS IN ADULT CARDIAC MUSCLE CELLS IN CULTURE

Asish C. Nag and Mei Cheng, Department of Biological Sciences, Oakland University, Rochester, Michigan 48063

INTRODUCTION

Several laboratories have successfully isolated and cultured adult cardiac muscle cells for periods of a few days to over a month [1,2,9,13-15,19]. It is evident from these studies that with extended time in culture, adult cardiac muscle cells undergo external and internal structural changes. Available metabolic data on cells in short-term culture (4-7d) indicate retention of _in vivo_ resting state properties [10], whereas those of the long-term culture are suggestive of the active state [4]. Adult cardiac muscle cells in long-term culture can undergo DNA synthesis and karyokinesis [1,3,14,17]. The expression of myosin heavy chain isoforms in these long-term cultured cells was found to be dependent on the concentration of thyroid hormone in the medium [18]. This report will discuss (1) the isolation and culture of adult rat cardiac ventricular muscle cells, (2) ultrastructural organization, (3) DNA synthesis and karyokinesis, and (4) the profiles of expression of myosin isoforms in these cells.

CELL CULTURE

Although single cardiac muscle cells can be isolated either from minced cardiac tissue treated with enzyme(s) or from intact heart perfused with enzyme(s), better preparations of cardiac myocytes are obtained from perfused hearts, which result in better yield of viable cells than that of minced preparations. Among different enzymes used for isolation of cells, collagenase is found to be essential for effective dissociation of the cardiac tissue into single-cell suspension (see review, Ref. 10). A mixture of 0.05% collagenase and 0.1% hyaluroindase has been used in our laboratory for isolation of cardiac myocytes from adult rat hearts. The heart was first perfused with CA^{2+}-free Joklik-modified medium (GIBCO) adjusted to pH 7.2-7.4. This was followed by perfusion with the above enzyme mixture in Joklik's medium (pH 7.2-7.4) for approximately 45 min., followed by a rinse with the same medium for approximately 5 min. The ventricle was then minced in Joklik's medium and shaken gently on ice bath for 5-7 min to release single cells. The cell suspension thus obtained was filtered and plated on collagen (type VII, sigma) or 2% gelatin-coated dishes, and cultured for 45 days as described previously [16,18]. Laminin did not produce results superior to those produced by collagen. Also, Fibronectin did not produce satisfactory results.

STRUCTURAL ORGANIZATION

Adult cardiac muscle cells undergo structural changes in long-term culture [12,14,15,20] while cells in short-term culture (4-7 d) [19] apparently maintain _in vivo_ structural organization. However, during the second week of incubation, the latter exhibit the same structural changes observed in the long-term culture. Jacobson and Piper [10] termed the above short-term culture the _rapid attachment model_, and the long-term culture the _redifferentiated model_.

Biology of Isolated Adult Cardiac Myocytes
William A. Clark, Robert S. Decker, and Thomas K. Borg, Editors

More than fifty percent of adult cardiac myocytes in long-term culture assumed oblong or round configurations during the first 10 days of culture. With progressive time in culture, most of the oblong or round cells spread out and take on various shapes. The rest of the cylindrical cells maintain an apparent cylindrical appearance while flattening out transversely [15]. Electron microscopy during the first 10 days of culture containing predominantly oblong or round cells showed disorganized myofibrils with interspersed mitochondria and disrupted sarcoplasmic reticulum and T-tubules. Autophagic vacuoles containing mitochondria and myofilaments were also observed. During second week and onward some cells resembled embryonic myocytes with fewer myofibrils, free myofilaments, small pleomorphic electron dense mitochondria, and many polysomes. Other cells contained closely-packed and well organized myofibrils, electron-dense pleomorphic mitochondria, and other cellular organelles as observed _in vivo_ or freshly-dissociated cardiac myocytes.

DNA SYNTHESIS AND KARYOKINESIS

Our earlier studies [14] have demonstrated that the adult cardiac myocytes in long-term culture regain the capacity for DNA synthesis. These findings were confirmed later by Claycomb and Bradshaw [3]. Our recent studies portrayed a detailed profile of DNA synthesis in adult cardiac myocytes during long-term culture [17]. Replication of DNA was followed by karyokinesis, as evidenced by the presence of mitotic apparatus in the myocytes (Fig. 1). During the early incubation period, cardiac myocytes showed fewer than 5% labeled cells. As the culture continued, the labeling index rose to a peak in the second week, showing approximately 23% labeled cells. The labeling indexes declined over the period of 30 days of culture, showing approximately 4% labeled cells at the end. In order to analyze what percentage of the total cell population became involved in DNA synthesis, cells were grown continuously for various time periods in the medium containing [^{3}H]-thymidine. Our studies showed that approximately 31% of cardiac myocytes regained the capacity to synthesize DNA during 30 days of culture.

EXPRESSION OF MYOSIN ISOFORMS

The profile of myosin isoforms expressed by the long-term cultured cardiac muscle cells differs from that of their counterparts _in vivo_ [18]. After seven days of culture in a serum-containing medium the adult rat cardiac myocytes contained a predominant isozyme V1, which was comparable to the isozyme profile of the ventricle. When culture of these cells was continued for 15-30 days, the myosin isozymes profile of these adult myocytes was the same as that of the embryonic ones that contained predominant isozyme V3 (Fig 2). The Ca^{2+}-ATPase activities of myosin isozymes in adult cardiac myocytes cultured 15-30 days were comparable to those of the embryonic ventricles. The myosin phenotype of these cultured cells seems to have a reflection of the switch in expression of the alpha and beta myosin heavy chain genes that are influenced by the low concentration of the thyroid hormone present in the culture medium. When we exposed these adult myocytes to the thyroid hormone (T_3 or T_4) in addition to the serum in the medium, the cells switched to the predominant V1 (Fig 3). It is known that thyroid hormone induces the synthesis of ventricular heavy chain alpha, which as a dimer forms the V1 myosin. As expected, thyroid hormone induced the synthesis of isozyme V1 and thus modulated the predominant fetal-type isozyme V3 in the adult cells cultured in the serum-containing medium to the adult type isozyme V1 in adult cells grown in serum-and thyroid hormone-containing medium.

In summary, adult cardiac muscle cells survive in culture conditions for a long period. The cultured myocytes undergo reversible dedifferentiation. The switching of the dedifferentiated state of myosin phenotype into the differentiated adult form depends on the thyroid hormone concentration of the culture medium. The cultured myocytes reinitiate DNA synthesis and karyokinesis.

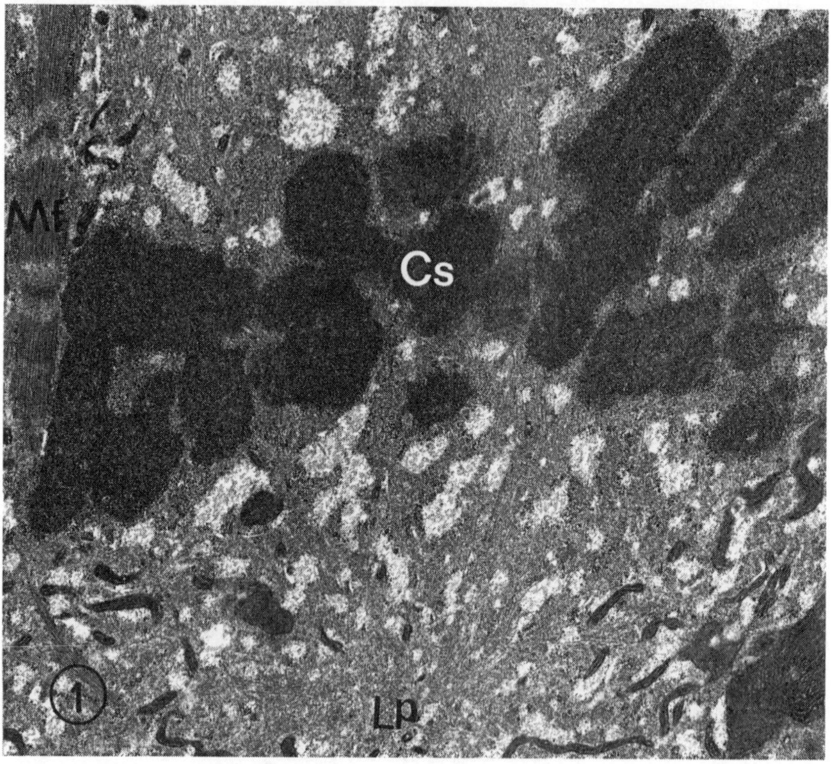

Fig. 1. Mitotic apparatus of an adult cardiac myocyte in a 12-day-old culture. Note the metaphase chromosomes (Cs) in the equatorial plate. Lp, lower pole of the mitotic spindle; Mf, myofibril. 11,250x.

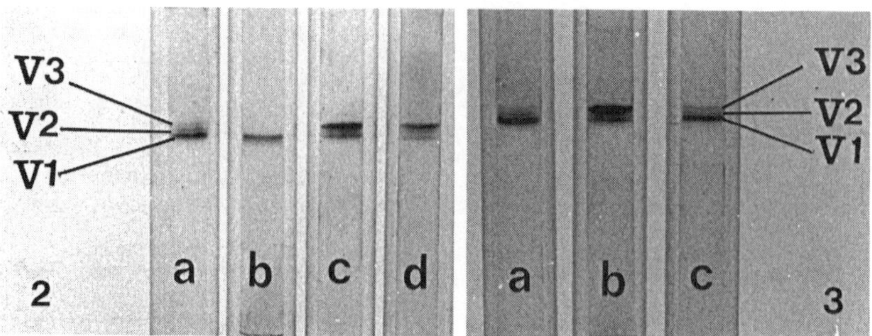

Fig. 2. Electrophoretic analysis of adult ventricular myosin, and long-term cultured adult cardiac ventricular muscle cell myosin: a) 350g rat ventricle; b) adult cardiac muscle cells after 7 days of culture in a serum-containing medium; c) adult cardiac muscle cells after 15 days of culture in a serum-containing medium; d) 18-day embryonic rat ventricle. (Reproduced from Nag & Cheng [18] with permission).
Fig. 3. Comparison of myosin isozymes between adult rat ventricle, cultured adult rat cardiac myocytes in a serum-containing medium, and adult cardiac myocytes cultured in a serum-containing medium supplemented with T_4: a) 350g rat ventricle; b) adult rat ventricular myocyte after 15 days of culture in a serum-containing medium; c) adult rat ventricular myocytes after 15 days of culture in a serum-containing medium supplemented with T_4. (Reproduced from [18] with permission).

ACKNOWLEDGMENTS

This work was supported by NSF Grant DCB 8709594 and American Heart Association of Michigan Grant-in-Aid.

REFERENCES

1. Cantin, M., Ballak, M., Benzeron-Magina, Srivastava, M.B.A., & Tautu, C. Science, 214, 569-570 (1981).
2. Claycomb, W.C. & Palazzo, M.C. Devel. Biol. 80, 466-482 (1980).
3. Claycomb, W.C. & Bradshaw, Jr. Devel. Biol. 99, 331-337 (1983).
4. Claycomb, W.C., Burns, A.H. & Shepard, R.E. FEBS Lett. 169, 261-266 (1984).
5. Everett, A.W., Sinha, A.H., Umeda, P.K., Jakovcic, S., Rabinowitz, M. & Zak, R. Bichemistry, 23, 1596-1599 (1984).
6. Gustafson, T.A., Markham, B.E. & Morkin, E. Biochem. Biophys. Res. Comm. 130, 1161-1167 (1985).
7. Hoh, J.F.Y., McGarath, P.A., & Hale, P.T. J. Mol. Cell. Cardiol. 10, 1053-1076 (1977).
8. Izumu, S., Nadal-Ginard, B., & Mahdavi, V. Science, 231, 597-600 (1986).
9. Jacobson, S.L. Cell struct. Funct. 2, 1-9 (1977).
10. Jacobson, S.L., & Piper, H.M. J. Mol. Cell. Cardiol. 18, 661-678 (1986).
11. Lompre, A.M., Nadal-Ginard, B., & Mahdavi, V. J. Biol. Chem. 259, 6437-6446 (1984).
12. Moses, R.L., & Claycomb, W.C. Am. J. Anat. 171, 191-206 (1982).
13. Nag, A.C., Fischman, D.A., Rabinowitz, M., & Zak, R. J. Cell Biol. 63, 238a (1974).
14. Nag, A.C., & Cheng, M. Tissue & Cell, 9, 419-438 (1981).
15. Nag., A.C., Cheng, M., Fischman, D.A., and Z.R. J. Mol. Cell. Cardiol. 15, 301-317 (1983).
16. Nag, A.C., Ingland, M., & Cheng, M. In vitro Cell. Devel. Biol. 21, 553-562 (1985).
17. Nag, A.C., & Cheng, M. Tissue & Cell, 18, 491-497 (1986).
18. Nag, A.C., & Cheng, M. Biochem. Biophys. Res. Comm. 137, 855-862 (1986).
19. Piper, H.M., Probst, I., Schwartz, P., Hutter, F.J., & Spieckermann. J. Mol. Cell. Cardiol. 14, 397-412 (1982).
20. Schwarzfeld, T.A., & Jacobson, S.L. J. Mol. Cell. Cardiol. 13, 563-575 (1981).

Protein Synthesis in Cultured Adult Rabbit Cardiac Myocytes

J. Haddad*, A.M. Samarel*, M.L. Decker*, M. Lesch*, and R.S. Decker* **
Department of Medicine (Cardiology)*, Cell Biology and Anatomy**,
Northwestern University Medical School, Chicago, IL 60611

INTRODUCTION

Pure populations of calcium tolerant, adult cardiac myocytes provide an attractive approach to investigate those factors that modulate the synthesis and degradation of contractile proteins and, ultimately, control cardiac mass. Although humoral, neural and physical factors are known to influence myocardial protein turnover in vivo [1,2,3], in perfused hearts [4] and in cultured embryonic and neonatal heart cells [5-10], only a few attempts have been made to directly study protein metabolism in freshly isolated [11,12] and cultured adult myocytes [13]. Whole animal infusions have supplied provocative data on the synthesis and degradation of total and myofibrillar proteins, but the complexity of in vivo isotope use complicates the interpretation of such studies [14]. Conversely, perfused hearts have generated an excellent measure of protein turnover but lack the stability required to study the proteolysis of long-lived proteins [3,4]. A variety of embryonic and neonatal myocyte cultures have also been employed to study protein metabolism; however, fractional rates of synthesis and degradation in these model systems [5,6,8,9] range from 6-10-fold greater than those values recorded in vivo [2,3], presently making direct comparisons with adult cells difficult, at best. Although protein synthesis and amino acid transport have been examined to some extent with freshly isolated myocytes, measurements of fractional synthesis rates and direct comparisons with whole animals have not been previously reported; therefore, the present experiments were conducted to compare and contrast protein synthesis in freshly isolated and cultured adult myocytes prepared from the hearts of New Zealand white rabbits.

MATERIALS AND METHODS

Isolated myocytes were prepared from 2 kg male rabbits by a modification of Powell's procedure [15], employing retrograde perfusion of collagenase (80 U/ml) and hyaluronidase (0.5mg/ml) in Krebs-Ringer bicarbonate buffer supplemented with 20 uM Ca^{2+}. Such preparations yielded 3 X 10^7 myocytes per heart which were plated onto laminin-coated petri dishes at a density of 85 $\pm$ 6 cells/mm^2 and cultured in Medium 199 plus 1 mM Ca^{2+} and 5% fetal calf serum [16]. Cytosine arabinoside (Ara-C) was added to some cultures (10 uM Ara-C) to suppress interstitial cell proliferation [10,16,17]. Interstitial cell cultures were prepared from the same hearts used to isolate myocytes and were cultured in the absence of Ara-C.

The fractional rate (K_s) of total protein synthesis (TP) and myosin heavy chain (MHC) synthesis was measured biosynthetically by labeling myocyte or interstitial cell cultures with 10 uCi/ml [4,5-^{3}H] leucine (leucine specific radioactivity $\simeq$ 2 X 10^5 DPM/nmol) for periods ranging from 30 min to 4 h at 37°C. Following incubation the medium was removed and retained and the cells were scraped from the plates with 10% trichloroacetic acid (TCA). TCA insoluble protein (TP) was collected by centrifugation and washed four times in 10% TCA before being extracted in ethyl ether. The precipitate was then hydrolyzed in 6 N HCl at 105°C for 24 hrs. MHC was prepared by extracting myocytes in low salt and then separating the proteins electrophoretically on an SDS 7-17% vertical slab gel. Gel bands containing MHC were identified by co-electrophoresis of adjacent purified standards and were cut from the gel and hydrolyzed in 6 N HCl at 105°C for 48h.

Biology of Isolated Adult Cardiac Myocytes
William A. Clark, Robert S. Decker, and Thomas K. Borg, Editors

Leucine specific radioactivity in the medium (F*) and TP (P*) was determined by direct radioassay following derivatization with [^{14}C] dansyl chloride and separation of amino acid derivatives by thin layer chromatography [3,6]. The specific activity of MHC was measured by isotope dilution [3]. The fractional rate of protein synthesis (K_s) was derived from Zilversmit's [18] equation:

$$dP^*/dt = K_s.F^* - K_d.P^*$$

where t is time (days), K_s and K_d are the fractional rates of synthesis (K_s) and degradation (K_d) and P* and F* are the specific radioactivities of leucine in the product (protein or MHC) and the precursor (medium), respectively. Since the labeling period in the present experiments was short relative to the half lives of cardiac protein [1,2,3,14], then F*>> P* and the calculation of K_s can be simplified by omitting $-K_dP^*$, resulting in an estimate of the fractional synthetic rate. After integration, the Zilversmit equation becomes:

$$K_s \cong P^*/F^*.t$$

RESULTS

Cultured myocytes and interstitial cells incorporated [^{3}H] leucine into TCA insoluble protein (TP) in a linear fashion after a short lag period. Figure 1 illustrates that myocytes cultured for varying intervals

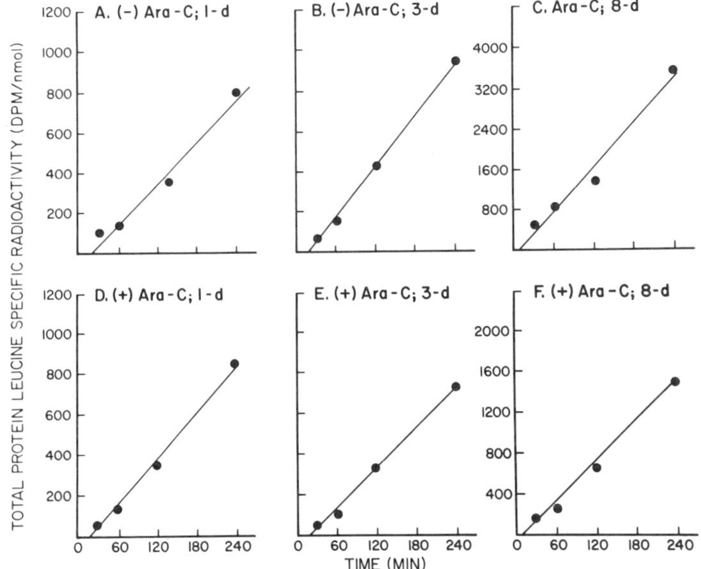

Figure 1. Incorporation of [3H] leucine into total cellular protein of cultured myocytes in the presence and absence of cytosine arabinoside. Data are representative experiments demonstrating linear rates of incorporation of [3H] leucine into total cellular protein following a brief lag period. Results for each experiment were subjected to least-squares analysis to determine the x-intercept of the best-fit line for leucine specific radioactivity vs. time for cultures maintained in the presence (+) and absence (-) of Ara-C (10 uM) for 1 day (Panels A and D), 3 days (Panels B and E) and 8 days (Panels C and F). Each point represents the mean of 4 determinations.

exhibited the same phenomena; moreover, exposure of the cells to Ara-C does not appear to alter this brief delay or, ultimately, influence P*. When the data for each experiment was subjected to linear regression analysis to obtain the X-intercept of the best-fit line for P* (vs. time), the lag period was found to be 15.1 ± 7.5 min (n = 10). Although these results demonstrated that labeled leucine rapidly equilibrated with intracellular leucyl t-RNA [5,6], the delay may imply some alteration in leucine transport or, perhaps, a block in the initiation of protein synthesis [4]. When similar cultures were "flooded" with a 20-fold excess of leucine (i.e., 200 uCi [^{3}H] leucine in 2 mM cold leucine) identical results were obtained, demonstrating that the lag does not reflect a diffusion barrier to leucine transport, *per se*. Furthermore, confluent interstitial cell cultures displayed similar kinetics for [^{3}H] leucine incorporation into TP.

When freshly attached cardiac myocytes were labeled with [^{3}H] leucine for 4 h *in vitro*, the fractional synthetic rate for TP was 3.2 ± 0.3%/d in the absence of Ara-C and 3.4 ± 0.3%/d in the presence of the anti-mitotic drug (Table I). Such observations conveyed the impression that Ara-C had no demonstrable effect upon myocyte protein synthesis over the duration of these experiments. Strikingly, these K_s values were significantly lower than the corresponding fractional rates measured during a 4 h infusion of labeled leucine *in vivo* [3], suggesting that isolation and culture of quiescent cardiac myocytes is accompanied by a marked suppression of myocyte specific TP synthesis. If culture was prolonged, the fractional rate remained depressed when compared to its *in vivo* counterpart, regardless of whether or not the cultures were supplemented with Ara-C (Table I).

By the fourth day *in vitro*, the fractional rate of synthesis for myocytes cultured in the absence of the anti-metabolite had almost tripled when compared to those cultured with Ara-C (5.9 ± 2.0 vs. 2.2 ± 0.4%/d, $P < 0.05$). Examination of these preparations by phase contrast microscopy revealed the presence of proliferating interstitial cells in cultures maintained in the absence of Ara-C, whereas those cultured with the drug displayed no evidence of non-myocytic cell division [10,16,17]. By the end of the first week *in vitro*, K_s values for cells maintained in the absence of Ara-C were considerably higher than those values obtained from either paired Ara-C-supplemented cultures or those fractional rates obtained from continuous *in vivo* infusions [3].

Table I. Effects of length of culture and cytosine arabinoside on fractional rates of total protein synthesis in cultured myocytes.

	0-d	1-d	2-d	3-d	4-d	8-d
(-) Ara-C	3.2±0.4	2.4±0.3	2.5±1.2	2.9±0.7	5.9±2.0	16.9±5.6
(+) Ara-C	3.4±0.3	2.6±0.3	2.3±0.7	2.0±0.3	2.2±0.4	5.0±0.1

Values are fractional synthetic rates (Ks, %/d) of total cellular protein in paired cultures of cardiac myocytes maintained in the presence (+) or absence (-) of cytosine arabinoside (10 uM, Ara-C). Values are means ± S.D. for 4 pairs of dishes within each group of cells grown for varying time periods (0-8d in culture). Data were analyzed by both 2-way and 1-way analysis of variance, where appropriate.

The sharply higher K_s values measured in cultures not receiving Ara-C appears related to the proliferation of non-myocytic cells. Day 4 cultures exhibited such cells randomly scattered amongst cardiac myocytes; by day 8 such cultures were almost completely overgrown by this rapidly dividing cellular population [16]. To explore this relationship somewhat further, confluent cultures of 8-day cardiac interstitial cells were labeled with [^{3}H] leucine in the presence or absence of Ara-C. Fractional rates of TP synthesis measured 20.9±6.6%/d and 21.3±2.6%/d (n = 4) for paired cultures supplemented with and without the antibiotic. These fractional rates were over six-fold greater than those values obtained from freshly isolated myocyte preparations, strongly supporting the contention that the presence of dividing non-myocytic cells and not the anti-mitotic agent was responsible for the elevated levels of protein synthesis in the older cultures (Table I). Conversely, the enhanced fractional rates measured in Ara-C-treated 8-day myocyte cultures could not be correlated with the appearance of proliferating interstitial cells, but may be associated with the dramatic spreading that cultured myocytes display at this juncture. Our present observations suggest that this event is accompanied by the remodeling of the contractile apparatus and a reorganization of the myocyte's cytoskeleton; processes which might be expected to alter rates of protein synthesis.

The fractional rates of MHC synthesis were assessed to develop a more accurate picture of the events that accompany remodeling of the myofibrillar apparatus (Table II). To our surprise K_s values for MHC isolated from myocytes cultured for 24 h were markedly suppressed, regardless of the presence (1.1±0.3/d) or absence (1.1±0.4%/d) of Ara-C. Even though it is clear that the anti-metabolite does not influence MHC synthesis, the K_s values obtained were 10-fold lower than those calculated from *in vivo* infusion experiments [19]. Such results suggested that isolation and culture of queiscent cardiac myocytes disproportionately inhibited the synthesis of MHC when compared to the more moderate decline in the K_s for TP. Moreover, prolonging culture for a week does not alter the fractional rate of MHC synthesis, even in the presence of Ara-C, demonstrating that the metabolic and functional "state" of the cultures was likely responsible for the inhibition of MHC and TP synthesis in cultured rabbit myocytes.

Table II. Effects of length of culture and cytosine arabinoside on fractional rates of myosin heavy chain synthesis in cultured myocytes.

	1-d	3-d	8-d
(-) Ara-C	1.1±0.4	0.4±0.1	1.4±0.4
(+) Ara-C	1.1±0	0.5±0.4	0.7±0.2

Values are expressed as in Table I.

DISCUSSION

The present investigation revealed that the isolation and culture of adult rabbit cardiac myocytes is associated with a significant suppression in the fractional rate of both TP and MHC synthesis. Furthermore, addition of Ara-C to the culture medium effectively prevented the proliferation of non-myocytic cells without further affecting protein synthetic rates. Nevertheless, other phenomena have been implicated in regulating protein synthesis in the heart, including (1) contractile function, (2) passive tension, (3) hormones and (4) neural inputs. The inhibition of contractility in cultured neonatal myocytes is accompanied by a significant suppression of TP synthesis and an even greater inhibition in MHC synthesis [8], supporting the present observations, and providing reasonable evidence linking the rate of TP and MHC synthesis with contractile function *in vitro*. Conversely, Kira *et al* [20] have reported that increases in myocardial wall tension produced greater effects on protein synthesis than could be accounted for by alterations in contractile function. Such results emphasize the importance of passive stretch and the development of isometric tension on the modulation of myocardial protein synthesis [21]. In addition to these mechanical parameters, several metabolic factors are well known effectors of protein synthesis, including hormones, amino acids, oxygen tension and oxidizable substrates [4]. Previous studies have demonstrated that insulin increases protein synthesis in cultured adult myocytes [11,12,13]. Preliminary studies from our laboratory indicate that insulin alone, or in combination with triiodothyronine stimulated an increase in the fractional rate of total myocyte protein synthesis by 20-30%, but was not sufficient to raise the K_s to values observed <u>in vivo</u> [3,19]. Future investigations must now address the role of each of these factors in regulating protein synthesis in cultured adult cardiac myocytes.

ACKNOWLEDGMENTS

These studies were supported in part by NHLBI grant HL33616, HL 34328 and a grant from the Oppenheimer Family Foundation. We appreciate the technical expertise of Ms. Lee-Chin Hsieh and thank Carole Becker and Belinda Berthold-Coichy for preparing the manuscript.

REFERENCES

1. A.F. Martin, J. Biol. Chem. 256: 964 (1981).
2. A.W. Everett, G. Prior, and R. Zak, Biochem. J. 194: 365 (1981).
3. M.S. Parmacek, N. Magid, M. Lesch, R.S. Decker and A.M. Samarel, Am. J. Physiol. (Cell Physiol.) 251: C727 (1986).
4. H.E. Morgan, D.E. Rannals, and E.E. McKee, In: Handbook of Physiology, R. Berne, ed. Am. Physiol. Soc. p. 945, Washington, D.C. 1979.
5. W.A. Clark, and R. Zak, J. Biol. Chem. 256: 424 (1981).
6. J. Airhart, J.A. Arnold, W.S. Stirewalt, and R.B. Low, Am. J. Physiol. (Cell Physiol) 243: C81 (1982).
7. P. Simpson, A. McGrath, and S. Savion, Circ. Res. 51: 787 (1982).
8. P. McDermott, M. Daood, and I. Klein, Am. J. Physiol. (Heart Circ.) 249: H763 (1985).
9. W.J. Carter, B.W.S. van der Weigden, and F.H. Faas, J. Mol. Cell Cardiol. 17: 897 (1985).
10. P. Libby, J. Mol. Cell Cardiol. 16: 803 (1984).
11. R. Kao, E.W. Christman, S.L. Luk, J.M. Krauhs, G.F.O. Tyers, and E.H. Williams. Arch. Biochem. Biophys,. 203: 587 (1980).
12. E.J. Walker, J.H. Burns, and J.W. Dow, Biochem. Biophys. Acta. 721: 280 (1982).
13. J. Eckel, G. van Echten, and H. Reinauer, Am. J. Physiol (Heart Circ.) 249: H212 (1985).
14. A.W. Everett and R. Zak, In: Degradative Processes in Heart and Skeletal Muscle. K. Wildenthal, ed., p. 31, Elsevier/North Holland Biomed. Press, Amsterdam, 1980.
15. T. Powell, D.A. Terrar, and V.M. Twist, J. Physiol. 302: 131 (1980).
16. J. Haddad, M.L. Decker, L-C. Hsieh, M. Lesch, A.M. Samarel and R.S. Decker, Am. J. Physiol. (Cell Physiol.). In Press, 1987.
17. R.L. Moses and W.C. Claycomb, Am. J. Anat. 164: 113 (1982).
18. D.B. Zilversmit, Am. J. Med. 29: 832 (1960).
19. A.M. Samarel, M.S. Parmacek, N.M. Magid, R.S. Decker, and M. Lesch, Circ. Res. 60: 933 (1987).
20. Y. Kira, P.J. Kochel, E.E. Gordon, and H. E. Morgan, Am. J. Physiol. (Cell Physiol.) 246: C247 (1985).
21. M.B. Peterson and M. Lesch, Circ. Res. 31: 317 (1972)

BIOSYNTHESIS AND REORGANIZATION OF LAMININ AND COLLAGEN TYPE IV IN ADULT CARDIAC MYOCYTES *IN VITRO*.

Louis Terracio*, Evy Lundgren**, Thomas K. Borg*, and Kristofer Rubin**.
*Departments of Anatomy and Pathology, University of South Carolina, School of Medicine, Columbia, SC 29208.
**Department of Medical and Physiological Chemistry, Uppsala University, Box 575, S-751 23 Uppsala, Sweden.

INTRODUCTION

The extracellular matrix (ECM) of the heart is a three-dimensional stress tolerant network that forms a continuum from the basement membrane (BM) and the cell surface to the interstitial collagens that interconnect the cellular components (1). The BM is a highly specialized structure of the ECM that underlies epithelial cells and surrounds muscle cells (2). Components of the BM are thought to mediate attachment of cells (3,4) and in conjunction with the cytoskeleton to dictate cell shape and polarity (5). We have previously shown that the BM components, collagen type IV (C IV) and laminin (LN) promote attachment, spreading and survival of adult cardiac myocytes *in vitro* (6). Although the synthesis and turnover of BM components has been studied in a number of cell types (7,8,9), it has not been investigated for adult cardiac myocytes. The present study was undertaken to determine if adult cardiac myocytes synthesize and/or remodel these BM components (C IV and LN) as they progress into culture.

MATERIAL AND METHODS

Cell culture

Cardiac myocytes were isolated from adult rat heart by retrograde perfusion with collagenase containing medium as previously described (10). The isolated myocytes were suspended in DMEM culture medium with 0.5 % BSA, plated in 12-well culture dishes (Costar) coated with 20 μg/ml of C IV (Bethesda Research Laboratories) or with 20 μg/ml of LN (11) and allowed to attach for 2 hours at 37°C. The attachment medium was removed and DMEM supplemented with 20 % fetal bovine serum (FBS), 10 μg/ml of ARA-C (Sigma) and antibiotics was added to the cells. The cell cultures were fed every other day with fresh medium.

Radioactive labelling

At various times in culture (1-14 days), the cells were washed three times with methionine-free DMEM (MF-DMEM) and incubated with 50 μCi/ml of ^{35}S-methionine (1330 Ci/mmole, Amersham) and 10 μCi/ml of ^{14}C-Glycine (58 mCi/mmole, Amersham) for 24 hours in MF-DMEM containing 50 μg/ml of sodium ascorbate and 50 μg/ml of β-amino-proprionitrile. After incubation the medium was removed, mixed with protease inhibitors and dialyzed against 0.15 M NaCl, 0.05 mM Tris-HCl, 0.2 % Triton X-100, pH 7.4 containing protease inhibitors.

Immunoprecipitation

Rabbit antibodies against C IV or LN were purified on Protein A-Sepharose (Pharmacia) and LN-Sepharose (LN coupled to Sepharose 4B; Pharmacia). The dialyzed cell culture media were incubated with 50 μg/ml of anti-C IV antibodies, 5 μg/ml of anti-LN antibodies or 50 μg/ml of

Biology of Isolated Adult Cardiac Myocytes
William A. Clark, Robert S. Decker, and Thomas K. Borg, Editors

preimmune IgG and precipitated using Protein A-Sepharose as a carrier (12). Precipitated proteins were analyzed by gradient SDS-PAGE (5-10%) and exposure to Fuji X-ray film at -70°C for 3 weeks.

Immunofluorescence

Freshly isolated myocytes, suspended in DMEM, were plated on glass coverslips coated with 20 μg/ml of C IV or LN. After 1 hour of attachment the cells were fed with DMEM supplemented as above. At various times from 1 hour to 14 days the cultures were washed with PBS, fixed with 2 % paraformaldehyde, washed with 0.1 M glycine and processed for routine immunofluorescence using the affinity purified anti-LN and anti-C IV antibodies.

RESULTS AND DISCUSSION

Metabolic labelling followed by immunoprecipitation showed the production of both LN and C IV by adult cardiac myocytes. Affinity purified anti-LN antibodies precipitated labelled protein bands from the cell culture medium with apparent M_r's in the region expected for LN (220 and 440 kD; Fig. 1 lane A). The anti-C IV antibodies precipitated labelled proteins from the cell media (Fig. 1, lane B) with apparent M_r's similar to the two C IV α-chains (170 and 185 kD). When the precipitated material was digested with a bacterial collagenase known to have a low amount of protease contaminants, both bands were digested indicated that precipitated material indeed was C IV. The anti-LN precipitated material was not affected by collagenase digestion.

Staining of freshly attached myocytes with anti-LN showed that this BM-antigen was present on the cell surface of the myocytes (Fig. 2a). The staining resulted in a uniform background interrupted by a more intense banding pattern indicative of the sarcomeric striations. Anti-C IV did not stain freshly attached myocytes indicating that the collagenase used to isolate the myocytes removed C IV from these cells (Fig. 2d). As the cells spread and progressed into culture, what appeared to be newly synthesized LN could be seen in the focal plane between the cells and the coverslip. The LN radiated into the cell processes and by 5-7 days resulted in a sarcomere-like distribution in many cells with linear striations into the cell processed (Fig. 2b). By 14 days in culture the LN fluorescence formed a dense layer under the cell that contained numerous circular non-fluorescent areas (Fig. 2c). Anti C IV staining showed a delicate honeycombed pattern in the spread cell processes (Fig. 2e) which persisted in many cells at 14 days _in vitro_ (Fig. 2f). The localization of LN in a banding pattern in both the freshly isolated and the cultured cells is significant in light of a recent investigation showing that LN binding proteins are linked to the cytoskeleton (13). The localization of LN near what appeared to be the Z-line of the myocyte places this BM component close to the site of vinculin internally (14) and interstitial collagen fibers externally (1).

SUMMARY

The data presented here indicate that adult myocytes do synthesize both LN and C IV as they progress into culture. Also these BM components are remodeled as the cells adapt to the culture environment. Since the BM is necessary for survival of adult myocytes _in vitro_, future studies will be important toward understanding the role of BM in heart cell function.

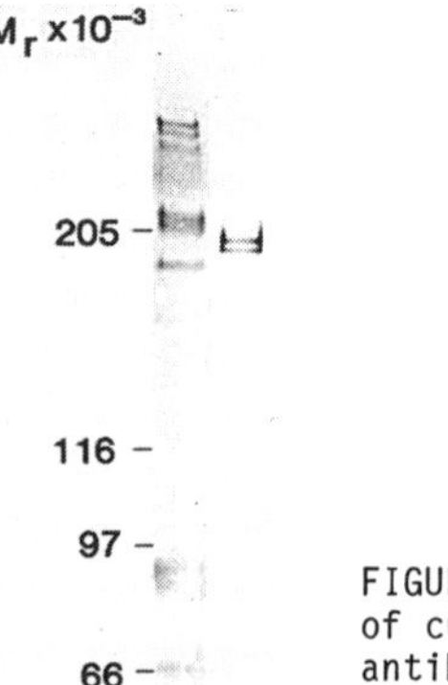

FIGURE 1. Immunoprecipitation of culture medium with anti-LN antibodies (A) and anti-C IV antibodies (B).

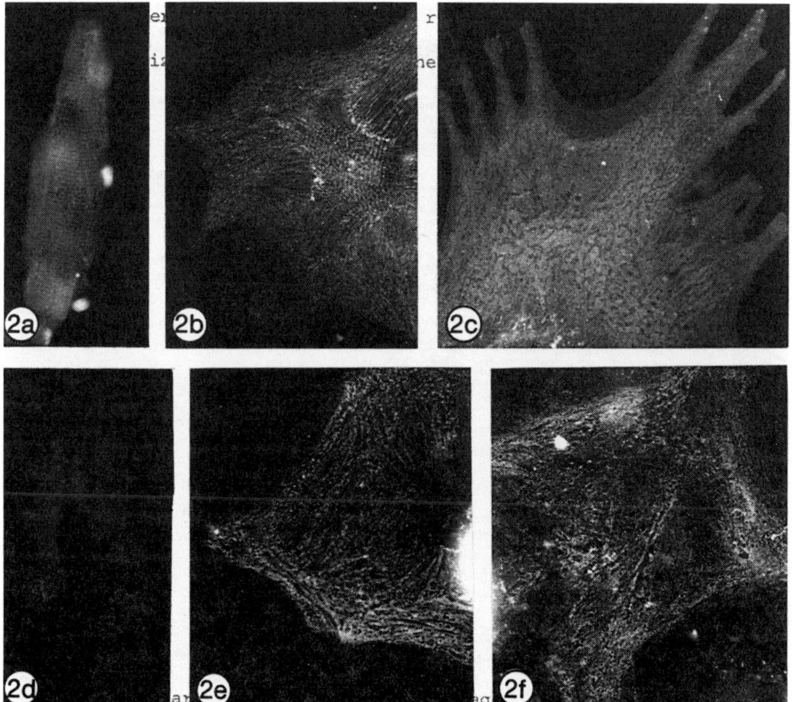

FIGURE 2. Immunofluorescence micrographs of adult cardiac myocytes, stained with anti-LN antibodies (a,b,c) and anti-C IV antibodies (d,e,f) after different times in culture.

ACKNOWLEDGEMENTS

This research was supported from grants from NIH HL-33656, HL-24935, HL-37669 and Swedish Medical Research Council 07466.

REFERENCES

1. T.K. Borg, L. Terracio, E. Lundgren and K. Rubin, in: Cardiac Morphogenesis. Ferrans, Rosenquist and Weinstein, eds (Elsevier 1985) pp. 69-77.
2. D.R. Abrahamson, J. Pathol. 149, 257-278 (1986).
3. J.D. Aplin and R.C. Hughes, Biochim. Biophys. Acta. 694, 375-418 (1982).
4. K.M. Yamada, S.K. Akiyama, T. Hasegawa, E. Hasegawa, M.J. Humphries, D.W. Kennedy, K. Nagata, H. Urushihara, K. Olden, and W-T. Chen, J. Cell. Biol. 28, 79-97 (1985).
5. K.M. Yamada, Ann. Rev. Biochem. 52, 761-799 (1983).
6. E. Lundgren, L. Terracio, S. Mårdh and T.K. Borg, Exp. Cell. Res. 158, 371-381 (1985).
7. U. Kühl, R. Timpl, K. and von der Mark, Dev. Biol. 93, 344-354 (1982).
8. M.J. Warburton, R. Kimbell, P.S. Rudland, S.A. Ferns, and R. Barraclough, J. Cell. Physiol. 128, 76-84 (1986).
9. D. Gospodarowicz, G. Greenburg, J.M. Foidart and N. Savion, J. Cell. Physiol. 107, 171-183 (1981).
10. E. Lundgren, T.K. Borg and S. Mårdh, J. Mol. Cell. Cardiol. 16, 355-362 (1984).
11. H.K. Kleinman, M.L. McGarvey, L.A. Liotta, P. Gehron-Robey, K. Tryggvason and G.R. Martin, Biochemistry 24, 6188-6193 (1982).
12. J.S. Rao, R.L. Beach and B.W. Festoff, Biochem. Biophys. Res. Comm. 130, 440-446 (1985).
13. R.L. Cody and M.S. Wicha, Exp. Cell. Res. 165, 107-116 (1986).
14. J.V. Pardo, J. D'angelo Siliciano and S.W. Craig, J. Cell Biol. 97, 1081-1088 (1983).

SUBCELLULAR REMODELING OF ADULT CARDIAC MYOCYTES IN CELL CULTURE

David G. Simpson*, Marlene L. Decker**, Robert S. Decker* **. Departments of Cell Biology and Anatomy* and Medicine**, Northwestern University Medical School, 303 E. Chicago Ave., Chicago, IL 60611

Quiescent adult rabbit cardiac myocytes undergo a significant subcellular reorganization during primary culture. The cylindrically shaped myocytes retain a rod-like configuration while gradually spreading on the culture substratum. Although the myocytes spread at heterogenous rates, the phenomena commences in a majority of cells within a few hours after attachment to laminin-coated surfaces. Early stages of spreading are characterized by the formation of lamellapodia-like processes in the regions of the cell associated with the remnants of the intercalated disks. Spreading is not restricted to this region however, and by the end of the first week in culture the lateral edges of the rods also exhibit evidence of spreading. As spreading progresses, the architecture of the myofibrillar apparatus and other elements that comprise the cytoskeleton is extensively remodeled. To study how spreading alters the structure of the contractile apparatus and several associated cytoskeletal proteins, an immunofluorescent approach was employed to visualize the relationships between the myofibrillar actin and representative cytoskeletal elements in these cardiac myocytes.

MATERIALS AND METHODS

Cardiac myocytes are obtained from New Zealand white rabbits by a protocol previously described [1]. The resultant cell suspension is plated onto laminin-coated coverslips and cultured in MEM plus 5% fetal calf serum supplemented with 10 um cytosine arbinoside. Coverslips are selected at intervals over a two week period and processed for indirect immunofluorescent microscopy. The actin specific probe, rhodamine phalloidin, is used as a marker for the myofibrillar apparatus and commercially available monoclonal antibodies are employed to localize beta tubulin (Amersham International, Arlington Hts., IL.) and vinculin (Miles Scientific,Naperville, IL.). Polyclonal antisera prepared against BHK 54 and 55 Kd proteins are donated by Dr. R.D. Goldman (Northwestern University, Dept. of Cell Biology and Anatomy). This antisera recognizes common epitopes on the intermediate filament proteins, desmin and vimentin. The distribution of each antigen is compared to the distribution of actin by double-label, indirect immunofluorescent microscopy. Fluorescently conjugated secondary antibodies are the products of Nordic Immunological Laboratories (Capistrano Beach, CA) and Kierkegard and Perry Inc. (Gaithersburg, MD).

RESULTS AND DISCUSSION

Polymers of actin are found in all cell types and comprise major structural components of the myofibrillar apparatus, the subcortical cytoskeleton and stress fibers. Aspects of cell motility, shape, and adhesion are believed to be dependent on the subcellular distribution of actin. The actin of cardiac myocytes is predominantly distributed within the myofibrils where it forms the thin filaments of the contractile apparatus. Throughout the first week of culture, the rhodomine-labeled phalloidin reveals that the myocytes display myofibrils that are in close apposition and full registry (Fig.1A). As the myocytes flatten markedly during the second week, the myofibrils are rearranged and appear to decline in number. This is accompanied by an increase in non-myofibrillar actin cables (Fig.1D). The contractile apparatus of neonatal heart cells [2] also undergoes a similar reorganization in culture, although these events occur in a considerably shorter time frame when compared to adult

Biology of Isolated Adult Cardiac Myocytes
William A. Clark, Robert S. Decker, and Thomas K. Borg, Editors

preparations. During the first 24 hrs. of culture, cell spreading is most evident at the intercalated disks (Fig.1F). The lamellapodia-like processes that originate from these areas exhibit a rhodomine phalloidin staining pattern that is consistent with the actin cables of the subcortical cytoskeleton. These cables often appear to display continuity with existing myofibrils and in a fraction of the spreading processes, phalloidin-positive sarcomeres seem to develop along the microfilaments (Fig.1C). Previous studies of cultured skeletal muscle myotubes suggest that nascent myofibrils may assemble along such actin cables [3]. Over the next three to five days, the lamellapodia-like processes enlarge and the lateral edges of the cells begin to exhibit evidence of spreading (Fig.1C). After two weeks in vitro the myocytes are extensively spread on the culture substratum and most cells reveal sparsely distributed myofibrils that intermingle with numerous stress-fiber-like actin cables. A sub-population of the fully spread myocytes also display a central core that is diffusely labeled by rhodamine phalloidin, suggesting the existence of an actin containing structure that appears distinct from the myofibrillar or stress-fiber-like actin (Fig.1D). The apparent reduction in the complexity of the myofibrillar apparatus may be correlated with several factors including: the loss of contractile function, alteration in neuronal and hormonal balance and minimal cell-to-cell contact. The development of stress fibers in cultured cells is often associated with the formation of adhesion sites with the substratum [4].

Vinculin is a sub-sarcolemmal protein that is closely associated with the cortical actin cytoskeleton and the inner leaflet of the lipid bilayer. In cultured fibroblasts, vinculin is located where actin stress fibers terminate in adhesion plaques. The subcellular distribution of vinculin implicates it in the formation of a macromolecular complex that mediates the attachment of the actin cytoskeleton to the plasma membrane [4]. However, the evidence supporting this hypothesis remains controversial [5,6]. Previous immunofluorescent studies with cardiac myocytes demonstrate that vinculin is a component of the fascia adherens junction of the intercalated disk as well as encircling the contractile apparatus along the costameres at the Z-lines [7]. The regular array of vinculin along the costameres suggests that this protein may be localized near the attachment site of the myofibrillar apparatus to the sarcolemma [7]. On day one of culture, the intercalated disks of the adult cardiac myocytes are intensely labeled by the anti-vinculin probes and the Z-lines are clearly discernible (Fig.1E). With the onset of spreading, the intensity of the fluorescent staining at the intercalated disks gradually diminishes and in the majority of cells, disappears entirely by the 7th day in culture. In such myocytes vinculin retains its normal Z-line location along the central myofibrillar core, but in the peripherally spread portions of the cell, vinculin staining loses its alignment along the costameres (Fig.1G). Anti-vinculin antibodies are also observed in regions where actin cables and myofibrils appear as continuous structures (Fig.1G). The significance of this staining pattern is unknown, but it may reflect a modification of the attachment site of the myofibril to the sarcolemma which develops in the absence of an intercalated disk. In fully spread myocytes, vinculin is distributed longitudinally along the stress fiber-like actin cables and the existing myofibrils (Fig.1H). The coordinated redistribution of vinculin with respect to the myofibrillar apparatus supports the hypothesis that this subsarcolemmal protein may be instrumental in the reorganization and/or assembly of contractile elements [8].

Desmin is a principle structural element of the Z- and intercalated disks of cardiac myocytes. Lazarides [9] speculates that desmin in the Z-disks acts to mechanically integrate the myofibrillar apparatus during the contractile cycle. Furthermore, Fuseler [10] suggests that intermediate

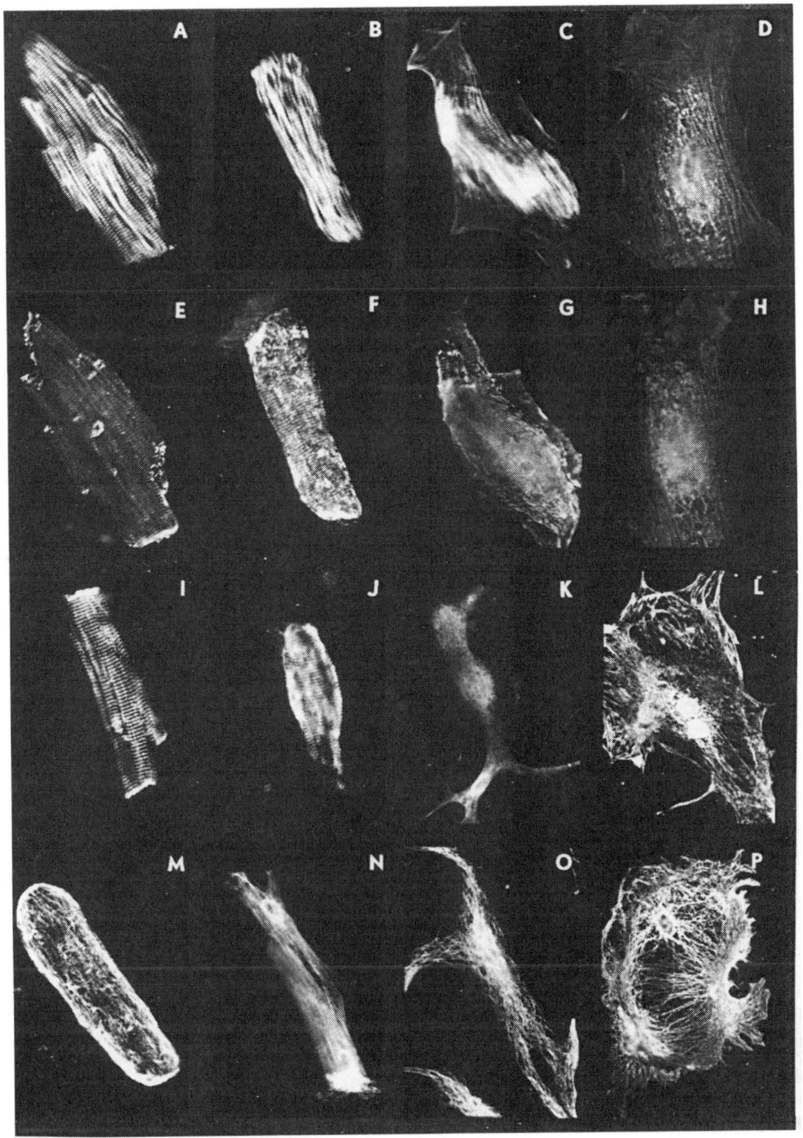

Figure 1. Cardiac myocytes cultured for 1 hr. (A,E,I,M), 1-3 days (B,F,J,N), 4-8 days (C,G,K,O) and 14 days (D,H,L,P). Actin (A,B,C,D), vinculin (E,F,G,H), desmin (I,J,K,L) and tubulin (M,N,O,P). Double immunofluorescent images of actin (A,B,C,D) and vinculin (E,F,G,H).

filaments provide a scaffolding for the assembly of myofibrils during embryogenesis. As the remnants of the intercalated disks are internalized during the first week in culture, desmin staining disappears, suggesting that it is degraded during the early phases of spreading (Fig.1I,J,K). The lamellapodia-like processes that develop in this region exhibit a filamentous pattern when stained with anti-desmin antibodies (Fig.1J). A similar filamentous network of desmin-containing structures replaces the Z-disk staining associated with the contractile apparatus. The redistribution of desmin from the Z-disks appears to be temporally related to the separation and subsequent reduction in the alignment of the myofibrillar apparatus. Myocytes cultured for two weeks disclose a diffuse network of intermediate filaments that do not exhibit any obvious spatial relationships with the remaining myofibrils (Fig.1L). Our present studies support the hypothesis that desmin may function to integrate and stabilize the myofibrillar apparatus [9].

Microtubules represent a third major cytoskeletal element whose role in the maintenance of myocytic organization is poorly understood. Microtubules are implicated in mediating intracellular organelle movement and in the regulation of cell shape [11]. In cultured skeletal muscle myotubes, Toyama [12] hypothesizes that microtubules interdigitate with myosin thick filaments during the assembly of sarcomeres. Freshly isolated cardiac myocytes attached to laminin-coated surfaces display microtubules that are arrayed parallel to the long axis of the cell with numerous transverse components visible in the sarcoplasm. These microtubules appear to form a network that subdivides the contractile apparatus (Fig. 1M). Like polymers of actin and intermediate filaments, microtubules appear to rapidly proliferate into the lamellapodia-like processes of actively spreading myocytes (DAYS 1-4, Fig.1N,O). The polymerized tubulin in these regions appears to originate from either preexisting microtubules or from microtubule organizing centers located near the proximal origins of the lamellapodia-like processes. Perinuclear microtubule organizing centers are nearly invisible in freshly prepared cells, but as the myocytes spread, vivid arrays of microtubules encompass both myocytic nuclei (Fig.1P). These regions often appear as nucleating sites for the microtubules found in the distal lamellapodia of the myocytes. After 14 days in culture myocytes exhibit elaborate arrays of microtubules that are not polarized with respect to the existing myofibrils or other cytoskeletal elements. The distribution of microtubules during the spreading process reaffirms the notion that this cytoskeletal system may be involved in the regulation of cell shape [11] and is not directly correlated with the reorganization of the myofibrillar apparatus.

CONCLUSION

Cultured adult cardiac myocytes offer a unique opportunity to study the structural and functional organization of the myofibrillar apparatus and related components of the cytoskeleton. The present investigation illustrates that an extensive and coordinated redistribution of these structural elements occurs as the myocytes spread in culture. There is evidence to suggest that the quiescent state of the cells is a significant contributing factor to the observed reorganization of the myofibrillar apparatus. The apparent decline in the number of myofibrils and the parallel reorganization of desmin in the Z-disks resembles the changes that occur during disuse atrophy of adult skeletal muscle tissue [13]. This implies that contractile function exerts a tonic influence on the structural integrity of the myofibrillar apparatus. Other factors which may contribute to the events described in the present study may include the absence of neuronal or hormonal input and the lack of the hemodynamic forces which are normally encountered in the intact heart. The effect of serum factors and the two dimensional environment in which the cells are maintained must also be considered. The principle advantage of this culture system is that it provides an avenue to directly study the effects of these variables on myofibrillar organization.

ACKNOWLEDGMENTS

This study is supported by U.S. Public Health Service grant HL33616. The authors express their appreciation to Melissa Green and Monica Behnke for technical assistance and to Debbie Bland and Belinda Berthold-Coichy for their help in preparing this manuscript. Our thanks to Mr. Robert Hughes (W. Nuhsbaum, Inc.) and Dr. J.C.R. Jones (Northwestern University, Dept. of Cell Biology and Anatomy) for sharing their technical expertise. D.G. Simpson is a recipient of a Lucille P. Markey Pre-Doctoral Fellowship in the Department of Cell Biology and Anatomy.

REFERENCES

1. J. Haddad, M.L. Decker, L-C. Hsieh, M. Lesch, A.M. Samarel, and R.S. Decker, Am. J. Physiol (Cell Physiol.). In Press, 1987.
2. B.T. Atherton, D.M. Meyer, and D.G. Simpson, J. Cell Science 86: 233 (1986).
3. P.B. Antin, S. Tokunaka, V. Nachmias, and H. Holtzer. J. Cell Bio. 102: 464 (1986).
4. B. Geiger, Biochimica et Biophysics Acta, 737: 305-341 (1983).
5. J. Wilkins, S. and Lin, Cell, 28: 83 (1982).
6. J. Wilkins, S. and Lin, J. Cell Bio. 102: 1085 (1986).
7. S. Craig, in: Cardiac Morphogenesis, V. Ferrans, G. Rosenquist and C. Weinstein, eds. (Elsevier, New York 1985) pp. 105-111.
8. A. Plugosz, P. Antin, V. Nachimias, and H. Holtzer, J. Cell Bio. 99: 2268 (1984).
9. E. Lazarides, Ann. Rev. Biochem 51: 219 (1982).
10. J.W. Fuseler, J.W. Shay, and H. Feit, Cell Mus. Motil 1: 205 (1981).
11. P. Dustin, in: Microtubules, P. Dustin ed. (Springer-Verlag, New York 1984) pp. 234-259, 322-345.
12. Y. Toyama, S. Forry-Schaudies, B. Hoffman, and H. Holtzer, Proc. Natl. Acad. Sci. USA 79: 6556 (1982).
13. S. Jacobson and H.M. Piper, J. Molec. Cell, Cardiol., 18: 661 (1986).

ULTRASTRUCTURAL ALTERATION OF CULTURED ADULT RAT VENTRICULAR CARDIAC MYOCYTES BY TPA AND DIACYLGLYCEROLS

R.L. MOSES and W.C. CLAYCOMB,*
Department of Anatomy,and Biochemistry and Molecular Biology*
LSU Medical Center, 1100 Florida Avenue, New Orleans,LA 70119

INTRODUCTION

Previous studies have established that adult rat ventricular cardiac muscle cells synthesize DNA when grown in culture. This DNA synthesis can be stimulated by the phorbol ester tumor promotor 12-0-tetradecanoyl-phorbol-13-acetate (TPA) as well as diacylglycerol (DAG). These compounds also stimulate protein accumulation. We, therefore, examined TPA- and DAG-treated adult myocytes in order to investigate the structural correlates of these altered biosynthetic capabilities. Control treatments included dimethyl sulfoxide (the TPA carrier), ethanol (the DAG carrier), and the α and β inactive TPA analogs.

MATERIALS AND METHODS

Ventricular cardiac muscle cells were isolated from adult (200-250g) female Holtzman rats and cultured according to previously published methods [1, 2]. Cells were treated with TPA (50 ng/ml) in DMSO (0.02%) or DAG (50μ g/ml) in ethanol (0.01%). Controls were treated with DMSO or ethanol at the same concentrations. Some cultures were exposed to the nontumor promotor phorbol ester α or β analogs. Treatments were for five days and were begun on the seventh day of culture.

Cultured ventricular muscle cells were processed for en face, in situ, transmission electron microscopy (TEM) as previously described [3]. Cells were fixed in glutaraldehyde, and postfixed in either osmium tetroxide or osmium ferrocyanide.

RESULTS

At the light microscopic level, the most obvious effect of TPA treatment was an increase in cell size (Fig. 1). Myocytes treated with DAG, DMSO, ethanol, or inactive phorbol ester analogs were the same size as control (untreated) cells.

Ultrastructural (TEM) examination of the TPA-treated myocytes demonstrated the chemical's disruptive effect on myofibril organization. Typically organized myofibrils were difficult to locate in TPA-treated cells. Myofilaments were scarce, and Z lines were diminished in frequency and of irregular morphology when present. Occasionally, T tubes were associated with these anomalous Z lines. Large collections of intermediate (10 nm) filaments were also frequently present in the cytoplasm. DAG-treated myocytes also possessed these ultrastructural cytoskeleton characteristics, although the disruption of typical myocyte cytoarchitecture was less complete in these cells. DMSO, ethanol, and the inactive α and β analogs had no effect on myocyte ultrastructure (compare Figs. 2 and 3) and resembled those described by us previously [1, 3]. TPA and DAG treated cells also frequently possessed leptomeres [4] (Fig. 3b). Intercalated discs and gap junctions were found between TPA- and DAG-treated cells.

Biology of Isolated Adult Cardiac Myocytes
William A. Clark, Robert S. Decker, and Thomas K. Borg, Editors

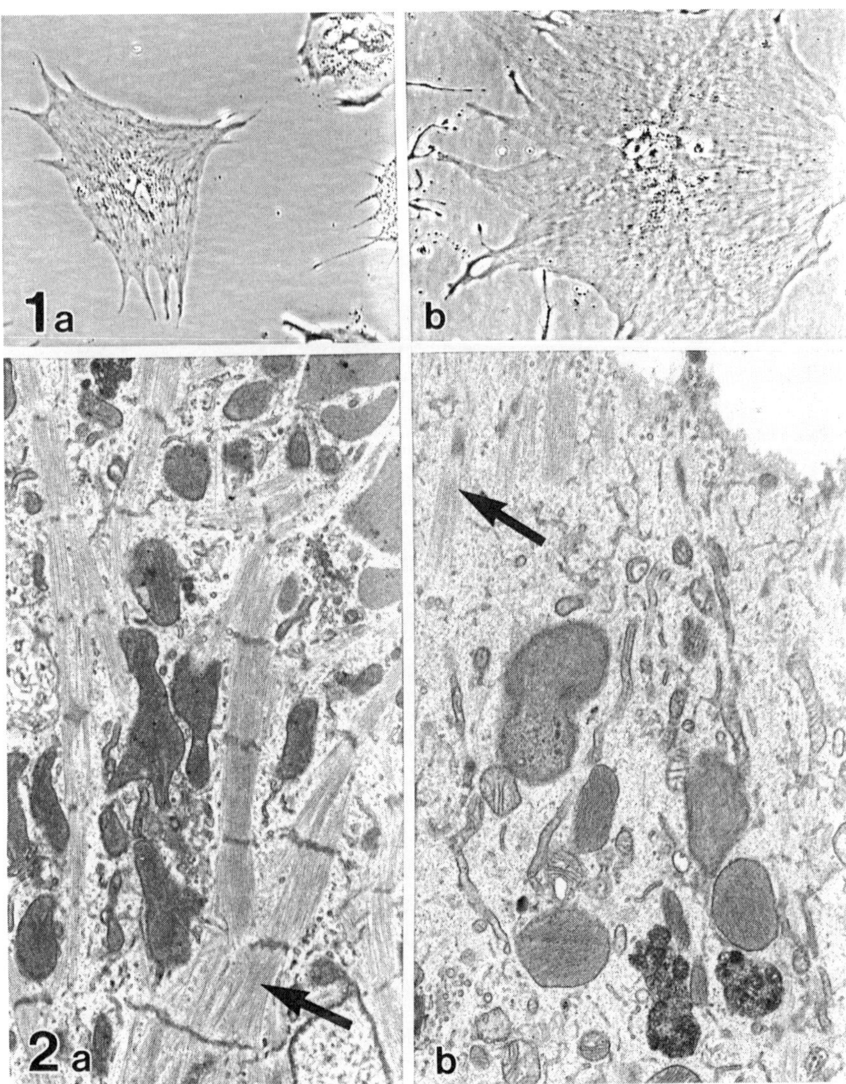

Figure 1. Light micrographs of control (a) and TPA-treated (b) cultured adult myocytes. Note the increased sized of the TPA-treated cell. (X140)

Figure 2. Electron micrographs of DMSO- (a) and DAG-treated (b) myocytes. Ethanol-treated myocytes (not illustrated), which served as the control for DAG, were similar to those treated with DMSO (the control for TPA, see Figure 3). Note the more regular sarcomeric organization in the control cell (arrow). Myofilament organization in the DAG-treated cell is minimal and irregular (arrow). (osmium ferrocyanide postfixation) (both micrographs X10,200)

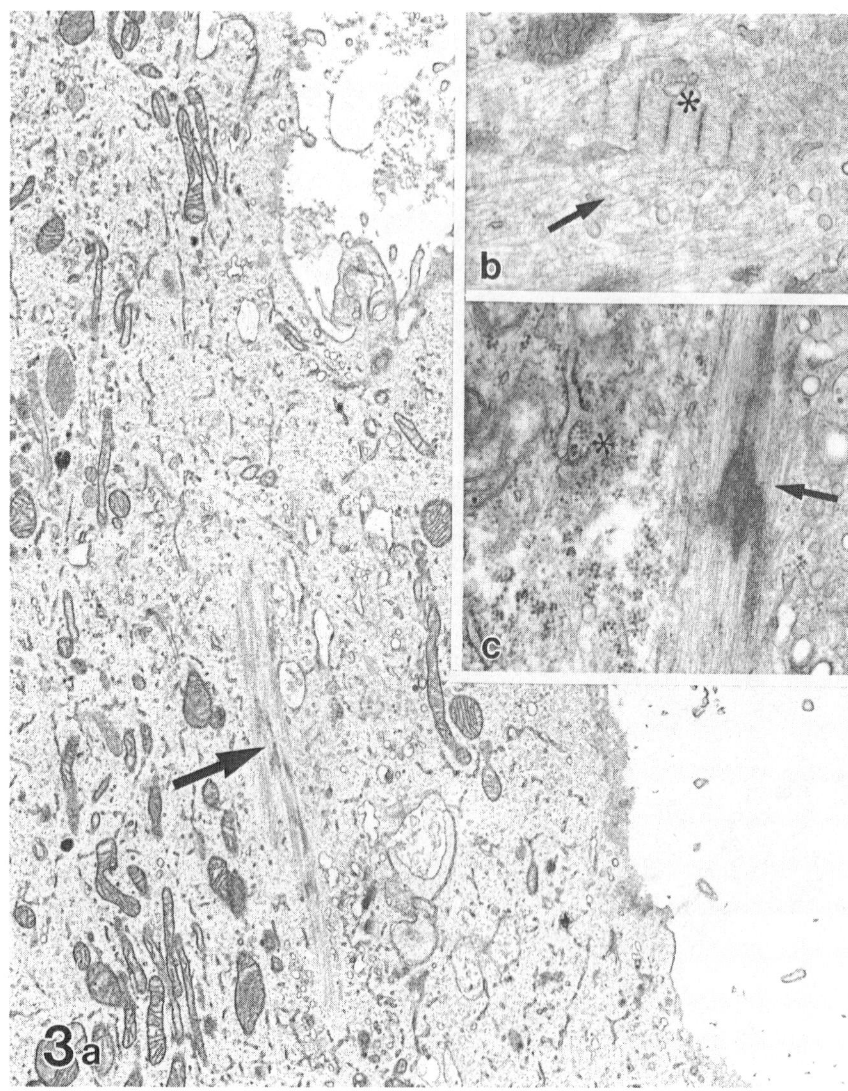

Figure 3. (a) Low power electron micrograph of TPA-treated myocytes. Note the absence of organized sarcomeres. The arrow indicates an area of minimal myofilament organization. (b) Region in a TPA-treated myocyte containing a leptomere (*) and numerous intermediate filaments (arrow). (c) Myofilament organization in a TPA-treated myocyte (arrow), and free polysomes and rough endoplasmic reticulum (*). (a,b; osmium ferrocyanide postfixation. c; osmium tetroxide postfixation) (a, X10,200; b, c, X21,400)

Both TPA- and DAG-treated myocytes contained large quantities of free ribosomes as well as numerous cisternae of rough endoplasmic reticulum (Fig. 3c). Golgi complexes were also well developed.

DISCUSSION

Our studies show that TPA induces myofibrillar disorganization in cultured adult rat ventricular cardiac myocytes in a manner similar to that observed in TPA-treated cultured skeletal myotubes [5]. The accumulation of intermediate filaments is not totally unexpected, since Holtzer and his coworkers have previously reported that TPA uncouples desmin synthesis from the synthesis of other muscle-specific proteins [6]. The increased frequency of leptomeres in TPA- and DAG-treated cultures may also reflect altered biosynthetic parameters.

Our biochemical studies have shown that TPA- and DAG-treated myocytes accumulate large amounts of protein [7, 8]. The morphological correlate of the synthetic capacity for this protein accumulation is the free polysomes and RER cisternae in the treated cells. The free ribosomes are probably involved in the production of both intermediate filaments and myofilaments [9]. The proteins synthesized on membrane bound ribosomes are more problematical and must await further investigation. Secretory granules, such as those described in cultured atrial myocytes [10 11], were not observed. Both TPA and DAG had similar effects on myocyte ultrastructure, as would be expected since the effects of both chemicals are mediated by protein kinase C.

In summary, our studies show that TPA and DAG induce similar ultrastructural disorganization in cultured adult rat ventricular muscle cells. This morphological plasticity should be useful in investigating cardiac muscle cell differentiation, growth, and proliferation.

This work was supported by NIH Grants HL 25873 and HL 35632.

REFERENCES

1. W.C. Claycomb and M.C. Palazzo, Develop. Biol., 80: 466-482 (1980).
2. W.C. Claycomb and N.G. Lanson, Jr., In Vitro, 20: 647-651 (1984).
3. R.L. Moses and W.C. Claycomb, Am. J. Anat., 164: 113-131 (1982).
4. R. Caesar, G.A. Edwards, and H. Ruska, Z. Zellforsch., 48: 698-719 (1958).
5. J. Croop, G. Dubyak, Y. Toyama, A. Dlugosz, A. Scarpa, and H. Holtzer, Dev. Biol., 89: 460-474 (1982).
6. H. Holtzer, S. Farry-Schaudies, P. Antin, G. Dubyak, and V. Nachmias, Adv. Exp. Biol. Med., 182: 179-192 (1985).
7. W.C. Claycomb, Biology of Isolated Cardiac Myocytes, W.A. Clark, T.K. Borg, and R.S. Decker, eds., Elsevier, in press.
8. W. C. Claycomb and R.L. Moses, submitted.
9. R.L. Moses and W.C. Calycomb, J. Ultrastruct. Res., 81: 358-374 (1982)
10. R.L. Moses and W.C. Claycomb, Am. J. Anat. 171: 191-206 (1984).
11. W.C. Claycomb and R.L. Moses, Exp. Cell Res., 161: 95-100 (1985).

VISUALIZATION OF MEMBRANE AND CYTOSKELETAL PROTEINS IN PERMEABILIZED ISOLATED ADULT CARDIAC MYOCYTES BY IMMUNOHISTOCHEMICAL AND MORPHOLOGICAL METHODS

D.A. MESSINA*, Y. ISOBE*, M. DELMAR**, AND L.F. LEMANSKI*
Departments of Anatomy and Cell Biology* and Pharmacology**, SUNY Health Science Center, Syracuse, NY 13210

INTRODUCTION

We are examining contractile/cytoskeletal/membrane protein relationships in the mammalian heart. Specifically, we are interested in the way in which myofibrils and related cytoskeletal elements interact with the sarcolemma. To accomplish these goals we isolated adult hamster and guinea pig cardiac myocytes permeabilized using 0.2% saponin and 0.5% Triton X-100. These methods of permeabilization were used to allow antibody access to cytoskeletal and myofibrillar proteins and are compared with one another for their usefullness in this study.

METHODS

Dissociation of Adult Guinea Pig and Hamster Heart Tissue

Single ventricular myocytes are obtained by enzymatic dissociation of adult guinea pig and hamster hearts according to Isenberg et al. [1]. Some modifications were necessary to accommodate the hamster perfusion, these included using 0.5 mg/ml of collagenase and 1 mg/ml of hyaluronidase for a 40 minute time period. After perfusion the ventricles were cut into pieces and the cells released by gentle agitation.

Permeabilization

Isolated cells were filtered through a nylon mesh and spun down using a Boekel hand-driven centrifuge to minimize cellular damage. The resulting pellet of cardiac cells was resuspended in HEPES buffer (70 mM KCl; 5mM $MgCl_2$, 3mM EGTA, 30mM HEPES and 0.25mM PMSF; pH=7.0) and distributed into two equivalent sized aliquots. One aliquot was treated with 0.2% saponin, in HEPES buffer and the other was treated with 0.5% Triton for 5 minutes. After rinsing 3 times with the same buffer, some cells were placed on poly-L-lysine (1 mg/ml) coated coverslips for light microscopic experiments while specimens for electron microscopy remained in suspension. Both specimens were then fixed with 2% formaldehyde for 5 minutes.

Immunohistochemistry

Permeabilized cells were incubated with 3% Carnation instant dry milk in HEPES buffer for 15 minutes to block non-specific staining. Specimens were incubated with anti-human red blood cell spectrin (Transformation Research, Inc.) or anti-porcine skeletal muscle α-actinin (Transformation Research, Inc.) diluted 20 fold and 30 fold, respectively for 3 hours, at room temperature, with agitation. After several rinses with the buffer, FITC conjugated goat anti-rabbit secondary (Miles; diluted 60 fold) or 5 nm colloidal gold conjugated goat anti-rabbit secondary (Janssen; diluted 4 fold) was applied for 3 hours. Silver enhancement was performed on colloidal gold stained cells using Janssen's kit after 5 minutes fixation with 2% glutaraldehyde.

Biology of Isolated Adult Cardiac Myocytes
William A. Clark, Robert S. Decker, and Thomas K. Borg, Editors

Thin-section Electron Microscopy

Dissociated cardiac myocytes were stained with anti-spectrin and colloidal gold conjugated secondary after permeabilization with Triton. These specimens were fixed with glutaraldehyde and osmium tetroxide. They were embedded in epoxy resin, then ultrathin-sectioned, and stained one minute each with lead citrate and uranyl acetate. Sections were viewed on a JEOL 100CX-II transmission electron microscope at 80 kV.

Deep-freeze Etching

For deep-freeze etching, isolated cardiac myocytes were permeabilized with saponin and immunostained with anti-spectrin and colloidal gold. After fixation with glutaraldehyde and osmium tetroxide, they were pelleted, and frozen by plunging them into liquid nitrogen cooled Freon 13 using 70% ethanol as a volatile cryoprotectant. The samples were transferred into a freeze fracture apparatus, fractured and deep etched for 5-10 minutes at -90°C. Replicas were made on a rotating stage with platinum at a shadowing angle of 20° and carbon at 90°. Replicas were cleaned with household bleach and examined with a JEOL 100CX-II electron microscope operated at 100 kV.

RESULTS AND DISCUSSION

Isolated adult guinea pig and hamster cardiac myocytes, permeabilized by treatment with saponin or Triton show excellent morphological preservation while maintaining easy access of antibodies to structural proteins. This methodology eliminates artifacts associated with conventional freezing/embedding and sectioning protocols and provides us with a 3-dimensional view of the subject matter. Cells can be immunohistochemically analyzed using light and electron microscopic means.

Cells permeabilized with saponin exhibited very little non-specific staining if they were incubated with our secondary antibody alone (fig. 1). The results obtained using our primary antibodies against spectrin and α-actinin are shown in figure 2. Anti-spectrin specifically stained Z-bands, intercalated discs and the sarcolemma of isolated cardiac myocytes treated with saponin, using either fluorescent (fig. 2a) or silver-enhanced gold (fig. 2b) labeling. In addition to Z-band and intercalated disc specific staining the anti-α-actinin antibody occasionally stained the M-lines (fig. 2c and d) of saponin treated cells.

Cells permeabilized with Triton show similar results to the saponin treated samples. In figure 3a, anti-spectrin antibody labels Z-bands, intercalated disc and perinuclear regions. Anti-α-actinin antibody (fig. 3b) exhibited a similar staining pattern seen in fig. 2. The use of saponin and Triton for permeabilizing isolated cardiac myocytes allows us to visualize spectrin and to analyze its distribution relative to the myofibrils. Spectrin label was found in Z-band and intercalated disc regions. Spectrin may be participating in myofibril organization by aligning adjacent myofibrils and anchoring them to the sarcolemma.

In order to view the relationship between spectrin and myofibrils

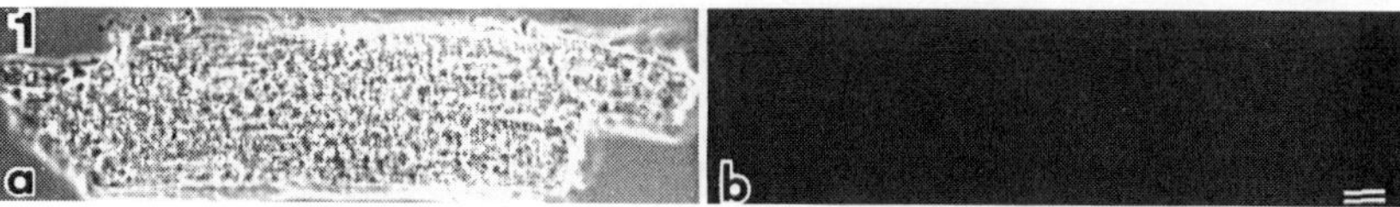

Fig. 1. Light micrographs of saponin treated cells. (a) phase contrast (b) stained with FITC-conjugated secondary antibody alone. Bar represents 10 μm.

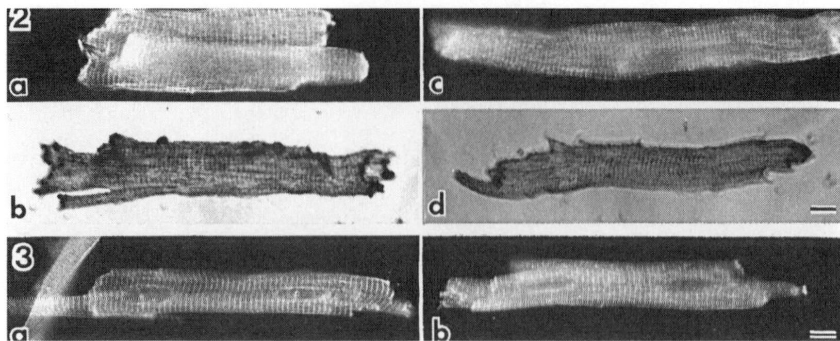

Fig. 2. Light micrographs of saponin treated cells. Stained with anti-spectrin antibodies using (a) FITC-conjugated secondary, (b) silver-enhanced colloidal gold-conjugated secondary. Stained with anti-α-actinin antibodies using (c) FITC-conjugated secondary, (d) silver-enhanced colloidal gold-conjugated secondary. Bar represents 10 μm.

Fig. 3. Light micrographs of Triton treated cells (a) stained with anti-spectrin antibodies or (b) stained with anti-α-actinin antibodies. Bar represents 10 μm.

with greater precision we analyzed isolated, adult, cardiac myocytes stained with spectrin antibody and gold-labeled secondary probes at the electron microscopic level. Triton treated, resin embedded and thin sectioned cells exhibit well-preserved filamentous structures while almost all membranes are removed. Colloidal gold tags representing the distribution of spectrin are found mainly around Z bands, associated with intermyofibrillar filaments and dense material (Fig. 4). The latter structures may represent the aggregation of the primary antibody.

Freeze-fracture, deep etching is performed on cells permeabilized with saponin and immunostained with anti-spectrin and colloidal gold to obtain a three-dimensional view of these relationships. The resultant replica (fig. 5) shows excellent preservation of myofibrils, intervening filamentous systems and residual membranous regions. The majority of the spectrin label is seen in the vicinity of filamentous structures at the level of the myofibrillar Z-band region, however, the membranes that

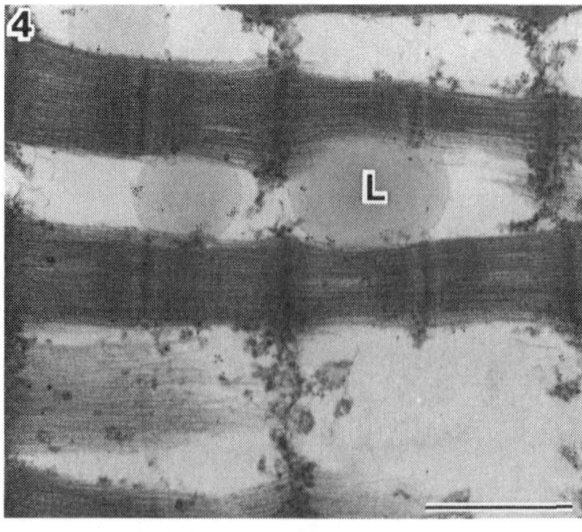

Fig. 4. Thin section electron micrograph of a Triton-permeabilized myocyte stained with anti-spectrin antibody and colloidal gold conjugated secondary antibody. Triton has removed membranous structures and leaves myofibrils intact. Gold particles are mainly associated with dense material located between myofibrils at the level of the Z-bands, and occasionally at the M-lines. Lipid droplets (L). Bar represents 1 μm.

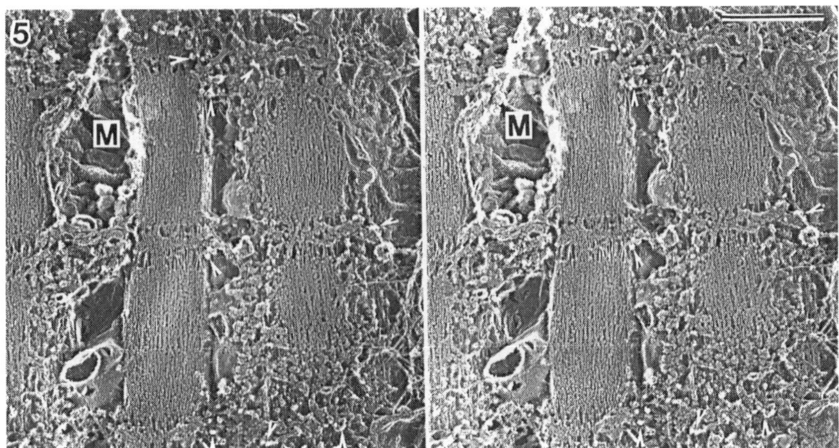

Fig. 5. Stereo micrographs exhibiting a freeze-fracture and deep etching image of a saponin treated cell. Membranous structures as well as myofibrils can be seen. Gold particles (arrowheads) indicating spectrin localization are found around Z-bands, between membranous residues (M). Bar represents 1 μm.

remain after treatment with saponin interfere with antibody access and our ability to view gold particles in surrounding areas. We are currently engaged in utilizing Triton X-100 to remove all membranous structures in order for us to view the gold particles more clearly.

Thus, it appears that permeabilized isolated adult hamster, and guinea pig cardiac myocytes provide an excellent model system to study cytoskeletal and myofibrillar interactions. Our use of spectrin antibody has revealed that spectrin is present between myofibrils, at the Z-band region, and adjacent to the sarcolemma at the intercalated disc region. These findings differ from previous studies of spectrin distribution in avian muscle where spectrin is limited to the cell membrane in areas overlying each Z-band [2-5]. Our cytoplasmic localization of spectrin in addition to its membrane position in mammalian cardiac myocytes may reflect differences between mammalian and avian myocytes. Interestingly, dystrophic avian skeletal muscle shows internal staining for spectrin [5]. Spectrin has also been found associated with cytoplasmic structures in mammalian brain tissue [6]. Spectrin, may participate in a wider range of cellular functions than previously proposed, especially in specialized cell types such as mammalian neurons and myocytes.

This work was supported by NIH grants HL32184 and HL37702 to LFL, HL29439 to MD, and grants from AHA to LFL and MD.

REFERENCES

1. G. Isenberg, U. Klockner, Pflugers Arch. 395, 6-18 (1982).
2. S.R. Goodman, I.S. Zagon, R.R. Kulikowski, Proc. Natl. Acad. Sci. 78, 7570-7574 (1981).
3. E.A. Repasky, B.L. Granger, E. Lazarides, Cell 29, 821-833 (1982).
4. W.J. Nelson, E. Lazarides, Proc. Natl. Acad, Sci. 80, 363-367 (1983).
5. E.A. Repasky, C.M. Pollina, M.M. Menold, M.S. Hudecki, Proc. Natl. Acad. Sci. 83, 802-806 (1986).
6. I.S. Zagon, R. Higbee, B.M. Riederer, S.R. Goodman, J of Neuroscience 6, 2977-2986.

CELL-SURFACE BOUND LAMININ MEDIATES ATTACHMENT OF ISOLATED ADULT MYOCYTES TO COLLAGEN TYPE IV

Evy Lundgren*, Louis Terracio**, Donald Gullberg*,
Thomas K. Borg** and Kristofer Rubin*.
* Department of Medical and Physiological Chemistry, Uppsala University, Box 575, S-751 23 Uppsala, Sweden.
** Departments of Anatomy and Pathology, University of South Carolina, Columbia, South Carolina, 29208.

INTRODUCTION

Recent investigations have increased the knowledge about cell-surface molecules involved in adhesion of cells to extracellular matrix (ECM) components (1). Cell-matrix interactions that can promote spreading and reorganization of the cytoskeleton most likely involve specific membrane bound receptors that directly or indirectly are connected with cytoskeletal proteins (2). The existence of such receptors has now been postulated for a number of ECM components such as fibronectin (3), laminin (4) and collagen (5,6).

The basement membrane that separates epithelial and endothelial cells from the underlying stroma and surrounds muscle cells (7) is a specialized structure of the ECM. The basement membrane components laminin (LN) and collagen type IV (C IV) have both been shown to mediate attachment of cells *in vitro* (4,8,9,10) and to influence growth and differentiation of several cell types in culture (11,12).

Interactions between LN and C IV have been demonstrated in several investigations (13,14,15). In cell adhesion experiments LN has been shown to mediate attachment of some epithelial cells to C IV (16).

In previous investigations we have reported that adult cardiac myocytes adhere readily to dishes coated with C IV or LN, weakly to fibronectin and not at all to interstitial collagen type I (C I). Only the basement membrane components C IV and LN promote survival and progression of the myocytes into high density cultures (12). This is in contrast to neonatal myocytes that also adhere to collagen types I, II, III, and V and to fibronectin (9). In this study we further examined the interaction between adult cardiac myocytes and C IV and LN.

MATERIALS AND METHODS

Adult rat cardiac myocytes were isolated as previously described (10). Isolated cells were washed and suspended in buffer A (136.9 mM NaCl, 4.7 mM KCl, 3.2 mM $MgSO_4 x 7H_2O$, 6.1 mM $CaCl_2 xH_2O$ and 50 mM HEPES) containing 0.5 % bovine serum albumin (BSA; Sigma). C IV was obtained from Bethesda Research Laboratories. LN (17), C I (18) and pepsin solubilized collagen type IV (pepsin-C IV; 19) were prepared as described.

Rabbit antibodies against C IV and LN were purified on protein-A Sepharose (Pharmacia) followed by laminin-Sepharose (laminin coupled to CNBr-activated Sepharose 4B; Pharmacia).

Multiwell dishes (16 mm, Costar) were coated overnight at 4°C with 20 µg/ml of C IV, pepsin-C IV, C I or LN diluted in buffer A. In experiments where attachment to collagen substrates was studied after incubation with LN, collagen-coated dishes were incubated with 1 % BSA in buffer A for 1 hour at 4°C, washed and incubated with various concentrations of LN for 4 hours at 4°C. The cells were plated at a density of 0.5-1 x 10^5 cells per well and allowed to attach for 1 hour at 37°C.

Biology of Isolated Adult Cardiac Myocytes
William A. Clark, Robert S. Decker, and Thomas K. Borg, Editors

The dishes were washed twice and the number of attached cells was determined using the method described by Landegren (20).

Antibodies against C IV or LN were incubated with freshly isolated myocytes in buffer A with 0.5% BSA for 20 minutes at 37°C. The cells were then plated in multiwell dishes coated with C IV or LN and plated either in the presence of antibodies or after the cells had been washed free from unbound antibodies.

RESULTS AND DISCUSSION

Adhesion of adult myocytes to ECM components

The basement membrane collagen (type IV) is different from interstitial collagens by having a globular, pepsin sensitive domain, denoted NC1 (21). Pepsin treatment of native C IV destroyed the ability of C IV to interact with adult myocytes. However, after incubation with soluble LN this substrate could promote attachment. Figure 1 shows attachment of adult myocytes to dishes that have been coated with C IV, pepsin-C IV, C I or left uncoated followed by coating with LN at different concentrations. These results indicate that collagen type IV contains binding sites for LN on the pepsin resistant part of the molecule. LN could not promote attachment of myocytes to C I. The interaction between LN and the different collagens was also studied in an enzyme linked immunosorbent assay (ELISA). LN bound to both native and pepsin treated C IV but with a lower affinity for the latter substrate (data not shown). The affinity of antibodies against NC1 (a generous gift from Dr. Brooks, Hoecht, West Germany) for the collagen substrates was also studied in ELISA. Anti-NC1 antibodies bound only to native C IV (data not shown) indicating that the globular domain had been digested during the pepsin treatment.

Several binding sites for LN have been demonstrated on the C IV molecule (14). A possible explanation for why cell-surface associated LN could not mediate attachment of LN to pepsin-C IV in this investigation while soluble LN promoted attachment to this substrate is that the binding site(s) remaining on C IV after pepsin treatment may have lower affinity for cell-surface bound LN compared to the LN binding sites on the native C IV.

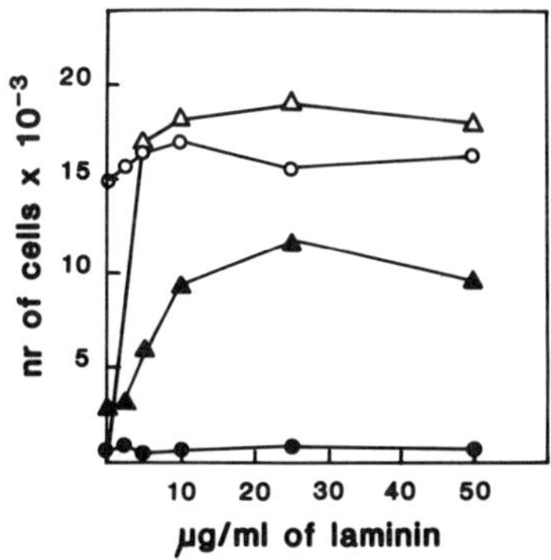

FIG 1. Attachment of myocytes to dishes initially coated with 20 µg/ml of C IV (○), pepsin-C IV (▲) or C I (●), then incubated with LN at the indicated concentrations. Attachment of myocytes to dishes coated with LN (△) at the indicated concentrations.

Effect of anti-laminin and anti-collagen type IV antibodies on attachment of adult myocytes

Affinity purified anti-LN antibodies inhibited attachment of myocytes to dishes coated with C IV (Fig. 2). This inhibition was seen both when the cells were plated in the presence of antibody (Fig. 2a) and when the cells were washed free of unbound antibodies prior to plating (Fig. 2b). This indicated that cell-surface bound LN mediated attachment of the myocytes to C IV. Attachment of adult myocytes to LN coated dishes was also inhibited by anti-LN antibodies but only at high concentrations (Fig. 2a) and this effect was not seen when the cells were washed prior to plating (Fig. 2b), indicating that the antibodies bound to the substrate and blocked the LN-myocyte interaction. Incubation of the myocytes with anti-C IV antibodies had no effect on either LN or C IV coated dishes (Figs. 2c and 2d).

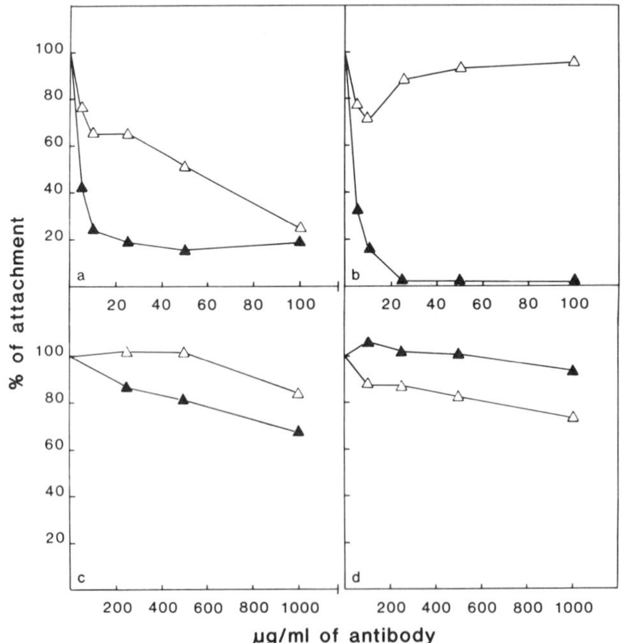

FIG. 2. Attachment of myocytes to dishes coated with LN (△) or C IV (▲) after incubation with anti-LN (a and b) or anti-C IV (c and d). The cells were either plated in the presence of antibodies (a and c) or after they were washed (b and d).

SUMMARY

The results of the present investigation demonstrate an interaction between collagen type IV and laminin and that cell surface bound laminin mediates attachment of adult cardiac myocytes to collagen type IV *in vitro*.

ACKNOWLEDGEMENTS

This research was supported from grants from NIH HL-33656, HL-24935, and HL-37669 and Swedish Medical Research Council 07466.

REFERENCES

1. J.D. Aplin and R.C. Hughes, Biochim Biophys. Acta 694, 375-418 (1982).
2. S.P. Sugrue and E.D. Hay, J. Cell Biol. 91, 45-54 (1981).
3. R. Pytela, M.D. Pierschbacher and E. Ruoslahti, Cell 40, 191-198 (1985).
4. K. von der Mark and U. Kühl, Biochim. Biophys. Acta 823, 147-160 (1985).
5. M. Kurkinen, A. Taylor, J.I. Garrels and B.L.M. Hogan, J. Biol. Chem. 259, 5915-5922 (1983).
6. K. Rubin, D. Gullberg, T.K. Borg and B. Öbrink, Exp. Cell Res. 164, 127-138 (1986).
7. D.R. Abrahamson, J. Pathol. 149, 257-278 (1986).
8. M. Aumailley and R. Timpl, J. Cell Biol. 103, 1569-1575 (1986).
9. T.K. Borg, K. Rubin, E. Lundgren, K. Borg and B. Obrink, Dev. Biol. 104, 86-96 (1984).
10. E. Lundgren, T.K. Borg and S. Mårdh, J. Mol. Cell. Cardiol, 16, 355-362 (1984).
11. H.K. Kleinman, R.J. Klebe and G.R. Martin, J. Cell Biol. 88, 473-485 (1981).
12. E. Lundgren, L. Terracio, S. Mårdh and T.K. Borg, Exp. Cell Res. 158, 371-381 (1985).
13. C.N. Rao, I.M.K. Margulies and L.A. Liotta, Biochem. Biophys. Res. Comm. 128, 45-52 (1985).
14. G.W. Laurie, J.T. Bing, H.K. Kleinman, J.R. Hassell, M. Aumailley and G.R. Martin, J. Mol. Biol. 189, 205-216 (1986).
15. A.S. Charonis, E.C. Tsilibary, T. Saku and H. Furthmayr, J. Cell Biol. 103, 1689-1697 (1986).
16. V.P. Terranova, D.H. Rohrbach and G.R. Martin, Cell 22, 719-726 (1980).
17. H.K. Kleinman, M.L. McGarvey, L.A. Liotta, P. Gehron Robey, K. Tryggvason and G.R. Martin, Biochemistry 24, 6188-6193 (1982).
18. K. Rubin, Å. Oldberg, M. Höök and B. Obrink Exp. Cell Res. 109, 413-422 (1987).
19. R. Timpl, H. Rohde, P. Genron Robey, S.I. Rennard, S.I. Foidart and G.R. Martin, J. Biol. Chem. 254, 9933-9937 (1979).
20. U. Landegren, J. Immunol. Methods 67, 379-388 (1984).
21. P.D. Yurchenco and H. Furthmayr, Biochemistry 23, 1840-1850 (1984).

A STUDY OF ADULT RAT ATRIAL MYOCYTE ATTACHMENT TO EXTRACELLULAR MATRIX COMPONENTS AND LONG TERM CULTURE

KATHRYN K. McMAHON
Department of Pharmacology, University of South Carolina School of Medicine, Columbia, South Carolina 29208

ABSTRACT

Adult rat atrial myocytes were isolated by a collagenase digestion of isolated atria in the absence of calcium ion. Calcium was slowly introduced to the cells before culturing by adding increasing proportions of the culture media to the isolation buffer. The ability of these cells to recognize and attach to extracellular matrix components was determined by a cell adhesion assay. The number of cells attached increased with time up to 4 hrs and was stable for at least 24 hr. The order of attachment to the extracellular matrix components was type III collagen = type IV collagen > fibronectin ≥ type I collagen > laminin. More cells attached when incubated at 37° C than when incubated at 24° C. Antibodies to type IV collagen and the collagen cell adhesion molecule (coll-cam) were detected to bind to cultured cells by immunofluorescence. Cultures have been maintained for up to two weeks. The rate of contraction and cyclic AMP levels of the cultured atrial cells were stimulated by forskolin and isoproterenol and inhibited by carbachol. The effects of carbachol were blocked by atropine.

INTRODUCTION

The atria has functions which differ from ventricle such as the synthesis and secretion of atrial natriuretic factor. Also the control of atria differs from that of the ventricles. For example, muscarinic cholinergic agonists directly control a K^+ channel in atria but not in ventricles [1]. This channel is, at least partially, responsible for muscarinic inhibition of heart contractile rate. These differences suggest that the atrial myocyte differs in many respects from the ventricular myocyte. Little work has been done with cultured atrial cells from adult animals. The work presented established isolation procedures and culturing conditions which allow maintenance for up to two weeks of adult rat atrial myocytes.

METHODS

Atria from 10 adult (150 to 200 g) animals were collected and minced in KRB-HEPES (KRB with 5 mM $NaHCO_3$ and 20 mM HEPES) at 24° C. The tissue was repeatedly digested in the presence of 100 U/ml collagenase (Worthington, type I) at 37° C for 10 min. Collected cells from each digestion were held at room temperature in the presence of 25% DMEM/F-12 media in KRB-HEPES. The third through seventh digests were combined and filtered across 10 μm nylon mesh and the ratio of media to KRB-HEPES increased to 1:1 before packing the cells by centrifugation. Cell viability and density were determined with trypan blue staining. Cells (0.5 ml) were plated on 24 well tissue culture plates at 1 X 10^6 cells/ml and cultured in the presence of 10% horse serum, 3% fetal bovine serum, 8 μg/ml in DMEM/F-12 media (Sigma). Extracellular matrix component coating of dishes was for at least 1 hr at 37° C. Cells were incubated for 24 hr for attachment studies and

Biology of Isolated Adult Cardiac Myocytes
William A. Clark, Robert S. Decker, and Thomas K. Borg, Editors

attachment was determined by the hexosaminidase assay of [2]. Contractile rates were determined by manual observation of cells at one minute intervals. For cyclic AMP experiments, cells were incubated at 37° C for 5 minutes in the presence of drugs dissolved in 0.5 ml of DMEM/F-12 media. The incubations were terminated by the addition of 0.25 ml of 0.8 M perchloric acid. The solution was removed for the radioimmunoassay determination of total cyclic AMP concentrations [3]. Following removal of the solution, cellular protein was suspended by incubating the precipitated protein in 0.075 ml of 1 N NaOH for 1 hr. Protein was determined by the method of Lowry [4].
Immunofluorescence of cells was done with FITC-liganded secondary antibodies [5].

RESULTS

Freshly isolated adult rat atrial cells had a rod shaped appearance (Figure 1) and were not spontaneously contracting. If cells were held on ice or supplemented media was abruptly introduced, cell survival and culturing was minimal. The average yield was 1 to 2 X 10^6 cells/atria. Cells in culture initially rounded up and then spread out with pseudopods at the periphery.

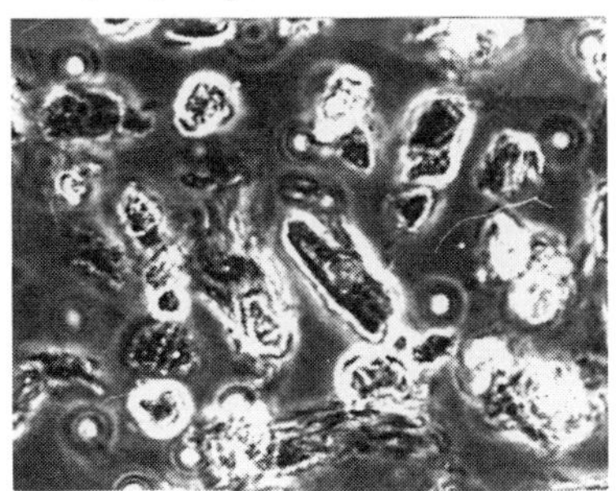

FIG. 1. Phase contrast micrograph of freshly isolated adult rat atrial myocytes.

TABLE I. Adult rat atrial cell attachment to extracellular matrix protein

Extracellular Matrix Component	% Cells Attached 10 μg/ml Component	20 μg/ml Component
Non-coated	0.7	
Laminin	1.1	1.5
Collagen I	2.1	3.9
Collagen IV	6.7	7.2
Fibronectin	3.9	4.6

Coating was overnight at 37° C. Attachment was for 24 hr. Cells were plated at 500,000/well. Similar results were seen in 5 experiments.

The percentage of plated cells which remain attached at 24 hr after plating was less one percent (Table I). Cellular attachment to dishes was improved by pre-coating the dishes with the extracellular matrix components types I,III, and IV collagen and fibronectin while laminin had only minimal effect on attachment (Table I). Attachment was dependent on the coating concentration of the components (Figure 2). Maximum attachment was seen by 4 hr and stable for at least 24 hr. A culturing temperature of 37° c allowed two times as many cells to attach as a temperature of 24° C. The maximum attachment was seen with 25 μg/ml of either type III or type IV collagen (Figure 2). This maximal level was equivalent to 14% of the cells plated. By immunofluorescence, both type IV collagen and collagen cell attachment molecules (coll-cam) were determined to be present in cells in culture for 5 days.

In 5 day old cultures, cells did spontaneously contract at very low rates (i.e.3 to 5 beats/min). The contraction rates were stimulated by 1 μM forskolin or 10 μM isoproterenol and inhibited by 10 μM carbachol (Figure 3). The effect of carbachol was blocked by 10 μM atropine. Likewise, cyclic AMP concentrations were increased by isoproterenol and forskolin and decreased by carbachol (Figure 4).

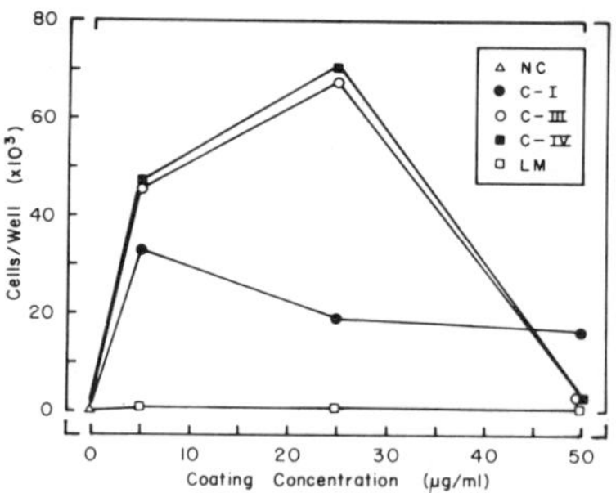

FIG 2. Attachment of adult rat atrial cells to varying concentrations of extracellular matrix components.

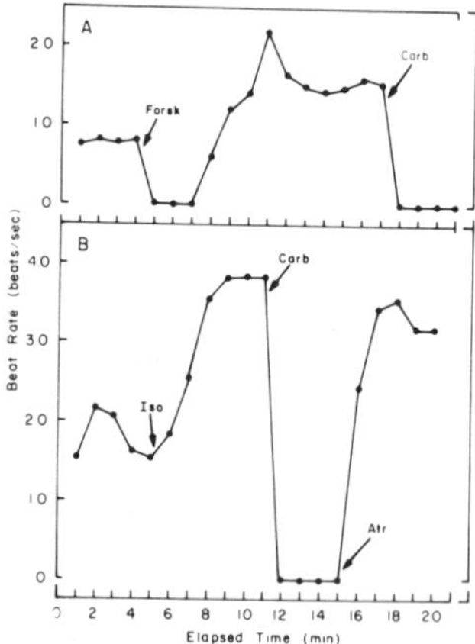

FIG 3. Control of contractile rate of cultured adult rat atrial cells by 1 μM forskolin, 10 μM isoproterenol, 10 μM carbachol and 10 μM atropine.

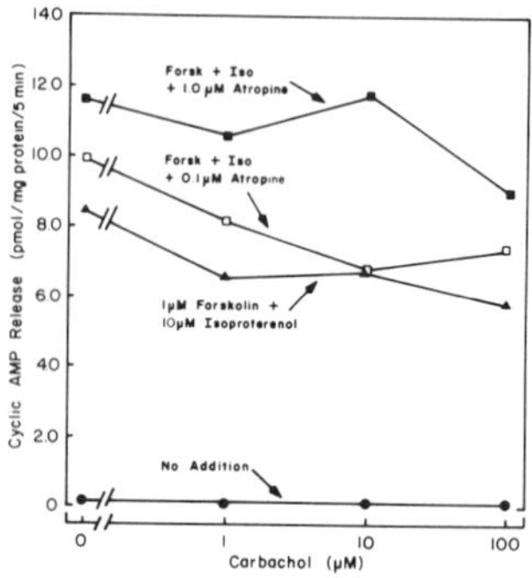

FIG. 4. Cyclic AMP production in cultured adult rat atrial cells in response to forskolin plus isoproterenol in the absence or presence of verying concentrations of carbachol and atropine.

DISCUSSION

The results demonstrate a method for isolation and culturing of adult rat atrial cells. These cells resemble ventricular cells visually during isolation and culture. Unlike adult ventricular cells, the adult atrial cells can be isolated without perfusion of the heart and so are relatively easily obtained. The percentage of attached cells is slightly lower than that seen with adult rat ventricular cells [5]. Cultures have been maintained routinely for one week and for as long as two weeks. It should be noted, however, that cells do continuously 'sluff off' during this time and are most reactive if used between day 3 to 7 of culture.

There is a significant difference noted between the attachment characteristics of the atrial cells from those reported for adult ventricular cells. The presence of laminin did not improve attachment of cells as is seen with ventricular cells [5]. Type I, III, and IV collagen and fibronectin do significantly improve attachment of cells in concentration-, time-, and temperature-dependent manners. Currently, it is not understood why the cells do not attach to laminin since there is type IV collagen attachment. The difference in atrial and ventricular cell attachment to laminin should provide a method for differential plating to separate atrial from ventricular cells.

The adult atrial cells in culture do respond appropriately to stimulating and inhibiting drugs in both contractile rate and cyclic AMP production. This suggests that this cultured cell preparation from adult atrial tissue can be used as a model for atrial cell function.

ACKNOWLEDGMENTS

The author is grateful for the insightful comments of Drs. Thomas Borg and Louis Terracio. This work is supported by the March of Dimes.

REFERENCES

1. Löffelholz, K. and Pappano, A.J. Pharmacology Reviews 37, 1 (1985).
2. Landegren, U., J. Immunol. Methods 67, 379 (1984).
3. Harper, J.F. and Brooker, G. J. Cyclic Nucleotide Res. 1, 207 (1975).
4. Lowry, O.H., Rosebrough, N.J., Farr, A.L. and Randall, R.J. J. Biol. Chem. 193, 265 (1951).
5. Borg, T.K., Rubin, K., Lundgren, E., Borg, K. and Öbrink, B. Developmental Biol. 104, 86 (1984).

CALCIUM METABOLISM AND KINETICS

STEVEN R. HOUSER
Department of Physiology, Temple University School of Medicine, 3400 N. Broad Street, Philadelphia, PA 19140

INTRODUCTION

The development of techniques for isolation of viable single cells from intact adult mammalian myocardium has allowed investigation of many aspects of calcium [Ca] homeostasis which previously could not be studied easily or directly in multicellular cardiac muscle preparations. The work presented at this symposium represents only a small sample of the new information which has been obtained during the past ten years from experiments in which isolated cells were used as the model preparation. Isolated myocytes are currently the preferred preparation for most studies of membrane [Ca] transport because the extracellular myocyte environment can be easily controlled and rapidly changed. This represents a major advantage over the multicellular preparations used previously because multicellular preparations contain diffusion-limiting extracellular spaces which restrict the movement of ions between the cell interior and the bulk phase of the bathing medium.

Isolated myocytes are also an extremely useful preparation for the study of voltage dependent ionic channels such as Ca channels. Recent studies conducted using isolated cardiocytes have shown that the kinetics of Ca channel activation and inactivation are much more rapid than suggested by studies conducted in multicellular cardiac muscle preparations (1). In addition, these studies suggest that there is more than one species of Ca channel in adult mammalian myocytes. The precise role of each of these putative Ca channels remains to be elucidated.

Carrier mediated Ca transport mechanisms (such as the Na/Ca exchanger) are also amenable to study in isolated cell preparations. The role of the Na/Ca exchanger in the control of both diastolic and systolic Ca is not yet clearly defined, and many laboratories are directing their research efforts in this area.

There have also been recent technical advances in the synthesis of Ca-sensitive fluorescent molecules. Specifically, Fura-2 and Indo-1 were introduced recently (2) and have been used to measure cytosolic [Ca] in single cardiac cells. The almost simultaneous development of single myocyte isolation techniques, "patch-type" (3) voltage clamp techniques, and Ca-sensitive fluorescent probes will undoubtably lead to studies which will provide a clearer

Biology of Isolated Adult Cardiac Myocytes
William A. Clark, Robert S. Decker, and Thomas K. Borg, Editors

understanding of excitation-contraction coupling mechanisms in the adult mammalian heart.

In the remainder of this "review of topics covered" I will summarize the major topics which were discussed at the symposium and will finish with a short discussion of some of the unresolved questions that require future study.

RECENT TECHNICAL ADVANCES

It is well known that in cardiac ventricular muscle, [Ca] increases dramatically during systole (4). It is this increase in cytosolic [Ca] that triggers the contraction of cardiac muscle. Until very recently, however, diastolic [Ca] and the systolic [Ca] transient were not easily measured in cardiac muscle. Most previous studies of the cardiac calcium transient have used either aequorin or Ca-selective microelectrodes. Aequorin is not very sensitive to Ca over the range of diastolic concentrations encountered in cardiac muscle, is difficult to calibrate, and usually must be injected with microelectrodes into many cells in the preparation in order to have an adequate signal (4). Ca-selective electrodes have their own set of problems, the most important of which is their slow temporal response, which limits their ability to follow the rapid changes in cytosolic [Ca] that can occur in cardiac muscle (5).

An important technical breakthrough occured when Roger Tsien and his collaborators (2) developed a new group of Ca-sensitive fluorecent probes. The novel aspect of these compounds is that they are synthesized in a Ca-insensitive, membrane permeable form by attaching acetoxymethylester groups to the Ca-sensitive parent compound. When these compounds diffuse into cells, however, these ester groups are cleaved by natural intracellular esterases, yielding the Ca-sensitive form of the molecule. This form is membrane impermeable, and becomes diffusion trapped within the cell. The most popular of these compounds are Fura-2 and Indo-1.

These Ca-sensitive fluorescent dyes have recently been used to study Ca homeostasis in cardiac myocytes. Numerous investigators presenting at the symposium used either Fura-2 or Indo-1 to measure cytosolic [Ca]. The specific data from these experiments can be found in the publications included in this book and will not be discussed in detail here. Instead, I thought it would be useful to point out the potential pitfalls involved in the use of these compounds so that first time users may save some time. The major problem with these compounds is that they can be extremely difficult to calibrate. This difficulty arises from the facts that 1) the dye can enter intracellular compartments such as mitochondria and sarcoplasmic reticulum. When collecting fluorecent light from the entire cell, it is therefore difficult to compute the fraction of the signal which is derived from the cytoplasmic compartment. 2) If too much dye is placed in the cell, Ca-insensitive fluorescent metabolites are often encountered. These produce an unquantified background signal which is not easily compensated for. These problems can be almost entirely avoided by judicious loading procedures. One such procedure is given in another chapter in this book entitled "A Technique to Measure Cytosolic [Ca] in Feline Ventricular Myocytes" and will not be discussed here. In addition, a recently published report by Li et al(6) was discussed at some length. This study showed that calibration of Fura-2 fluorescence signals required an in-vivo calibration technique. This technique uses deenergized myocytes in the calibration procedure to produce reliable maximum fluorescence signals. The consensus of those at the symposium was that reliable calibration procedures have yet to be fully developed. The most useful calibration techniques will those which may be performed once, and which will then be applicable to other cells to be studied. This would eliminate the need to perform time consuming in vivo calibrations on every myocyte.

A few laboratories have developed techniques for simultaneously recording intracellular [Ca] (with fluorescent dyes), membrane electrophysiological properties and myocyte contractions. This should be a powerful approach for studies of excitation-contraction coupling in adult mammalian cardiac myocytes. A description of one such approach was presented by Capogrossi et al at this symposium. The basis of the approach is that red light is used to view and then quantify (videoanalytical technique) the rate and magnitude of myocyte contraction. The red light did not interfere significantly with the blue wavelengths of the Ca-sensitive dye, Indo-1, that was used in their experiments. Similar approaches are being used currently by Barry (7) and duBell and Houser (8).

ENERGY METABOLISM AND CYTOSOLIC [Ca]

The role of cytosolic [Ca] in ischemic and anoxic myocardial injury has been of interest to cardiac physiologists for many years. This topic was addressed in many of the presentations at the symposium and some interesting new information was given. Cobbold and Li (see papers from this session) presented data demonstrating that depletion of cellular ATP stores, respectively, with either anoxia or metabolic inhibitors, was not immediately associated with large elevations of resting cell [Ca]. This was true even if ATP was depleted to the point at which myocytes went into a contracture or rigor state. One possible reason for the small changes in cytosolic [Ca] during this period was offerred by Haworth, who presented data showing that Ca influx is reduced during this time period. Along these same lines, Silverman (from Lakatta's laboratory at NIH/NIA) showed that as rat myocytes become ATP depleted during anoxia, action potential durations shorten, and cells eventually become inexcitable. These electrophysiological changes probably result from the opening of ATP sensitive potassium channels of the type recently decribed by Noma (9), and discussed in another paper by Weiss. The studies presented thus show that there are a host of compensatory cellular responses which occur during anoxia and which act to limit the extent of Ca loading during anoxia. It appears that if cells are reoxygenated before there has been a substantial rise in cytosolic [Ca], myocytes go through a transient phase of Ca overload (probably secondary to the sodium loading that takes place during anoxia) but are eventually able to restore cytosolic [Ca] to normal levels. Studies of this nature should eventually lead to a better understanding of the role of altered intracellular Ca in cell injury and death following cardiac anoxia and/or ischemia.

EXCITATION-CONTRACTION COUPLING

Much of the focus of the presentations and the subsequent discussions in this session centered on research concerning excitation-contraction coupling. Of particular interest were studies which examined whether or not Ca influx through voltage dependent membrane channels is the trigger for Ca release from the sarcoplasmic reticulum (SR). Presentations (included in this book) by Weir, Cannell, Talo and Isenberg all addressed this issue to a certain extent. The consensus of these presentations was that Ca current induces SR Ca release in a variety of adult mammalian preparations. There was serious debate, however, concerning whether or not other mechanisms are involved in triggering SR Ca release and loading SR Ca stores.

The source of the Ca which loads the SR was discussed following several of the talks. Gil Weir presented data which supported the notion that the Na/Ca exchange mechanism is able to transport Ca into the cell over the voltage range of the cardiac action potential plateau. This Ca could be involved in direct activation of the myofibrils as well as in loading the SR for release during subsequent beats. Isenberg also presented interesting data along these same lines. His experiments in rat myocytes showed that when micropipettes contained Na in the filling solution, depolarizations to positive membrane potentials (+30 or above) caused large phasic contractions and Ca transients. When filling solutions did not contain Na, depolarizations to these same potentials caused little or no contraction. These results suggest that the Na/Ca exchanger can move Ca into the cell when the membrane voltage is depolarized to inside positive values. The phasic nature of the Ca transients and twitches observed under these conditions (Na in the cytosol) suggests that the Ca was derived from a rapidly releasable pool such as the SR. Therefore, the Ca entry via the Na/Ca exchanger appears to load the SR. These ideas require further investigation.

An interesting question that came up at this symposium and has been discussed previously in the literature is whether or not mechanisms other than Ca influx via "L type" (10) Ca channels is capable of inducing Ca release from the SR. One possibility is that the release process is voltage dependent. Cannell presented evidence that this might be the case. He described experiments in which Ca transients were observed at membrane potentials below the threshold for activation of the Ca current. Another explanation for this finding is that Ca influx through "T type" Ca channels (which activate over this voltage range) may also be able to induce Ca release from the SR. No direct evidence for this hypothesis was presented at the symposium. Houser did show that a TTX-insensitive inward current was activated over this voltage range (-60 to -30 mV), for which Na (rather than Ca) was the current carrier. The possibility that SR Ca release may be triggered by inward current through voltage dependent channels other than L type calcium channels therefore deserves consideration in future experiments. Another possible trigger for SR Ca release at membrane potentials at which the classical Ca current is small or absent is Ca influx via the Na/Ca exchanger. Therefore, Ca influx via the Na-Ca exchanger may also play a role in the contractions produced by voltage steps to positive membrane potentials (such as those that occur during the normal action potential). These ideas also need to be evaluated critically in future experiments. Isolated myocytes will be the preparation best suited for such experiments because both intra- and extracellular Na and Ca concentrations must be carefully controlled.

UNRESOLVED QUESTIONS AND FUTURE DIRECTIONS

There are many areas in which work is still required to clarify our understanding of how cardiac cells control cytosolic [Ca] during both systole and diastole. It is beyond the scope of this discussion to try to present an exhaustive list of all of these areas. Therefore, only those which were topics of discussion at this symposium will be discussed here.

It is always important to keep in mind that isolated myocytes are a relatively new experimental preparation. It is therefore important to carefully evaluate the characteristics of the preparation before it is used in hypothesis testing. Along these lines, Kim and Smith presented data showing that in isolated guinea pig myocytes, cytosolic Ca is only stable for a few hours following isolation. After a few hours, cells begin to Ca overload and exhibit abnormal mechanical properties.

An area in which some progress has been made but where much more is required is in the development of techniques for the measurement of isometric tension in single adult mammalian cardiocytes. The problem is primarily one of finding a way to reliably attach myocytes to recording probes. This problem deserves attention.

Finally, a topic which was frequently discussed at the symposium was the source of the Ca which activates the myofilaments during normal contraction. While much work is currently being performed in this area, there is still no consensus as to the fraction of activator Ca which enters from the extracellular space via voltage activated channels or the Na-Ca exchanger, versus the fraction which is released from intracellular stores (primarily the SR). Particularly little is known about the source of activator calcium for excitation-contraction coupling in human myocardium. This is an important question which will hopefully be answered in the forseeable future.

SELECTED REFERENCES

1. G. Isenberg and U. Klockner, Am. J. Physiol. 345, H891-H896 (1983).
2. G. Grynkiewicz, M. Polnie and R. Y. Tsien, J. Biol. Chem. 260, 3440-3450 (1985).
3. O. P. Hamill, A. Marty, E. Neher, B. Sakmann, and F. J. Sigworth, Pflug. Arch. 391, 85-100 (1981).
4. J. R. Blinks, W. G. Wier, P. Hess, and F. G. Prendergast, Prog. Biochem. Mol. Biol. 40, 1-114 (1982).
5. D. Amman, P. C. Meier, W. Simon, In : Detection and Measurement of Free Ca^{2+} Ions in Cells (Elsevier Press, North Holland, Amsterdam, 1979). pp. 117-127.
6. Q. Li, R. A. Altschuld, and B. T. Stokes, Biochem. Biophys. Res. Com. 147, 120-126 (1987).
7. O. Kohmoto, and W. H. Barry, Physiologist 30(4), 201, 1987.
8. W. H. duBell and S. R. Houser, Circulation 76, 472 (1987).
9. A. Noma, Nature 35, 147-148 (1983).
10. B. Nilius, P. Hess, J. B. Lansman, and R. W. Tsien, Nature 41, 443-446, (1985).

MEASUREMENT OF SPONTANEOUS AND ELECTRICALLY STIMULATED Ca^{2+} TRANSIENTS IN SINGLE RAT VENTRICULAR MYOCYTES.

JONATHAN R. MONCK, KUMPEI KOBAYASHI, ÓLAF BJÖRNSSON AND JOHN R. WILLIAMSON
Department of Biochemistry and Biophysics, University of Pennsylvania, Philadelphia PA 19104.

INTRODUCTION.

The importance of the cytosolic free Ca^{2+} concentration in the regulation of cardiac contractility has been well established [1]. However, the details of the mechanisms involved in controlling cellular Ca^{2+} fluxes are not fully understood. The cardiac ventricular myocyte is a useful model for studying calcium homeostasis [2], however, interpretation of the results from bulk cells in suspension is made difficult by cellular heterogeneity. This can be overcome by using the fluorescent Ca^{2+} indicator fura-2 [3] which, because of its high fluorescence yield, can be used in conjunction with videomicroscopy to measure the Ca^{2+} concentration in single cells [4]. A property of some isolated cardiac myocytes is that they exhibit spontaneous contractile waves in the unstimulated state [5], which have been shown to be due changes in the cytosolic Ca^{2+} concentration [6]. In this study, localized Ca^{2+} changes in single spontaneously contracting fura-2 loaded myocytes are compared with the Ca^{2+} transient induced by electrical stimulation.

METHODS.

Ventricular myocytes were isolated from rat hearts as previously described [2]. Cells were loaded with fura-2 by incubating cells with 5nmol of fura-2/AM per mg dry wt of cells for 10 min and then plated on to glass coverslips for use in a Dvorak cell chamber. The fluorescence images were collected using a Nikon Fluor 20x objective attached to a Nikon Optiphot microscope equipped for epifluorescence, and the images were analyzed with a Joyce/Loebl Magiscan 2A computer as described elsewhere [7]. Excitation wavelengths were selected with narrow bandpass filters (340nm or 380nm, 10nm half bandpass) and the emitted fluorescence collected between 470 and 600nm. The results are presented as the fractional change in 340nm excited fura-2 fluorescence or as the Ca^{2+} concentration calculated as described elsewhere [7].

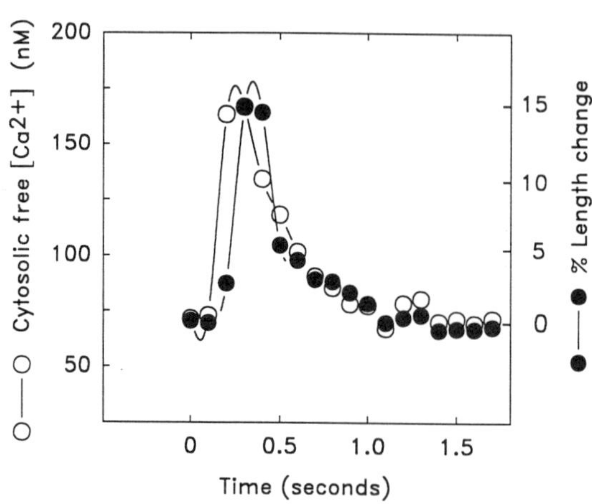

FIG. 1. Comparison of time courses for the Ca^{2+} transient and contraction of a myocyte induced by electrical stimulation. Fluorescence images of myocytes were collected at 100ms intervals during stimulation with a square wave pulse (100V, 10ms). The Ca^{2+} concentration was calculated from the fluorescence of fura-2 excited at 340nm.

Biology of Isolated Adult Cardiac Myocytes
William A. Clark, Robert S. Decker, and Thomas K. Borg, Editors

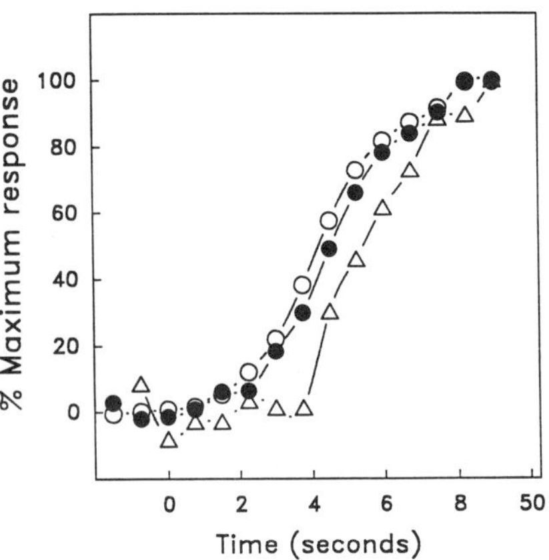

FIG. 2. Comparison of Ca^{2+} concentration changes determined from the fluorescence of fura-2 excited at 340nm and 380nm. A myocyte was stimulated with a depolarizing concentration of KCl (60mM). The Ca^{2+} concentration changes, which were calculated from the 340nm (●) and 380nm (○) signals during successive stimulations, and length change (△) are expressed as percentage of maximum changes to facilitate comparison.

RESULTS AND DISCUSSION.

Electrically induced calcium transients in single myocytes.

Fluorescence images of fura-2 loaded myocytes excited with 340nm light were collected during stimulation with a square wave pulse (100V, 10ms duration). Figure 1 shows the time courses of the changes in fluorescence intensity, integrated over the whole cell area, compared with the change in cell length. The decrease in cell length shows a similar time course, but follows the increased Ca^{2+} concentration with a slight delay. The same relationship also held after treatment with isoproterenol, but both the Ca^{2+} increase and the length change had an increased magnitude and returned to resting levels more rapidly (data not shown).

A potential problem with single wavelength measurements is that a change in the morphology of the cell during contraction might alter the measured fluorescence independently of a change in the Ca^{2+} concentration. Fura-2 has the property that an increase in Ca^{2+} concentration gives an increase in fluorescence when excited at 340nm and a decrease when excited at 380nm [3], whereas a contraction artifact would change both signals in the same direction. Figure 2 compares the Ca^{2+} concentration calculated from the 340nm and 380nm fluorescent signals using the single wavelength method [7], with contraction during stimulation with a depolarizing concentration of KCl. The good correlation between the values from both wavelengths indicates that contraction artifacts must be minimal under these conditions. This is probably because fluorescence is monitored using low power microscopy which has a relatively deep depth of focus, so that the volume from which the fluorescence is being monitored contains the myocyte during the whole of the excitation-contraction cycle. In other experiments using the 380nm light to excite the fura-2, similar, but inverted, changes in fluorescence were observed upon stimulation electrically or with caffeine. In addition, in myocytes with high fura-2 or quin2 loads, which totally inhibit contraction, transient increases in fura-2 fluorescence were still seen, although in these cases the peak height and rate of recovery of the Ca^{2+} transient were reduced due to the buffering action of the indicator. Therefore, the change in 340nm fluorescence can be attributed to an increase in the cytosolic free Ca^{2+} concentration and not to a contraction artifact.

Calcium concentration changes during spontaneous contractions.

In a preparation of Ca^{2+}-tolerant myocytes there is a small population of cells that undergo spontaneous contractions. These are characterized by contractile waves that propagate along the myocyte at a rate of 100μm/s [4]. Fig. 3A shows the time course of the fluorescence change averaged over the whole cell during a spontaneous contraction. The transient has a different shape from that of the electrically induced transient (compare Fig. 3A with Fig. 1). In the spontaneous contraction, the Ca^{2+} change is localized, beginning at one end of the cell (area (a) in the schematic in Fig. 3) and moving along the cell (towards area (h)). Comparison of the fluorescence change for just one region (area (e) as shown in Fig. 3B) with the electrically stimulated transient (Fig. 1) shows similar kinetics. Fig. 4 shows the Ca^{2+} transients for all eight of the regions of the myocyte as defined in Fig. 3. The Ca^{2+} increase occurs first in area (a) and has returned to resting values in this region by the time the transient in area (h) has reached a maximum. The transients all reach a similar peak height and decay with a half-time of around 200ms, which suggests that the wave is self-propagating rather than merely diffusion of Ca^{2+} down a concentration gradient. These results are consistent with a mechanism such as Ca^{2+}-induced Ca^{2+} release as suggested for Ca^{2+} oscillations in Purkinje fibres [9].

Conclusions.

Fluorescence videomicroscopy of fura-2 loaded cardiac myocytes was used to measure transient changes in Ca^{2+} concentration and cell length simultaneously. The single wavelength method used has the potential problem

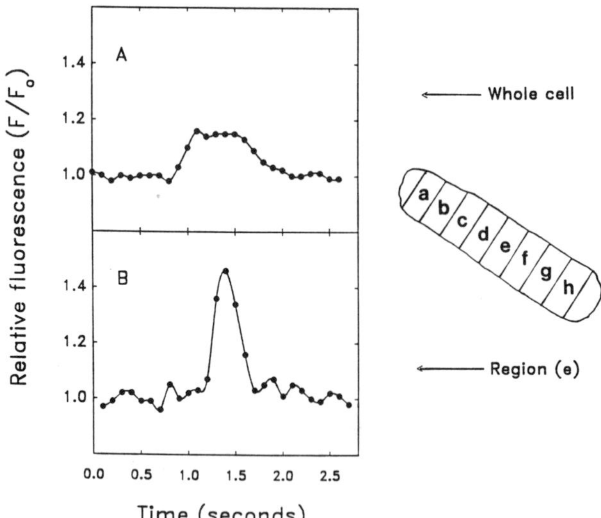

FIG. 3. Fura-2 fluorescence changes during a spontaneous contraction. Fluorescence images of a myocyte were collected every 100ms during a spontaneous contraction which began at one end of the cell (area (a) as illustrated in the scheme) and propagated along the cell (to area (h)). The fluorescence intensity was integrated (A) over the whole cell area and (B) over a localized region of the cell (area (e)).

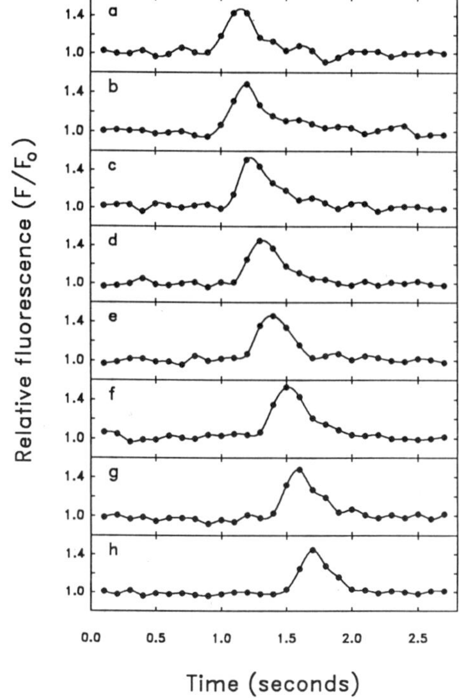

FIG. 4. Comparison of fluorescence changes in different areas of the cell during a spontaneous contraction. Panels (a) - (h) represent the time courses of fluorescence changes occuring in localized parts of the cell as defined in the scheme in Fig. 3.

of artifacts due to contraction and has a limited temporal resolution using a SIT camera video imaging system. The alternative use of a photomultiplier improves the temporal resolution, but cannot detect spatially localized changes or simultaneously monitor length changes. However, provided that potential artifacts due to contraction are considered, quantitative measurements can be made from video images using the single wavelength method. Thus, it has been possible to demonstrate the close correlation between the Ca^{2+} transient and contraction of the myocyte and to show that the localized changes in Ca^{2+} concentration during a spontaneous contraction exhibit similar kinetics to the electrically induced Ca^{2+} transient.

REFERENCES.

1. A. Fabiato, Am. J. Physiol. 245, C1-C14 (1983).
2. A.P. Thomas, M. Selak and J.R. Williamson, J. Mol. Cell. Cardiol. 18, 541-545 (1986).
3. G. Grynkiewicz, M. Poenie and R.Y. Tsien, J. Biol. Chem. 260, 3440-3450 (1985).
4. R.Y. Tsien and M. Poenie, Trends Biochem. Sci. 11, 450-455 (1986).
5. A.A. Kort, C. Capogrossi and E.G. Lakatta, Circ. Res. 57, 844-855 (1985).
6. W.G. Wier, M.B. Cannell, J.R. Berlin, E. Marban, and W.J. Lederer, Science 235 325-328 (1987).
7. J.R. Monck, E.E. Reynolds, A.P. Thomas and J.R. Williamson, J. Biol. Chem., submitted.
8. A. Fabiato, J. Gen. Physiol. 78 457-497 (1987).
9. W.G. Wier, A.A. Kort, M.D. Stern, E.G. Lakatta and E. Marban, Proc. Natl. Acad. Sci. 80 7367-7371 (1983).

X-ray microprobe analysis of elemental distribution in isolated guinea-pig ventricular myocytes shock-frozen under voltage-clamp conditions

MARIA FIORA WENDT-GALLITELLI* AND GERRIT ISENBERG+
*Institute of Physiology II, University of Tübingen, Gmelinstraße 5, D-74 Tübingen 1; +Institute of Physiology, University of Cologne, Robert-Koch-Straße 39, D-5 Köln 41, Federal Republic of Germany

INTRODUCTION

Excitation-contraction coupling in heart muscle is mediated by short lasting intracellular calcium transients. This activator-calcium stems mainly from intracellular stores (sarcoplasmic reticulum, SR). Extracellular calcium which enters through the sarcolemma via the calcium inward current (I_{Ca}) or the sodium, calcium-exchanger (Na^+,Ca^{2+}-exchanger) is considered to be a rather minor source of the activator calcium. But it is required to fill the intracellular stores and to trigger the release process.
Although the amount of calcium-entry (I_{Ca}) via calcium inward current during the action potential can be defined by voltage-clamp experiments, the intracellular routes of this calcium are absolutely inaccesible by means of electrophysiological methods. But calcium concentrations in subcellular compartments such as sarcoplasmic reticulum, mitochondria, sarcolemma and cytoplasma can be measured by x-ray microanalysis. Minimal detectable concentrations (total mass fraction of an element in the analyzed volume) are presently in the range of 0.5 mmol Ca/kg dry weight (d.w), which corresponds, for instance in the cytoplasma, to 70-80 µmol Ca/kg wet weight (w.w.).

We have now adapted the methods of quick-freezing to isolated ventricular myocytes under the conditions of the voltage-clamp. We undertook this further development since we are convinced that the combination of the voltage-clamp and x-ray microprobe analysis can lead to information concerning the fate of the calcium-ions which have been transferred from the extracellular to the intracellular space by the calcium inward current.

METHODS

A patch pipette served for both the transfer of the cell from the chamber to a special silver holder as well as for the electrophysiological measurements. The silver holder was hand-made, the tip of its taper was opened electrolytically and covered with a thin pioloform film. Having selected a myocyte with clear cross-striation, the GΩ seal was built but without disrupture of the patch of the membrane. The cell was lifted from the bottom of the chamber to the holder and placed on the transparent pioloform film. Intracellular contact was then established by rupturing the patch of the membrane. After checking that the intracellular stimulation induced normal action potentials (130 mV, 260 ms at 36°C, 3.6 mmol/l Ca), the voltage clamp circuit was switched on. Pulses depolarizing from -45 to -5 mV evoked net membrane currents which were largerly determined by the Ca inward current. The elicited shortening of the unloaded cells could be visualized on the monitor of a TV-microscope.
Then, keeping the holder with the cell absolutely still, the chamber and the microscope were slid away horizontally (Fig.1). The horizontal movement stopped after 110 ms, before the vertical movement of the coolant started and the preparation contacted the coolant (undercooled propane at -198°C).
After freezing the holder was transferred under liquid nitrogen and mounted on the cryoultramicrotome, where ultrathin cryosections were cut at -140 to -160°C, freeze-dried and (when not lost during one of the several tricky preparative steps) finally analyzed in the electron microscope equipped with a full-quantitative energy-dispersive Link-System.

Biology of Isolated Adult Cardiac Myocytes
William A. Clark, Robert S. Decker, and Thomas K. Borg, Editors

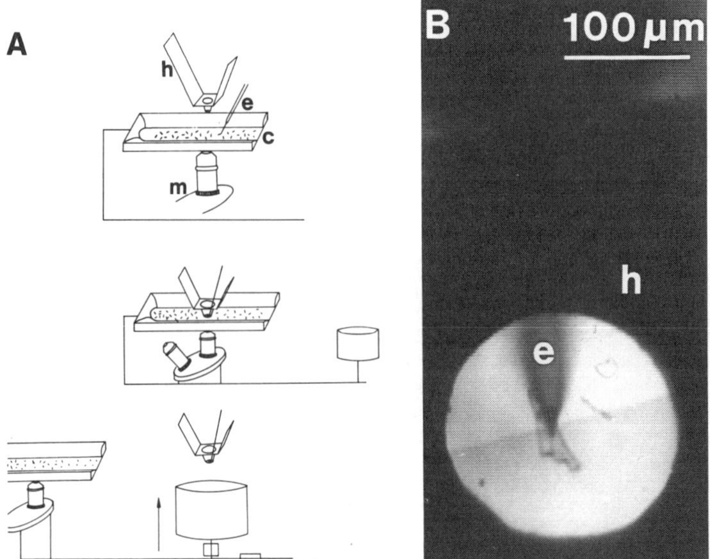

Fig. 1(A) Schematic of the set up for transferring and freezing the myocyte. On the top, arrangement of the microscope (m), holder (h), chamber (c) and patch-electrode (e). In the middle the myocyte has been transferred to the holder. On the bottom, microscope and chamber have been moved away, the coolant is moving up to the holder with the cell.
Fig.1(B). A myocyte has been transferred with the patch-electrode from the chamber to the silver-holder (photographs from the TV-screen). e = electrode; h = holder.

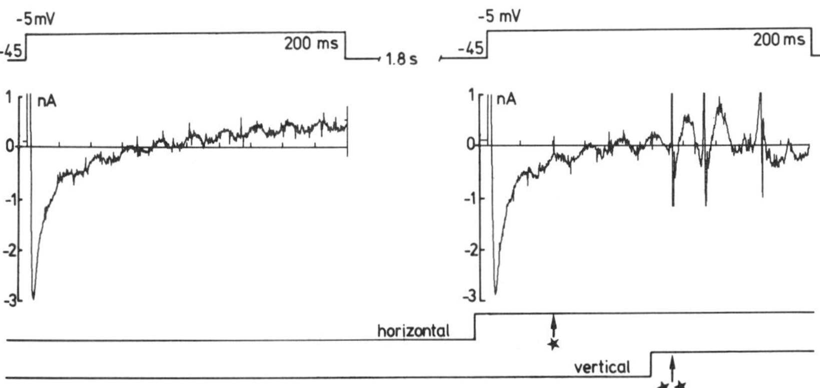

Fig. 2 shows the membrane currents from one isolated myocyte as recorded before (left) and during (right) shock-freezing. 200 ms long pulses were applied at 0.2 Hz. Note that the start of the horizontal movement (*) does not disturb the cell. The impact of the cell with the coolant (**) evoked large current artifacts.

RESULTS AND DISCUSSION

In fig. 3 the excellent preservation of cell structures is documented in a cell which was freeze-substituted after shock-freezing . In the superficial 5 microns of the cell no distorsions of myofilaments are recognizable and cross-bridges reveal normal periodicity. Mitochondria and t-tubuli have normal morphology.

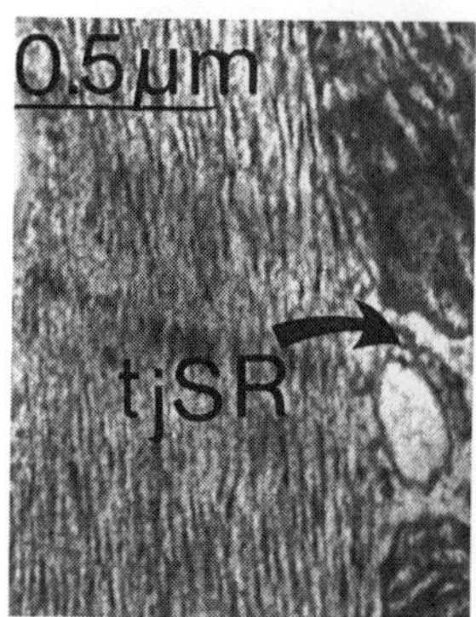

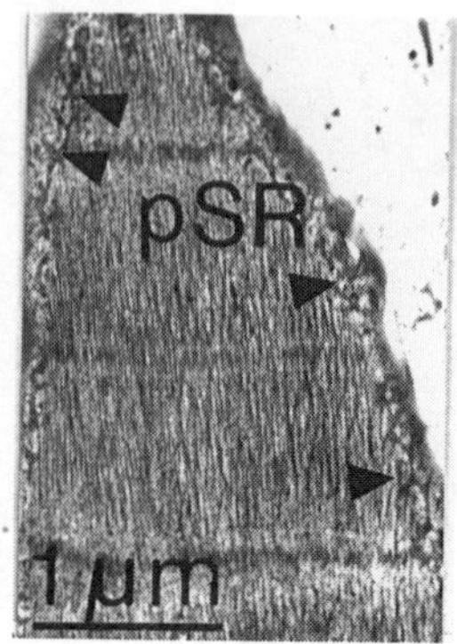

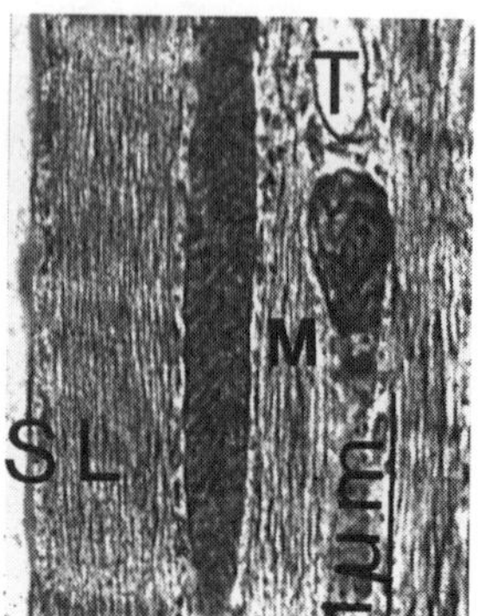

Fig. 3. Longitudinal section of a myocyte freeze-substituted after shock-freezing. M= mitochondria; TjSR= junctional SR (curved arrow) adjacent to t-Tubuli (T); SL= cell border with peripheral SR (pSR, arrowhead).

With an analyzing beam focussed to 50 nm diameter we could analyze the elements in the following compartments: (1) the <u>cytoplasma</u>: the electron beam was located in the space occupied by the filaments. (2) The <u>cell border:</u> the electron beam was deformed astigmatically to a spot of 10 nm width and 1 µm length, and it was placed as close as possible on to the inner side of the surface membrane. The concentrations sum up from elements bound to the inner side of the sarcolemma, from elements stored in those parts of the junctional SR that were closely attached and elements of the cytoplasma close to the cell border. (3) <u>Junctional sarcoplasmic reticulum</u> adjacent to t-tubuli. Finally (4) the <u>mitochondria</u>.

We analyzed the influence of Ca-entry on the Ca-concentration of the compartments. In the first experiment, as a control, myocytes were frozen after prolonged rest (at least 20 min).
At rest the calcium concentrations in all compartments were below the limit of detection (Fig. 4, upper row).
In the second experiment cells were frozen at the peak of contraction, after contractility was potentiated with a serie of 5 short pulses of 200 ms.
In the cell frozen at the peak of contraction after a train of 5 short pulses Ca could now be measured in all compartments. 0.5 mmol/kg d.w. in the cytoplasma corresponds to 125 µmol/kg w.w.. This Ca exceeded the 73 mol/kg w.w. which entered through the plasmalemma during the last pulse. The increment of Ca was calculated on the basis of the charges transferred by the current as a function of the duration of depolarisation and the cell volume. But this cytoplasmic Ca measured by microanalysis is less than the total Ca-increment due to the 5 pulses. This can be partly due to Ca-extrusion from the cell. Partly is certainly due to an accumulation of Ca in intracellular stores, which is revealed by microanalysis.

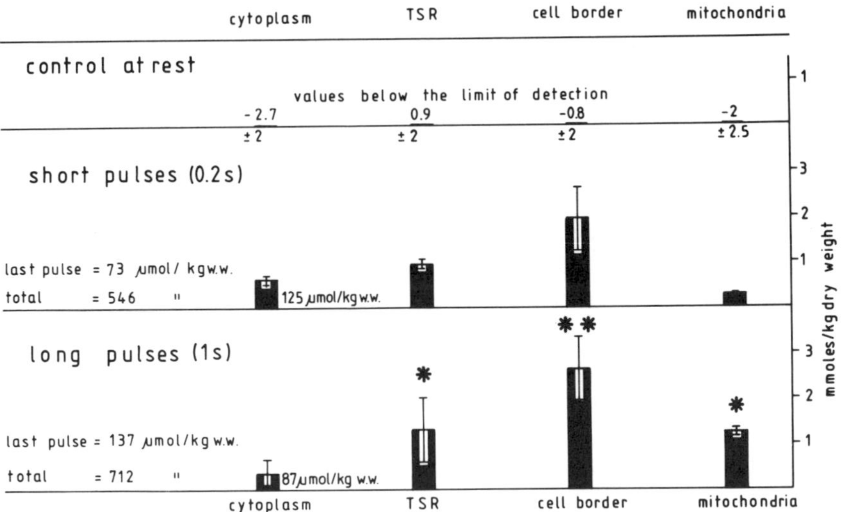

Fig. 4. Total Ca-concentrations in cytoplasma, TjSR, cell border and mitochondria as measured by microprobe (columns) and total Ca-increment (D[Ca]) as calculated from the duration of depolarisation and the cell volume .

In the third experiment contractility was potentiated by a train of 4 long pulses of 1 second. The myocytes were then shock-frozen at the end of the long pulse (800 ms after start of depolarisation). During the long pulse, the cell had almostly relaxed. This is in line with the result that 800 ms after start of the pulse, only 87 µmol/kg w.w. Ca were detected on the cytoplasma by microanalysis. This concentration is less than the calcium increment of 137 µmol due to the last pulse and is also less than the total increment due to the sum of the four pulses. Thus, at this time Ca seems to have moved from the cytoplasma and to have been accumulated in SR (to 1.4 ± 1 mmol Ca/ kg d.w.) and in mitochondria and, probably to some extent, extruded from the cell. The cytosolic Ca-concentration was at this point also less than the 125 µmol detected in the cytoplasma during contraction after short pulses. This is not surprising, since 800 ms after start of the pulse, the cell is practically relaxed, parallel to the intracellular stores having accumulated Ca.

In conclusion:

(1). This method make it possible to quantitate total Ca in compartments of single isolated cells under defined voltage-clamp conditions.

(2). Ca-entry regulates the Ca-load of the cells.

(3). Long pulses load the cell compartments with higher Ca amounts compared to short pulses.

(4). During contraction total cytoplasmic Ca is higher than during relaxation.

CYTOSOLIC FREE Ca^{2+} IN SINGLE CARDIOMYOCYTES: EFFECTS OF ANOXIA AND REOXYGENATION

PETER COBBOLD, ASHLEY ALLSHIRE
Department of Human Anatomy and Cell Biology, University of Liverpool, P.O. Box 147, Liverpool L69 3BX, U.K.

Healthy, rod-shaped, isolated rat ventricle myocytes undergo shortening and rounding-up a few minutes after exposure to metabolic inhibition or glucose-free hypoxia. We have previously shown, using aequorin in poisoned cells that cytoplasmic free Ca^{2+} ($[Ca^{2+}]_i$) rises after shortening has occurred [1]. Here we show that, likewise, glucose-free anoxia induces shortening of the myocyte prior to any rise in $[Ca^{2+}]_i$ above the resting level.

Our key findings [2] may be summarised as;

(i) Glucose-free anoxia in normal $[Ca^{2+}]_o$ medium (1mM) did not cause any prompt rise in $[Ca^{2+}]_i$.

(ii) Shortening occurred after 35-130 minutes, varying from cell to cell.

(iii) No significant rise in $[Ca^{2+}]_i$ occurred at shortening.

(iv) $[Ca^{2+}]_i$ started to rise a minute or so after shortening; there was little variability form cell to cell suggesting a close temporal relationship between shortening and the rise of $[Ca^{2+}]_i$.

(v) The rise in $[Ca^{2+}]_i$ was gradual, reaching 1μM c. 3-5mins after the rise began; 5 minutes later $[Ca^{2+}]_i$ reached c. 3μM at which point exhaustion of aequorin ended the recording. No further shape changes occurred during this rise in $[Ca^{2+}]_i$.

(vi) Reoxygenation of the myocyte had different effects on $[Ca^{2+}]_i$ and cell shape according to $[Ca^{2+}]_i$ at the time of reoxygenation:

(a) Reoxygenation when $[Ca^{2+}]_i$ was c. 1 to 1.5μM led to a c. 10-20s long fall in $[Ca^{2+}]_i$ followed by a period of large amplitude oscillations (see figure A) which ceased after c. 3-5 min, whereupon $[Ca^{2+}]_i$ fell back to close to normal resting levels. The cell showed isotropic squirming movements at a frequency similar to the $[Ca^{2+}]_i$ oscillations.

(b) Reoxygenation of cells in which $[Ca^{2}]_i$ had reached 1.5 to 3μM induced similar effects to above, but $[Ca^{2+}]_i$ often showed incomplete recovery after the oscillatory period, undergoing a second rise 5-20 minutes later. At this point the cells were rounded-up and often showed large blebs of the surface membrane.

(c) Reoxygenation of cells in which $[Ca^{2+}]_i$ was above 3μM led to prompt rounding-up of the shortened cell, bleb formation and lysis. $Ca^{2+}]_i$ showed at best a temporary slowing of the rise. Stern et al [3] have noted that the fate of a cell upon reoxygenation depended on the time since shortening (T_2) and not on the time

Biology of Isolated Adult Cardiac Myocytes
William A. Clark, Robert S. Decker, and Thomas K. Borg, Editors

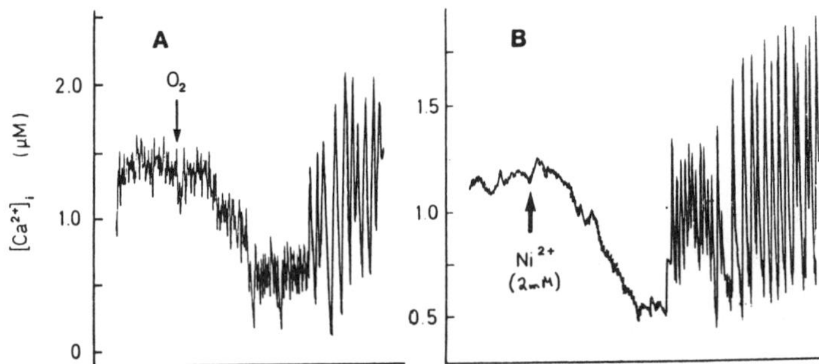

since imposition of anoxia. From our data we now know that their 'T_2' period is the period in which $[Ca^{2+}]_i$ is steadily rising.

(vii) In experiments carried out in nominally Ca-free medium, or medium containing 100μM added Ca, $[Ca^{2+}]_i$ did not rise after the cells shortened. Reoxygenation did not induce either oscillation of $[Ca^{2+}]_i$ or movement of the cells.

(viii) The route for a presumed influx of Ca into a shortened myocyte was investigated in cells poisoned with cyanide (2mM) and 2-deoxyglucose (5mM) [4]. Ni^{2+} (2mM) Co^{2+} or Mn^{2+}, applied when $[Ca^{2+}]_i$ had reached c. 1μM caused a fall in $[Ca^{2+}]_i$ shortly followed by large amplitude oscillations (figure B), a phenomenon reminiscent of that induced by reoxygenation (fig A). Verapamil (10μM) penta-vanadate (0.5mM), and amiloride (0.1mM) had no effect on the rate of the $[Ca^{2+}]_i$ rise. If Ca_o was removed during the $[Ca^{2+}]_i$ rise, $[Ca^{2+}]_i$ fell to a stable low level, rising rapidly upon restoration of Ca_o to about the same level that would have been predicted if Ca_o had never been removed. This suggests a progressive loss of the set-point for $[Ca^{2+}]_i$ the set point treading steadily towards higher values independently of the $[Ca^{2+}]_i$ history of the cell. So a progressively greater saturation of intracellular storage capacity, which would be expected to depend on the $[Ca^{2+}]_i$ history, is unlikely to explain the steady rise in $[Ca^{2+}]_i$. Rather we suspect a progressive perturabion of the influx-efflux balance across the sarcolemma. Our dissection of the mechanism must embrace parameters such as rising $[Na^+]_i$ through loss of the Na,K-ATPase activity and hence Ca-Na exchange, partial reversal of the Ca pump, Ca channels such as i_{si} and receptor-linked channels, and so forth.

(ix) The fall and oscillations of $[Ca^{2+}]_i$ induced by either reoxygenation (fig A) or extracellular Ni^{2+} (fig B) were abolished in cells treated with caffeine (5mM), although caffeine itself appeared not to alter the time course of shortening or the subsequent $[Ca^{2+}]_i$ rise during anoxia. It seems likely that the $[Ca^{2+}]_i$ oscillations depend upon a functional sarcoplasmic reticulum mechanism for Ca uptake and release. We surmise that caffeine-sensitive oscillatory release of Ca may occur in cells in which $[Ca^{2+}]_i$ had been rising for several minutes to c. 1µM or more, which would promote loading of the SR with sequestered Ca, and in which a reduction in $[Ca^{2+}]_i$ suddenly occurs, either by restoration of ATP-dependent Ca pumping (as in reoxygenation) or by blockade of a Ca influx across the sarcolemma (as with Ni^{2+}). The oscillations can be an order of magnitude longer than normal contraction transients, can rise to several micromolar $[Ca^{2+}]_i$, and could conceivably be the cellular process underlying the uncoordinated mechanical activity of the oxygen paradox. Their mechanism needs further investigation.

How does metabolic inhibition induce shortening of the myocyte and the subsequent rise in $[Ca^{2+}]_i$? Shortening is clearly independent of $[Ca^{2+}]_i$. [1,2,]. We hypothesize that rigor complex formation promotes activation of the myosin S-1 ATPase [5]. to bring about the shortening of the cell. Importantly, Holubarsch et al [6] implicate rigor processes in generating tension in the ischaemic heart, paralleling the conclusions of Ventura-Clapier and Vassoort [7]. We have presented a hypothesis [8] that, as the cell shortens, the activity of the myosin S1-ATP-ase rises, leading to a raised consumption of ATP. We postulate that this causes a sudden fall in ATP (or more correctly in phosphorylation potential) as the cell shortens which results in a perturbation of Ca homeostasis thereby offering a possible causal link for the close temporal relationship we have observed. Measurements of ATP, or rigor complex formation, continually in single cells will be central for testing our hypothesis that the $[Ca^{2+}]_i$ rise follows a precipitous fall in ATP as the cell undergoes shortening.

REFERENCES

(1) Cobbold PH, Bourne PK (1984) Nature (Lond) 312 444-446.

(2) Allshire et al. (1987) Biochem. J.244 381-385

(3) Stern et al (1985) Circ. Res. 56 899-903.

(4) Allshire A, Piper H. Cuthbertson R, Cobbold P. Biochem Soc. Trans (in press)

(5) Bremel RD, Weber A (1972) Circ. Res. 51 777-786.

(6) Holubarsch et. al. (1982) Circ. Res. 51 777-786.

(7) Ventura-Clapier R, Vassoort G. (1931) J. Mol. Cell. Cardiol 13 551-561.

(8) Allshire A. Cobbold P. in "Adult Cardiac Myocytes" eds Piper HM, Isenberg G. CRC Press (in press)

Supported by British Heart Foundation grant 84/45.

AEQUORIN MEASUREMENTS OF CYTOSOLIC FREE Ca^{2+} IN SINGLE CARDIOMYOCYTES :TECHNIQUES.

PETER COBBOLD, ASHLEY ALLSHIRE
Department of Human Anatomy and Cell Biology
University of Liverpool, P.O. Box 147, Liverpool L69 3BX, U.K.

Aequorin is a 21Kd photoprotein whose luminescence is triggered by Ca^{2+} ions. We have previously described procedures for its use in single mammalian cells [1]. Here we outline improvements to the technique which have led to its use in heart cells [2,3], liver cells [4] and chromaffin cells [5].

(i) Single collagenase-isolated myocytes were picked up in a c.60µm-bore pipette and transferred to a pool of medium containing 1% agarose (Sigma VII) held at 37°C in a 0.1mm path-length flat glass capillary. The capillary, covered in liquid paraffin (mineral oil) was held on a rectangular piece of coverslip (see [1]). After positioning the cell parallel to the agarose/oil interface within c. 50-100µm of the end of the capillary, the coverslip was held at 5°C for c. 4 minutes to gel the agarose.

(ii) To microinject aequorin the coverslip was attached with a silicon grease film to the free end of a piezoelectric bender element [1], and the cell viewed with x40 objective and 15 x eyepieces of a Nikon Diaphot inverted microscope with cut-away stage [1]. After dimpling the equator of a cell with the pipette tip, a reversing switch caused the bender element to impale the cell on the pipette tip. Raising the gas pressure behind the short column of aequorin in the pipette tip allowed a roughly calibrated volume of aequorin solution to be injected, totalling c. 1% of the cell's volume.

(iii) Aequorin, supplied by Dr. J.R. Blinks, was dissolved to c. 150mg ml^{-1} in EDTA-HEPES (10mM pH 7.0) and stored at -70°C in glass tubules immersed under liquid paraffin. Aliquots of c. 0.2µl were dialysed twice-weekly against (mM) KCl (Spectroscopy grade) 150, PIPES 1, EGTA 0.025, EDTA 0.1, DTT 1 pH 7.4 (in double-glass distilled water), in a c. 3mm length of Biorad Biofiber 50A microdialysis tubule held in a Pt-wire hook and plugged with short columns of liquid paraffin. Dialysis was carried out for 4-6 hours at room temperature. The dialysed aequorin, now c. 70-100 mg ml^{-1}, was placed as a droplet under oil (light liquid paraffin, BDH) on the surface of a tissue culture polystyrene dish, and stored at -70°C until use.

Biology of Isolated Adult Cardiac Myocytes
William A. Clark, Robert S. Decker, and Thomas K. Borg, Editors

(iv) Borosilicate micropipettes of electrophysiological tip size (resistance c. 10MΩ when filled with 3M KCl) were pulled and promptly tip-filled with aequorin by simply immersing the tip for c. 10s in the liquid paraffin and then in the droplet of dialysed aequorin, under visual control by stereomicroscope. The oil breaks the surface tension around the pipette tip, allowing aequorin to enter by capillarity. The filled pipette was promptly fitted to a gas-tight holder on a Leitz micromanipulator. Gas pressure of c. 10-60psi (.5-4atm) was used to expel the aequorin, which forms a column only 50-100μm long in the pipette tip, and offers little resistance to flow (unlike back-filled pipettes).

(v) The aequorin luminescence from the cell was recorded by placing the cell under a cooled, low-noise photomultiplier [1]. A modified apparatus which allows the cell shape to be recorded at intervals was built for anoxia studies [3]. This apparatus was similar to that in (1) except that the base of the cell chamber was cut away to provide a window for a x40 LWD microscope lens. The chamber was moved across the lens field of view by electric motors, and a focussing lens mount (Ealing), again friction-driven by an electric motor, provided remote focus. The separation of the top of the cup from the photomultiplier was increased to allow inclusion of a 1mm plastic optical fibre coupled to a near infra-red diode to provide a light source for microscopy. A remotely-activated air-driven shutter was also fitted, to protect the tube during inspection of the cell. The image of the cell was captured by a CCD camera (Pulnix) and videotaped for subsequent photography of the monitor. Suprisingly sarcomeres were easily detected, despite the crude illumination.

(vi) Anoxic medium needs rigorous preparation to achieve a sufficiently low pO_2 around a single, solitary cell [3]. Glucose-free Ringer (mM; NaCl 125, KCl 2.6, KH_2Po_4 1.2, Mg SO_4 1.2,$CaCl_2$ 1.0, HEPES 10, pH 7.4) was bubbled with O_2-free N_2(O_2< 5ppm). 200ml portions supplemented with 1.5μM resazurin (Sigma), as redox indicator, and 0.83mM cysteine were autoclaved then kept under O_2-freeN_2 at positive pressure. The resazurin dye oxidizes to a pink colour at c. 2 x 10^{-10} atmO_2; coloured solutions were discarded. The medium was piped to the chamber under the photomultiplier in c. 0.5mm bore stainless steel tubes articulated with short lengths of butyl xx rubber tubing.

(vii) The photomultiplier signal was captured as single photoelectron pulses from an amplifier-discriminator (C601, E.M.I.) by a Sirius (Victor) microcomputer and DIO card (EDC Photomic), and binned at 20 samples $^{-1}$. When aequorin discharge was complete the computer performed off-line signal normalisation (background subtraction, computation of rate of comsumption of remaining aequorin) and calibration against _in vitro_ measurements of aequorin consumption in Ca-EGTA buffers, as before [1-4].

The technique is not as fearsome as commonly believed. The success-rate of the injections is between 50 and 100%. Microinjection is now a trivial part of the whole procedure, requiring only c. 5 minutes per cell. The costs of instrumentation (and its complexity) are an order of magnitude lower than for fluorescent Ca indicators.

REFERENCES

(1) Cobbold, P.H. et.al. (1983) J. Cell Sci. 61 123-136.

(2) Cobbold, P.H., Bourne P.K. (1984) Nature 312 444-446.

(3) Allshire, A. et. al. (1987) Biochem. J. 244 381-385.

(4) Woods, N,M. et. al. (1986) Nature 319 600-602.

(5) Cobbold, P.H. et.al. (1987) FEBS Lett. 211 44-48.

Supported by British Heart Foundation, the Wellcome Trust and M.R.C.

CATION AND MEMBRANE POTENTIAL ALTERATIONS IN ENERGY DEPLETED CARDIAC MYOCYTES

QIAN LI***, RUTH A. ALTSCHULD*, BRUCE A. BIAGI** AND BRADFORD T. STOKES**
Departments of *Physiological Chemistry and **Physiology, *Division of Cardiology, and Biophysics Program***, The Ohio State University, Columbus, Ohio 43210

INTRODUCTION

In cardiac cells, more than fifty percent of cellular energy production at rest is used to maintain appropriate ionic gradients across the plasmalemma and subcellular membranes. Disturbance of energy supply can result in severe imbalance of cation homeostasis within the cell. The present study utilizes single cardiac myocytes as a model to characterize alterations in cytosolic Ca^{2+} under ATP-depleted and subsequent reenergized conditions. We have previously demonstrated that myocytes show heterogeneous responses in $[Ca^{2+}]_i$ during rapid deenergization [1]. In particular, the rate of Ca^{2+} increase in energy depleted cells can be altered by changes in extracellular Ca^{2+}, Na^+ and K^+ during the depletion process. Recovery of the cells from energy depletion depends on the degree of calcium accumulation as well as the duration of ATP depletion.

METHODS

Adult Sprague Dawley rat heart myocytes were isolated as previously described [2]. Subsequent to isolation, cells were diluted to approximately 50,000/ml in a HEPES buffer. Fura-2 loading and $[Ca^{2+}]_i$ measurements of individual cells were as described in [1,3]. Double-barreled Na+-selective microelectrodes were made according to Biagi et. al [4], with substitution of the sodium cocktail (Fluka; sodium cocktail 71176) in the ion-selective barrel. Other methodological details are found elsewhere [1-4].

RESULTS AND DISCUSSION

Previous experiments from this lab [1] have revealed that intracellular free calcium increased when cellular ATP was depleted rapidly by respiratory inhibition and uncoupling. In these experiments, cytosolic Ca^{2+} accumulation was found to be primarily dependent on influx from the extracellular space rather than on release from intracellular calcium stores (e.g. SR and mitochondria), since the absence of extracellular Ca^{2+} abolished the increase in $[Ca^{2+}]_i$. The rate of $[Ca^{2+}]_i$ increase, however, differed considerably from cell to cell even when the same deenergization protocol was used. The elevation of $[Ca^{2+}]_i$ was also affected by protocols that should increase intracellular sodium concentration. Alterations in intracellular sodium could therefore play a role in the rapidity with which an energy depleted cell takes up calcium.

The possible pathways for Ca^{2+} influx would include the Ca^{2+} channel and the Na/Ca exchanger. The inadequacy of Ca^{2+} channel phosphorylation in ATP-depleted cells makes the contribution of this pathway relatively of less importance as a mechanism for the Ca^{2+} influx. Alternatively, movement of Ca^{2+} via the Na/Ca exchanger across the cell membrane in either direction seems to be dependent on the Na gradients that are maintained by a normally functioning Na/K ATPase transport system. Impaired pump function caused by energy depletion is likely to result in $[Na^+]_i$ accumulation and $[K^+]_i$ loss. The subsequent dissipation of Na^+ gradient can in turn induce Ca^{2+} entry through the exchanger [5]. A further test of this hypothesis

Biology of Isolated Adult Cardiac Myocytes
William A. Clark, Robert S. Decker, and Thomas K. Borg, Editors

would require direct measurement of intracellular Na^+ activities under these conditions.

As illustrated in Fig. 1, a double-barreled Na^+-selective microelectrode was used to follow membrane voltage (V_m) and intracellular sodium activity (a_{Na}). Initially, we examined the response of the cell to a low potassium (0-K) challenge in order to demonstrate a reversible inhibition of the Na/K pump. As shown, during the rapid change to 0-K, the cell quickly depolarized. This was accompanied by a significant increase in sodium activity that resolved itself after the re-establishment of normal bath conditions. The cell was next treated with amytal and CCCP as described in [1]. A gradual elevation in a_{Na} is evident after deenergization. Sodium activities in different cells ranged from 20-80 mM after 5 min of these conditions. Such variations in sodium activity may explain our previous finding of heterogeneous intracellular hypercalcia after energy depletion [1]. Removal of amytal/CCCP 10 min later enabled ATP production and reversal of the Na^+ increase, presumably by recovery of the Na/K pump. It is clear that the rapid alterations in membrane voltage are not directly associated with the slow changes that occur in intracellular sodium activity. Similar patterns of alteration in membrane potential have been measured with single barrel electrodes thus establishing that these fluctuations are not a consequence of the double-barrel electrode technique. It would appear, therefore, that these shifts in membrane voltage reflect changes in relative membrane permeabilities and/or electrogenic transport systems. In summary, our measurements of ionic activities clearly demonstrate that energy depletion results in significant increases in intracellular sodium that are accompanied by reproducible voltage patterns which reflect remarkable alterations in surface membrane properties.

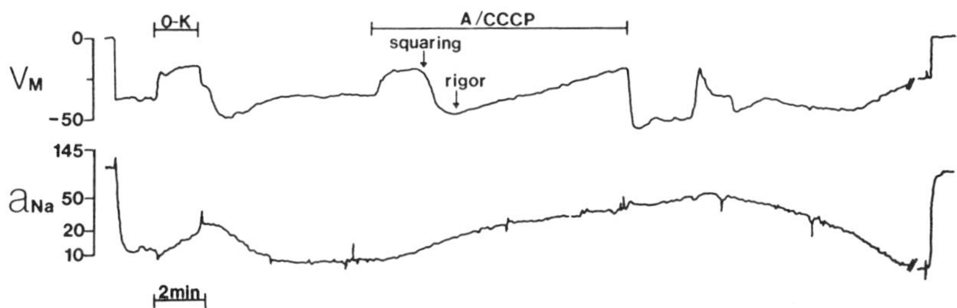

Fig. 1. Alterations of membrane potential (Vm) and Na^+ activity (a_{Na}) measured with a double-barrel Na^+-selective microelectrode. The cell was perfused with Krebs Henseleit buffer containing 1 mM Ca^{2+} and 6 mM K^+. Extracellular K^+ was removed during the 0-K period to inhibit Na/K ATPase. 3 mM amytal (A) and 2 uM CCCP were added to the perfusate (A/CCCP) to deenergize the cell.

An example of one pattern of change in $[Ca^{2+}]_i$ that may occur after ATP depletion is shown in Fig. 2. Cells were deenergized as in Fig. 1 and free Ca^{2+} levels determined by fura-2 microscopy. We speculate that the rapid increase in $[Ca^{2+}]_i$ that occurs after ATP depletion is associated with a high rate of Na^+ accumulation in these cells. Reenergization (by washout of amytal and CCCP) in these hypercalcic cells induced cellular disruption as indicated by a transition of the cell from a striated squared shape (rigor) to a disorganized round form. The partial recovery in calcium presumably is the result of the re-establishment of the Na^+ gradient and thus exchanger function or the reactivation of the sarcolemmal calcium-dependent ATPase.

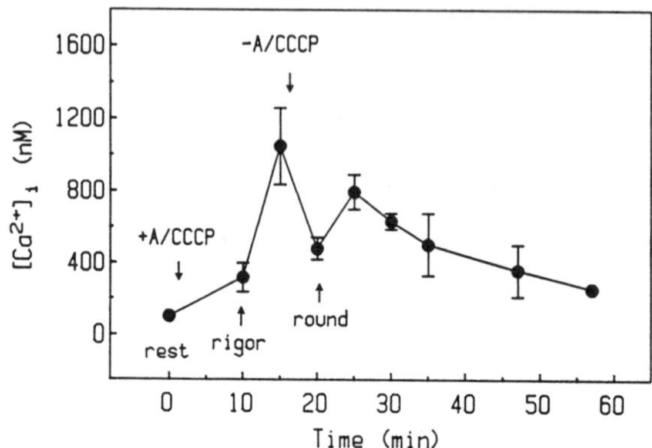

Fig. 2. Hypercalcia induced by cellular ATP depletion and cellular disruption by subsequent reenergization. $[Ca^{2+}]_i$ levels were determined by fura-2 fluorescence ratio at 350 and 380 nm. These cells became Ca^{2+} loaded when the same amytal/CCCP protocol as Fig. 1 was applied. Restoration of respiration led to hypercontracture (round) of these cells.

Other cells (with presumably slow Na^+ accumulation) show different patterns in $[Ca^{2+}]_i$ increase after deenergization (Fig. 3). As shown, only a minor increase occurred in these two groups of cells illustrated after energy depletion. One group (solid diamonds) that was energy depleted for the same period of time as those in Fig. 2, went into contracture (rigor) with little hypercalcia. When amytal and CCCP were removed, they retained their sarcomeric organization and ability to contract. If, however, in the other population (open diamonds), the oxidative phosphorylation was not restored (by removal of A/CCCP) until 40 min after the onset of contracture, cellular deterioration occurred even though the free calcium level was low (as compared to Fig. 2). Hypercontracture (round) was followed by a large increase in free calcium. We predict that degradation of the nucleotide pool during the prolonged ATP depletion resulted in depressed ATP production when oxidative phosphorylation is restored [2]. Under these prolonged exposure conditions, the recovery of the Ca^{2+} and Na/K ATPases would not be sufficient to re-establish the cation gradients of the cell. It is clear that temporal alterations in intracellular electrolytes and other metabolic pools are therefore both of importance in determining intracellular calcium activities during deenergization and recovery.

In summary, intracellular Na^+ increases as a result of sodium pump inhibition after rapid ATP depletion. The elevated $[Na^+]_i$ induces Ca^{2+} influx via the Na/Ca exchanger and regulates the rate of Ca^{2+} accumulation. Inhibition of oxidative phosphorylation and glycolysis results in heterogeneous responses in $[Na^+]_i$ and $[Ca^{2+}]_i$ in the same population of cells. Recovery and survival from cellular energy depletion insult depends on both calcium overload and the duration of ATP depletion. Future experiments will investigate the nature of accompanying voltage alterations and the role of other metabolites in the pathological process.

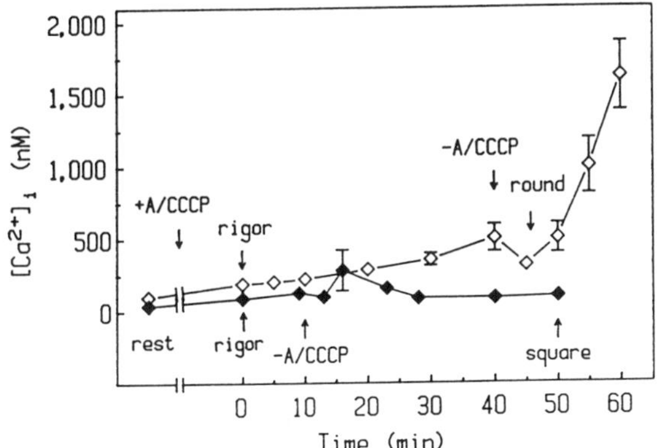

Fig. 3. Dependence of cell recovery on the duration of ATP depletion. Cellular structure and low Ca2+ levels (solid diamonds) could be preserved by early restitution of energy production (-A/CCCP at 10 min). In spite of the relative low $[Ca^{2+}]_i$, however, washout of amytal/CCCP after prolonged ATP removal (at 40 min) could also precipitate hypercontractrue and Ca^{2+} overload.

ACKNOWLEDGMENTS

These studies were supported in part by grants-in-aid from the Central Ohio Heart Chapter, Inc., United States Public Health Services Grant H136240 and National Institutes of Health Grant NS 10165. We wish to thank Ms. Ellen Patricia for skillful assistance in preparing Na^+ electrodes.

REFERENCES

1. Q. Li, R.A. Altschuld, and B.T. Stokes, Am. J. Physiol., Submitted (1987).
2. R.A. Altschuld, L.M. Gamelin, R.E. Kelley, M.R. Lambert, L.E. Apel, and G.P. Brierley, J. Biol. Chem., In Press (1987).
3. Q. Li, R.A. Altschuld, and B.T. Stokes, Biochem. Biophys. Res. Comm. 147, 120-126 (1987).
4. B. Biagi, M. Sohtell, and G. Giebisch, Am. J. Physiol. 241, F677-F686 (1981).
5. J.P. Reeves, Curr. T. Mem. 25, 77-127 (1985).

CONTROL OF Ca AND Mn INFLUX IN ISOLATED ADULT RAT HEART CELLS

ROBERT A. HAWORTH, ATILLA B. GOKNUR, HERBERT A. BERKOFF
Department of Surgery, University of Wisconsin Clinical Science Center, 600 Highland Avenue, Madison, WI 53792, USA

INTRODUCTION

An understanding of the control of Ca fluxes across the sarcolemma is vital to an understanding of excitation contraction coupling, contractile function, and cell dysfunction in a variety of pathological conditions. Isolated adult heart cells in suspension offer new possibilities for studying this control, using ^{45}Ca and intracellular Ca-sensitive dyes. We have recently investigated the role of ATP depletion as a controller of Ca fluxes, and found that it inhibits cellular Ca influx even under conditions of severe Na loading [1]. In addition we have developed an assay for the Ca channel using ^{54}Mn uptake which can be applied to cells stimulated to beat in suspension [2]. This assay allows us to rapidly measure Ca channel activity which is characteristic of the whole population of cells for any given condition.

METHODS

Cells were isolated as previously described [3], and resuspended in experimental medium containing 118 mM NaCl, 4.8 mM KCl, 25 mM HEPES, 1.2 mM KH_2PO_4, 1.2 mM $MgSO_4$, 1 mM $CaCl_2$ (unless otherwise stated), 5 mM Na pyruvate, 11 mM glucose, 2 mM sucrose, 1μM insulin, adjusted to pH 7.4 with NaOH. Suspensions were maintained aerobic at 37° by equilibration with air.

Measurement of intracellular Ca levels using quin2 and indo1, measurement of cell Na with ^{22}Na, and ATP analysis were as described [1] uptake was measured as described in [2].

RESULTS

When ^{45}Ca was added to cells in a medium containing 1mM Ca a rapid labelling of the cells was observed which quickly leveled off (Fig. 1). Addition of rotenone (4μM) plus FCCP (2μM) caused a reduction in ATP levels from 17.08±2.26 to 0.63±0.11 nmol/mg after 8 min. By this time the amount of rapidly exchangeable Ca had dropped by 1.65±0.10 nmol/mg (Fig. 1). If ^{45}Ca was added to cells which were already ATP depleted, its uptake reached a plateau at this new lower level (Fig. 1). However, on addition of the Ca ionophore A23187 (1.5 μg/ml) a massive Ca influx was induced (Fig. 1). This shows that even though the cells were ATP depleted they were capable of excluding the extracellular Ca. This observation caused us to investigate the effect of ATP depletion on the rate of Ca influx.

The measurement of the effect of ATP depletion on the rate of Ca influx in heart cells is complicated by the fact that ATP depletion inhibits the Na pump, causing intracellular Na buildup which will tend to potentiate Ca entry. To overcome this we have measured the rate of Ca entry into cells in suspension which are equally Na loaded by ouabain treatment but which differ in their ATP content. To load cells with Na, ouabain (1 mM) was added and cells were incubated at 37°C for 30 min. This resulted in a rise of intracellular Na from 16.8±1.5 mM to 93.9±5.8 mM as measured with ^{22}Na. If the metabolic poisons oligomycin (36.4 μM) and iodoacetate (0.91 mM) were added 15 min after ouabain, the cellular Na level 15 min later was 95.3±4.2 mM, not significantly different from that of cells incubated with ouabain alone. ATP levels, however, were reduced by over 90%.

Biology of Isolated Adult Cardiac Myocytes
William A. Clark, Robert S. Decker, and Thomas K. Borg, Editors

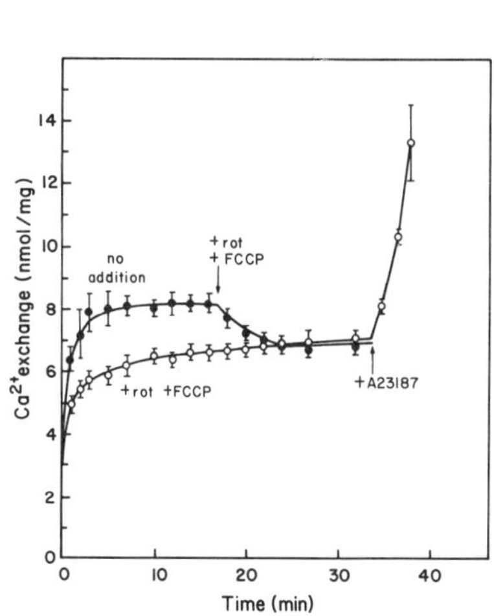

Figure 1. Ca exchange by normal & ATP depleted cells. Cells were in experimental medium containing 1 mM, and ^{45}Ca was added at time zero.

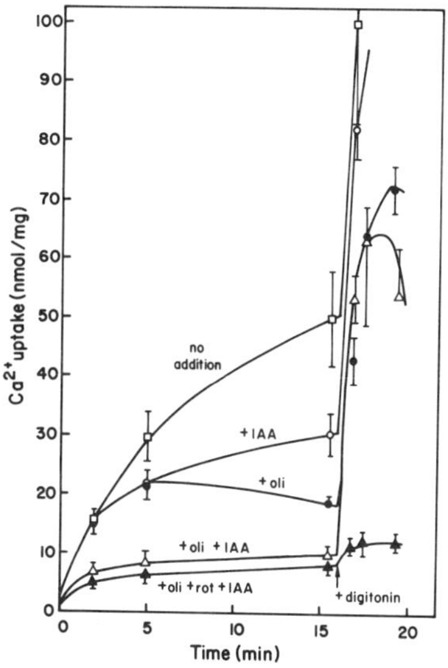

Figure 2. Inhibition of Ca influx in Na-loaded cells by ATP depletion, measured by ^{45}Ca (by permission of the American Heart Association, Inc.)

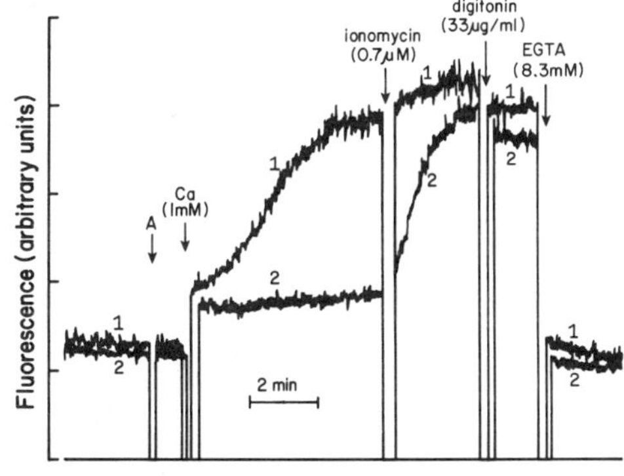

Figure 3. Inhibition of Ca influx in Na-loaded cells by ATP depletion, measured by quin2. Curve 1: cells with ATP; curve 2: ATP-depleted cells.

When cells loaded with Na were given 1 mM Ca containing ^{45}Ca, a massive Ca uptake resulted (Fig. 2). If the cells also were ATP depleted with oligomycin plus iodoacetate, Ca uptake was strongly inhibited, even though on disrupting the sarcolemma with digitonin (22 μg/ml) a large mitochondrial Ca uptake was still possible (Fig. 2). In cells treated with oligomycin or iodoacetate alone, ATP levels at the time of Ca addition were no different from control, and the initial rate of Ca uptake was the same as in cells without oligomycin or iodoacetate (Fig. 2). This suggests that

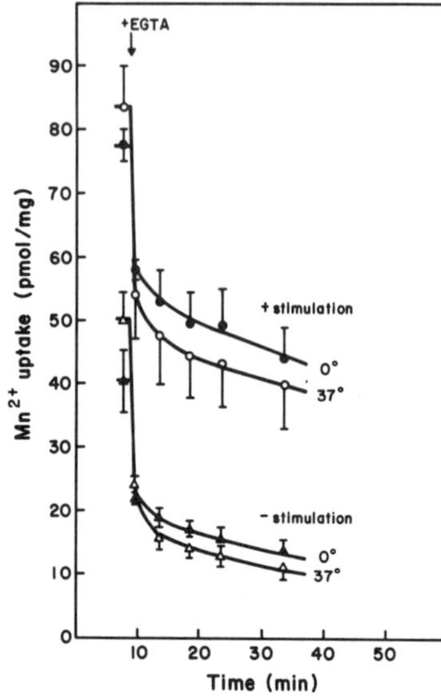

Figure 4. Promotion of ^{54}Mn uptake by electrical stimulation. Cells treated with isoproterenol were stimulated to beat for 5 min at 2 Hz. (Reproduced from the Journal of Molecular and Cellular Cardiology with permission).

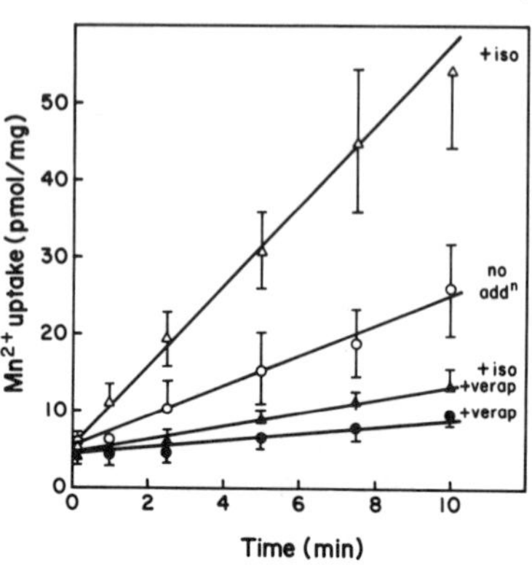

Figure 5. Effect of isoproterenol and verapamil on cellular Mn uptake. Cells were stimulated at 2 Hz for the times and conditions shown, and the Mn remaining 20 min after EGTA addition was measured. (Reproduced from the Journal of Molecular and Cellular Cardiology a with permission).

the effect on Ca uptake rates was a result of ATP depletion rather than a direct effect of the inhibitors. Oligomycin or iodoacetate alone did have an effect on Ca uptake at later times (Fig. 2). This could be related to the compromised ability of these cells to maintain ATP levels after Ca addition, or to their having some effect on the ability of mitochondria to accumulate Ca. The rate of Ca entry into these cells was then examined by measuring the rate of increase of fluorescence on addition of 1 mM Ca to Na-loaded cells containing quin2 [4]. Cells in experimental medium without Ca were loaded with quin2 by incubation with 30 µM quin2-AM for 30 min at 37°, resulting in a cellular uptake of 3.4$\pm$0.3 nmol quin2/mg protein. The cells were washed twice. To load cells with Na, ouabain (1mM) was then added and cells were incubated at 37^{o} for 30 min. Fig. 3 shows that in cells with ATP (curve 1), fluorescence increased sigmoidally over five minutes to near saturation, while in ATP-depleted cells (curve 2), the fluorescence hardly increased at all. The step increase in fluorescence after Ca addition in both samples corresponds to Ca binding to residual extracellular quin2, as revealed by the ability of Mn^{2+} to immediately quench it. Calculation of intracellular Ca values after 5 min, using a Mn quench cycle [1] after the method of Rink and Pozzan [4], gave values of 1727$\pm$832 nM for cells with ATP and 9$\pm$5 nM for ATP-depleted cells. Addition of ionomycin, a Ca ionophore, resulted in a rapid rate of rise in intracellular Ca in ATP-depleted cells (Fig. 1). It is therefore clear that ATP depletion results in a very strong inhibition of the rate of Ca entry, such that a large sarcolemmal Ca gradient can be maintained.

Since the massive Ca uptake requires Na loading we conclude that it is mostly carried by the Na/Ca exchanger. Caroni and Carafoli [5] have given evidence that activation and deactivation of Na/Ca exchange activity in sarcolemmal vesicles is controlled by a calmodulin-regulated kinase and phosphatase. Such a system could well account for the inhibition of Ca uptake observed here. This control of Ca influx by ATP could well be of relevance to reperfusion-induced injury after a period of ischemia, which is associated with a large calcium uptake [6].

One of the major determinants of contractile force is the excitation-dependent influx of Ca through the Ca channel. Measurement of Ca channel activity in single cells by voltage clamp techniques has been achieved in recent years [7,8]. We have sought a method for measurement of Ca channel activity in cell suspensions which would be rapid and give a measure characteristic of the whole suspension for any given condition. Isolated adult heart cells are normally quiescent but can be stimulated to beat in suspension [9]. The measurement of excitation-dependent rates of Ca influx are, however, problematic. The rate of Ca influx by Na loaded cells is readily measured with ^{45}Ca, because the conditions are rigged to promote influx and retard efflux. In cells without ouabain, however, the extent of ^{45}Ca labelling is rather small (Fig. 1). Influx rates are hard to measure, because the systems for Ca removal from the cell are so active. On the other hand, Mn uptake by the whole heart is almost unidirectional and is verapamil sensitive, indicating its usefulness as a probe of Ca channel activity [10]. We have therefore investigated the use of ^{54}Mn uptake as a probe of Ca channel activity in isolated cells in suspension.

Cells in suspension with 1 mM Ca plus 5µM ^{54}Mn showed a biphasic Mn uptake pattern: a rapid phase, followed by slow phase [2]. The rapid phase was rapidly removable by EGTA and was temperature-insensitive. The Mn remaining after EGTA addition could be released by digitonin plus A23187, suggesting it is intracellular [2]. When cells were treated with isoproterenol (1 µM) and stimulated to beat in suspension for 5 min at 2Hz, the intracelluar Mn pool was greatly increased (Fig. 4). The amount of Mn remaining 20 min after EGTA addition depended linearly on the length of time the cells were stimulated (Fig. 5). This indicates that the rate of Mn efflux was very low. The rate of Mn influx was strongly stimulated by the isoproterenol treatment, and was inhibited by 10 µM verapamil (Fig. 3). Nitredipine (10 µM) gave a similar degree of inhibition. This Mn uptake thus shows a pharmacology characteristic of the Ca channel, indicating that it can be used to measure such in isolated adult heart cells stimulated to beat in suspension.

REFERENCES

1. Haworth RA, Goknur AB, Hunter DR, Hegge Jo, Berkoff HA. Circ. Res. 60:586-594 (1987).
2. Haworth RA, Goknur AB, Berkoff HA. J. Mol. Cell. Cardiol., accepted for publication.
3. Haworth RA, Hunter DR, Berkoff HA. J. Mol. Cell. Cardiol., 12:715-723 (1980).
4. Rink TJ, Pozzan T. Cell Calcium. 6:133-144 (1985).
5. Caroni P, Carafoli E. Eur. J. Biochem. 132:451-460 (1983).
6. Bourdillon PD, Poole-Wilson PA. Cardiovasc. Res. 15:121-130 (1981).
7. Isenberg G, Klockner V. Pflug. Arch. 395:30-41 (1982).
8. Lee KS, Tsien RW. Nature. 297:498-501 (1982).
9. Haworth RA, Hunter DR, Berkoff HA, Moss RL. Circ. Res. 52:342-351 (1983).
10. Hunter DR, Haworth RA, Berkoff HA. J. Mol. Cell. Cardiol. 13:823-832 (1981).

THE RELATIONSHIP BETWEEN THE CYTOSOLIC Ca^{++} TRANSIENT AND CELL LENGTH DURING THE TWITCH IN SINGLE ADULT CARDIAC MYOCYTES

HAROLD A. SPURGEON, GUNTHER BAARTZ, MAURIZIO C. CAPOGROSSI, STEFANO RAFFAELI, MICHAEL D. STERN, AND EDWARD G. LAKATTA
Laboratory of Cardiovascular Science, Gerontology Research Center, National Institute on Aging, National Institutes of Health, Baltimore, MD 21224

INTRODUCTION

The recent development of fluorescent Ca^{++} indicators [1] that are sensitive to $[Ca^{++}]$ as low as that expected to be found in cardiac muscle in diastole and that can be loaded into cardiac myocytes, without disrupting the sarcolemma, has presented a new opportunity to address questions of excitation-contraction coupling in the heart. We have used one of these new probes, i.e. Indo-1 and a newly developed apparatus that can simultaneously record cytosolic Ca^{++} (Ca_i) and cell length in single adult cardiac myocytes [2] to determine the temporal relationship of the Ca_i transient and contraction during the twitch with particular emphasis on the slow phase of relaxation.

METHODS

Left ventricular myocytes were obtained from 2-6 month old rats by retrograde perfusion of the aorta with a low-Ca^{++}, collagenase bicarbonate buffer as previously described [3]. Following the dissociation procedure cells were resuspended in Hepes buffer of the following composition in mM: 137 NaCl, 1.2 $MgSO_4 \cdot 7H_2O$, 5 KCl, 20 HEPES, 16 D-glucose; $CaCl_2$ 1 mM was varied between 0.25 and 30; pH 7.4 ± 0.05. Loading of Indo-1 AM into single cardiac myocytes was done at 23°C in a chamber on the stage of the microscope according to a recently described method which utilizes Indo-1 AM dissolved in dimethylsulfoxide and mixed with fetal calf serum and a dispersing agent, Pluronic F-127 [4]. Cells were stimulated to twitch by field depolarization with electrodes placed in the bathing fluid [3]. All experiments were done at 23°C. Indo-1 fluorescence was excited by epi-illumination with 10 μsec flashes of 350 ± 10 nm light at repetition rates of up to 250 Hz. Indo-1 emission was collected by paired photomultipliers to measure simultaneously spectral windows of 411 ± 20 nm and 481 ± 25 nm selected by bandpass interference filters. The fluorescence emission from each flash was collected by a pair of fast integrator sample-and-hold circuits of custom design under the control of a VAX 11/730 computer which, for each flash, calculated the ratio of Indo-1 emission at the two wavelengths as a measure of Ca_i. Cell length was measured from the bright-field image of the cell by an optical edge tracking method using a photodiode array with a 5 msec time resolution. The VAX computer calculated cell length and the contractile parameters that relate to the twitch. By using red light (700-750 nm) for the bright-field image and a dichroic mirror to transmit the fluorescent light (380-550 nm) and reflect the red light, length and Ca_i measurements were obtained simultaneously without cross-talk.

RESULTS AND DISCUSSION

Indo-1, as well as the other fluorescent Ca^{++} indicators [1], can buffer the Ca_i transient and the contractile response of the cell to changes in Ca_i. However it is possible to find loading conditions that minimize this problem [2]. Figures 1A and 1B show the time course of a rested twitch before and 1 hour after exposing the cell to 4 μM Indo-1 AM

Published 1988 by Elsevier Science Publishing Co., Inc.
Biology of Isolated Adult Cardiac Myocytes
William A. Clark, Robert S. Decker, and Thomas K. Borg, Editors

for 90 sec. Note that prior to Indo-1 loading a slow phase of relaxation, which is typical of unloaded myocytes at this temperature, is present. It has not been determined whether this slow phase of relaxation is due entirely to a passive "restoring force" intrinsic to the anatomic structure of the myocyte or whether a slow decrease in Ca_i could be involved in the restoration of cell length to its resting level. Following Indo-1 loading there was a small decrease in maximal twitch amplitude but the maximum shortening velocity, the rate of relaxation and in particular the slow phase of relaxation were similar for both contractions (Figure 1A). In Figure 1B the contractions from Figure 1A have been normalized to their peak amplitude to facilitate comparison of their shapes. Figure 1C shows, in the same cell as in Panels A and B, how the temporal changes in Ca_i and cell length are related to each other, and in particular demonstrates that there is a slow decrease in Ca_i which parallels the slow tail of relaxation. A similar slow phase of relengthening in cultures of chick embryonic heart cells [5-7] has been related to changes in Ca_i in preparations loaded with Indo-1 AM [8]. Thus, these and the present results suggest that a passive restoring force may not be the sole or even the major determinant of the slow phase of relaxation in unloaded cardiac myocytes. To further examine the potential roles of passive restoring forces and Ca_i in determining the slow phase of relaxation we used the β-adrenergic agonist, isoproterenol.

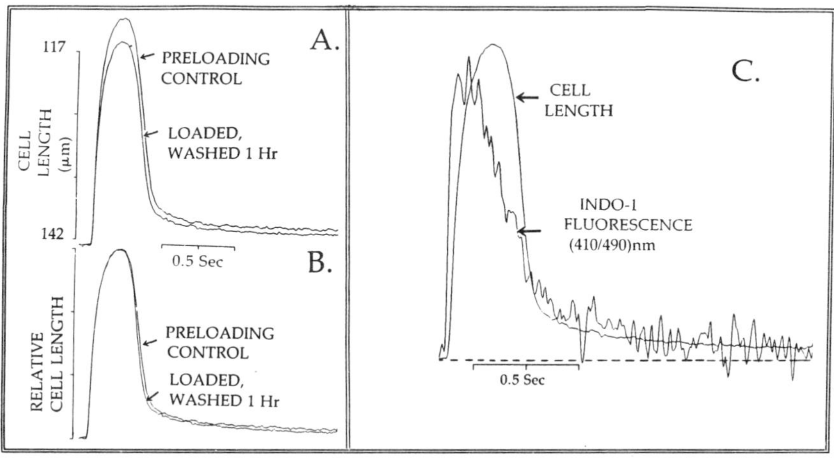

Figure 1. Effect of a 90 sec period of loading with Indo-1 AM on cell length and Ca_i in a representative single adult cardiac myocyte. Indo-1 loading was done on the stage of the microscope and rested contractions were obtained prior to and after exposure of the myocyte to the indicator. A) Cell length during a twitch in control and 1 hour after removal of Indo-1 AM from the bathing medium. B) Same twitches as in Panel A normalized to the same maximal twitch amplitude. C) Same cell as in Panel A after Indo-1 loading. Note the slow tail of relaxation of cell length and Ca_i.

It is known that β-adrenergic stimulation enhances twitch amplitude and reduces twitch duration in rat myocardium [9] and single cardiac cells [10]. It has not been established, however, whether β-adrenergic stimulation can alter the slow phase of relaxation in single rat myocytes. Figure 2A shows a twitch and the Ca_i transient in a representative rat myocyte before and after addition of 0.1 μM isoproterenol. Isoproterenol increases the rate of rise of Ca_i, decreases its time to peak and enhances its decay, both the early phase and particularly the slow phase. These events are reflected in an increase in velocity and extent of twitch shortening, a decrease in time to peak shortening, and a reduction in relaxation time, including that of the slow tail. In addition, in accordance with a previously described effect of β-adrenergic stimulation to decrease Ca_i in the absence of membrane depolarization [11] isoproterenol decreased the resting ratio of Indo-1 fluorescence.

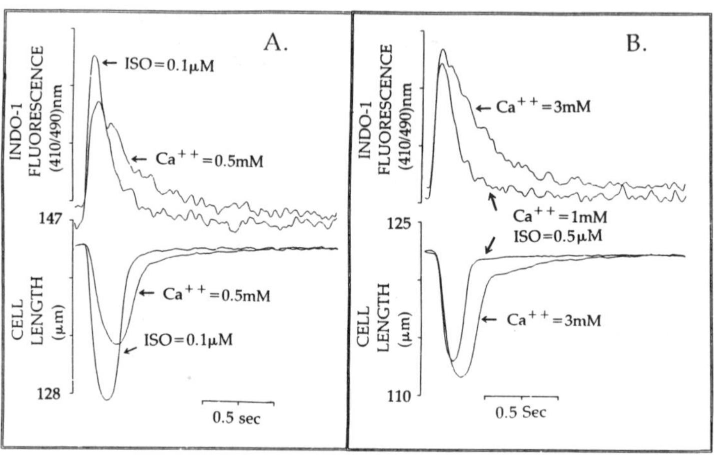

Figure 2. A. Change in Ca_i and cell length during stimulation at 0.2 Hz in the steady state in 0.5 mM Ca_o before and after addition of 0.1 μM isoproterenol (see text for details). B. Changes in Ca_i and cell length during stimulation at 0.2 Hz in the steady state either in 1.0 mM Ca_o and 0.5 μM isoproterenol or in 3 mM Ca_o without isoproterenol (see text for details).

In order to elucidate whether isoproterenol accelerated the slow phase of relaxation by affecting passive mechanical restoring forces via an increase in twitch amplitude rather than by accelerating Ca_i removal after the twitch we compared the Ca_i and contractile transients during a twitch in 3 mM Ca_o to those of similar amplitude generated by isoproterenol in 1 mM Ca_o in the same myocyte. Figure 2B shows that the marked effect of β-adrenergic stimulation to accelerate the rapid and slow phases of relaxation of Ca_i and cell length under these conditions is qualitatively similar to that observed in Figure 2A. Thus, the marked effect of β-adrenergic stimulation to accelerate the decay of the contractile transient cannot be attributed to its effect to enhance the magnitude of a passive restoring force on the basis of an increase in twitch amplitude. Rather, the enhanced rate of the slow relaxation phase that accompanied the larger twitch amplitude must be attributable to the concomitant accelerated removal of Ca^{++} from the cytosol.

In conclusion, we have used a novel system to study the relationship between Ca_i and contractile motion during a twitch and how this is affected by β-adrenergic stimulation. Our results show that a slow tail of relaxation exists in unloaded adult single cardiac myocytes and is accompanied by a slow decay of the Ca_i transient that elicits the twitch. β-Adrenergic stimulation shortens the slow tail of relaxation and this is associated with a more rapid return of Ca_i to a lower resting value. Thus, the well known effects of β-adrenergic stimulation on the time course of the twitch can be accounted for by its effects to abbreviate the time course of the Ca_i transient. While restoring forces are required to return the cell to its slack length following contraction, these do not appear to be completely passive in nature. Rather the removal of Ca_i appears to be a mechanism that determines both the early and late phase of relaxation in unloaded cardiac cells.

REFERENCES

1. G. Grynkiewicz, M. Poenie, and R.Y. Tsien, J. Biol. Chem. 260, 3440-3450 (1985).
2. H.A. Spurgeon, M.D. Stern, S. Raffaeli, R. Hansford, A. Talo, E.G. Lakatta, and M.C. Capogrossi, in preparation.
3. M.C. Capogrossi, A.A. Kort, H.A. Spurgeon, and E.G. Lakatta, J. Gen. Physiol. 88, 589-613 (1986).
4. Poenie, M., J. Alderton, R. Steinhardt, and R. Tsien, Science 233, 886-889 (1986).
5. W.T. Clusin, Proc. Natl. Acad. Sci. USA 77, 679-683 (1980).
6. W.T. Clusin, J. Physiol (London) 320, 149-174 (1981).
7. D.S. Miura, S. Biedert, and W.H. Barry, J. Mol. Cell. Cardiol. 13, 949-961 (1981).
8. H.-C. Lee and W.T. Clusin, Biophys. J. 51, 411a (1987).
9. T. Guarnieri, C. R. Filburn, G. Zitnik, G.S. Roth, and E.G. Lakatta, Am. J. Physiol. 239, H501-H508 (1980).
10. M.C. Capogrossi, B.A. Suarez-Isla, and E.G. Lakatta, J. Gen. Physiol. 88, 615-633 (1986).
11. S.-S. Sheu, V.K. Sharma, and M. Korth, Biophys. J. 49, 350a (1986).

THE VOLTAGE DEPENDENCE OF THE MYOPLASMIC CALCIUM TRANSIENT IN GUINEA PIG VENTRICULAR MYOCYTES IS MODULATED BY SODIUM LOADING

GERRIT ISENBERG*, HAROLD SPURGEON, ANTTI TALO**, MICHAEL STERN, MAURIZIO CAPOGROSSI, AND EDWARD LAKATTA
Laboratory of Cardiovascular Science, Gerontology Research Center, National Institute on Aging, National Institutes of Health, Baltimore, MD 21224; Present Addresses: *Department of Applied Physiology, University of Cologne, West Germany; **Department of Biology, University of Turku, Finland

INTRODUCTION

Depolarization induced Ca influx can be attributed to sarcolemmal Ca^{2+} channels or to Na-Ca exchange. Both can contribute to the excitation induced myoplasmic Ca^{2+} transient but depend on membrane potential in different ways: Ca^{2+} channels have a bell-shaped voltage dependence, with a maximum around +10mV [1]; the Na-Ca exchanger in contrast, depends exponentially on membrane potential [2], and also exhibits a dependence on cytosolic $[Na^+]$, (Na_i). In the experiments discussed here, we assessed the voltage dependence of the myoplasmic Ca^{2+} transient in single ventricular guinea pig myocytes in the presence and absence of Na^+ in the patch pipette.

METHODS

Myocytes were isolated from guinea pig (300g) hearts by retrograde perfusion at 37°C with a solution containing collagenase and a low $[Ca^{2+}]$ as previously described [3] and were subsequently bathed in Hepes buffer containing in mM NaCl 136.9, KCl 5, Hepes 20, dextrose 15, $MgSO_4$ $7H_2O$ 1.2, at pH 7.4. and 23°C. Cells were then loaded with the acetoxymethyl ester of the fluorescent Ca^{2+} probe, Indo-1,4μM for 10 minutes as described in detail elsewhere [4]. Changes of cytoplasmic $[Ca^{2+}]$ (ΔCa_i) were monitored as changes in the ratio of Indo-1 fluorescence 410/490nm as described in the preceding paper [5]. Contraction was measured via a video edge monitor detector as described previously [3]. The degree of Indo-1 loading achieved via the 10min loading procedure was sufficient to permit the detection of the excitation induced ΔCa_i during each twitch without averaging or filtration. However, this degree of Indo-1 loading buffered Ca_i sufficiently to reduce the twitch amplitude and to prolong its relaxation time [5]. Whole cell membrane current [1] was measured with patch electrode (2-3 MΩ resistance) filled with 150mM KCl, 10 mM Hepes/KOH, pH 7.4 (20μM EGTA) with or without 10mM NaCl. Following one minute of rest, cells were stimulated with 10 pulses once every 2 seconds. Steady state was usually achieved within 6 pulses.

RESULTS

Measurements with Na free pipettes. Figure 1 shows the steady state response of a guinea pig ventricular myocyte to a 200 ms voltage step from -50 to 0mV. The step induces a net inward current (I_{Ca}), that quickly activates to a peak and inactivates, and upon repolarization rapidly deactivates. Following the initiation of I_{Ca}, Ca_i increases from the resting level as indicated by an increase in the ratio of Indo-1 fluorescence. We interpret the initial portion of this Indo-1 transient to reflect rapid Ca-release from the sarcoplasmic reticulum (SR) as it (1) exhibits beat to

Published 1988 by Elsevier Science Publishing Co., Inc.
Biology of Isolated Adult Cardiac Myocytes
William A. Clark, Robert S. Decker, and Thomas K. Borg, Editors

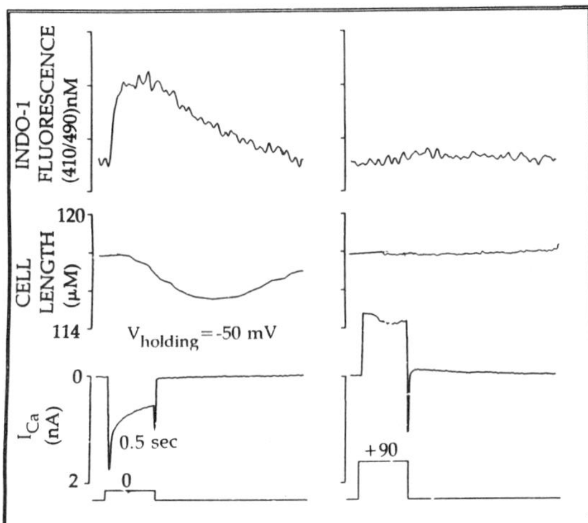

Fig. 1. Voltage clamp steps from -50mV to 0 (left panel) elicits an inward current (lower), a calcium transient, measured as a change in Indo-1 fluorescence at 410/490 nM (top), and a contraction (middle panel) in a representative myocyte without NaCl added to the patch pipette. A clamp to +90mV in the same cell (right panel) fails to elicit an inward current, a rapid increase in Ca_i or a twitch.

beat increase prior to achieving steady state following stimulation from rest in the absence of substantial beat to beat alterations in I_{Ca}, and (2) is markedly reduced in amplitude and prolonged by Ryanodine (results not shown). The figure also shows that depolarization to +90mV which does not elicit a net inward current does not trigger a rapid increase in Ca_i or contraction. (In most but not all cases the repolarization following depolarization to strong positive potentials causes a Ca-influx through a short lasting tail current and an increase in Ca_i as already described by other studies [6]).

Figure 2 shows the voltage dependence of the peak I_{Ca}, the ΔCa_i and its maximum rate of $d\Delta Ca_i/dt_{max}$ (inward current is plotted in the upward direction for comparison with voltage dependence of Ca_i parameters). I_{Ca} reaches threshold at approximately -30mV and increases with more positive potentials until a maximum is reached at about +10mV. At more positive potentials, the current amplitude falls and is approximately zero above +50mV. That the shape of the voltage dependence of the Ca-current, ΔCa_i and $d\Delta Ca_i/dt_{max}$ during the clamp step resemble each other suggests that Ca-influx through voltage operated sarcolemmal Ca-channels is a determinant of the voltage dependent gradation of the Ca_i transient.

<u>Measurements with Na loaded pipettes</u>. Na_i has been estimated to be about 7mM in resting cardiac preparations [7]. In experiments in cells voltage clamped with patch-electrodes of 1-2μm in diameter, a rapid equilibration of the cytosol with the constituents of the electrolyte filling the patch-electrode can occur. If the pipette solution is free of Na^+ as it was in Figures 1-2, the Na_i can be diluted to low levels. Since Ca-influx via Na,Ca-exchange is Na_i dependent, experiments in Figure 2 may have artifically underestimated its potential impact on the Ca_i-signal. We thus studied other cells with pipettes to which 10mM NaCl was added. For brevity, we call these myocytes "Na^+-loaded myocytes", though this designation is not intended to indicate Na^+ "overloaded".

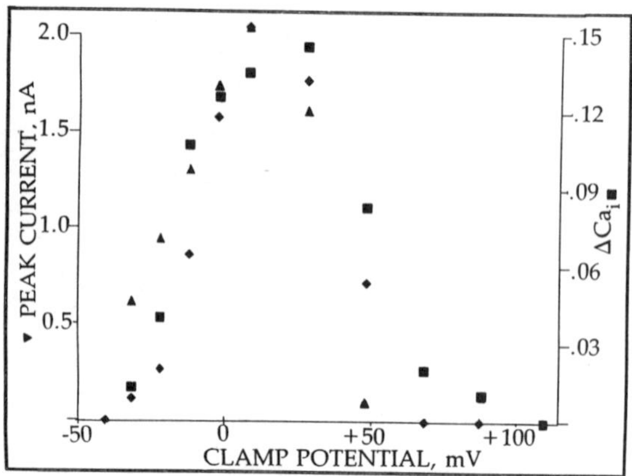

Fig. 2. The voltage dependence of Ca current (▲), cystolic Ca^{2+} transient (ΔCa_i), measured as in Fig. 1 (■), and the maximum rate of rise of the rapid upstroke of the Ca_i transient (CF Fig.1 left panel) $d\Delta Ca_i/dt_{max}$ (◆) in a cell without NaCl added to the patch pipette.

Figure 3 shows membrane current, Ca_i, and contraction as recorded from a representative Na^+-loaded cell in response to clamp steps to +25 and +100mV. The calcium current is not altered significantly by Na loading, i.e. its peak value and time-integral as well as its i-v curve are similar to those of cells represented by Figure 2 (result not shown). Na loaded cells generally had larger contractions and Ca_i-transients compared to cells studied in the absence of pipette Na^+. A major difference between Na-loaded and Na-free cells was observed at clamp steps to strong positive potentials. Figure 3 shows that a step to +100mV, produces an increase in Ca_i which is larger but lacks the initial rapid rate of rise than that obtained in the same cell at +25mV, during which Ca-influx through the Ca-channels would be substantial.

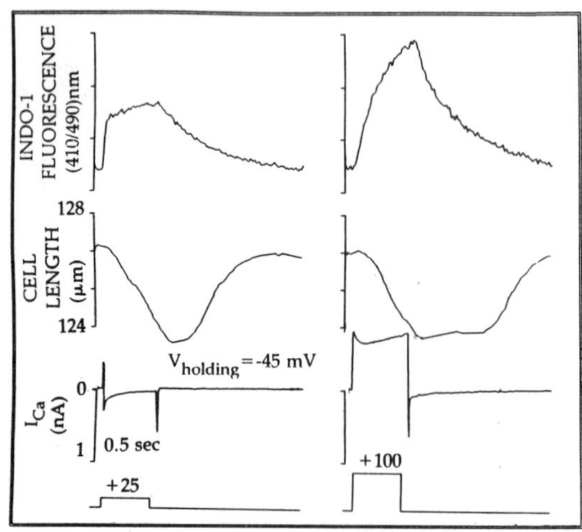

Fig. 3. Left, depolarization from -45mV to +25mV of a cell containing 10mM NaCl in the patch pipette, elicits a calcium current, a rapid rise in Ca_i, measured as in Fig. 1, and a contraction. Right depolarization to +100mV in the same cell does not elicit a net inward current and the Ca_i transient increases at a much slower rate but to a greater extent.

The voltage-dependence of the peak Ca_i transient (ΔCa_i) in Na-loaded myocytes increases monotonically with membrane potential (Fig. 4).

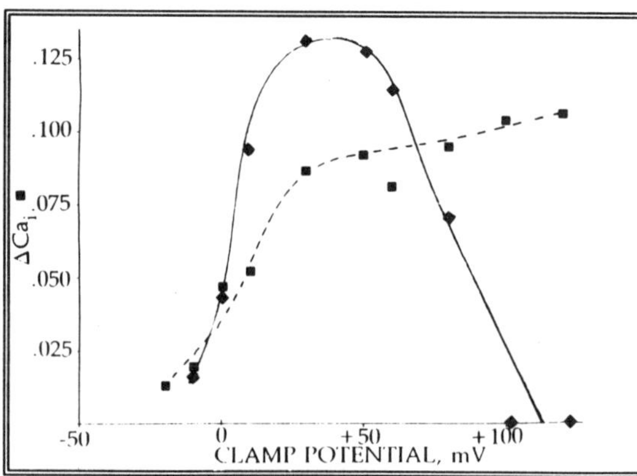

Fig. 4. The voltage dependence of the Ca_i transient ■, and its initial maximum rate of rise ◆, in a myocyte in which 10mM NaCl has been added to the patch pipette. While the latter exhibits a bell-shaped voltage dependence, the former does not (in contrast to cells in which NaCl is omitted from the patch pipette, Cf Fig. 2)

An exponential dependence of Ca-influx on membrane potential via Na-Ca exchange would be expected on the basis of theoretical considerations [5] and experimental evidence [2]. However, at voltages at which Na-Ca is operative but at which I_{Ca} is markedly reduced, the dΔCa/dt is markedly reduced (Fig. 4). Since we interpret the rapid rise in Ca_i to reflect a contribution of SR-Ca release to the Ca-signal, that the voltage-dependence of dΔCa/dt in Na-loaded cells is bell-shaped would indicate that SR Ca^{2+} calcium release in these cells, as in those in which NaCl was not added to the pipette, requires a very rapid Ca^{2+} trigger [8] which can be provided by Ca channels but not by Na-Ca exchange. The results in Figs. 3 and 4 are consistent with the hypothesis that Ca derived from the extracellular space via Na,Ca-exchange can produce only a slow increase in cytosolic Ca^{2+}.

CONCLUSION

The present experiments are compatible with the notion that in the absence of I_{Ca}, Ca-influx through the Na-Ca exchanger cannot trigger a rapid and an initially large SR Ca release from the holding potentials employed but can during depolarization contribute a slower component to the Ca_i transient, the extent of which increases with Na_i and with the amplitude and duration of depolarization.

REFERENCES

1. G. Isenberg and U. Klöckner, Pflügers Arch. 395, 30-41 (1982).
2. J. Kimura, S. Miyamae, and A. Noma, J. Physiol. 384, 199-222 (1987).
3. M.C. Capogrossi, A.A. Kort, H.A. Spurgeon, and E.G. Lakatta, J. Gen. Physiol. 88, 589-613 (1986).
4. M. Poenie, J. Alderton, R. Steinhardt, and R. Tsien, Science 233, 886-889 (1986).
5. M.C. Capogrossi, H.A. Spurgeon, S. Raffaeli, M.D. Stern, and L.G. Lakatta in: Biology of Isolated Adult Cardiac Myocytes, W.A. Clark, R.S. Decker, and T.K. Borg, eds. (Elsevier, New York 1988).
6. L. Barcenas-Ruiz and W.G. Wier, Circ. Res. 61, 148-155 (1987).
7. W.B. Im and C.O. Lee, Am. J. Physiol. 247, C478-C487 (1984).
8. A. Fabiato, J. Gen. Physiol. 85, 247-289 (1985).

$[Ca^{2+}]_i$-TRANSIENTS, MEASURED WITH FURA-2, IN ISOLATED GUINEA-PIG VENTRICULAR MYOCYTES

WIER, W.G., BARCENAS-RUIZ, L., AND D.J. BEUCKELMANN
The Deparment of Physiology, University of Maryland, School of Medicine, 660 West Redwood St., Baltimore, MD 21201

ABSTRACT

In order to study some of the cellular processes that are important in excitation-contraction coupling, we studied the voltage-dependence of changes in $[Ca^{2+}]_i$ in single, voltage-clamped guinea-pig ventricular myocytes. The cells were loaded with fura-2 (salt) directly by superfusion with the pipette used for "whole-cell recording." To study the processes governing Ca^{2+}-release from sarcoplasmic reticulum (s.r.) we examined the voltage-dependence and pharmacology of membrane currents and $[Ca^{2+}]_i$-transients elicited by pulse depolarization from a holding potential of -40 mV. The results support the theory that the Ca^{2+}-current triggers or induces the release of Ca^{2+} from the s.r., in accordance with the theory of Ca^{2+}-induced release of Ca^{2+} (CICR). To study Na/Ca exchange, release of Ca^{2+} from s.r. was abolished with ryanodine (10μM) and entry of Ca^{2+} through surface membrane Ca^{2+}-channels was blocked with verapamil (10μM). Under these conditions, depolarizations elicted slow increases in $[Ca^{2+}]_i$, with the level being reached at the end of a 1.5 sec depolarization depending approximately exponentially on voltage.

INTRODUCTION

The use of fluorescent Ca^{2+}-indicators, such as fura-2 [1], to measure $[Ca^{2+}]_i$ in single cardiac cells [2] has many potential advantages over previously available methods [3]. These include the facts that inhomogeneities of $[Ca^{2+}]_i$ can be observed directly (by digital imaging microscopy), that measurement and identification of specific membrane currents is far more reliable than in multicellular preparations, and that the intracellular and extracellular mileau can be controlled far better. Thus the relationship between $[Ca^{2+}]_i$ and specific membrane currents and membrane voltage can be characterized much more reliably than in the past.

The basic features of $[Ca^{2+}]_i$-transients in voltage-clamped guinea-pig ventricular myocytes were revealed first in the experiments of Barcenas-Ruiz and Wier [9]. The patterns of voltage-dependence of the fluorescence transients elicited by pulse depolarization, by repolarization and by pulse depolarization in the presence of verapamil and ryanodine were all distinct from each other. The data obtained in these studies supported strongly certain concepts on the origins of the $[Ca^{2+}]_i$-transients, as discussed below. In the present work we have extended their initial observations by calibrating the fluorescence signals in terms of $[Ca^{2+}]_i$, more extensively, and we have devised additional experimental protocols to study Na/Ca exchange in more detail.

Some of the important issues with which we have been concerned are: 1) the mechanism of the release of Ca^{2+} from the sarcoplasmic reticulum, (is it Ca^{2+}-induced release of Ca^{2+} [4,5,6] or is there a voltage-dependent component?), and 2) What part of the $[Ca^{2+}]_i$-transient might be due to Na/Ca exchange, rather than to Ca^{2+}-entry or Ca^{2+}-release? To study the

Published 1988 by Elsevier Science Publishing Co., Inc.
Biology of Isolated Adult Cardiac Myocytes
William A. Clark, Robert S. Decker, and Thomas K. Borg, Editors

first issue, we observed the pharmacology and voltage-dependence of the $[Ca^{2+}]_i$-transients and the verapamil-sensitive currents. We found, first, that Ca^{2+}-release from the sarcoplasmic reticulum can occur upon repolarization, under conditions when a "tail" of Ca^{2+} current occurs. Second, the voltage-dependence of the $[Ca^{2+}]_i$-transient and the verapamil sensitive current is essentially identical. We suggest that these observations support the theory of Ca^{2+}-induced release of Ca^{2+}. We have also investigated voltage-dependence and electrogenicity of the Na/Ca exchange. In this case, we blocked interfering ionic current and entry and release of Ca^{2+} by ion-substitutions and pharmacologically, thus isolating the changes in Ca^{2+} and currents that result from Na/Ca exchange. The results support the concept that Na/Ca exchange is electrogenic and voltage-dependent [7,8].

METHODS

The methods for voltage-clamping the single cells and for the recording of fura-2 fluorescence from them were similar to those described in detail previously (2,9). The cells were loaded over 5-15 minutes by internal perfusion with a "whole cell patch microelectrode" (1.8-3.5 Mohm).

For the experiments in which we investigated the mechanism of Ca^{2+}-release from the s.r. the procedures and external and internal solutions were as reported already in [9].

For the experiments on Na/Ca exchange, the electrode was filled (in mM) with: fura-2, 0.070 (Molecular Probes, Junction City, OR, Lot:6H); CsCl, 130; $MgCl_2$, 2; NaCl 10; Hepes (sodium salt), 10 (pH=7.2). The cells were superfused with a Tyrode's solution containing (in mM) $CaCl_2$, 2.5; NaCl, 135; CsCl, 10; $MgCl_2$, 1; NaH_2PO_4, 0.33; Dextrose, 10; Hepes, 10; TEA, 10; verapamil, 0.01; ryanodine, 0.01; (pH = 7.3 with NaOH). Thus, interfering potassium (K^+) currents were blocked by substituting impermeant ions (Cs^+ and TEA). Ca^{2+}-channel blockers (verapamil) and ryanodine [10] blocked the interfering changes in $[Ca^{2+}]_i$ that result from entry of Ca^{2+} through surface membrane Ca^{2+}-channels and release and uptake of Ca^{2+} by the sarcoplasmic reticulum (s.r.).

All experiments were performed at room temperature, which was usually 21°C.

$[Ca^{2+}]_i$ was calculated from the ratio of fluorescence emission at 510 nm elicited with illumination at 380nm to that elicited by illumination at 360 nm. The method of calibration of the fura-2 signals was essentially that reported by Barcenas-Ruiz and Wier [9].

RESULTS

The basic features of $[Ca^{2+}]_i$-transients in voltage-clamped guinea-pig ventricular myocytes were revealed first in the experiments of Barcenas-Ruiz and Wier [9]. The patterns of voltage-dependence of the fluorescence transients elicited by pulse depolarization by repolarization and by pulse depolarization in the presence of verapamil and ryanodine were all distinct from each other. The data obtained in these studies supported strongly certain concepts on the origins of the $[Ca^{2+}]_i$-transients, as discussed below.

The rapidly rising $[Ca^{2+}]_i$-transients (Fig. 1, and Fig. 2 of [9]) elicited by pulse depolarization are almost certainly dominated by Ca^{2+} released from the s.r., since they are reduced strongly by ryanodine, when Ca^{2+}-current is present (see Fig. 4 of ref. [9]). The mechanism may be Ca^{2+}-induced release of Ca^{2+} (CICR) since the voltage dependence is similar to that of the Ca^{2+}-current (Fig. 1B).

$[Ca^{2+}]_i$-transients elicited by repolarization ("tail transients") also

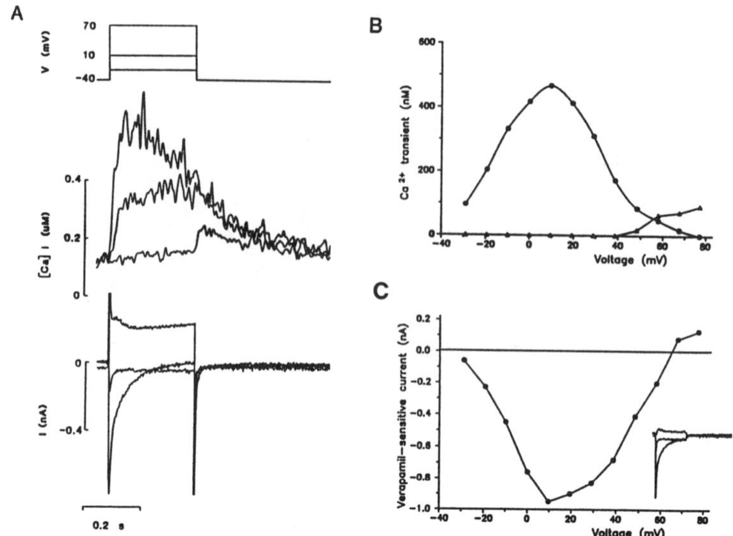

FIG. 1. Voltage-dependence of $[Ca^{2+}]_i$-transients in guinea-pig ventricular myocyte. **(A)** The three sets of recordings are, from top to bottom, membrane voltage, $[Ca^{2+}]_i$, and membrane current. The holding potential was always -40 mV and depolarizing clamp pulses 300 msec in duration were given. **(B)** Voltage-dependence of the $[Ca^{2+}]_i$-transient measured 100 msec after depolarization (circles), and upon repolarization (triangles; "tail transients). **(C)** Voltage-dependence of verapamil sensitive current. Inset shows the same currents as in (A), after the current remaining in verapamil had been subtracted.

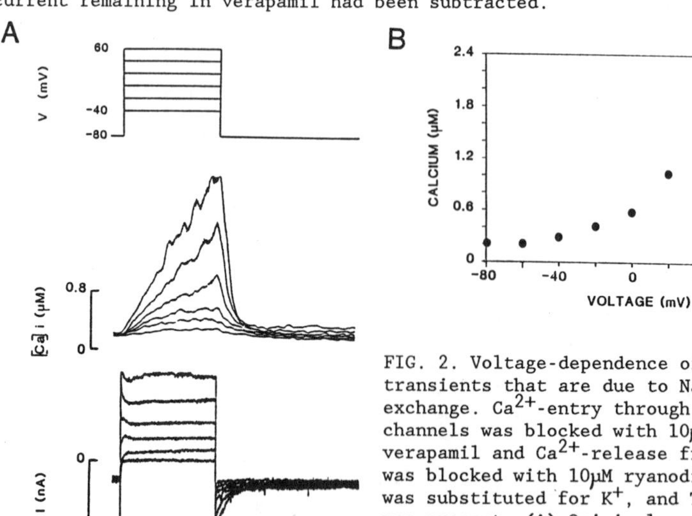

FIG. 2. Voltage-dependence of $[Ca^{2+}]_i$-transients that are due to Na/Ca exchange. Ca^{2+}-entry through Ca^{2+}-channels was blocked with 10µM verapamil and Ca^{2+}-release from s.r. was blocked with 10µM ryanodine. Cs^+ was substituted for K^+, and TEA (10mM) was present. **(A)** Original recordings of $[Ca^{2+}]_i$ and membrane currents that were elicited by step depolarizations as shown schematically in the top traces. **(B)** Plot of $[Ca^{2+}]_i$, measured at the end of the depolarizing pulse, as a function of the voltage of that pulse.

probably arise from CICR. Repolarization from positive potentials elicits a large, instantaneous, inward Ca^{2+}-current ("tail") during the time taken by Ca^{2+}-channels to deactivate. Nevertheless, it is unlikely that the "tail transients" arise from Ca^{2+}-current directly because ryanodine abolishes "tail transients" but does not abolish Ca^{2+}-current. Thus, tail transients [9] probably arise from Ca^{2+} released from the s.r., and the mechanism must be CICR since the release occurs upon repolarization, not depolarization. The increase in the "tail transient" over the range of 40 mV to 80 mV (Fig. 1B) could be accounted for by one or a combination of three possible mechanisms 1) an increased "trigger", i.e. increase in the tail of Ca^{2+}-current, which would result from a decrease in the Ca^{2+}-dependent inactivation of Ca^{2+}-current [11] during the preceding pulse, 2) an increased availability in the s.r. of Ca^{2+} to be released; this would result from less having been released during the preceding pulse, or 3) by an increased availability of the release mechanism itself, as a result of a decrease in the putative Ca^{2+}-dependent inactivation of Ca^{2+}-release [5] that occurs during the pulse. These possibilities above are supported, but not distinguished, by the observation that the "tail transient" appears and increases only as the $[Ca^{2+}]_i$-transient on which it is superimposed decreases (Fig. 1B). Observation of "tail transients" with digital imaging microscopy revealed that they are spatially uniform, distinct from the spontaneous, unphysiological, spatially inhomogeneous "waves" of $[Ca^{2+}]_i$, also attributed to CICR, that can be observed in a subpopulation of isolated cardiac cells. Thus we believe that these "tail transients" are a clear demonstration of CICR in an intact cell under physiological conditions; tail transients arise from a rapid, spatially homogeneous release of Ca^{2+}, from the s.r., that does not depend on depolarization.

In the presence of ryanodine [10, 12] and verapamil, (Fig. 2A) $[Ca^{2+}]_i$-transients elicited by pulse depolarization are unlikely to arise either from Ca^{2+}-entry through surface membrane Ca^{2+}-channels (Ca^{2+}-channels blocked and wrong voltage dependence) or from Ca^{2+}-release from the s.r. Therefore, one possible candidate is Ca^{2+}-entry via Na/Ca exchange. The voltage dependence is similar to that observed for Na/Ca exchange currents [13,14] when a similar holding potential is used.

REFERENCES

1. Grynkiewicz, G., Poenie, M., Tsien, R. Y. 1985. J. Biol. Chem. **260**: 886-889.
2. Wier, W. G., Ccannell, M. B., Berlin, J. R., Marban, E., and Lederer, W. J. 1987. Science. **235**: 325-328.
3. Blinks, J.R., Wier, W.G., Hess, P., Prendergast, F.G. 1982.
4. Fabiato, A. 1985a. J. Gen. Physiol. **85**: 198-246.
5. Fabiato, A. 1985b. J. Gen. Physiol. **85**: 247-289.
6. Fabiato A., 1985c. J. Gen. Physiol. **85**: 291-320.
7. Difrancesco, D., Noble, D. 1985. Phil. Trans. R. Soc. Lond. B. **307**, 353-398
8. Barcenas-Ruiz, L., Beuckelamnn, D. J., Wier, W. G. 1987a. J. Physiol. (Abstr.)
9. Barcenas-Ruiz, L., Wier, W. G. 1987. Circ. Res. **61**: 148-154.
10. Sutko, J. L., Kenyon, J. L. 1983. J. Gen. Physiol. **82**: 385-404.
11. Lee, K.S., Marban, E., Tsien, R.W. 1985. J. Physiol. (Lond.) **364**:395-411
12. Marban, E., Wier, W.G. 1985 **56(1)**: 133-138.
13. Hume, J., R., Uehara, A. 1986a. **87**: 833-856.
14. Hume, J., R., Uehara, A. 1986b. J. Gen. Physiol. **87**: 857-844.

THE RELATIONSHIP OF CALCIUM CURRENT, SARCOPLASMIC RETICULUM FUNCTION AND CONTRACTION IN SINGLE RAT VENTRICULAR MYOCYTES EXCITED IN THE RESTED STATE

ANTTI TALO,* HAROLD A. SPURGEON, AND EDWARD G. LAKATTA
Laboratory of Cardiovascular Science, Gerontology Research Center, National Institute on Aging, National Institutes of Health, Baltimore, MD 21224; *Present Address: Department of Biology, University of Turku, 20500 Turku, Finland

INTRODUCTION

The availability of Ca^{++}-tolerant single cardiac myocytes with intact sarcolemmal function has intensified an interest in studies of mechanisms of cardiac excitation contraction coupling. Such studies have begun to test a hypothesis regarding Ca^{++} induced Ca^{++} release from the sarcoplasmic reticulum (SR). A possible role of the Ca^{++} channel current as a trigger for SR Ca^{++} release is a key feature of this hypothesis that had been generated in myocytes in which the sarcolemma had been removed [1]. A dependence of contraction or of the myoplasmic [Ca^{++}] on Ca^{++} currents has already been described in single guinea pig, and cat ventricular cells [2-5]. Here, we report on this relationship in single rat myocytes in the rested state, which unlike other species, exhibits the strongest twitch contraction that can be achieved with a given experimental milieu, presumably due to a maximum state of SR Ca^{++} loading [6]. Thus, in rat myocytes in the rested state, sarcolemmal currents associated with an action potential would be expected to elicit the maximum SR Ca^{++} release.

METHODS

Single ventricular myocytes were prepared from rat (250-500 g) hearts by retrograde aortic perfusion with buffer solution containing collagenase and a low free [Ca^{++}] at 37°C as described previously [7]. Following isolation myocytes were suspended in a physiologic salt solution containing in mM: NaCl 136.9, KCl 5, Hepes 20, dextrose 15, $MgSO_4 \cdot 7H_2O$ 1.2, pH 7.4 at 26°C. Petri dishes containing cells were placed on the stage of an inverted microsocope (Leitz Diavert). Whole cell currents were measured by the patch-clamp technique [8] using Dagan 8800 amplifier. Electrodes drawn of borosilicate glass had a resistance less than 3 MΩ when filled by 150 mM KCl, 10 mM Hepes and 5 μM EGTA, pH 7.2. Following the formation of a gigaseal the cell was lifted up by the electrode, which was positioned in the center of the cell. Myocyte length at rest and during stimulated contraction was quantitated by projection of the cell image on a photodiode array (Reticon RC100B/10246) which was scanned at 5 msec intervals. Current, voltage and cell length were displayed on an oscilloscope and a chart recorder and stored on a tape for further analysis. Holding potential of -40 or -45 mV was used to inactivate sodium and transient outward currents. Inward Ca^{++} current was measured as a nitrendipine -sensitive current.

RESULTS AND DISCUSSION

Records of current and contraction representative of those measured in present study are shown in Figure 1.

Published 1988 by Elsevier Science Publishing Co., Inc.
Biology of Isolated Adult Cardiac Myocytes
William A. Clark, Robert S. Decker, and Thomas K. Borg, Editors

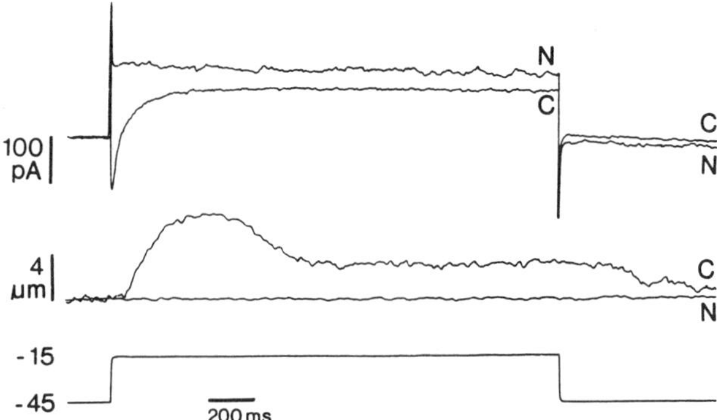

Figure 1. Transient changes in current (top), and cell length (middle) in response to a +30 mV voltage step from -45 mV (lower) in control (C) and following addition of 1 µM nitrendipine (N) in a representative rat myocyte bathed in 1.0 mM Ca^{++} at 26°C. Pipette resistance was 2 MΩ. The amplitude of the inward current was measured from the peak of the inward current to the steady state level prior to nitrendipine plus the steady shift in outward direction after nitrendipine.

Nitrendipine abolishes both inward current and contraction. The time course of the inhibition of the Ca^{++} current by nitrendipine was paralleled by that of the contractile inhibition (results not shown). Similar results (not shown) were obtained using verapamil (1 µM), Cd^{++}, Mn^{++} or Ni^{++} (1 mM). It might be argued, though, that Ca^{++} channel inhibitors listed above somehow have an effect to alter the intracellular Ca^{++} homeostasis, e.g. to interfere with Na/Ca exchange [9] or to deplete the SR of its Ca^{++} load, and that the failure for the depolarization to elicit a contraction in the presence of these inhibitors is due to this effect rather than to Ca^{++} channel inhibition. To examine the latter possibility, advantage can be taken of the ability of rat myocyte to exhibit spontaneous SR Ca^{++} release in the absence of stimulation, the occurrence of which produces spontaneous contractile waves [6]. The presence and frequency of this form of SR Ca^{++} release depend on the extent of cell and thus SR Ca^{++} loading [6,7]. It has previously been shown in intact resting rat muscle that spontaneous SR Ca^{++} release can persist at the same frequency in the presence of verapamil or nitrendipine as in the absence of drug [10,11]. Additionally, in the present study of single rat myocytes that exhibit contractile waves at rest, nitrendipine, while abolishing the Ca^{++} current and contraction, fails to alter the wave frequency. Thus, we interpret the result of Figure 1 to indicate that the Ca^{++} channel current that occurs with depolarization is essential for excitation-contraction coupling, and that depolarization of the sarcolemma, per se, from this holding potential is insufficient to produce a twitch.

Figure 2 illustrates the average dependence of the nitrendipine-sensitive current and contraction magnitude on the voltage for 6 different cells. The shape of the current-voltage relationship in Figure 2 is similar to that measured previously in rat myocytes in studies in which the Ca^{++} current had been selectively measured [12,13]. Both current and contraction exhibit a threshold at potentials just positive to -40 mV, and both increase in magnitude to test potentials of about zero mV. The maximum contraction in these cells averaged 16 ± 1.2% of resting cell length, which is near to the maximum contraction that single unloaded rat myocytes can achieve even in the absence of an attached patch pipette [6]. The figure shows that a current which is a small percentage of the maximum current triggers a sizable contraction (e.g. contraction has reached about 80% of its maximum at 25 mV whereas the current is 40% of its maximum measured value. This result is compatible with an hypothesis that over the range of clamp potentials from threshold to about -20 mV the Ca^{++} current relates to the contraction as a "trigger" function. This may not be a unique interpretation, however. The further increase in current at steps to more positive potentials than -10 mV does not elicit substantial further increases in the contraction and thus could serve to Ca^{++} load the cell.

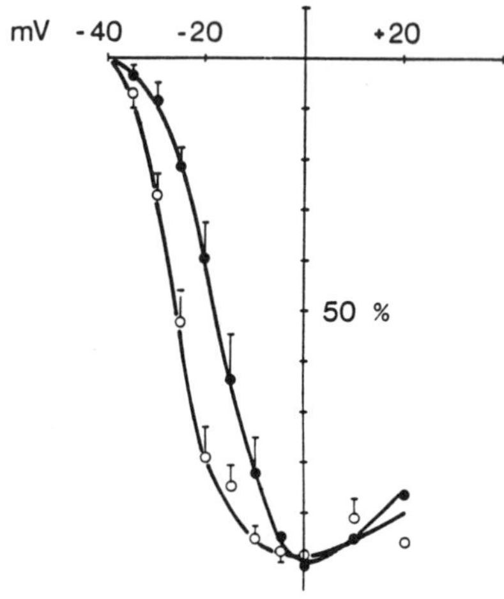

Figure 2. The average voltage -dependence of contraction and nitrendipine-sensitive current for 6 rat myocytes bathed in $[Ca^{++}]$ of 1.0 mM at 26°C and rested for 30 sec between voltage clamp steps. Current and contraction are normalized to the maximum value in each cell which, respectively, averaged 780 ± 75 pA and 16 ± 1.2% rest cell length. ● = I_{Ca}: is the Nitr.-sensitive current as explained in Figure 1, o is contraction amplitude, n = 6 ± SE Vh = -45 mV.

The magnitude of the currents that elicit near maximum twitches in the present or previous studies are likely not sufficient to increase the cytosolic Ca^{++} to an extent or at a rate sufficient to produce a twitch [14]. This is consistent with the interpretation placed on the results in Figures 1 and 2, i.e. that the Ca^{++} current is a trigger for the release of Ca^{++} from an intracellular store. That this intracellular store is the SR is suggested by the experiment in Figure 3. The major point of the figure is that ryanodine, while not attenuating the peak Ca^{++} current, abolishes the contraction. This effect of ryanodine in rat myocytes can be attributed to its ability to markedly deplete the SR Ca^{++} load [15]. Two noteworthy features of the ryanodine effect on current are (1) that the peak amplitude is not decreased and (2) the "apparent" inactivation is altered. This latter effect may result from the abolition by ryanodine of an inward current related to SR Ca^{++} release due possibly to Na/Ca exchange [16]. Another remarkable feature of Figure 3 is that depolarization to -25 mV which could elicit a twitch and a sustained contraction prior to ryanodine, cannot, in the presence of ryanodine, even elicit sustained "tonic tension." This suggests that an appreciable level of tonic activation of the myofilaments by depolarization to this level requires intact SR Ca^{++} release [17], and that continual "low grade" SR Ca^{++} release supports tonic tension under this condition [16].

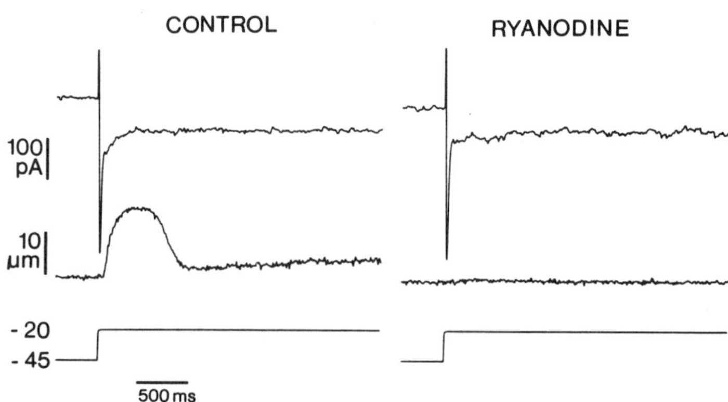

Figure 3. A recording of the effect of ryanodine (2 µM) on the inward current and contraction in response to a voltage step from -45 mV to -20 mV in a representative rat myocyte in the rested state for 30 seconds. Microelectrode resistance was 2.0 MΩ. Cell was bathed in Hepes buffer containing 1.0 mM Ca^{++} at 26°C.

CONCLUSION

From the results presented in Figures 1-3 we conclude that the contraction elicited by depolarization of rat cardiac myocytes in the rested state results from Ca^{++} release from the SR that is not due to the depolarization per se, but is triggered by sarcolemmal Ca^{++} channel activation.

REFERENCES

1. A. Fabiato and F. Fabiato, J. Physiol. 249. 469-495 (1975).
2. B. London and J.W. Krueger, J. Gen. Physiol. 88, 475-505 (1986).
3. L. Barcenas-Ruiz and W.G. Wier, Circ. Res. 61, 148-155 (1987).
4. S.R. Houser, A. Bahinski, W.H. duBell, V. Duthinh, H.A. Hartmann, R.B. Kleiman, and C. Philips, Abstracts of the NHLBI International Workshop, Biology of Isolated Adult Cardiac Myocytes, D-9 (1987).
5. G. Isenberg, Zeitschrift fur Naturforschung Teil C. 37, 502-512 (1982).
6. M.C. Capogrossi, B.A. Suarez-Isla, and E.G. Lakatta, J. Gen. Physiol. 88, 615-633 (1986).
7. M.C. Capogrossi, A.A. Kort, H.A. Spurgeon, and E.G. Lakatta, J. Gen. Physiol. 88, 589-613 (1986).
8. P.O. Hamill, A. Marty, E. Neher, B. Sakmann, and F.J. Sigworth, Pflugers Archiv. 395, 6-18 (1981).
9. J. Kimura, S. Miyamae, and A. Noma, J. Physiol. 384, 199-222 (1987).
10. M.D. Stern, A.A. Kort, G.M. Bhatnagar, and E.G. Lakatta, J. Gen. Physiol. 82, 119-153 (1983).
11. A.A. Kort and E.G. Lakatta, Circ. Res. 54, 396-404 (1984).
12. A.M. Brown, K.S. Lee, and T.J. Powell, J. Physiol. 318, 455-477 (1981).
13. M.R. Mitchell, T. Powell, D. A. Terrar, and V.W. Twist, Proc. R. Soc. Lond. B. 219, 447-469 (1983).
14 A. Fabiato, Am. J. Physiol. 245, C1-C14 (1983).
15. R.G. Hansford and E.G. Lakatta, J. Physiol. 390, 453-467 (1987).
16. A. Fabiato, J. Gen. Physiol. 85, 189-246 (1985).
17. A. Talo, H.A. Spurgeon, and E.G. Lakatta, Manuscript in preparation.

VOLTAGE DEPENDENT CHANGES IN INTRACELLULAR CALCIUM IN SINGLE CARDIAC MYOCYTES MEASURED WITH FLUORESCENT CALCIUM INDICATORS

J. R. BERLIN, M. B. CANNELL* AND W. J. LEDERER
Department of Physiology, University of Maryland School of Medicine, Baltimore, MD 21201 and *the Department of Pharmacology, University of Miami School of Medicine, Miami, FL.

INTRODUCTION

Depolarization of heart muscle leads to the development of a transient increase in intracellular calcium ion concentration ($[Ca^{2+}]_i$) which activates contraction. Although it is not known how depolarization of heart muscle cells leads to the $[Ca^{2+}]_i$ transient, recent work has tended to favor two distinct explanations. In an elegant series of experiments, Fabiato [1] has suggested that calcium influx via sarcolemmal ion channels can activate the release of calcium from the large intracellular calcium store, the sarcoplasmic reticulum (SR). An alternative explanation for which there is little direct support in heart muscle is based on work carried out in skeletal muscle. Schneider and Chandler [2] suggested that sarcolemmal charge movement may be linked to calcium release by the proteins spanning the gap between the SR and the sarcolemma. We have carried out experiments examining the voltage-dependence of the calcium current and the $[Ca^{2+}]_i$ transient to see if such experiments would illuminate this issue. While we have found some data consistent with "calcium induced calcium release", we have also noted results that are not readily explained by the simplest view of calcium-induced calcium release (CICR).

METHODS

Rat cardiac ventricular myocytes, isolated by an enzymatic procedure, were placed in an experimental chamber mounted on the stage of an inverted microscope [3] and superfused with a modified Tyrode's solution at 32-35°C. The microscope was modified to contain fused silica optics and an epifluorescent illuminator which could select between ultraviolet light of 340 nm and 380 nm wavelength with 10 nm interference filters [4,5].

Quiescent myocytes were voltage-clamped by a single patch electrode technique. The electrode filling solution contained an intracellular salt solution which included 30 uM of the potassium salt of Fura-2. The fluorescence of the cell at 505 nm was recorded from a 10 um diameter region of the cell with a photomultiplier tube [6]. Intracellular calcium ion concentration, $[Ca^{2+}]_i$, was calculated by dividing fura-2 fluorescence recorded during illumination with 340 nm light by that recorded during 380 nm illumination (after subtraction of appropriate background fluorescence). This fluorescence ratio was converted to calcium concentration using an <u>in vitro</u> calibration curve [7]. Details of the methods presented have been published elsewhere [6].

RESULTS AND DISCUSSION

Figure 1 shows the voltage dependence of the calcium current (D-600 sensitive component of I_{si}) and the $[Ca^{2+}]_i$ transient. I_{si} activated around -40 mV and reached half maximal amplitude at -22 mV (-18 $\pm$ 1.4 mV; mean $\pm$ S.E.M. of 6 experiments). Peak I_{si} was recorded between -10 and 0 mV but more positive depolarizations produced I_{si} of smaller amplitude. Detectable increases in $[Ca^{2+}]_i$ occurred when the cell was depolarized to -50 mV and reached half maximal amplitude at -38 mV (-30 $\pm$ 1.7 mV). Between -20 and +20 mV, the $[Ca^{2+}]_i$ transient was of maximum amplitude and relatively insensitive to changes in depolarization potential. Depolarization beyond +30 mV produced a $[Ca^{2+}]_i$ transient of smaller amplitude during the pulse. That the voltage dependence of the $[Ca^{2+}]_i$

Biology of Isolated Adult Cardiac Myocytes
William A. Clark, Robert S. Decker, and Thomas K. Borg, Editors

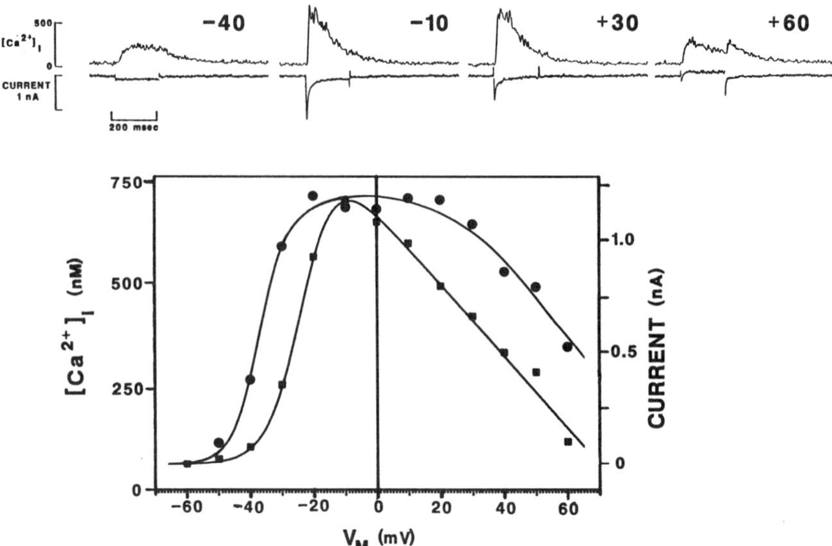

Fig. 1. Voltage dependence of I_{si} and the $[Ca^{2+}]_i$ transient. The top 3 panels show the $[Ca^{2+}]_i$ and I_{si} for depolarizations from -60 mV to -40, -10, +30 and +60 mV (left to right). I_{si} is a difference current obtained by subtracting current recorded in the presence of 25 uM D-600 from that recorded during a control period. In this, and all other figures, 30 uM TTX was present during the entire experiment. The bottom panel shows I_{si} amplitude (squares) and peak $[Ca^{2+}]_i$ (circles) as a function of depolarization potential. The curve drawn through the current data was fit with a modified Boltzmann equation (E_{rev} = +70 mV, V_h = -23 mV, k = 5.4). The curve through the $[Ca^{2+}]_i$ data was drawn by eye. (from [6], with permission).

transient was significantly different than the voltage dependence of I_{si} demonstrates several points: (1) The recorded increases in $[Ca^{2+}]_i$ are not simply the result of calcium influx via I_{si}. Thus, SR calcium release is functional in these cells and not inhibited by the injection of fura-2. (2) The relatively small effect of increasing I_{si} (between -20 and 0 mV) on the amplitude of the $[Ca^{2+}]_i$ transient suggests that the increase in $[Ca^{2+}]_i$ produced by a depolarizing pulse is largely the result of calcium release from the SR. (3) If D-600 sensitive I_{si} triggers calcium release from the SR, only a small fraction of total current is required to initiate SR release.

Depolarization to +60 mV produced a $[Ca^{2+}]_i$ transient during the pulse and an aftertransient with repolarization. At an even more positive potential (+100 mV), no change in $[Ca^{2+}]_i$ occurred during the pulse but an aftertransient of $[Ca^{2+}]_i$ was produced on repolarization (Fig. 2). This result could be explained in the framework of the CICR mechanism if Ca^{2+} entry during the pulse (near E_{Ca}) is insufficient to trigger Ca^{2+} release from the SR. The repolarization transient could also be explained by the calcium tail current activating Ca^{2+} release. An alternative explanation for this result, however, is that at very positive potentials, the SR calcium release channel rapidly enters an inactivated state so that a $[Ca^{2+}]_i$ transient is prevented. On repolarization, Ca^{2+} release could occur as the channel returns through the open state.

The dependence of the $[Ca^{2+}]_i$ transient on I_{si} was studied further by examining the effect of depolarization duration on the size of the $[Ca^{2+}]_i$ transient (Fig. 3). The cell was depolarized from -54 to -24 mV so that a submaximal $[Ca^{2+}]_i$ transient was produced. Short depolarizations decreased the size of the $[Ca^{2+}]_i$ transient, even when peak I_{si} was reached by the end of the pulse (for the 10 and 20 msec depolarizations). This result points out clearly that the level of I_{si} at its peak does not determine the size of the $[Ca^{2+}]_i$ transient (see also Fig. 1). Additional features of the dependence of the $[Ca^{2+}]_i$ transient on depolarization duration are:

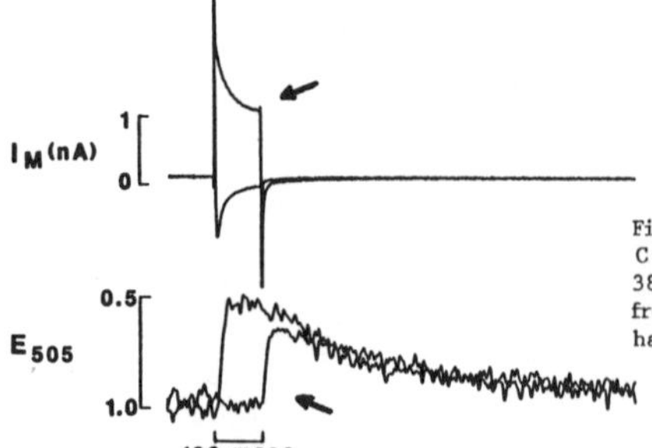

Fig. 2. Depolarization to very positive potentials. Current (upper panel) and fluorescence (excitation 380 nm, emission 505 nm) records for depolarizations from -60 mV to +10 and +100 mV (noted with arrows) have been superimposed. (from [6], with permission).

(1) After approximately 40 msec, $[Ca^{2+}]_i$ begins to decrease from the peak level even if the cell is still depolarized. This feature has previously been reported in voltage-clamped Purkinje fibers which had been injected with the calcium indicator, aequorin [8]. (2) The rate of decline of $[Ca^{2+}]_i$ is faster when the membrane is repolarized. (3) With long depolarizing pulses, $[Ca^{2+}]_i$ does not decline to resting levels but is maintained at an elevated concentration (data not shown). In some experiments, $[Ca^{2+}]_i$ even begins to slowly increase again, similar to the voltage- and sodium-dependent tonic tension observed in Purkinje fibers [9].

In the CICR model, Ca^{2+} entering via I_{si} binds to a site that activates Ca^{2+} release from the SR. The tendency towards positive feedback in this mechanism is prevented by Ca^{2+} slowly binding to an inhibitory site which prevents further release [1]. The model could explain the depression of the $[Ca^{2+}]_i$ transient by brief depolarizations, if occupancy of the activator site is decreased when I_{si} is terminated following repolarization. However, when repolarization does stop the rise in $[Ca^{2+}]_i$, Ca^{2+} is already being released from the SR. As a result of this release, the $[Ca^{2+}]_i$ around the activator sites will depend not only on the contribution of Ca^{2+} from I_{si}, but also on Ca^{2+} from the SR. Our calculations [6] suggest that the flux of Ca^{2+} from the SR is at least an order of magnitude greater than that of I_{si}. Therefore, once initiated, the SR rather than I_{si} should dominate the $[Ca^{2+}]$ around the activator site. An alternative explanation for the depression of the $[Ca^{2+}]_i$ transient by early repolarization (even when maximal I_{si} is observed) is that $[Ca^{2+}]_i$ increases more rapidly around the inhibitory site after repolarization. During the few milliseconds that I_{si} deactivates following repolarization, Ca^{2+} flux through the

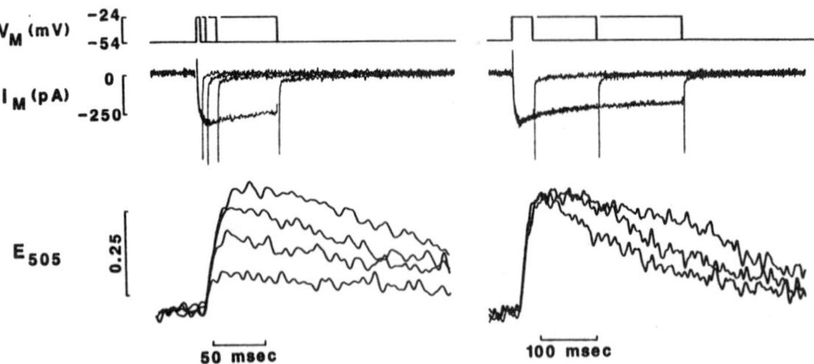

Fig. 3. Effect of depolarization on the $[Ca^{2+}]_i$ transient. The panels (top to bottom) are voltage, current and fluorescence (excitation 380 nm, emission 505 nm). The cell was depolarized from -54 to -24 mV for 100 msec every 1.5 sec. Every fourth depolarization, the duration of the depolarizing pulse was varied. The left hand panels display depolarizing pulses of 5, 10, 20 and 80 msec duration. The right hand panels show 40, 160 and 320 msec depolarizations. (from [6], with permission).

channel would be expected to transiently increase because of an increase in the electrochemical gradient for Ca^{2+} entry. However, the small augmentation of this flux on repolarizing from -24 to -54 mV (less than 20% assuming E_{Ca} is +90 mV) and its short duration are hard to reconcile with the profound depression of the $[Ca^{2+}]_i$ transient. In addition, as shown in Fig. 1, increases in the size of I_{si} produced an increase rather than a decrease in the size of the transient. Thus, the duration dependence of the $[Ca^{2+}]_i$ transient is not easily explained by CICR. This raises the possibility that repolarization may directly inhibit Ca^{2+} release from the SR.

SUMMARY

We have examined the relationship between the calcium current, I_{si}, and the $[Ca^{2+}]_i$ transient. The magnitude and timecourse of the $[Ca^{2+}]_i$ transient is dependent on both the voltage and the duration of the depolarizing clamp pulse. In addition, the size of the $[Ca^{2+}]_i$ transient is not simply related to I_{si} amplitude. These results could be explained by either a CICR mechanism or a mechanism in which SR Ca^{2+} release is controlled directly by sarcolemmal potential. Neither mechanism can easily explain all of the results. It is possible, however, that both calcium and voltage are modulators of SR Ca^{2+} release.

REFERENCES

1. A. Fabiato, J. Gen. Physiol. 85, 291-320 (1985).
2. M.F. Schneider and W.K. Chandler. Nature. 242: 244-246.
3. M.B. Cannell and W.J. Lederer, Pfluegers Arch. 406, 536-639 (1986).
4. W.G. Wier, M.B. Cannell, J.R. Berlin, E. Marban, and W.J. Lederer, Science 235, 325-328, 1987.
5. M.B. Cannell, J.R. Berlin, and W.J. Lederer in: Cell Calcium and the Control of Membrane Transport, L.J. Mandel and D.C. Eaton, eds. (Rockefeller University Press 1987) pp. 202-214.
6. M.B. Cannell, J.R. Berlin, and W.J. Lederer, Science In Press.
7. G. Grynkiewicz, M. Poenie, and R.Y. Tsien, J. Biol. Chem. 260, 3440-3450 (1985).
8. W.G. Wier and G. Isenberg, Pfluegers Arch. 392, 284-290 (1982).
9. D.A. Eisner, W.J. Lederer, and R.D. Vaughan-Jones, J. Physiol. 335, 723-743 (1984).

TEMPORAL VARIATION IN CONTRACTILE STATE AND $[Ca^{++}]_i$ IN ISOLATED ADULT RAT AND GUINEA PIG CARDIAC MYOCYTES

DONGHEE KIM AND THOMAS W. SMITH
Harvard Medical School and Brigham and Women's Hospital, Boston, MA 02115

INTRODUCTION

Isolated adult cardiac myocytes are useful in the study of cardiac muscle biochemistry, physiology and pharmacology at the cellular and molecular level. The advantages of using isolated cells over intact tissue include more accurate measurement of the movements and levels of various ions that affect the contractile function of heart cells, due to an environment that is relatively free of extracellular and intracellular space ambiguities, and the presence of a single predominant cell type. Many investigators have employed isolated adult heart cells for electrophysiological and ion flux studies. However, it is not certain whether single cardiac myocytes prepared by enzymatic digestion retain all the physiologic properties that are exhibited by intact muscle. Studies performed by Capogrossi et al.(1) in single enzymatically dissociated adult rabbit and rat cardiac myocytes suggested that the rate- and Ca-dependent changes in contractile amplitude were similar to those observed in intact tissues. In the experiments described below, we studied in detail the contractile behavior and associated changes in cytosolic free Ca ($[Ca^{++}]_i$) in response to various agents known to alter the rate and extent of cell shortening and relaxation. We used enzymatically dissociated isolated single ventricular myocytes from adult rats and guinea pigs.

METHODS

Cell Isolation

Male Sprague-Dawley rats(250-350 g) were anesthetized with diethyl ether and hearts placed in bicarbonate-buffered physiologic medium. Hearts were perfused via aorta with bicarbonate-buffered medium (37°C) containing 118 mM NaCl, 4.7 mM KCl, 1.25 mM $CaCl_2$, 1.20 mM $MgSO_4$, 1.20 mM KH_2PO_4, 25 mM $NaHCO_3$ and 15 mM glucose. Hearts were then perfused with buffer containing 0.05% collagenase and 0.03% hyaluronidase. The ventricular muscle was cut into pieces and placed in a flask with the above enzyme solution containing 0.002% trypsin. The flask was shaken gently at 37°C for 25 min. Tissue pieces were then transferred to Ca-free enzyme buffer with 2.0% bovine serum albumin added and mechanically dissociated by gentle pipetting. The isolated myocytes were filtered through Nitex mesh and collected in a centrifuge tube. The isolated myocytes were resuspended in 1.2 mM Ca^{++} solution and kept in a 95% O_2/5% CO_2 atmosphere. Cells used for $[Ca^{++}]_i$ and contractility measurements were attached to 12 mm glass coverslips coated with collagen C.

Contractility

A 12 mm circular glass coverslip with attached myocytes was placed on the stage of an inverted phase contrast microscope and perfused with HEPES-buffered physiological solution containing 5 mM HEPES, 0.6 mM $CaCl_2$, 4.0 mM KCl, 140 mM NaCl, 0.5 mM $MgCl_2$ and 11 mM glucose (pH 7.35, 37°C). The cells were electrically stimulated using a platinum electrode. Light-dark contrast at the edge of the cell provided a marker for measurement of the amplitude of motion. Movement of cells was monitored using a video motion detector that provides new position data every 16 msec, and the amplitude signal from the detector together with its first derivative(velocity) were relayed to a recorder (Honeywell).

Biology of Isolated Adult Cardiac Myocytes
William A. Clark, Robert S. Decker, and Thomas K. Borg, Editors

$[Ca^{++}]_i$ Measurement

Intracellular free Ca ($[Ca^{++}]_i$) of single cardiac myocytes was measured using the Ca-sensitive fluorescent dye, fura-2, as described previously(2). The glass coverslip with attached fura 2-loaded cells was placed in a perfusion chamber on the stage of the microscope (Nikon) and perfused with oxygenated HEPES-buffered solution at 37^oC. The microscope was attached to a SPEX fluorolog 2 instrument whose excitation wavelength were 340 nm and 380 nm and emission wavelength 505nm. The two excitation wavelength were made to alternate once every 20 msec. Cells were electrically stimulated at desired frequencies using platinum electrodes, and contractions were visually confirmed before, during and after each experiment. After equilibration of the baseline fluorescence signal from one cell, the cell was perfused with a test drug and the change in fluorescence signal was continuously monitored. At the end of an experiment, background autofluorescence from a cell not loaded with fura 2 was subtracted from the original signals. To calibrate the signals to represent actual $[Ca^{++}]_i$ values, the cell was perfused with medium containing ionomycin (2.5 uM) and digitonin (6 ug/ml) to obtain the maximum fluorescence, and then perfused with Ca-free medium with 5 mM EGTA to obtain the minimum fluorescence signal. Using the equations provided by Grynkiewicz et al.(3), the 340nm/380nm fluorescence intensity ratio was transformed into $[Ca^{++}]_i$ values.

RESULTS AND DISCUSSION

Isolated cardiac myocytes were incubated in oxygenated bicarbonate-buffered physiologic solution (pH 7.35) at room temperature until use. The amplitude of cell shortening of cells 1-3 hr after isolation ranged from 1-3 um in 0.6 mM Ca medium when electrically stimulated at 1.5 Hz. Figure 1 shows the $[Ca^{++}]_o$-dependent changes in contractile amplitude. When cells incubated for 3-4 hr were studied, the range of contractile amplitude was 2-6 um in 0.6 mM Ca medium and the concentration effect curve for Ca shifted to the left compared to that observed in cells that were 1-3 hr old. At longer incubation periods (4-6 hr), the contractile amplitudes of most of the cells were greater than 6 um. Thus progressive increases in contractile amplitude were present with increasing periods of time after cell isolation. Using cells 1-3 hr old, we studied the frequency-dependent changes in amplitude of cell motion. In rat ventricular cells, increasing the frequency of stimulation from 12 to 180 per min in severalsteps caused a progressive decline in the contraction amplitude. In contrast, increasing the frequency

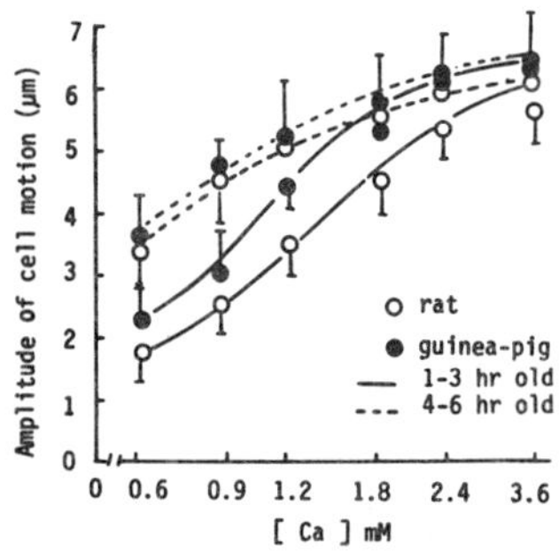

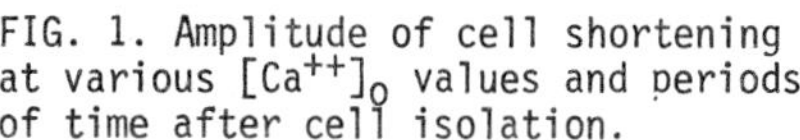

FIG. 1. Amplitude of cell shortening at various $[Ca^{++}]_o$ values and periods of time after cell isolation.

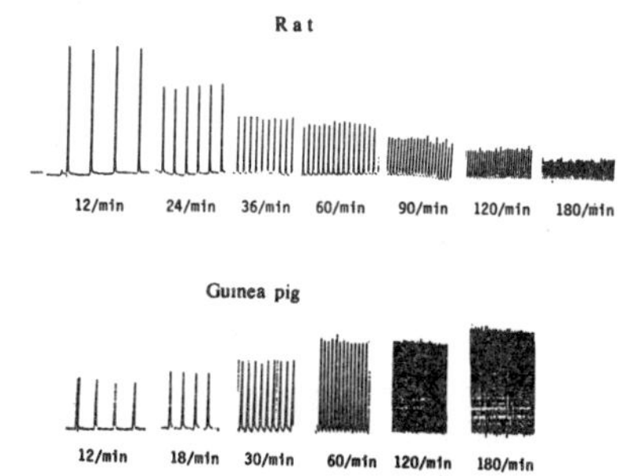

FIG. 2. Frequency-dependent changes in the amplitude of cell shortening.

of stimulation caused a progressive increase in the contraction amplitude in guinea-pig ventricular myocytes (figure 2). These changes are similar to those observed in intact rat or guinea-pig heart muscle and indicate that the processes responsible for the positive and negative staircase phenomena are retained in isolated heart cells.

We next examined the contractile responses to ouabain, isoproterenol, Bay k 8644, isobutylmethylxanthine (IBMX) and nifedipine. As illustrated in Fig. 3, cells with contractile amplitudes in the 1-3 um range in 0.6 mM Ca medium exhibited contractile responses very similar to those observed in intact cardiac tissue. For example, ouabain, Bay k 8644 and IBMX produced increases in the rate of shortening and the rate of relaxation with minimal changes in the time to peak shortening. Isoproterenol increased the rates of shortening and relaxation and also decreased the time to peak shortening, similar to responses in intact tissue. The Ca channel antagonist nifedipine reduced rates of both shortening and relaxation as well as the amplitude of cell shortening in a concentration-dependent manner. In cells with initial amplitudes of shortening in the 4-6 um range, the contractile responses to a given drug were variable and unpredictable. For example, in these cells propranolol or nifedipine produced an increase, no change or a decrease in the amplitude of cell shortening. The percent increase in the amplitude of cell shortening produced by ouabain or isoproterenol was small compared to that observed in cells with initial amplitudes in the 1-3 um range, presumably due to the already augmented amplitude of contraction and incipient Ca overload.

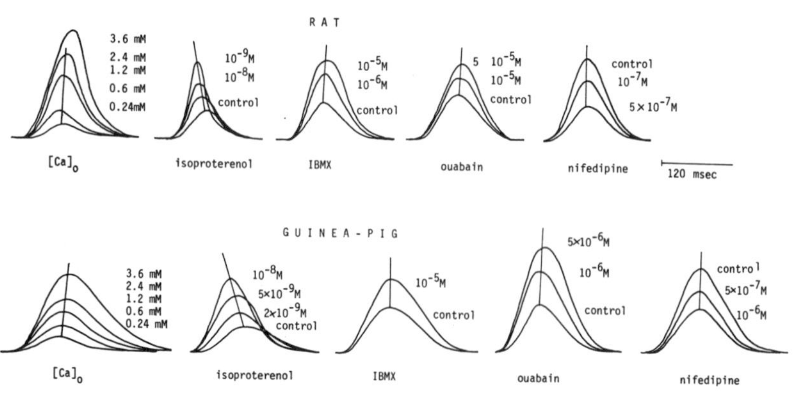

FIG. 3. Contractile responses to various positive and negative inotropic agents.

The progressive increases in amplitude of cell shortening with increasing periods of time after cell isolation occurred even in oxygenated medium with or without supplementation with fetal calf serum or necessary nutrients. The increase in contraction amplitude with time suggests that internal Ca stores may be increasing slowly, thus leading to an enhanced intracellular Ca transient in myocytes isolated according to the method described. Therefore, we measured the changes in $[Ca^{++}]_i$ using the fluorescent dye fura 2 in cells beating at 0.5 Hz. As shown in Figure 4, in cells with amplitudes of 1-3 um range, individual contractions were associated with a Ca transient. Since fura 2 may be partly compartmented, these $[Ca^{++}]_i$

values may not accurately reflect actual $[Ca^{++}]_i$. In response to ouabain, isoproterenol and Bay k 8644, systolic $[Ca^{++}]_i$ rose. Nifedipine and lowering of Ca_o diminished only the systolic $[Ca^{++}]_i$ with no demonstrable effect on diastolic $[Ca^{++}]_i$. In cells with amplitudes of 4-6 um range, both the resting and peak $[Ca^{++}]_i$ were significantly elevated compared to those in cells with 1-3 um amplitude. $[Ca^{++}]_i$ increased further in response to isoproterenol or Bay k 8644. These findings indicate that isolated cardiac myocytes become progressively Ca overloaded several hours after cell isolation by the techniques used in these studies, producing irregular and unpredictable responses to agents that alter contractile state. One must therefore be cautious and take into account the heterogeneity of cell properties, both among cells and with time, in the planning and analysis of experiments with isolated cardiac myocytes.

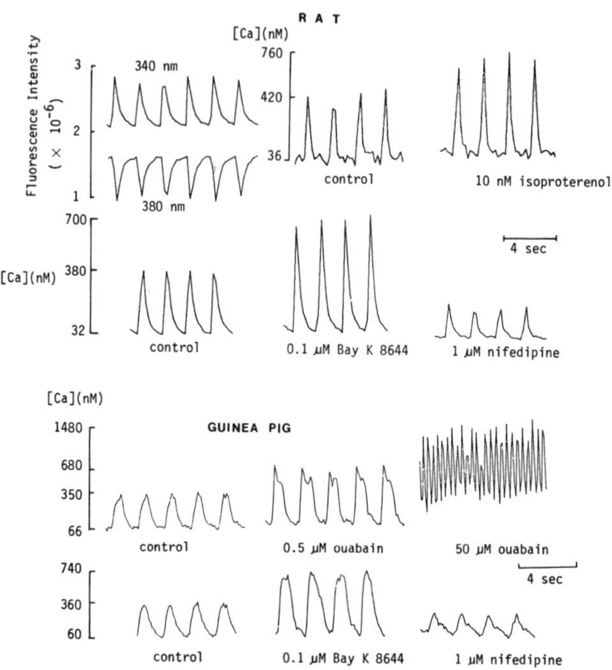

FIG. 4. Cytosolic free Ca^{++} as measured by the fura 2 fluorescence ratio.

REFERENCES

1. M.C. Capogrossi, A.A. Kort, H.A. Spurgeon, and E.G. Lakatta. J. Gen. Physiol. 88, 589-613 (1986).
2. D. Kim, E.J. Cragoe Jr., and T. W. Smith, Circ. Res. 60, 185-193 (1987).
3. G. Grynkiewicz, M. Poenie, and R.Y. Tsien, J. Biol. Chem. 260, 3440-3450 (1985).

BIOPHYSICS OF THE ISOLATED CELL

PAGE A.W. ANDERSON, M.D.* AND ROY L. WHITE, Ph.D.+
Departments of Pediatrics and Physiology, Duke University Medical Center,* Durham, North Carolina 27710 and Department of Neuroscience, Albert Einstein College of Medicine,+ Bronx, New York 10461

The isolated myocyte has been used to study many aspects of cardiac structure and function because the single cell possesses a number of advantages. Its lack of diffusion limitations and its freedom from the extracellular matrix and cell-to-cell connections allow simpler interpretation of biophysical data than is possible with the more complex multicellular preparation. These advantages have led to the development and application of techniques for measuring sarcomere dynamics, membrane currents, and cytosolic calcium concentrations in the single cell, and to studies of activation and contraction in, and effects of development and pharmacological agents on, the isolated cell.

The following are among the aspects of the single cell preparation that were considered at this meeting: cell damage, myocyte heterogeneity, effects of development, experimental techniques, the sarcomere shortening waveform, and membrane properties.

Cell Damage

Cardiac tissue is subjected to various procedures in order to yield isolated myocytes. These procedures, which usually include treatment by enzymes having proteolytic activity, have the potential for damaging the cells and altering their properties. At the same time, studies of the isolated myocyte are based on the implicit assumption that the cells are intact and that they exhibit the same cellular properties that they had in situ in the intact myocardium. When this assumption is justified, the response to an experimental perturbation or treatment would characterize the intrinsic properties of the cell in-situ; for example, functional differences observed among groups of isolated cells obtained from hearts of animals of different ages would be manifestations of the cell properties in-situ, rather than age-dependent differential sensitivity of the cells to tissue processing and cell treatment.

Studies of isolated myocytes are also based on the assumption that the isolation procedures do not result in favoring the survival of a certain subset of cells over another. The validity of this assumption may be difficult or impossible to ascertain, and bears on the applicability of the results of experiments on isolated cells to the population of cardiac myocytes from which the test myocytes were presumed to have been sampled (see Cell Heterogeneity).

A further bias, but one which is presumably under the control of the investigator, occurs when cells are selected to be used in an experiment. Random selection of cells to guard against bias is not always employed. In fact, investigators frequently consciously select cells that have particular properties that, in their opinion, make these cells especially suitable for a particular experiment. For example, early electrophysiological studies of single cells suggested that the larger myocytes were preferable because they appeared more robust [1]. Implied in this selection is the reasonable assumption that membrane properties are not a function of cell size. However, measurement of membrane properties may be adversely affected by such factors as deep clefts in the cell surface [2]. Also cell heterogeneity in the expression of protein isoforms such as Na/K-ATPase [3] may affect these properties and may (or may not) be related to cell size.

Biology of Isolated Adult Cardiac Myocytes
William A. Clark, Robert S. Decker, and Thomas K. Borg, Editors

Cell isolation techniques have now improved to the point where apparently undamaged single cells can be obtained in large numbers (over 10,000,000 cells from one rat heart, Wittenberg). Although such yields are striking, cells that are considered intact in one study often may not be so considered in another: What is considered intact depends on the criteria used and on the purpose of the experiment.

The tests and criteria used in the evaluation of cell intactness have evolved with time. The criteria that were used in the early studies, e.g., failure to take up trypan blue and quiescence in physiological calcium concentrations, are no longer sufficient when the experiment requires that the membrane systems that modulate cell calcium be intact and interact normally. Many of the studies presented at this meeting showed evidence that the cells survived the disaggregation process intact, based on the similarity of the responses of the isolated cell to those of the tissue (such as the effects of changing extracellular calcium, adrenergic receptor response, etc.) Other criteria used were all-or-none mechanical response to electrical stimulation, resting potentials near those of cells in situ, the retention of specific membrane properties, e.g., the slow inward calcium current, and homogeneous and reproducible sarcomere shortening. It is apparent from the papers presented at this meeting that a wide variation in the amount of cell shortening exists in the unloaded cell. This raises the question of whether a standard can be developed that defines the extent of shortening in a normal cell. Clearly, cell shortening depends on a range of factors that will vary among experiments, including cell type, extracellular ionic concentrations, temperature, pacing rate, et cetera.

By combining different experimental techniques in the characterization of the cell, comparing the physiological and ultrastructural characteristics of the same cell, for example, the sensitivity of the screening process for detecting cell damage is increased. By monitoring cell shortening and intracellular calcium concentration (using fura-2) Kim and Smith found that cell shortening, resting intracellular calcium, and the calcium transient increase after about 3 hours following isolation, indicating excessive calcium loading in these cells. This change was accompanied by a deterioration in the response of these cells to changes in extracellular calcium concentration, ouabain, isoproterenol, nifedipine, and isobutylmethylxanthine. Cells that did not show evidence of calcium overload responded to these agents like intact tissue. It may be presumed that the increased resting free calcium concentration in the calcium-overloaded cells would result in a shorter-than-normal resting sarcomere length, thus providing a simple test for identifying such cells.

Although the study of Kim and Smith does not provide a relationship between rest sarcomere length and resting cytosolic calcium concentration, its findings indicate that the cell's ability to control intracellular calcium deteriorates with time following isolation which can result in enhanced sarcomere shortening. On the other hand, Nassar et al. described ultrastructural damage to the Z-lines of isolated cells which was associated with weak sarcomere contractions. These observations indicate that degeneration of cell function can occur following isolation and, therefore, the investigator should ensure, as far as possible, that such deterioration does not confound the results of the investigation.

The physiological and biochemical effects of the enzymes used to isolate the cardiac myocyte were examined by Dowell and Tarr. Sarcomere shortening and magnesium- and calcium-activated myofibrillar ATPase and creatine kinase activities in myocytes from hearts of 3-week-old and 9-week-old rats isolated using either collagenase or protease were compared. Although the integrity of the cells, as judged by quiescence in calcium, appeared to be unaffected by replacing collagenase with a non-specific protease, sarcomere shortening and myofibrillar ATPase and creatine kinase activities were affected in an age-dependent manner: In cells isolated using protease, the peak velocity of sarcomere shortening was greater in cells from 3-week-old than 9-week-old hearts. The opposite was found in cells isolated using collagenase: sarcomere shortening velocity was greater in myocytes from the 9-week-old heart than 3-week-old. In myofibrils from cells isolated using protease from the 9-week-old heart, ATPase and creatine kinase activities were markedly reduced compared to myofibrils from collagenase-isolated cells of the same age. The myofibrillar ATPase and creatine kinase activities of myofibrils prepared from the 3-week-old heart did not depend on the enzyme used to isolate the cells.

These findings suggest, among other possibilities, that the enzymes used to isolate cells can alter the contractile proteins while leaving the cells' calcium control systems intact. Moreover, the effects of these enzymes can depend on the developmental age of the cells. In order to guard against using experimental results from cells that have received this kind of damage, it must be ascertained that the structure and function of the cells used are the same as those of the cells in situ.

Evidence of damage to myofilament structure was found in some rabbit myocytes in the study by Nassar et al. The Z-discs appeared damaged and the amount and velocity of sarcomere shortening were small, yet the systems for controlling cytosolic calcium appeared intact (see below). These data and those of Dowell and Tarr demonstrate that cells that survive isolation with their membranes intact may have sustained damage to the contractile system, as indicated by structural, biochemical, and functional markers.

The integrity of the isolated calcium-tolerant quiescent myocyte from the rabbit was tested in the study by Nassar et al. using physiological perturbations that modulate intracellular calcium concentration and sarcomere shortening. For example, the pattern of stimulation was altered by introducing an extrasystole into the basic pacing rate. The cells responded normally and demonstrated restitution of contractility and post-extrasystolic potentiation. These characteristics of cardiac muscle are associated with corresponding changes in cytosolic calcium concentration [4].

Altering the pattern of stimulation revealed another group of cells that showed evidence of subtle damage. By all the criteria so far mentioned, these cells appeared normal: they were quiescent in physiological extracellular calcium concentrations (1 to 3 mM), stimulation at a constant interval resulted in uniform and reproducible sarcomere shortening, sarcomere shortening was altered appropriately by changes in extracellular calcium concentration, and the ultrastructure of the isolated cell was normal. Yet when an extrasystole was elicited, these cells responded abnormally: spontaneous, non-uniform, chaotic sarcomere shortening followed the extrasystole. The regional variations in the chaotic sarcomere shortening is similar to the oscillations in calcium described in the spontaneously contracting isolated cell [5] and in the calcium-overloaded multicellular preparation [6]. It is likely that these cells, although overloaded with calcium, were able to control cytosolic calcium under regular stimulation conditions, but that the system was not able to cope with a further increase in cell calcium brought about by the extrasystole. The condition of calcium overload may be due to abnormalities in sarcolemmal function or in the function of the sarcoplasmic reticulum. Wittenberg has suggested that although calcium overload may occur with cell isolation, cells can extrude the excess calcium and recover with time.

The possibility of various forms of cell damage and their potential effects on the experimental results must be considered and resolved by the investigator. Even when very strict criteria were applied for cell intactness, the studies presented at this meeting demonstrate that isolated cells can be obtained that fulfill these criteria. This confirms the value of the single cell as a viable preparation for cardiac muscle studies.

Experimental Techniques

By applying several experimental techniques in the study of the same cell, different forms of complementary data can be obtained. For example, Houser et al. characterized the electrical and mechanical properties of isolated feline ventricular myocytes by measuring simultaneously, in the same cell, membrane potential, calcium current, cell length, and cytosolic calcium concentration. The acquisition of such data from the same cell enables the investigator to describe different aspects of the systems that control excitation and contraction and to explore the molecular basis of these systems and their modulation by different variables.

Other approaches make use of the experimenter's ability to control the extracellular and intracellular ionic environment of the isolated cell. Studies that focused on membrane properties exploited this: the intracellular environment was altered, e.g., by dialyzing the cell with CsCl and EGTA while the extracellular medium was constituted with TEA with or without replacement of calcium with magnesium, barium, or cadmium, in order to eliminate or block currents that were not of interest and that would have complicated the interpretation of the results. Although considered here, the experimental manipulations of the single cell are best appreciated by reading the text of these papers.

Several techniques for monitoring sarcomere dynamics were used in the investigations presented at this meeting, e.g.: 1) Light diffraction of the cell attached to a coverslip (Haworth et al.) was used to measure sarcomere length (determined from the position of the first-order diffraction peak, as initially used to describe sarcomere motion during the contraction of living cardiac tissue, [7]); 2) An edge detector to measure cell shortening and relengthening (Krueger et al., and Houser et al.); 3) Phase contrast microscopy and video recording of the cell image, from which sarcomere length measurements were made using a video micrometer (Nassar et al.) A variety of such approaches for measuring changes in sarcomere length are discussed in the chapter by Krueger.

Roos and Taylor used an altogether different approach to measure sarcomere length and contraction dynamics in the isolated cell. The myocytes were imaged digitally, and the data processed to enhance and quantitate striation positions. In essence, a bright-field image of the myocyte was projected onto a photodiode array, digitally acquired, stored, and processed. The analysis included background subtraction, digital filtering, gray-scale manipulation, convolutions, histograms, and false-color reading.

Each of these approaches has advantages, limitations, and inherent assumptions. Thus, depending on the purposes and the expertise of the investigator, the approaches used to measure sarcomere length will be different in different laboratories.

Sarcomere Shortening and Re-extension

The studies by Haworth et al., Krueger et al., and Nassar et al. demonstrate that the level of contractility, i.e., the extent to which cytosolic calcium is increased with activation, is a major factor in the control of sarcomere shortening. The relationship between cytosolic calcium and the amount of sarcomere shortening is demonstrated by the effects of manipulations such as changes in the pattern of stimulation and in the extracellular calcium concentration, and exposure to isoproterenol and ryanodine. In the rabbit myocyte, increasing extracellular calcium concentration enhances sarcomere shortening; altering the pattern of stimulation causes cytosolic calcium and sarcomere shortening to be modulated from beat to beat. An extra stimulus interpolated in the regular pacing pattern elicits a contraction that has a smaller amount and velocity of sarcomere shortening than that of the contraction at the basic rate. Sarcomere shortening in the following contraction is potentiated.

The amount of sarcomere shortening during a contraction depends on the cytosolic free calcium concentration, the sensitivity of the myofilaments to calcium, and the internal load against which the sarcomeres contract. The amount of sarcomere shortening was found to be linearly related to the velocity of sarcomere shortening in two single cell studies: Haworth et al. found that in the rat myocyte the contractions had to have the same duration for this relationship to hold while Nassar et al. did not find this requirement in the rabbit myocyte.

The peak velocity of sarcomere re-extension was also found to be related linearly to the amount of sarcomere shortening in the intact cell and, therefore, to the level of cytosolic calcium during contraction (Krueger et al., Nassar et al., and [8]). In addition, the slope of this relationship was affected by the extracellular calcium concentration [8] suggesting that peak velocity of sarcomere re-extension, and therefore the rate at which calcium is removed from the cytosol, depends on extracellular calcium concentration. To separate the effects of activation from the analysis of sarcomere re-extension, Krueger et al. analyzed re-extension velocity as a function of sarcomere length. Relaxation had two exponential phases, both independent of the time of repolarization. The first and most rapid phase was limited by the sarcoplasmic reticulum rate of uptake of calcium. The second phase of relengthening appeared to be independent of this process. This finding suggests that the second phase determines the diastolic tone of the myocardium.

Myocyte Heterogeneity

A frequent assumption is that cells from the same ventricle have the same properties. A large number of studies indicate that heterogeneity in cell function exists in cells from the same heart and from the same ventricle. For example, in the intact myocardium, cell-to-cell variation in myosin isozyme content has been found [9,10]. This variability was confirmed in a study of isolated adult rat myocytes [11]. Variability in the expression of troponin T isoforms has also been found in isolated adult rabbit myocytes [12]. At this meeting, evidence for heterogeneity in cell function was provided by Nassar et al. The velocity and amount of sarcomere shortening was found to vary among intact cells from the same heart. Marked morphological variability was also found among these cells, e.g., a two-fold difference in cell length (all of these cells were found, upon examination under the electron microscope, to be single cells) and in the rat myocytes described by Wittenberg et al. [13].

Heterogeneity in biochemical function was demonstrated in the study by Smith et al. Comparing right ventricular myocytes and those isolated from different regions of the left ventricle demonstrated a regional variation in creatine kinase activity. The presence of variability among myocytes in the isoform expression of other proteins is suggested by the study of Porterfield et al. Two classes of binding sites for ouabain were found in isolated myocytes. These results are consistent with those of Charlemagne et al. [3], who identified in isolated myocytes two isoforms of the alpha catalytic subunit of Na/K-ATPase. It would seem likely that the isoform expression of the alpha subunits would vary from cell to cell. Consequently, the physiological and pharmacological properties would also be expected to vary from cell to cell.

The variation in morphological and physiological properties and in the isoform expression of contractile and membrane proteins in myocytes from the same species, and, indeed, from the same heart, indicate that cell heterogeneity is a common property of mammalian myocardium. Such heterogeneity must be considered in isolated cell studies and in understanding the function of the intact heart. It should be pointed out that the heterogeneity observed in these myocytes would appear to bestow upon the myocardium the ability to respond to a wide variety of work loads, and allow it to adapt more easily to disease processes.

Developmental Changes in Sarcomere Dynamics

The effects of development on sarcomere dynamics are considered in several studies of the rat heart. Two studies (Tarr and Dowell, Haworth et al.) appear, on first glance, to provide results that are contradictory. Tarr and Dowell found that the amount and velocity of sarcomere shortening were enhanced in myocytes from the older rat heart while Haworth et al. found that sarcomere shortening was greater in myocytes from the younger rat. The apparent contradiction can be attributed to the differences in the ages studied. Tarr and Dowell used rats at 3 weeks and 9 weeks of age while Haworth et al. compared rats at 5-6 weeks and 8-9 months. An increase in sarcomere shortening velocity from 3 weeks to 9 weeks of age is not likely to be related to changes in myosin ATPase isoforms, as the alpha isozyme is predominantly expressed at this stage of development [14]. An increase in the expression of the beta isozyme occurs with aging in the rat [14] and could contribute to the slower shortening observed in myocytes from the 9-month-old rat.

As discussed above, the velocity of sarcomere shortening depends on the cytosolic calcium concentration during activation and on the sensitivity of the myofilaments to calcium. Haworth et al. found that although the linear relationship between the amount and velocity of sarcomere shortening was the same for myocytes at both stages of development, myocytes from the younger rats required a lower extracellular calcium concentration for comparable amounts of sarcomere shortening. In another species (rabbit), the developmental increase in the amount and velocity of sarcomere shortening has been discussed in relationship to the maturational changes in the restitution of contractility and the differentiation and organization of the sarcoplasmic reticulum [2]. These studies support the notion that maturational changes occur in the control of calcium made available during activation. Thus, developmental changes in the modulation of cytosolic calcium are likely to contribute significantly to maturational changes in myocardial contractility.

Developmental changes in the sensitivity of the myofilaments to calcium may also occur. Maturational changes in the isoform expression of the thin filament regulatory proteins, troponin T and troponin I, have been observed in the mammal [15-17]. In view of the observations that in fast skeletal muscle, troponin T isoform expression was found to be related to the sensitivity of the myofilaments to calcium [18] and that in cardiac muscle, troponin T expression has been found to affect myofibrillar ATPase [19], it is not unreasonable to suggest that developmental changes in cardiac troponin T isoform expression may contribute to maturational changes in sarcomere shortening and myofibrillar ATPase [20].

Membrane Properties

Several attributes of the single cell preparation (the lack of significant barriers to diffusion and hormonal influences and its amenability to membrane potential and intracellular environment control) were utilized in investigating sarcolemmal function in many of the studies presented here.

The basis and treatment of dysrhythmias were considered in studies of the Na channel. Hill et al. have previously demonstrated that batrachotoxinin A (BTXB) binds specifically to a sarcolemmal site which has the characteristics of the Na channel. An advantage of this toxin is that it activates the channel so that agents that inhibit Na channel opening or that displace BTXB from its binding site can be assessed using standard pharmacological approaches. The steric requirements for type 1 agent binding to the Na channel were examined using stereoisomeric pairs of type 1 antiarrhythmic agents. The conformations of the asymmetric carbons in the common structure appear important for drug binding and suggest that at least two stereo-specific domains are present on the receptor associated with the Na channel. Further, these receptors may be associated with the part of the Na channel protein located in the hydrophobic region of the membrane.

Delmar et al. used the single cell as a model for Wenckebach by studying the recovery of excitability, i.e., post-repolarization refractoriness, in guinea pig ventricular myocytes. Analyses of the voltage changes using computer simulations showed a correlation between the recovery of excitability and the time-dependent deactivation of the repolarizing outward current. They concluded that frequency-dependent activation failure follows from a basic membrane property inherent to the isolated myocyte rather than a consequence of tissue disaggregation and isolation of the cell.

The mechanisms that control cell calcium were studied by introducing a prolonged rest period in the pacing pattern and examining the calcium currents and the calcium transients in the contractions following the rest. At physiological holding potentials, Bers and Hess found a positive staircase in the peak calcium current, while at holding potentials of −40 or −50 mV, a negative calcium current staircase was noted. This positive staircase is consistent with the beat-dependent fall in extracellular calcium concentration and the contractile staircase observed in the multicellular preparation [21]. In isolated cat myocytes, Houser et al. found the calcium transient also to have a positive staircase. These staircases in cytosolic calcium and in the calcium current are probably related. However, the relative contributions of each of the sources to the calcium that results in the staircase in sarcomere shortening and in force remain to be determined.

The range of techniques that can be applied to studying membrane function is exemplified further by the study of Weiss. Single channel recordings were obtained from cells whose sarcolemma was made permeable at one end by exposure to saponin, and from excised inside-out patches. An ATP-sensitive K channel was activated when intracellular ATP fell. Sufficient local ATP to suppress the channel was thought to be generated in some of the excised patches. The success of glycolysis in regulating this cardiac ATP-sensitive K channel and the excised patch findings suggest that key glycolytic enzymes are located in the membrane or cytoskeleton in close proximity to the K channels.

Bahinski and Gadsby studied the current-voltage relationship of the Na/K pump in guinea-pig ventricular myocytes under conditions that cause the pump to run backwards (large concentration gradients for Na and K, and low ATP/ADP ratio). The Na/K pump current was determined under voltage clamp conditions as the difference between the inward currents with and without pump inhibition by strophanthidin. The inward current was strongly voltage dependent and there was no clear evidence of negative slope conductance in the current-voltage relationship, suggesting a Na/K pump reaction cycle with one voltage-dependent step which may be located at the Na binding step.

SUMMARY

The studies presented at this meeting demonstrate the range of questions that can be addressed using the isolated adult ventricular myocyte preparation and the range of experimental manipulations that are possible with this preparation. They demonstrate that the isolated cell preparation can be used to test hypotheses through the acquisition of new data that are not available from other cardiac preparations.

ACKNOWLEDGEMENTS

This work was supported in part by NIH Grants HL20749 and HL33680.

REFERENCES

Papers presented at this meeting are referred to by author and found in the text of this summary.

1. C.O. Lee, D.Y. Uhm, and K. Dresdner, Science 209, 699-701 (1980).
2. R. Nassar, M.C. Reedy, and P.A.W. Anderson, Circ. Res. 61, 465-483 (1987).
3. D. Charlemagne, E. Mayoux, M. Poyard, P. Oliviero, and K. Geering, J. Biol. Chem. 262, 8941-8943 (1987).
4. W.G. Wier and D.T. Yue, J. Physiol. 376, 507-530 (1986).
5. W.G. Wier, M.B. Cannell, J.R. Berlin, E. Marban, and W.J. Lederer, Science 235, 325-328 (1987).
6. C.H. Orchard, D.A. Eisner, and D.G. Allen, Nature 304, 735-738 (1983).
7. R. Nassar, A. Manring, and E.A. Johnson, Physiological Basis of Starling's Law of the Heart, Ciba Foundation Symposium 24, 57-91 (1974).
8. R. Nassar and P.A.W. Anderson, Biophys. J. 51, 465a (1987).
9. B.R. Eisenberg, J.A. Edwards, and R. Zak, Circ. Res. 56, 548-555 (1985).
10. S. Sartore, L. Gorza, P. Bormioli, L.D. Libera, and S. Schiaffino, J. Cell. Biol. 88, 226-233 (1981).
11. J.-L. Samuel, L. Rappaport, J.-J. Mercadier, A.-M. Lompre, S. Sartore, C. Triban, S. Schiaffino, and K. Schwartz, Circ. Res. 52, 200-209 (1983).
12. R. Nassar, M.E. Moore, and P.A.W. Anderson, Biophys. J. 51, 329a (1987).
13. B.A. Wittenberg, R.L. White, R.D. Ginzberg, and D.C. Spray, Circ. Res. 59, 143-150 (1986).
14. A.M. Lompre, J.J. Mercadier, C. Wisnewsky, P. Bouveret, C. Pantaloni, A. D'Albis, and K. Schwartz, Dev. Biol. 84, 286-290 (1981).
15. P.A.W. Anderson, G.E. Moore, and R.N. Nassar, J. Mol. Cell. Cardiol. 19(Suppl IV), S.21 (1987).
16. L. Saggin, S. Ausoni, L. Gorza, S. Sartore, and S. Schiaffino, J. Mol. Cell. Cardiol. 19(Suppl IV), S.21 (1987).
17. R.J. Solaro, J. Lee, J. Kentish, and D.G. Allen, J. Mol. Cell. Cardiol. 19(Suppl IV), S.60 (1987).
18. P.W. Brandt, M.S. Diamond, B. Gluck, M. Kawai, and F. Schachat, Carlsberg Res. Commun. 49, 155-167 (1984).
19. L.S. Tobacman and R. Lee, J. Biol. Chem. 262, 4059-4064 (1987).
20. T. Nakanishi and J.M. Jarmakani, Am. J. Physiol. 246, H615-H625 (1984).
21. D.M. Bers, Am. J. Physiol. 244, H462-H468 (1983).

EFFECTS OF PERINATAL DEVELOPMENT ON THE CONTRACTILE PERFORMANCE OF ISOLATED RAT CARDIAC MYOCYTES.

MERRILL TARR, RUSSELL T. DOWELL
Department of Physiology, University of Kansas Medical Center,
Kansas City, Ks 66103

INTRODUCTION

Cardiac function during perinatal development has been investigated in the intact animal using the rat as an experimental animal [1]. When indices of heart contractile performance were determined *in situ*, a substantial enhancement in the rate of left ventricular pressure development (dP/dt) occurred from the time of weaning until early adulthood. Because left ventricular dP/dt has been shown to reflect the contractile state of the myocardium which, in turn, is related to the enzymatic rate of ATP hydrolysis by cardiac myofibrils [2], the presence of enhanced ATPase activity in cardiac myofibrils purified from left ventricles of adult rats suggested a potential subcellular correlate for the functional responses observed. Nevertheless, *in situ* heart contractile performance is influenced by heart rate, loading conditions, and neural/humoral status such that subcellular explanations for developmental enhancement of cardiac performance remain speculative. On the other hand, if developmentally related enhancement in contractile performance were demonstrated in isolated cardiac myocytes of weanling and adult hearts, then more compelling subcellular mechanisms could be hypothesized. Therefore, the present experiments were conducted to evaluate contractile performance in cardiac myocytes isolated from left ventricles of weanling and adult rats. Subsequently, purified myofibrils were prepared from isolated myocytes and analyzed for ATPase enzymatic activity.

METHODS

For the preparation of isolated cardiac myocytes, weanling and adult rats were killed by a blow to the head. The heart was excised and placed in a beaker of heparinized saline. Retrograde perfusion of the excised heart with a collagenase enzyme solution allowed heart muscle and nonmuscle cells to be disaggregated [3]. Cardiac myocytes were separated from nonmuscle cells by gravity in room temperature buffers which were nominally calcium free. Final cell suspensions were made by gradually increasing the calcium concentration in the resuspending buffer until a final concentration of 1 mM calcium or 3 mM calcium was obtained. Aliquots of cardiac myocytes were used to obtain purified cardiac myofibrils. Myofibrillar adenosine triphosphatase (ATPase) activity was measured as previously described [3].

Intracellular potentials of single cells were measured using whole cell recording techniques with patch pipettes [4] filled with 150 mM KCl. To elicit action potentials, the cells were stimulated with a 10 msec depolarizing constant current pulse applied at a rate of 0.1 Hz. Conventional bright field light microscope techniques were used to view the cell and the sarcomere pattern within the cell, and these images were recorded on videotape. The time course of changes in cell length and sarcomere length during a contraction-relaxation cycle were analyzed using the stop frame (pause mode) capability of the videotape recorder in combination with a double TV cursor [5]. The time resolution of the length changes was 1/60th of a second. For sarcomere length determinations, the length occupied by 10 sarcomeres was determined and an average sarcomere length was calculated. The rate of length change (cell and sarcomere) was determined for each time

Biology of Isolated Adult Cardiac Myocytes
William A. Clark, Robert S. Decker, and Thomas K. Borg, Editors

interval during a contraction and the maximum rate of shortening was used for analysis purposes. The average of the maximum rate of shortening obtained from five contractions was taken as the value representative of the peak velocity of shortening (cell and sarcomere) for a given cell. Similarly, the average of the extent of shortening obtained from five contractions was used to calculate a representative value for the percent change in length (cell and sarcomere).

RESULTS

Typical recordings of the time course of sarcomere shortening during action potential elicited contractions are shown in Figure 1. This figure demonstrates some consistent findings regarding the contractile performance of myocytes derived from 3 week and 9 week old rats. First, both the velocity and extent of sarcomere shortening were greater in the 9 week myocyte then in the 3 week myocyte. Second, the duration of the contraction was markedly shorter in the 3 week myocyte. Although not shown, there was good agreement between the time course of sarcomere shortening (as derived from a population of 10 sarcomeres) and the time course of overall cell shortening. There was also good agreement between the percent change in sarcomere length and percent change in cell length.

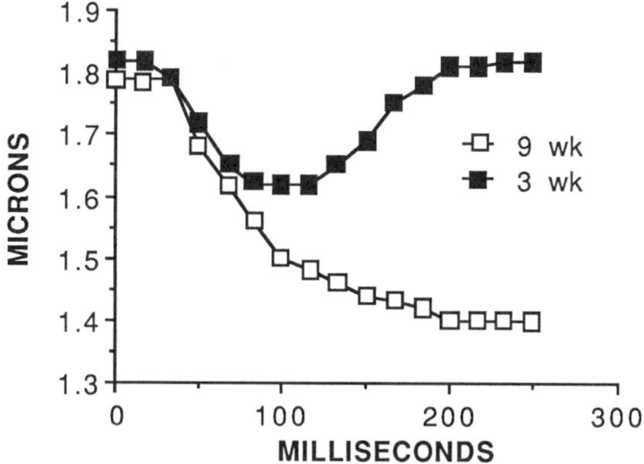

FIG. 1. Sarcomere length vs time during contractions in 3 week and 9 week myocytes bathed in 3 mM calcium.

Figure 2 presents a summary of the results regarding sarcomere performance in 3 week and 9 week myocytes placed in either 1 mM or 3 mM extracellular calcium. The left part of this figure gives the percent change in sarcomere length during contraction; the right part of this figure gives the peak velocity of sarcomere shortening. As would be expected, for both 3 week and 9 week myocytes an increase in extracellular calcium resulted in an increase in both the extent and velocity of sarcomere shortening. But at both calcium concentrations the 9 week myocyte had a greater extent of sarcomere shortening. The percent sarcomere shortening in 1 mM calcium was 10.6 $\pm$ 0.6 (n=6) for the 3 week myocyte compared to 13.8 $\pm$ 0.4 (n=6) for the 9 week myocyte. In 3 mM calcium the values were 12.5 $\pm$ 1.4 (n=7) and 19.5 $\pm$ 0.9 (n=12), respectively. The 9 week myocyte also had a higher velocity of sarcomere shortening than did the 3 week myocyte at both calcium concentrations. The velocity (μm/sec) of sarcomere shortening in 1 mM calcium was

3.3 ± 0.2 for the 3 week myocyte compared to 4.6 ± 0.2 for the 9 week myocyte. In 3 mM calcium the values were 4.0 ± 0.5 and 6.1 ± 0.6, respectively.

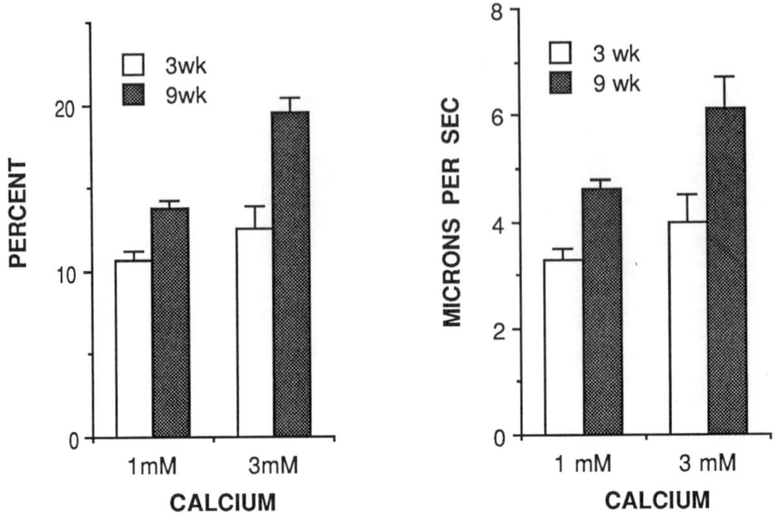

FIG. 2. Sarcomere shortening and sarcomere velocity in 3 week and 9 week myocytes. Mean values and one standard error are presented.

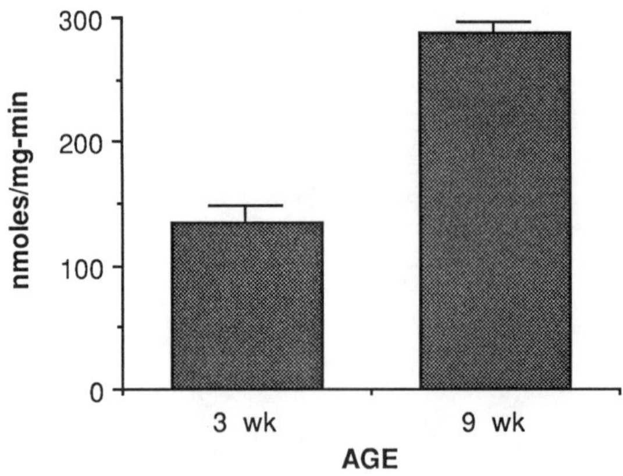

FIG. 3. Myofibrillar ATPase activity in 3 week and 9 week myocytes. Mean values and one standard error are presented.

Figure 3 presents the magnesium-activated ATPase activity of myofibrils derived from 3 week and 9 week myocytes. It is apparent that 9 week myocytes had higher myofibrillar ATPase activity than did the 3 week myocytes (288 ± 8 compared to 134 ± 14).

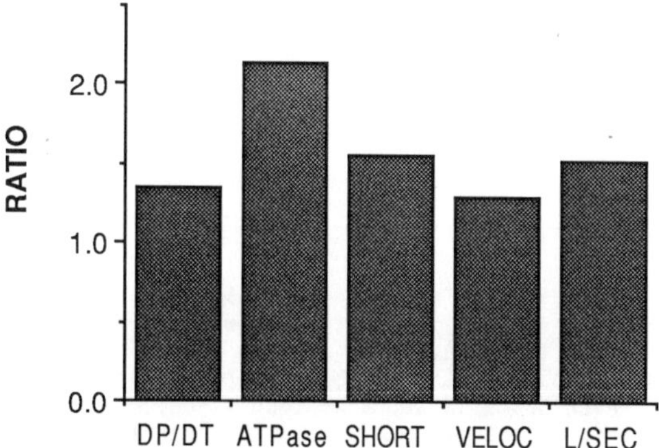

FIG. 4. Ratios (9 week/3 week) for the rate of left ventricular pressure development in intact rat hearts (DP/DT), and from isolated myocytes the myofibrillar ATPase activity (ATPase), percent sarcomere shortening (SHORT), peak velocity of sarcomere shortening (VELOC), and the peak velocity of overall cell shortening in initial lengths per sec (L/SEC): extracellular calcium of 3 mM.

Figure 4 gives the ratios (9 week/3 week) for various parameters related to contractile performance in either intact heart tissue or the isolated myocyte. It is apparent that the ratio was greater than unity for each of these parameters. Also, there was good agreement between the increase in contractile performance during perinatal development as measured in the intact heart (rate of pressure development) and in the isolated myocyte (velocity and extent of shortening).

DISCUSSION

The results presented in this paper demonstrate that the individual rat myocyte shows improved contractile performance during normal development of the heart. Such a finding indicates that the improved contractile performance of the heart which occurs during perinatal development is related to increased contractile performance at the cellular level.

ACKNOWLEDGEMENTS

This research was supported by NIH grant HL33677.

REFERENCES

1. R.T. Dowell, Mechanisms of Ageing and Development 25, 307-321 (1984).
2. B.B. Hamrell and R.B. Low, Pflugers Arch. 377, 119-124 (1978).
3. A.F. Cutilletta, M.C. Aumont, A.C. Nag, and R. Zak, J. Mol. Cell. Cardiol. 9, 399-407 (1977).
4. O.P. Hamill, A. Marty, E. Neher, B. Sakmann, and F.J. Sigworth, Pflugers Arch. 39, 85-100 (1981).
5. M. Tarr, J.W. Trank, and P. Leiffer, Circ. Res. 48, 189-200 (1981).

CONTRACTILE FUNCTION OF ISOLATED RAT AND HUMAN HEART CELLS

ROBERT A. HAWORTH, ATILLA B. GOKNUR, HERBERT A. BERKOFF
Department of Surgery, University of Wisconsin Clinical Science Center, 600 Highland Avenue, Madison, WI 53792

INTRODUCTION

Isolated adult heart cells offer new opportunities for the investigation of contractile function at the cellular level. In recent years several different methods have been applied to the measurement of contractile function in unloaded single adult heart cells: cell video image analysis [1], which has a 32msec time resolution; monitoring fluctuations in scattered light intensity [2], which is simple but cannot be calibrated in terms of sarcomere dynamics; cell edge position detection [3], which has a 1 msec time resolution but requires an independent measure of sarcomere length; and laser light diffraction [4], with which the contractile function of isolated adult rat heart cells were first measured. An advantage of using laser light diffraction is that sarcomere dynamics are measured directly. We have adapted this method by interfacing a photodiode array, which detects the diffraction pattern, with a microcomputer. This enables us to measure contractile function and sarcomere length in quite a large number of cells relatively easily, while maintaining their viability in a perfusion chamber.

Using this device we have investigated the contractile function of cells from young (5-6 week) and mature (8-9 month) rats, under a variety of contractile conditions [5]. We also show here some preliminary measurements on human cells isolated from failing hearts of transplant recipients.

METHODS

Rat heart cells were isolated as previously described [6]. Either female retired breeders (8-9 months) or young unbred female rats (5-6 weeks) were used. Cells were isolated from hearts of transplant recipients by a similar procedure, except that a branch of the left anterior descending artery was cannulated and a chunk of tissue (about 30 gm) perfused by the branch was excised, instead of using the whole heart. Also, tissue perfusion was with medium without added Ca throughout, and 1 mg collagenase/ml was used. Informed consent of all patients was obtained.

Cells were resuspended in a medium containing 118 mM NaCl, 4.8 mM KCl, 25 mM HEPES, 1.2 mM KH_2PO_4, 1 mM $CaCl_2$ (unless otherwise stated), 5mM Na pyruvate, 11 mM glucose, 1 μM insulin, 2 mg/ml bovine serum albumin (fraction V, fatty acid free), penicillin (50 I.U./ml), streptomycin (50 μg/ml), and basal Eagle medium amino acids (Flow labs). The medium was adjusted to pH 7.4 with NaOH.

Cells were attached to coverslips coated with laminin (4 μg/cm^2) and incorporated into a perfusion chamber on the microscope stage maintained at 25°. The chamber contained electrodes with which the cells could be stimulated to beat. Details of the perfusion chamber and of the data processing are given elsewhere [5].

RESULTS

The periodic structure of the sarcomere causes very strong first order diffracted peaks when single adult heart cells are illuminated with laser light (Fig. 1). Since the distance between peaks is inversely

Biology of Isolated Adult Cardiac Myocytes
William A. Clark, Robert S. Decker, and Thomas K. Borg, Editors

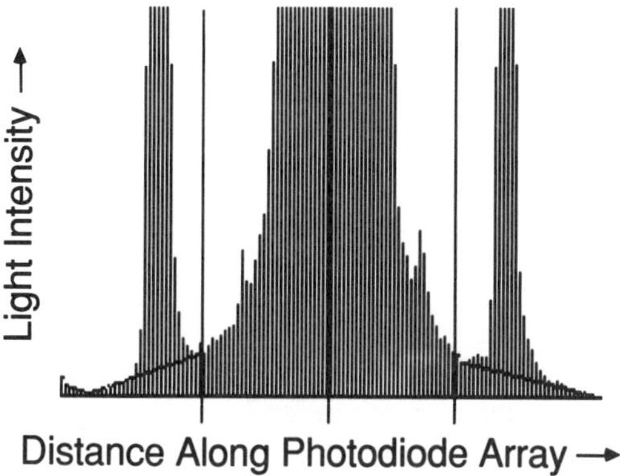

Fig. 1. Diffraction pattern from a single adult rat heart cell, as detected by 128 photodiode linear array. (By permission of American Journal of Physiology).

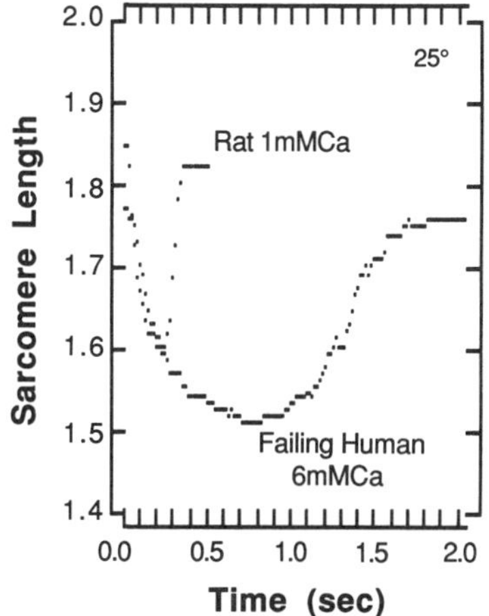

Fig. 2. Comparison between rested state contractions of rat and failing human single heart cells.

Cells were attached to cover slips and incorporated into a perfusion chamber where they could be maintained for up to eight hours. Attachment did not appear to affect the velocity or extent of cell shortening (data not shown). Fig. 2 shows the time course of sarcomere length changes after stimulation of a normal rat cell and a failing human cell at 25°. Data in this figure was taken every 16msec to accommodate the beat duration of the human cell. There is clearly a vast difference in beat duration between rat and human. Part of this undoubtedly reflects a difference in beat duration related to heart size. It could well also reflect the fact that the cells were from failing hearts: a prolongation of contraction duration and of intracellular Ca transients has been proportional to the sarcomere length, cell contraction can be followed by measuring the time course of changes in peak position. In our system, peak positions are calculated on line from array data collected every 4msec after stimulation of a cell. observed in trabeculae carnae from such hearts [7]. Such differences should be measurable when we isolate cells from control human hearts, which has yet to be done. In addition, the contractile properties of these cells may reflect deterioration or selection during isolation. The isolation procedure is not yet optimized, and the yield of Ca tolerant cells is low. Even so, some properties of these cells are evident: isoproterenol shortens the contraction duration considerably and slightly enhances the extent of shortening, while extra Ca increases the extent of shortening without affecting contraction duration (Table I).

The contractile function of cells isolated from young (5-6 week) and mature (8-9 month) rat hearts has also been compared. These cells when stimulated repetitively show a negative staircase [8]. We found that the negative staircase was less marked in cells from the younger rats (Fig. 3).

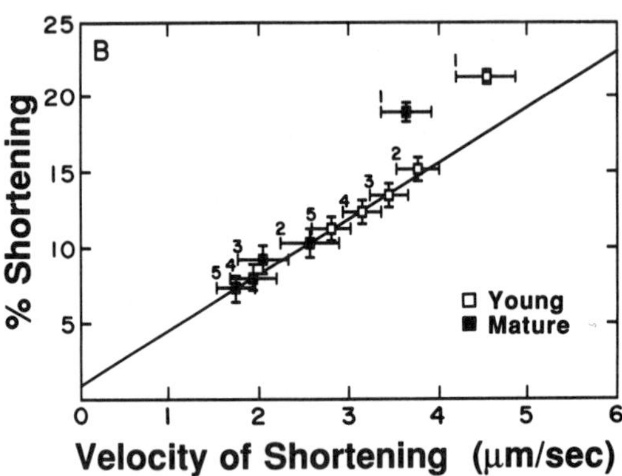

Fig. 3. Extent and velocity of contraction of young and mature rat heart cells. Cells were stimulated five times at 1 Hz at 25°, in medium containing 2 mM Ca. Data is mean ± SEM from 18 cells. (By permission of American Journal of Physiology).

If the medium contained 1 mM Ca instead of 2 mM Ca, the negative staircase was more marked, such that cells from young rats in 1 mM Ca beat like

Table I. Rested state contraction parameters of single cells from failing adult human hearts.

	Time to half relaxation (sec)	Shortening (%)
3 mM Ca	1.46±0.36	6.70±3.94
3 mM Ca and isoproterenol	0.84±0.14**	9.10±2.93*
6 mM Ca	1.40±0.32	11.36±3.91**

Values shown are mean ± SD from 24 cells from three hearts failing subsequent to ischemic heart disease. Significant differences: * $p < 0.05$, ** $p < 0.001$ with respect to 3 mM Ca values by t-test. This data does not include 3 cells which did not beat when stimulated, in 3 mM Ca. Rested state contractions were measured at 25°. Resting sarcomere length was 1.817 ± 0.061 μm in 3 mM Ca.

those from mature rats in 2 mM Ca [5]. At 25° (as in Fig. 3) the rested state contraction was of significantly longer duration than subsequent beats. For beats of similar duration (beats 2 to 5, Fig. 3), there was a proportionality between the velocity and extent of contraction. These data suggest to us that the differences in contractile function between young and mature cells are related to differences in Ca metabolism. Using our Mn uptake assay for Ca channel activity we found that such activity was not significantly greater in the young cells than in the mature cells, though the mean value was 20% higher [9]. On the other hand, Fabiato has observed that cells from young rats require less Ca to release Ca from the sarcoplasmic reticulum, suggesting that in older cells the same Ca trigger would release less Ca [10]. This could explain why more extracellular Ca is required in the mature cells for a given contractile strength.

REFERENCES

1. Capogrossi MC, Kort AA, Spurgeon HA, Lakatta EG. J. Gen. Physiol. 88:589-613 (1986).
2. Mitchell MR, Powell T, Terrar DA, Twist VW. J. Physiol. 364:113-130 (1985).
3. London B, Krueger JW. J. Gen. Physiol. 88:475-505 (1986).
4. Krueger JW, Forletti D, Wittenberg BA. J. Gen. Physiol. 76:587-607 (1980).
5. Haworth RA, Griffin P, Saleh B, Goknur AB, Berkoff HA. Am. J. Physiol., Heart Physiology, scheduled for publication in Dec. 1987 issue.
6. Haworth RA, Hunter DR, Berkoff HA. J. Mol. Cell. Cadiol. 12:715-723 (1980).
7. Gwathmey JK, Copelas L, MacKinnon R, Schoen FJ, Feldman MD, Grossman W, Morgan JP. Circ. Res. 61:70-76 (1987).
8. Fabiato A. J. Gen. Physiol. 78:457-497 (1981).
9. Haworth RA, Goknur AB, Berkoff HA. J. Mol. Cell. Cardiol., accepted for publication.
10. Fabiato A. Fed. Proc. 41:2238-2244 (1982).

CONTRACTILE AND BIOCHEMICAL PROPERTIES OF RAT CARDIAC MYOCYTES ISOLATED USING NONSPECIFIC PROTEASE

RUSSELL T. DOWELL, AND MERRILL TARR
Department of Physiology, University of North Carolina, Chapel Hill, N.C. 27514; Department of Physiology, University of Kansas Medical Center, Kansas City, Kansas 66103

INTRODUCTION

Isolated cardiac myocytes represent an ideal experimental preparation in which to determine the intrinsic cellular properties of the heart. The contractile characteristics of isolated muscle cells can be measured in the absence of confounding influences such as loading conditions, neural status, and humoral or ionic fluctuations. Cellular and subcellular metabolic correlates are also obtainable from isolated myocytes, thus, mechanisms responsible for modulating cardiac performance can be identified. Enzymatic digestion of cardiac tissue is the most common method for preparing myocytes for experimentation, and varying concentrations of collagenase/hyaluronidase have been espoused depending upon the particular requirements of the experimental protocol. The strengths and weaknesses of a number of disaggregation methodologies have been reviewed [1]; however, a persistent problem with proteolytic enzyme methods for cardiac myocyte disaggregation is the variability of results depending upon the supplier of enzyme and/or the variation which accompanies different lots from the same supplier. To avoid this complication, a cardiac myocyte disaggregation method employing nonspecific protease has been developed by Mitra and Morad [2]. In our ongoing studies of cardiac myocytes during normal heart development, we encountered periodic inconsistency in both yield and viability of cells prepared using collagenase/hyaluronidase. Preliminary observations using nonspecific protease disaggregation procedures indicated a subjective improvement in yield and viability of cells; however, a systematic comparison of cellular properties was required. The present studies were conducted to provide a comparative, quantitative evaluation of cardiac myocyte properties when disaggregation was by either collagenase/hyaluronidase or nonspecific protease.

METHODS

Weanling (3 weeks post-birth) and adult (9 weeks post-birth) rats were killed by a blow to the head. The heart was then rapidly excised and placed in a beaker of heparinized saline. Following aortic cannulation, retrograde perfusion of the heart was acomplished using a recirculating system as previously described [3]. Perfusion conditions were identical except for the disaggregating enzymes employed. Collagenase/hyaluronidase was used in one series of experiments while nonspecific protease (Sigma, Type XIV) was substituted for hyaluronidase in a second series of experiments. Following enzyme disaggregation, myocytes were separated from nonmuscle cells by gravity in room temperature buffers that are nominally calcium free. During the end stages of cell preparation, myocytes were exposed to gradually increasing concentrations of calcium until final suspensions of cells were made using buffer containing 3 mM calcium.

Biology of Isolated Adult Cardiac Myocytes
William A. Clark, Robert S. Decker, and Thomas K. Borg, Editors

The contractile performance of single cells was evaluated by determining the extent and velocity of sarcomere shortening as the cell contracts in the absence of external load. Stimulation frequency for weanling and adult myocytes was 0.1 Hz in conjunction with a stroboscopic illumination, closed circuit TV-video tape system. Recording and data analysis techniques for sarcomere kinetic studies were those previously employed [4,5].

In parallel experiments, purified myofibrils were prepared from isolated myocytes. Subsequently, myofibrillar enzymatic activities for adenosine triphosphatase (ATPase) and creatine kinase (CK) were measured. Magnesium-activated myofibrillar ATPase activity (MgATPase) was assayed in a free calcium concentration of 1 mM. Calcium-activated myofibrillar ATPase (actomyosin ATPase) was measured in the presence of 10 mM calcium under conditions similar to those used for purified myosin. Creatine kinase enzyme activity in purified myofibrils was measured using kinetic assay procedures [6].

RESULTS

On the basis of subjective appearance, cardiac myocytes isolated using nonspecific protease were consistently superior in yield and overall viability. Myocytes disaggregated using collagenase/hyaluronidase demonstrated a significant enhancement in contractile performance as a function of perinatal development (Figure 1). In contrast, myocytes disaggregated using collagenase/

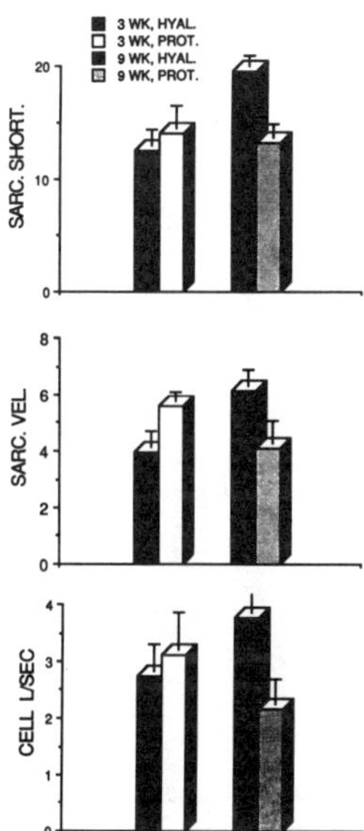

Figure 1. Contractile properties of weanling (3 WK) and adult (9 WK) myocytes disaggregated by collagenase/hyaluronidase (HYAL.) or protease (PROT.). Sarcomere shortening (%), sarcomere shortening velocity (uM/SEC), and cell shortening velocity (L/SEC) values are mean and standard error for three preparations of each type.

protease exhibited a divergent functional response. Contractile function was somewhat enhanced by protease disaggregation in weanling myocytes, but markedly decreased in adult myocytes.

The biochemical measurements related to cardiac myocyte contractile performance are shown in Figure 2. As previously described, myofibrillar MgATPase activity is enhanced during perinatal development; however, the magnitude of enhancement is blunted in myofibrils prepared from adult myocytes disaggregated with protease. Because different disaggregation protocols could influence myofibrillar ATPase activity by influencing either the thick filament, thin filament, or both, it is interesting to consider the AM ATPase and CK results. When assayed under conditions reflecting the myosin ATPase activity of the thick filament, there is no evidence of preferential or differential influence of protease disaggregation on myosin enzymatic activity. In contrast, the myofibrillar CK enzymatic activity mirrors the enzyme activity observed in myofibrillar MgATPase. Thus, it appears that the differential influence of protease disaggregation is a function of actions taking place within the complete contractile protein unit rather than disturbances occurring within the myosin molecule.

DISCUSSION

Previous studies in the intact heart have documented a developmentally related increase in cardiac functional performance which is correlated with enhanced ATPase activity of contractile protein [7]. The present experiments in myocytes isolated from

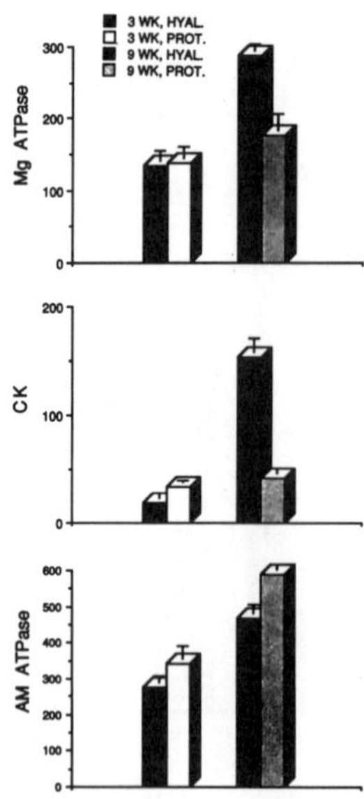

Figure 2. Myofibrillar biochemical measurements related to myocyte contractile properties. Enzyme activities are nmole/mg protein/min.

weanling and adult hearts confirm the cellular/subcellular basis for enhanced contractile function. However, it is clear that the functional status of the myocyte may be related to events involving the complete contractile protein structural unit and cannot be ascribed solely to the enzymatic status of the myosin molecule.

In view of the results presented in Figures 1 and 2, it may be hypothesized that the myofibrillar component of the phosphorylcreatine shuttle mechanism [8] plays a regulatory role in cardiac myocyte contractile performance. Elevated CK enzymatic activity could be responsible for parallel enhancement in myofibrillar ATPase activity by local regeneration of contractile substrate (ATP). This effect would occur independently from prevailing myosin ATPase activity. In turn, cardiac contractile function would then be closely correlated with myofibrillar MgATPase. The differential and selective alteration of myofibrillar CK activity by proteolytic disaggregation in hearts of weanling and adult rats may provide a useful experimental means for testing this hypothesis.

ACKNOWLEDGEMENT

Supported by National Institutes of Health grants HL28456 and HL33677.

REFERENCES

1. B.B. Farmer, M. Mancina, E.S. Williams, and A.M. Watanabe. Life Sciences. 33:1-18, (1983).
2. R. Mitra and M. Morad. Am. J. Physiol. 249:H1056-H1060, (1985).
3. R.T. Dowell, J.L. Haithcoat, H.M. Thirkill, and W.K. Palmer. Am. J. Physiol. 246:H197-H206, (1984).
4. M. Tarr, J.W. Trank, and K.K. Goertz. Circ. Res. 52:161-169, (1983).
5. M. Tarr, J.W. Trank, and K.K. Goertz. Circ. Res. 54:58-64, (1984).
6. R.T. Dowell and A.F. Martin. Can. J. Physiol. Pharmacol. 63: 627-629, (1985).
7. R. T. Dowell. Mech. Ageing and Develop. 25:307-321, (1984).
8. S.P. Bessman. Ann. Rev. Biochem. 54:831-862, (1985).

TIME COURSE OF ELECTROPHYSIOLOGICAL PROPERTIES AND CONCENTRATION OF SODIUM AND POTASSIUM IN CULTURED ADULT RAT CARDIAC MYOCYTES

STUART L. JACOBSON, ALEXANDER E. JUHASZ, AND ADRIAN SCULPTOREANU
Department of Biology, Carleton University, Ottawa, Canada, K1S 5B6

INTRODUCTION

Single cardiac myocytes isolated from adult animals provide a preparation whose utility is not limited by the usual problems encountered with intact tissue [1]. Notwithstanding improvements in the quality of isolated myocytes, problems of isolation damage and of inadequate vital support from suspending media still limit the range and duration of experiments for which these cells are useful. Cell culture can provide a milieu that promotes repair of lesions and that can support a near normal stable cellular state for prolonged periods [1].

In culture the morphology of myocytes depends, among other things, on the culture substratum and on whether serum is used to supplement culture media. In the absence of serum, on substrata coated with a component of the extracellular matrix [2,3] or treated with fetal bovine serum [4], cells attach rapidly and maintain their elongated *in situ* morphology for several days. Subsequently, they either detach from the substratum and degenerate or flatten and spread laterally. On other substrata [5-7] serum must be present for cells to establish in culture. Once established, they persist for several weeks to months. In this case, cells round up during the first few days in culture, gradually losing their myotypic order. They attach then to the substratum, flatten and spread polymorphically outward, apparently redifferentiating and developing new cytoskeletal components and myotypic features [8]. Rounding and spreading of these cells is asynchronous over the population in a culture so that during the first 2 weeks, cells in various developmental stages coexist there [9].

A good deal is known about the timecourse of redifferentiation at the light and electron microscopic level [8-11]. The timecourse of changes in electrophysiological properties of these cells has received only limited attention, however [12,13]. It is known that from about 2 to 4 weeks in culture, some cells, selected from those in a sample that could be impaled with a microelectrode, have a transmembrane potential difference (E_m) in the normal *in vivo* range [12]. However, the *mean* E_m of *all* cells of a sample of cells impaled is less than expected for cells *in vivo* [13].

We examined the electrophysiological properties and their timecourse in redifferentiating cells for the first 11 weeks in culture and have measured intracellular concentrations of sodium (Na) and potassium (K) in an effort to better understand the genesis of the measured potentials. Some of the results of these measurements are reported here.

MATERIALS AND METHODS

Isolation and culture of cells: Cardiac myocytes from Sprague-Dawley male rats were isolated and established in culture according to a modification [14] of the method of Jacobson, 1977 [7]. Some cultures were treated with 10 μM cytosine 1-β-D arabinofuranoside (ARA) for the first 7 days in order to virtually eliminate non-myocytes.

Electrophysiological measurements: Intracellular glass microelectrodes were used to measure electrical activity of cardiac myocytes in cultures from the time of plating to 11 weeks. Cells at all morphological stages

Biology of Isolated Adult Cardiac Myocytes
William A. Clark, Robert S. Decker, and Thomas K. Borg, Editors

were examined. Techniques used have been described elsewhere [13].

Measurement of Na and K: Concentration of intracellular sodium ($[Na]_i$) and potassium ($[K]_i$) was determined in samples of newly isolated myocytes and in myocytes in culture for up to 5 weeks. Concentrations were calculated from the relation:

$$[I]_i = ([I]_t - V_e/V_t \ [I]_e) (1 - V_e/V_t)^{-1}$$

where $[I]_i = [Na]_i$ or $[K]_i$; $[I]_t$ = concentration of intra- plus extracellular Na or K measured in a cell sample, respectively, by atomic absorption or flame emission spectroscopy; $[I]_e$ = the measured concentration of Na or K in the extracellular medium of the sample; V_e = extracellular volume of the sample determined by measuring the concentration of ^{35}S in the extracellular medium after addition of a known amount of $H_2{}^{35}SO_4$; V_t = the total volume of the sample determined by measuring the concentration of ^3H in the sample after addition of a known amount of ^3H_2O. Newly isolated cells: Cell samples for analysis of $[Na]_i$ and $[K]_i$ consisted of (8 to 10) X 10^4 calcium tolerant myocytes along with hypercontracted calcium intolerant cells. After addition of ^3H and ^{35}S isotopes, cells were layered on silicone oil (General Electric SF1250) and spun for 20 sec. at 10^4G. Cells were stripped of excess extracellular fluid as they passed through the oil and formed a pellet. The pellet was transferred to acid (reagent grade Nitric, BDH Chemicals nr. 45004) and was solubilized in it, forming a clear solution that was diluted and analyzed for Na and K. Cultured Cells: Cells were cultured on plastic coverslips (Lux Thermonox, Miles Labs. nr. 5412). Three to 6 coverslips, each with about 2 X 10^4 myocytes, were incubated in medium 199 (M199) containing the ^3H and ^{35}S isotopes. Coverslips were then rinsed briefly in Na-ion-free saline (with the same concentrations of isotope plus sucrose added to maintain isotonicity with the M199) and immersed in silicone oil (General Electric SF1265) to displace excess extracellular fluid. Following immersion in the oil, nitric acid was injected below the oil phase, displacing it and immersing the coverslips with their adherent cells in the acid. The adherent cells were solubilized by the acid, and the resulting clear solution was diluted and analyzed for Na and K.

RESULTS AND DISCUSSION

Electrophysiology: Electrophysiological properties of the approximately 275 myocytes studied depend upon their morphological state and to a lesser degree upon whether they have a significant population of non-myocytes in culture with them. Cells at all stages are capable of producing action potentials (AP) in response to depolarizing stimulation. In newly isolated and spread cells, but not in round cells, AP are accompanied by a synchronous contraction. The maximum rate of depolarization ($+\dot{V}_{max}$) of AP from cells at all stages increases monotonically with increasingly negative E_m. At E_m of -80 mV the mean values of $+\dot{V}_{max}$ for AP stimulated from newly isolated, round, and spread cells are respectively, 198 ± 7, 212 ± 18, and 64 ± 9 V/s. Spontaneous AP are usual only in spread cells. None of the round cells studied and only 3 percent of newly isolated cells, but 65 percent of spread cells produced spontaneous AP. These AP are accompanied by synchronous contractions.

When the resting potential (RP) of quiescent myocytes or most negative (diastolic) potential of spontaneously contractile myocytes is plotted as a function of time in culture (not shown), the data are scattered but nonetheless show a trend. Resting potential becomes more negative and diastolic potential less negative with increasing time in culture. When the values for RP *and* diastolic potential are considered together (E_m), a clear relationship emerges. The mean E_m of newly isolated, round, and spread cells are, respectively, -46 ± 4, -25 ± 4, and -47 ± 1 mV. In cultures not treated with ARA, myocytes sit amongst non-myocytes and have a mean E_m of -42 ± 2, significantly (P=.04) lower than the value for cells in ARA-treated cultures.

The histogram of Figure One shows the distribution of mean E_m for each cell stage. The solid bars are SEM and the dashed bars indicate the range of values in each sample. Mean E_m decreases as cells round up, reaches a minimum value at the round stage and then, as cells spread, rises to the same value as that in newly isolated cells. Values of mean E_m are lower than *in vivo*, but both the population of newly isolated and of spread cells (29 - 77d) have cells with E_m in the *in vivo* range.

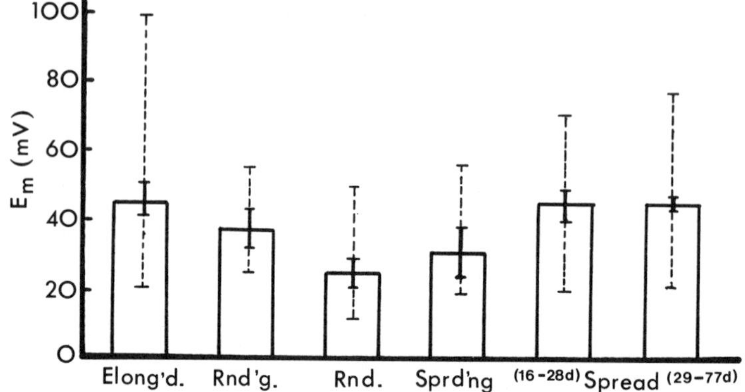

Figure One: Distribution of membrane potential of cells in culture versus morphological stage. This cell sample includes spontaneously active and quiescent myocytes in cultures treated with ARA. Stages from left to right: elongated (newly isolated), rounding, round, spreading and fully spread 16 to 28, and 29 to 77 days in culture. Solid bars are SEM. Dashed bars are range of measured potentials.

Concentration of Na and K: The histogram of Figure Two shows values (±SEM) of $[Na]_i$ and $[K]_i$ determined for groups of cultures whose ages correspond to those at which most cells are elongated (ie., newly isolated), round, spreading, or spread. After about 8 days in culture

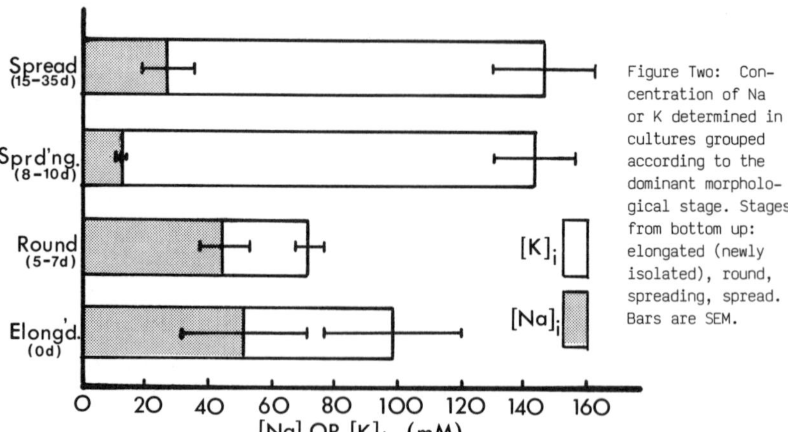

Figure Two: Concentration of Na or K determined in cultures grouped according to the dominant morphological stage. Stages from bottom up: elongated (newly isolated), round, spreading, spread. Bars are SEM.

(ie., for spreading and spread cells), values of $[Na]_i$ and $[K]_i$ in these groups approach those given in the literature for cat papillary muscle [15], (ie., 43 ± 5 and 162 ± 3); left ventricle of the rat [16], (ie., 30 ± 5 and 151 ± 2); and isolated cat ventricle myocytes [17], (ie., 17 ± 1 and 134 ±1). Prior to 8 days in culture, values for $[Na]_i$ are considerably higher, and for $[K]_i$, lower than normal values.

Factors Determining E_m : Values observed for E_m should, to a first approximation, depend on intra- and extracellular concentrations of Na and K, as well as membrane permeability to Na, (P_{Na}) and to K, (P_K). Taken together, the data for E_m , and $[Na]_i$ and $[K]_i$ suggest that, before 8 days in culture, the low *mean* E_m could result from the abnormal distribution of Na and K and/or abnormal membrane permeabilities. After the initial 8-day period, the distribution of Na and K appears to be normalized, and the still present lower than normal mean value of E_m likely arises from a perturbation of values of P_{Na} and/or P_K. The continued increase of mean E_m with time in culture and the eventual appearance of some spread cells with normal RP suggest that values of membrane permeability tend toward normal with increased time in culture but do so at a rate that lags the normalization of values of $[Na]_i$ and $[K]_i$.

ACKNOWLEDGEMENTS

We thank Ms. Irmgard Messmer for technical assistance in preparing and maintaining the cell cultures, and Mr. Cliff Wilson and personnel of the Carleton Science Technology Centre for help with design and fabrication of instrumentation. Some of the data presented here comprise parts of theses submitted by A.E.J. and A.S. to the Carleton University Faculty of Graduate Studies and Research. This work was supported by an operating grant to S.L.J. from the Heart and Stroke Foundation of Ontario.

REFERENCES

1. S.L. Jacobson and H.M. Piper, J. Mol. Cell. Cardiol. 18, 661, 1986.
2. E. Lundgren, L. Terracio, T. Borg and S. Mardh, Exp. Cell. Res. 158, 371, 1985.
3. G. Cooper, IV, W.E. Mercer, J.K. Hoober, P.R. Gordon, R.L. Kent, I.K. Lauva and T.A. Marino, Circ. Res. 58, 692, 1986.
4. H.M. Piper, I. Probst, P. Schwartz, F.J. Hütter and P.G. Spieckermann, J. Mol. Cell. Cardiol. 14, 397, 1982.
5. A.C. Nag, M. Cheng, D.A. Fischman and R. Zak, J. Mol. Cell. Cardiol. 15, 301, 1983.
6. W.C. Claycomb and N. Lanson, Jr., In Vitro 20, 647, 1984.
7. S.L. Jacobson, Cell Structure and Function 2, 1, 1977.
8. J.-X. Guo, S.L. Jacobson and D.L. Brown, Cell Motility and the Cytoskeleton 6, 291, 1986.
9. T.A. Schwarzfeld and S.L. Jacobson, J. Mol. Cell. Cardiol. 13, 563, 1981.
10. R.L. Moses and W.C. Claycomb, J. Ultrastruct. Res. 81, 358, 1982.
11. R.L. Moses and W.C. Claycomb, Am. J. Anat. 171, 191, 1984.
12. C.F. Meier, Jr., G.M. Briggs and W.C. Claycomb, Am. J. Physiol. 250, H731, 1986.
13. S.L. Jacobson, C.B. Kennedy and G.A.R. Mealing, Can. J. Physiol. and Pharmacol. 61, 1312, 1983.
14. S.L. Jacobson, M. Banfalvi and T.A. Schwarzfeld, Basic Res. Cardiol. 80,[Suppl 1], 79, 1985.
15. E. Page, J. Gen. Physiol. 46, 201, 1962.
16. E. Page and E. Gross-Page, Circ. Res. 22, 435, 1968.
17. L.H. Silver and S.R. Houser, Am. J. Physiol. 248, H614, 1985.

HIGH SPEED DIGITAL IMAGING OF RAT CARDIAC MYOCYTE CONTRACTILE DYNAMICS

KENNETH P. ROOS* AND STUART R. TAYLOR**
*American Heart Association, Greater Los Angeles Affiliate, Cardiovascular Research Laboratory, UCLA School of Medicine, 10833 Le Conte Avenue, Los Angeles, CA. 90024-1760; and
**Department of Pharmacology, Mayo Foundation, Rochester MN. 55905.

INTRODUCTION

To understand contractile events at the sarcomere level, it is important to accurately resolve distances among clearly defined striations not blurred by rapid motion, to measure them objectively, and to thereby obtain information that can be directly related to contractile dynamics at the molecular level. When such data are digitized at high speed, it becomes possible to extract the maximum information in space, time and frequency domains through subsequent computer processing. The analysis, quantitation, and interpretation of cardiac muscle contractile dynamics at the cellular and sub-cellular level is usually limited by deficiencies in the available technology. Twitches and spontaneous contractions have already been recorded from myocytes by visible light microscopy and light diffractometry using cine film [1-2], TV [1-6], and single line CCD or photodiode detection systems [1-2, 8-11]. All of these systems have limitations acquiring and processing rapidly changing sub-cellular events: cine films cannot easily be measured accurately, precisely and objectively; standard TV systems have slow, fixed acquisition rates; and single-line solid state systems can only measure a narrow strip from a possibly non-uniform 2-D image. Here, we describe a new approach, that can be integrated with other data collected simultaneously, to rapidly acquire, store, process and quantitatively analyze a series of 2-D images from a complete contraction/relaxation cycle.

METHODS

Ca^{2+}-tolerant myocytes were isolated using standard Langendorff retrograde coronary perfusion of adult (250 gm) rat hearts; they were treated with 1% collagenase for 25-35 minutes at 37°C [10-11]. Isolated cells were maintained at room temperature (23°C) in oxygenated Tyrode's solution containing 0.25 mM calcium at pH 7.2. The Ca^{2+} was raised to 2.0 mM before an experiment. Single myocytes were selected under the microscope from an aliquot of cells using rigorous criteria [10,11]. The selected myocytes were electrically stimulated with single pulses (0.4 ms) after periods of rest or paced at 1 to 2 Hz. Stimuli were applied via a cathode inside a micropipette placed under the microscope objective.

Myocytes were imaged through a 40X (Numerical Aperture, N.A. = 0.75) or a 63X (N.A. = 1.20) water immersion objective coupled to an ordinary visible light microscope (Carl Zeiss, Thornwood, NY). Brightfield images were projected without another image forming lens directly onto a 128 X 128 array of silicon photodiodes (EG&G Reticon #MC9128, Sunnyvale, CA.). Data were acquired, stored and subsequently processed by a digital imaging system (Figure 1), configured by Microtex Inc. (Cambridge, MA.). Sequences of 40 to 46 full frames were acquired at 50 to 175 Hz; longer sequences of partial frames could be obtained at rates up to 500 Hz [12]. The start of each sequence of images was synchronized with the delayed output of a stimulator to capture a complete myocyte contraction/relaxation cycle. The array was positioned for its field of view to cover from 20 X 20 μm to 50 X 50 μm of each cell. This magnification provided a sufficient number of pixels per striation covering the full width and 20%-50% of the length (10 to 25 sarco-

Biology of Isolated Adult Cardiac Myocytes
William A. Clark, Robert S. Decker, and Thomas K. Borg, Editors

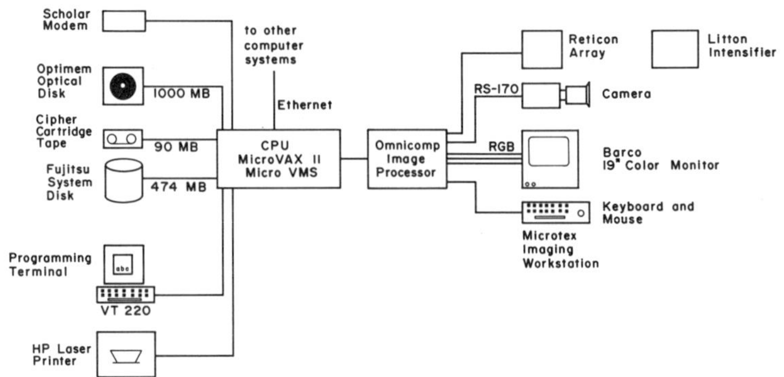

Fig. 1. CAMERA CENTER: An integrated high speed digital imaging system.

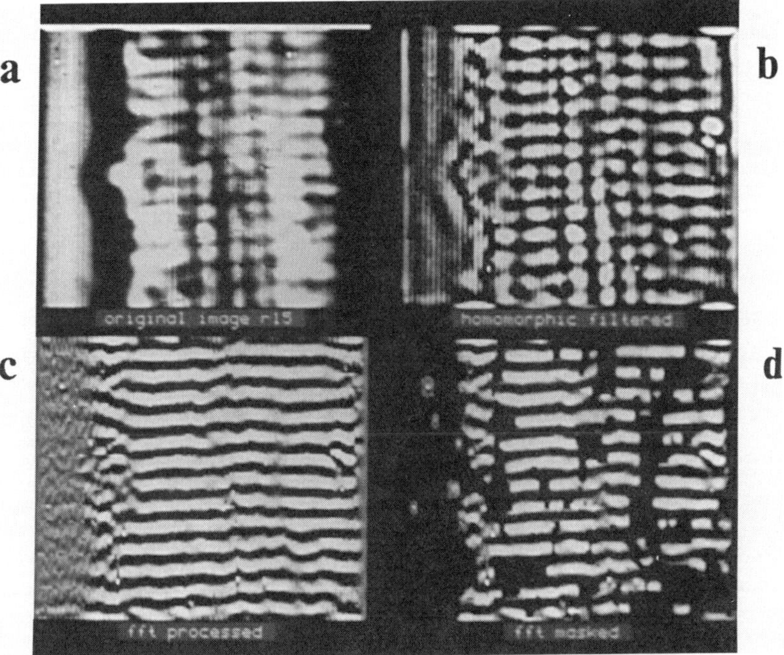

Fig. 2. Digital Processing of a Myocyte Image: The upper-left panel (a) is the original brightfield image of resting myocyte #870323R15. The upper-right panel (b) is the background subtracted and homomorphic filtered image. The lower-left panel (c) is the FFT processed image which is masked for regions of highest contrast in (d) the lower-right panel.

meres) of most myocytes. In addition, the ability to use the full N.A. of each objective and digitally remove the scattered light, produced a very thin (<0.5 μm) optical section through each cell.

Images were first stored on magnetic disk and then on tape for later analysis. Each frame of data was processed in several ways to first enhance striations, then to trace sharp edges around areas of comparable intensity. This made it possible to define uniform regions and accurately measure the striation spacing in given locations as they moved about during contraction. These procedures were performed interactively via the Microtex workstation, and custom designed image processing software. Images were enhanced for display and analysis by digital background subtraction, homomorphic filtering, fast Fourier transform (FFT) processing, gray scale manipulation (thresholding and clipping), convolutions, histogram normalization and false color rendering. Figure 2 illustrates the enhancement obtained with these approaches applied to the original brightfield image of a myocyte (Fig. 2a). Figure 2b is the background subtracted and homomorphic filtered image; low and high frequency noise are reduced substantially. Figure 2c is the FFT processed image; additional low frequency noise and the longitudinal stripes are eliminated. Figure 2d masks the FFT processed image leaving only the highest contrast portions of the striation pattern for unbiased quantitative analysis. Striation periodicity was measured to determine uniform regions and select longitudinal sections along the length of the cell to be re-displayed, using analytical tools similar to those previously detailed [9-11]. The inclusion of artifacts owing to aliasing and non-striated material invisible in the unprocessed images was minimized during analysis by side-by-side display of an original and same image after processing. The data shown here do not contain such artifacts.

RESULTS AND DISCUSSION

Sixty-four image sequences obtained from 29 myocytes provided the results on which this report is based. Figure 3 shows the relationship between average striation periodicity versus time in a regions a few sarcomeres long when this myocyte was stimulated at 1 Hz for an extended period. This myocyte contracted 22% from 1.89 μm to 1.55 μm. The maximum rates of shortening and relaxation were similar. But relaxation was slightly faster than shortening in this example: shortening = 3.17 l/s; and relaxation = 3.42 l/s. Cells rested for 2 minutes or more before stimulation shortened further (up to 28% L_o) than paced cells. These myocytes demonstrated the characteristic negative staircase relationship. After an initial fast relaxation, there was an extended period of much slower relaxation in all cells. Relaxation of entire cardiac myocytes is similar to relaxation of single skeletal muscle cells [1]. However, sarcomere shortening and lengthening can occur simultaneously during the rapid exponential phase of relaxation in skeletal muscle, which makes the physical basis of relaxation difficult to assess. We did not see such heterogeneity in a small group of relaxing sarcomeres in myocytes (Fig. 3). Hence, relaxation measured by our present method can be evaluated with confidence on the assumption that the rates reflect contractile dynamics in a uniform sub-cellular region.

These findings are qualitatively similar to those previously reported by several investigators using alternative approaches [1,3-4,7-8,11]. But the present results are based on the analysis of data collected at high speed, enhanced to a greater degree and with greater objectivity, and analyzed with more reproducible measurement tools. These results include quantitative information on selected regions from the same 2-D area and provide information on the dynamics of shortening and relaxing myocytes not previously available. VHS video recordings of processed contractions are available for viewing from either author's laboratory.

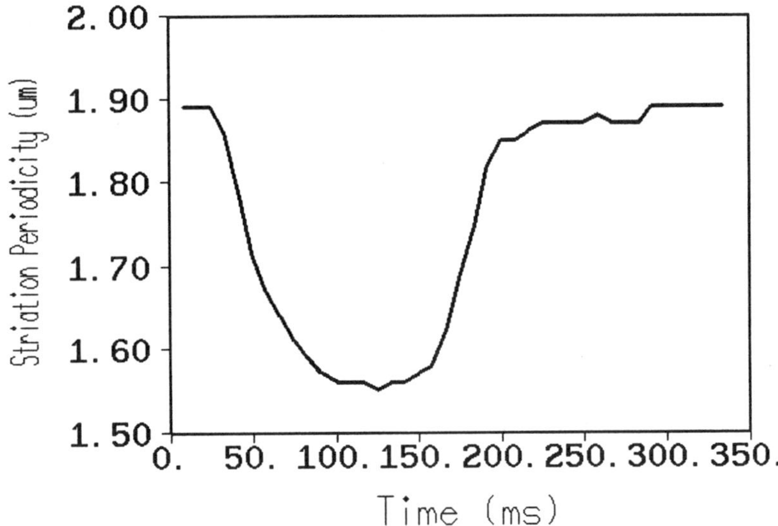

Fig. 3. Contractile Dynamics: The change in average striation spacing (in µm) is plotted over the time course (in ms) of a twitch contraction from an 11 striation long longitudinal segment of cell #870323R16 paced at 1 Hz.

ACKNOWLEDGEMENTS

We thank Chris Bliton, Bradford Lubell, Mark Patton, and Laurel Wanek for their analytical, programming, and technical assistance with this project. These studies were funded by USPHS NHLBI HL-29671 to KPR; USPHS NS/AM-22369, CA 42286, and NSF DMB-8503964 to SRT.

REFERENCES

1. J.W. Krueger, D. Forletti, and B.A. Wittenberg, J. Gen. Physiol. 76:587-607 (1980).
2. J.W. Krueger, and B. London, in: Contractile Mechanisms in Muscle, G.H. Pollack and H. Sugi, eds., (Plenum Press, New York, 1984) pp. 119-134.
3. M.C. Capogrossi, A.A. Kort, H.A. Spurgeon, and E.G. Lakatta, J. Gen. Physiol. 88:589-613 (1986).
4. N.M. DeClerck, V.A. Claes, and D.L. Brutsaert, J. Mol. Cell. Cardiol. 16: 735-745 (1984).
5. G. Rieser, R. Sabbadini, P. Paolini, M. Fry, and G. Inesi, Am. J. Physiol. 236:C70-C77 (1979).
6. M. Tarr, J.W. Trank, and P. Leiffer, Circ. Res. 48:189-200 (1981).
7. A.F. Leung, J. Muscle Res. Cell Motil. 4:485-502 (1983).
8. C.M. Philips, V. Duthinh, and S.R. Houser, IEEE Trans. Biomed. Eng. BME-33:929-934 (1986).
9. K.P. Roos, Biophys. J. 49:44-46 (1986).
10. K.P. Roos, Biophys. J. 52:317-327 (1987).
11. K.P. Roos, and A.J. Brady, Biophys. J. 40:233-244 (1982).
12. L.A. Helland, J.R. Lopez, S.R. Taylor, G. Trube, and L.A. Wanek, Proc. N.Y. Acad. Sci., in press (1987).

PHYSIOLOGY AND ULTRASTRUCTURE OF THE INTACT ISOLATED VENTRICULAR MYOCYTE

RASHID NASSAR*, MARY C. REEDY+, and PAGE A.W. ANDERSON*≠.
Departments of Physiology*, Anatomy+ and Pediatrics≠; Duke University.

INTRODUCTION

Large variations in cell size, rest sarcomere length, amount and velocity of sarcomere shortening, and action potential configuration have been observed in isolated adult ventricular myocytes [1-3]. Understanding the sources of this variability is important in evaluating experimental results from these preparations. The large differences in the physiological properties among cells from the same heart may result from intrinsic, in-situ differences, or from cell damage. Intrinsic differences have important implications for the organization and function of the intact tissue. Further, if intrinsic differences reflect structural and molecular variation, the single cell should be especially useful in studying how these variations affect cell characteristics. In contrast, variability that is a result of damage would render experimental results from single cell studies suspect. In this paper, we examine both the sarcomere dynamics and the ultrastructure of isolated myocytes.

METHODS

We isolated ventricular myocytes (n=72) from 3-4 month-old rabbits. Criteria for studying a cell were: 1) quiescence in physiological $[Ca]_o$, 2) electrically excitable, 3) all-or-none response with uniform sarcomere shortening. The methods are described in detail elsewhere [4].

RESULTS AND DISCUSSION

Cell dimensions varied over a large range (Fig. 1): length 147 ± 27 µm (mean ± s.d.), cross-sections 23 ± 9 µm by 17 ± 6 µm. LV and RV cells did not differ significantly. Serial sections of 27 cells showed all preparations, including those > 200 µm in length, to be single cells.

Cell structure. Few cells had a simple shape. Electron microscopy showed pod-like protrusions and prominent indentations and grooves, particularly in larger cells. Some cells had longitudinal clefts, several micrometers deep, which, in a given section, caused the cell to appear branched or as two cells before narrowing so that the sarcolemmal layers were in close apposition over a relatively long distance. Among cells from the same heart, the larger and more complex cells had longer contraction durations (Fig. 1), but when all cells were included, no such correlation was found. Smaller cells had the simplest shape, and are, therefore, generally the best for electrophysiological and mechanical studies.

The ultrastructure of cells in intact myocardium was well preserved in the isolated cells. An exception was a group of cells in which peak sarcomere shortening velocity ($\dot{s}$) was < 0.5 µm/s and amount of shortening (Δs) was < 0.15 µm. In those cells, although the Z-lines appeared irregular and "moth-eaten," the cell coat, including the glycocalyx, was intact and the intercalated discs retained their specialized characteristics. Moreover, the Ca-controlling systems were intact: the responses to perturbations in $[Ca]_i$ were normal (see below). Isolated cells with normal resting and action potentials have been shown to incorporate during disaggregation extracellular markers that can pass through the nexus

Biology of Isolated Adult Cardiac Myocytes
William A. Clark, Robert S. Decker, and Thomas K. Borg, Editors

(personal communication, RL White). One could speculate that transient openings to extracellular space at the time of cell separation allow $[Ca]_i$ to rise to a level that activates specific Ca-dependent cell proteases which would disrupt the myofilaments. These cells provide new criteria for cell damage.

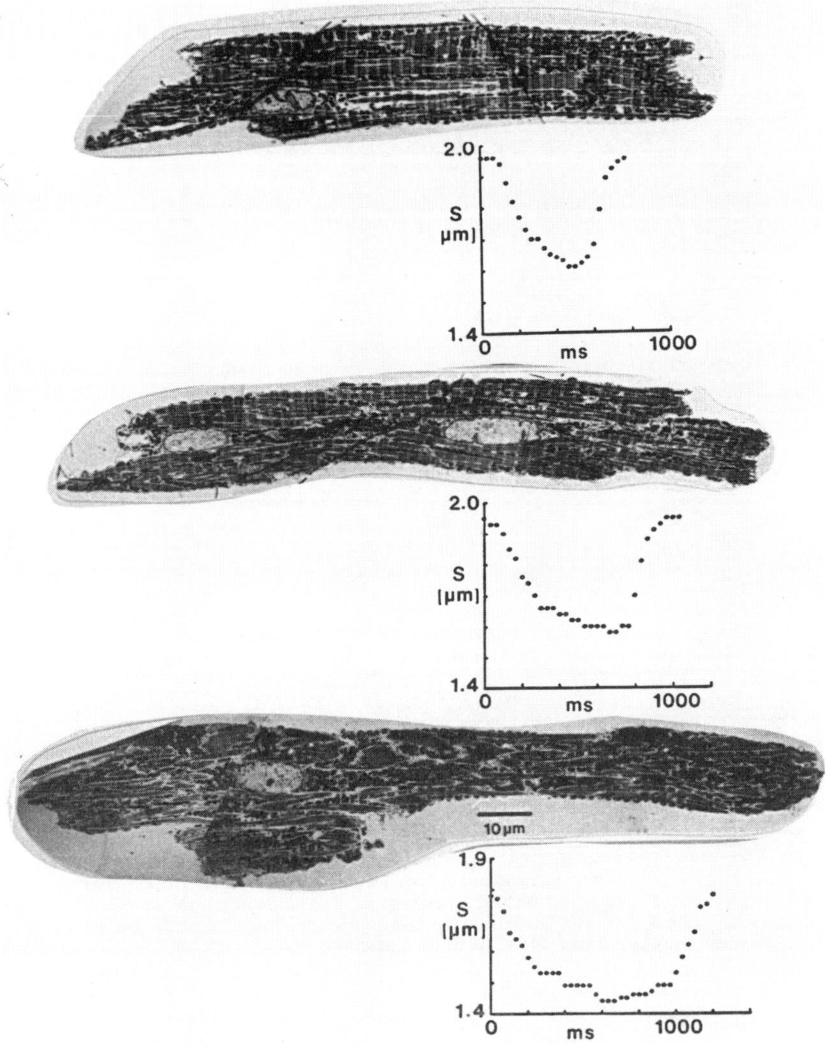

FIG. 1. Central sections and sarcomere shortening waveforms from three cells obtained from the same heart. (10-µm bar indicates scale).

In cells that had been paced for over 30 min, the mitochondrial matrix density and the number and size of the lipid droplets appeared to decrease. Transverse tubules and junctional sarcoplasmic reticulum (JSR) profiles were well preserved. The abundant corbular SR profiles had foot processes similar in appearance to those of JSR, suggesting that the Ca-release channel found in JSR [5] is present in corbular SR.

Rest Sarcomere Length (s_o) ranged from 1.75 to 2.09 μm (mean 1.87 $\pm$ 0.06 μm). s_o was uniform throughout the cell, except in damaged cells and in some larger cells where small regional differences were found (e.g., 1.84 to 1.92 μm). RV and LV cells did not have significantly different s_o. $[Ca]_o$, over the range studied, did not affect s_o. Cells having s_o < 1.75 μm, which included some cells with abnormal Z-lines, were considered damaged even when they passed our physiological criteria.

Sarcomere Shortening under Steady-State Conditions. The sarcomere contraction waveform elicited by a constant stimulus interval (4 s) consisted of a delay (81 $\pm$ 29 ms) followed by a phase of shortening (Δs, 0.3 $\pm$ 0.05 μm, 2 mM $[Ca]_o$, at room temperature) to a sustained peak which varied in height and duration among cells (Fig. 1), and in the same cell when the pattern of stimulation was altered (see below). Sarcomere re-extension usually had a fast onset, and was synchronous throughout the cell. Some cells exhibited the two marked phases of re-extension described by Krueger et al. [6]. Cell shortening was proportional to sarcomere shortening.

Over a large portion of cell shortening, $\dot{s}$ was approximately constant even in the double overlap region (Fig. 1) [6]. At 2 mM [Ca], $\dot{s}$ ranged from 0.53 to 3.1 μm/s (1.5 $\pm$ 0.6 μm/s) and did not differ between RV and LV cells. In large complex cells, where s_o varied slightly from region to region, sarcomere shortening was uniform throughout the cell. The velocity of sarcomere re-extension ($\dot{r}$) was usually greater than $\dot{s}$ and varied from 0.5 to 3.8 μm/s (1.8 $\pm$ 0.7 μm/s).

Changing $[Ca]_o$ from 0.5 to 3.0 mM increased Δs and $\dot{s}$. Further increase in $[Ca]_o$ did not significantly change shortening. Raising $[Ca]_o$ between two beats usually enhanced Δs and $\dot{s}$ in the next beat, but in some cells this increase was gradual. Changing $[Ca]_o$ did not significantly affect s_o, the delay, nor the contraction duration.

Isoproterenol (0.15 μM) increased Δs, $\dot{s}$, and $\dot{r}$ while the delay and the duration decreased significantly. Raising the temperature from 23°C to 37°C decreased Δs and the contraction duration while $\dot{r}$ and $\dot{s}$ were unaffected.

Effect of Changing the Pattern of Stimulation. Introducing an extrasystole during pacing at a constant rate was a stringent test for revealing damage to the membrane systems that control $[Ca]_i$. In some Ca-tolerant cells with normal s_o, $\dot{s}$, Δs, and $\dot{r}$, an extrasystole was followed by spontaneous, nonsynchronous, chaotic sarcomere shortening (Fig. 2). Upon returning to the constant pacing rate, the cell again responded normally. Repeating the pacing pattern often resulted in irreversible shortening.

This abnormal response in otherwise normal cells demonstrates an inability to control perturbations in $[Ca]_i$. The chaotic sarcomere shortening is consistent with gradients in $[Ca]_i$ described in spontaneous myocytes [7] and in Ca-overloaded tissue [8]. It suggests the SR is unable to contain further Ca due to SR damage or Ca overload from sarcolemmal damage.

Most cells did not exhibit this abnormal behavior. They retained the in-situ properties of post-extrasystolic potentiation and restitution of contractility: 1) Δs and $\dot{s}$ were smallest in the extrasystole elicited at the shortest interval following the previous contraction (t_1); 2) in the post-extrasystole $\dot{s}$, $\dot{r}$, and Δs were potentiated; 3) potentiation was a function of t_1: the shorter t_1, the greater the potentiation.

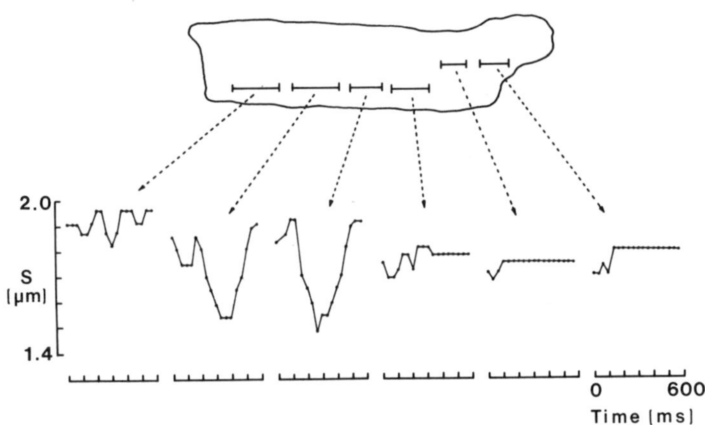

FIG. 2. Sarcomere shortening in different regions of a "defective" cell from the same contraction following an extrasystole. The cell responded normally at a constant pacing rate in 2 and 3 mM $[Ca]_o$.

The combined physiological and ultrastructural approaches revealed subtle damage to the contractile apparatus and Ca-control systems of some cells. Cells that manifested one form of damage did not necessarily show evidence of the other.

The many cells which passed all our criteria for intactness had a wide range of characteristics. This indicates that cell heterogeneity is a basic myocardial property and reflects in-situ properties. The heterogeneity in size, physiological response, and the ability of these cells to modulate their function result in distributed differences in cell properties. Such heterogeneity should give the myocardium great malleability in responding to loading, disease, and aging.

ACKNOWLEDGEMENTS

This work was supported in part by NIH grants: HL 33680, HL 20749, and HL 12486.

REFERENCES

1. SP Bishop and JL Drummond, J Mol Cell Cardiol. 11, 423-433 (1979)
2. T Watanabe, LM Delbridge, JO Bustamante, and TF McDonald, Circ Res. 52, 280-290 (1983)
3. JW Dow, NGL Harding, and T Powell, Cardiovasc Res. 15, 549-579 (1981)
4. R Nassar, MC Reedy, and PAW Anderson, Circ Res. 61, 465-483 (1987)
5. M Inui, A Saito, and S Fleischer, Biophys J. 51, 369 (1987)
6. JW Krueger, D Forletti, and BA Wittenberg, J Gen Physiol. 76, 587-607 (1980)
7. WG Weir, MB Cannell, JR Berlin, E Marban, and WJ Lederer, Science 235, 325-328 (1987)
8. CH Orchard, DA Eisner, and DG Allen, Nature 304, 735-738 (1983)

SEPARABILITY OF RELAXATION INDICES IN ISOLATED VENTRICULOCYTES

JOHN W. KRUEGER, BARRY LONDON, AND GERARD SICILIANO
The Albert Einstein College of Medicine, 1300 Morris Park Ave, Bronx, N.Y. 10461

ABSTRACT

Single unattached cardiac muscle cells shorten the same but relengthen 4-6X faster than intact muscle. This means that relengthening of the cell is the origin of the restoring force in the isolated muscle preparation. Linear relations between the velocity of relengthening and sarcomere length reveal two discrete exponential phases of relaxation which appear to be separable and independent from contractility. Only the latter phase influences diastolic properties, and it appears independent of the normal sequestration of calcium by the sarcoplasmic reticulum.

INTRODUCTION

Relengthening in the unattached heart cell is independent of extracellular elements and minimally influenced by any altered sensitivity to calcium by cross-bridges formation. Thus several features of relengthening in cardiac myocytes provides some ways to examine the mechanisms which controls relaxation and filling of the heart.

METHODS & RESULTS

Single, intact, cardiac cells were isolated enzymatically from the ventricles of Guinea Pigs using techniques described elsewhere [1]. The cells were placed on a small chamber filled with Hepes-buffered physiological solution, and viewed with an inverted microscope at 34 ^{o}C. The cells were electrically stimulated to contract via an extracellular micopipet. Shortening and relengthening was measured 500 to 1000 times per second using a precision edge detector [1]. In practice, the device detects changes in sarcomere length to less than 0.01 um/sarcomere, or 0.5%.

Origin of Restoring Forces in Cardiac Muscle: Unattached cells shorten and relengthen independently of the uncertain influence of surrounding tissue *in situ*. The extent and time course of shortening resembles that seen in intact muscles. Since the striations buckle in the passively shortened heart cell, the force which relengthens the muscle could originate within the cell [2]. But is the cell the sole origin of the restoring force in cardiac tissue? For example, a persistent yet untested assumption is that shortening distorts extracellular elements *elastically* in muscle. This would give rise to forces which should i) increase the speed of muscle relengthening, ii) slow shortening, and iii) increase the ratio of lengthening to shortening velocities when the dynamics of the sarcomere in intact heart muscles are compared to that

Biology of Isolated Adult Cardiac Myocytes
William A. Clark, Robert S. Decker, and Thomas K. Borg, Editors

in the unattached single cell.

Enzymatically isolated cells were bathed in 1.0< [$CaCl_2$] <3.0 mM to bracket the uncertain [Ca^{2+}] at the cell surface within muscle. Shortening speed was varied by altering stimulus rate (0.1 to 3hz). The maximum velocity of relengthening and shortening were always about equal, as is seen in Figure 1.

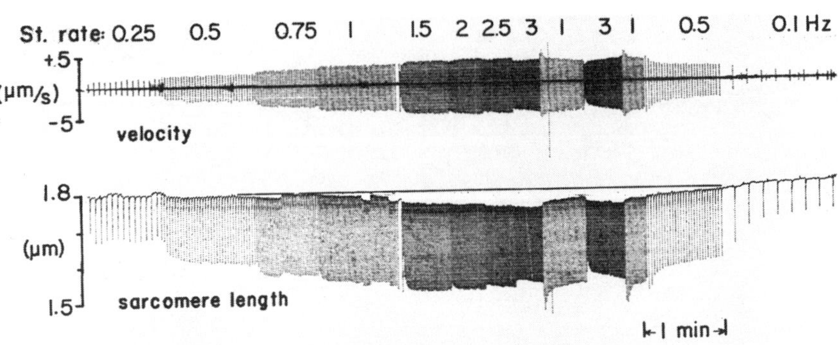

FIG 1. The influence of stimulus rate on the velocity of sarcomere motion in an isolated cardiac cell ([$CaCl_2$] = 2mM). The ratio of the respective speeds of relengthening and shortening in all cells ranged between 1.04 ± 0.24 in 1 mM $CaCl_2$ (59 cases) and 0.74 ± 0.28 in 2 ≤ [$CaCl_2$]< 3mM (30 cases). (The abrupt shifts represent a recording artifact.)

It is well known that the speed of muscle relengthening slows at the very low loads [3] at which unattached cells function. In Guinea Pig right ventricular trabeculae, the velocity of shortening and relengthening of the sarcomere approaches 2.4 and 0.4 L/s, respectively, while their ratio is 1/6 at zero load. (The [$CaCl_2$] was 2.0 mM.) With comparable stimulus rates, shortening speed in the isolated cell was comparable (2.25 L/s ± 1.08 SD) yet the relengthening ratio was not (0.93 ± 0.20, N = 16). Since unattached cardiac muscle cell relengthens fully 4 to 6 times <u>more rapidly</u> than intact muscle, the restoring force in muscle must reflect the determinants of relengthening of the isolated cell.

<u>Two Exponential Phases of Cellular Relaxation</u>: Initial length shortened when single cells were stimulated at physiologic rates [4]. This 'preshortening' was stable and reversible when stimulation was slowed or stopped (Figure 1), and so slowed or delayed relengthening would affect the diastolic properties of cardiac muscle. However, the relation between relaxation and diastole isn't clear. In unattached cells, the changes in the maximum speed of relengthening parallel both the maximum speed and extent of shortening (Figure 1). Consequently, relaxation dynamics are not easily separated from changes in internal load and intracellular calcium release. However, whenever velocity is linearly related to length, relengthening can be characterised by a constant equal to the slope, m, of the velocity-length relation

as shown in Figure 2. The slope of the linear phase of the relengthening trajectory can be related to a rate constant, since the general solution to the equation $d(SL)/dt = m(SL)+b$ results in an exponential, $SL(t) = e^{(mt+b)}$. Sarcomere relengthening can be approximated by two such phases.

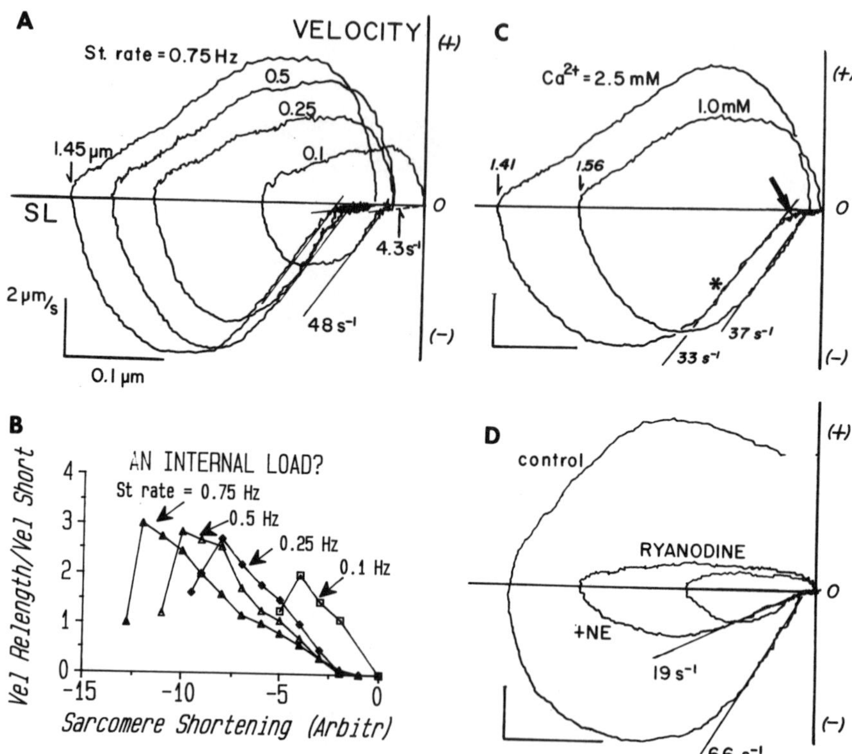

FIG. 2. Computer displays of the velocity-length trajectories in isolated cardiac cells. Initial sarcomere length occurs at right in all panels, and velocity of shortening is denoted as (+).

The peak velocity of relengthening depends upon sarcomere length as well as upon contractility. In contrast, the slope of the velocity-length trajectory appears largely independent of internal shortening, sarcomere dynamics, and calcium release (Figure 2A & C). Addition of 2-5 uM Ryanodine revealed that the first phase is limited by the intracellular reuptake of calcium (Figure 2D), an effect which is not restored by addition of norepinephrine. Under these conditions, stimulus rate still reversibly decreases initial sarcomere length. The length-dependence of the ratio of the velocity of relengthening to shortening for the cell in Figure 2A is also shown in Figure 2B. Its slope appears to be fairly linear, as expected for the influence of a length-dependent internal load which resists shortening of the sarcomere in the isolated cell.

Relengthening was also re-examined in voltage-clamped cells which are internally dialyzed as studied previously [1]. Both i) the rate constant of early relaxation and ii) the onset of late relaxation are independent of repolarization and the degree of prior shortening. This further localizes the first phase of cell relengthening to intracellular components, and it shows that the transition between each phase of relaxation is independent of the variable time course of membrane repolarization [5].

DISCUSSION

Relengthening in the isolated muscle preparation could be altered by interstitial ion accumulation, viscosity, or extracellular elements, but we show that these factors can only serve to slow the reextension which originates in the cell. A comparable inflection in the velocity-length trajectories also occurs in isotonically relengthened muscle (Refer to Figure 3, reference [6]). Like the unattached cell, the peak velocity of isotonic relengthening in cardiac muscle [6] is increased by calcium, but in the cell the slope of the velocity-length trajectory is unchanged. One possibility is that shortening and calcium have little direct influence on the rate of calcium reuptake under conditions where the complicating effect of cross-bridge formation is minimized. Our results provide direct evidence for the functional role of at least two separate phases of relaxation, but only the latter appears to be physiologically relevant to diastole. Specifically, the basis of the late phase of relengthening and, consequently, diastolic tension, reflects the cellular readjustment to the Ca^{2+} accumulated during the heart beat rather than the incomplete sequestering of Ca^{2+} by a ryanodine sensitive intracellular pool. The important feature of the velocity trajectories in the isolated cell is that the relaxation mechanism can be examined under conditions where it may be separated from changes due to calcium release.

Acknowledgements: Supported, In part, by HL21325 (NIH), T32 GM 7288 (NIGMS), and the Martin Fund. We thank Robert Smith, Nadine Stram, and Hong Zhao for assistance.

REFERENCES

1. B. London and J. Krueger, J. Gen. Physiol. 88, 475-505 (1986).
2. J.W. Krueger, D. Forletti, and B. Wittenberg, J. Gen. Physiol. 76, 587-607 (1980).
3. B.E. Strauer, Am. J. Physiol. 224, 431-434 (1973).
4. G. Isenberg, Z. Naturforsch. 37c, 502-512 (1982).
5. W.T. Clusin, J. Physiol. 320, 149-174 (1981).
6. J.E. Strobeck, A.S. Bahler, and E.H. Sonnenblick, Am. J. Physiol. 229, 646-651 (1975).

THE INFLUENCE OF REST PERIODS ON CALCIUM CURRENTS AND CONTRACTIONS IN ISOLATED VENTRICULAR MYOCYTES FROM GUINEA-PIG AND RABBIT HEARTS

DONALD M. BERS* AND PETER HESS**
*Division of Biomedical Sciences, University of California, Riverside, CA 92521;
** Department of Physiology, Harvard Medical School, Boston, MA 02115

INTRODUCTION

In rabbit and guinea-pig ventricular muscle the insertion of a period of rest leads to a reduction of the first post-rest contraction [1,2]. The decline of developed force as a function of rest duration is often referred to as "rest decay". The first post-rest contraction (B1) appears to depend importantly on SR Ca release and rest decay may reflect in part the loss of SR Ca during quiescence. Post-rest contractions in rabbit and guinea-pig ventricle are depressed by caffeine and ryanodine, which would be expected to strongly inhibit SR Ca uptake and/or release [2,3]. However, in both rabbit and guinea-pig ventricular muscle twitches during steady state stimulation are only modestly depressed by maximal concentrations of caffeine and ryanodine. These results are in contrast to rat ventricular muscle where caffeine and ryanodine strongly suppress steady state as well as post-rest twitches [2,4]. These results have been interpreted to suggest that contractile force in rabbit and guinea-pig ventricle can be largely supported by Ca influx [2]. In the presence of caffeine or ryanodine, the recovery of twitches back to the steady-state level is monotonically increasing (i.e. like a staircase) and positive force-frequency relationships are observed (even in rat ventricle).

Transient extracellular Ca depletions indicative of Ca influx have been measured with extracellular Ca microelectrodes and these Ca_o depletions also increase monotonically after rest and with increasing frequency in rabbit ventricle [5]. These results suggest that a "staircase" of Ca influx may occur and be responsible for the increase or staircase of tension observed in these tissues (especially when SR function is inhibited).

Voltage-dependent Ca channels are likely to be the major route of Ca entry during the action potential under normal conditions. Most reports of Ca current in multicellular preparations have indicated a decrease of I_{Ca} with stimulation from rest or upon increasing frequency [6-8], although increases have also been reported [9,10]. These studies, however, were mostly done at either relatively positive holding potentials or under conditions where concurrent outward current changes complicate the interpretation of the results.

In the present study of isolated ventricular myocyte, we have examined 1) the post-rest recovery of contractions and 2) changes in Ca current following a rest period.

METHODS

Ventricular myocytes were dissociated from guinea-pig and rabbit hearts using coronary perfusion with collagenase and hyaluronidase, both as described by Lee and Tsien [11] and Langer et al. [12] with similar results. Cell shortening was assessed using a video edge-detection system [13]. In the experiments where cell shortening was measured the extracellular medium contained (in mM) NaCl 140, KCl 6, $CaCl_2$ 2, $MgCl_2$ 1, glucose 10, HEPES 5 at pH 7.4 equilibrated with 100% O_2. Myocytes were stimulated by platinum electrodes on either side of the cell. at 0.5 Hz.

Myocytes were also voltage-clamped using the whole cell variation of the patch-clamp technique. The cells were dialyzed by patch pipets (1-4 MΩ) containing 135 mM CsCl, 5 mM EGTA and 10 mM HEPES, pH 7.5. Sometimes 1 mM $MgCl_2$ and ATP were included in the pipet, but the results were basically unchanged. Calcium currents (I_{Ca}) were recorded with the cells in a medium containing 135 mM tetraethylammonium chloride, 2-5 mM $CaCl_2$ and 10 mM HEPES, pH 7.5. Voltage clamp pulses (200 msec duration, 0.5 Hz) were initiated from various holding potentials (-40 to -80 mV) to various clamp potentials. Clamp pulses to 0 or +10 mV produced the largest inward Ca current transients.

Biology of Isolated Adult Cardiac Myocytes
William A. Clark, Robert S. Decker, and Thomas K. Borg, Editors

RESULTS AND DISCUSSION

After brief rest periods (5-60 sec) in rabbit ventricular myocytes the first contraction (B1) was usually larger than the second post-rest contraction (B2). Subsequent contractions increased progressively and returned to the steady-state level. This is illustrated in the upper panel of Fig. 1. After longer rest intervals of 2-5 min, the first contraction is usually smaller than B2 and the recovery of twitches from rest is usually monotonically increasing. The lower panel in Fig. 1 illustrates this characteristic in the same cell as the upper panel. When SR Ca release was inhibited by caffeine or ryanodine B1 was smaller than B2 and the entire post-rest recovery of contractions increased monotonically back to steady-state. These patterns of shortening observed in the isolated rabbit myocytes were very similar to the patterns of twitch force observed in intact ventricular strips under nearly isometric conditions. Additionally, the post-rest contraction characteristics of guinea-pig and rabbit ventricular myocytes were quite similar. Experiments with extracellular Ca microelectrodes in intact rabbit ventricular strips have also suggested that Ca influx associated with individual contractions increases monotonically after a rest [2].

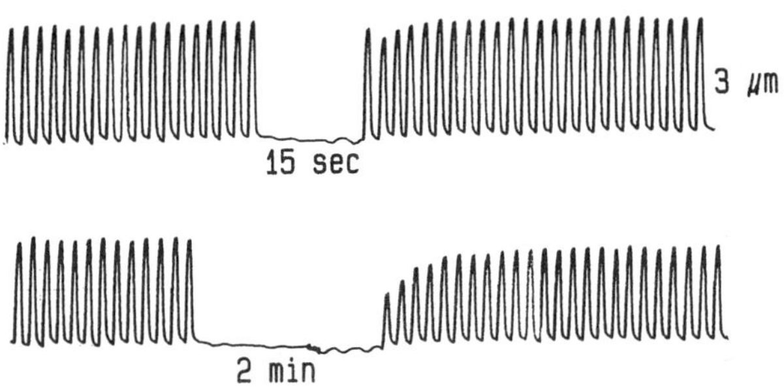

Figure 1. Shortening in an isolated rabbit ventricular myocyte with interposed rest periods of 15 sec (top) and 2 min (bottom) during 0.5 Hz stimulation at 23°C. Recording speed was reduced during part of the 2 min rest.

In order to examine how changes in Ca current may contribute to this post-rest staircase, voltage clamp experiments were performed in isolated myocytes. In order to measure Ca currents with reasonable accuracy, the ionic conditions are drastically altered from the above and this must be considered when comparing these results. At more negative holding potentials (-80 & -70 mV), rest intervals (5-300 sec) resulted in a positive I_{Ca} "staircase". That is, peak I_{Ca} at B1 was less than steady state and increased monotonically back toward steady state. This is illustrated in Fig. 2 where the lower panel shows the current traces for clamp pulses just prior to a 30 sec rest (SS) at the first post-rest clamp pulse (B1) and the second (B2). The upper panel shows peak current values for consecutive clamp pulses surrounding this 30 sec rest. The arrows indicate when small hyperpolarizing pulses were applied (for leak subtraction, not shown) and resulted in an extra two sec between pulses. This brief pause is sufficient to partially induce the I_{Ca} staircase.

At more positive holding potentials (-40 or -50 mV) these rest intervals resulted in a negative I_{Ca} "staircase", where I_{Ca} at B1 is greater than steady state followed by a monotonic decline back to steady state. This is illustrated in Fig. 3. Again, it can be seen that the short pauses for collecting leakage currents for subtraction (at arrows in upper panel) are sufficient to partially induce the negative I_{Ca} staircase. It can also be seen that there is little difference in the negative I_{Ca} staircase when the rest period is increased from 30 sec to 2 min. At intermediate holding potentials (-50 or -60) there is often no effect of such rest periods. The negative I_{Ca} staircase may be attributable to recovery from inactivation during the rest. The positive I_{Ca} staircase is less simply

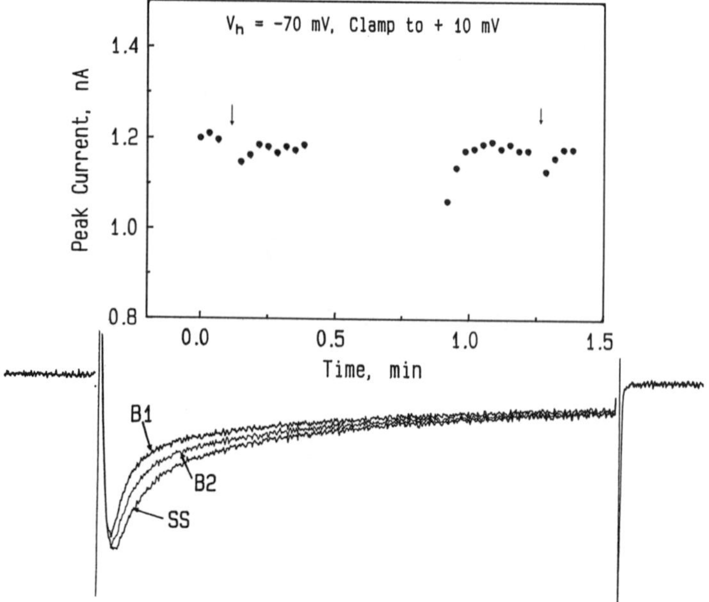

Figure 2. Ca currents recorded from a guinea-pig myocyte during 200 msec clamp pulses from a holding potential (V_h) of -70 mV to +10 mV prior to 30 sec rest (SS) and at the first two post-rest pulses (B1 and B2). These records have been leak subtracted. The graph shows peak I_{Ca} values for the pulses around this rest period (see text).

explained. However, such a positive I_{Ca} staircase at physiological membrane potentials might contribute to the contractile staircase observed when such cells are stimulated after longer rests or in the presence of caffeine or ryanodine. This positive I_{Ca} staircase may also contribute to the apparent staircase in Ca influx seen in the Ca microelectrode experiments cited above [2,5].

Recently Lee [14] has reported a similar staircase of I_{Ca} in guinea-pig ventricular myocytes at higher frequency (~ 2 Hz) and characterized clamp potential dependence of this phenomenon (from a holding potential of -90 mV). Miller and Houser [15] have also recently reported a similar holding potential dependence of post-rest Ca currents induced by depolarizing voltage clamp pulses in cat ventricular myocytes. While Figs. 1 and 2 of the present study show good temporal correlation, it should again be noted that the experimental solutions are not the same and the myocytes in Fig. 2 were not contracting, due to internal dialysis with 10 mM EGTA. The timecourse of the currents in Fig. 3, when scaled, were exactly superimposable. The first post-rest current trace in Fig. 2 exhibited a slightly shorter time to peak than did the currents at B2 or steady-state. This agrees with recent results of Lee [14].

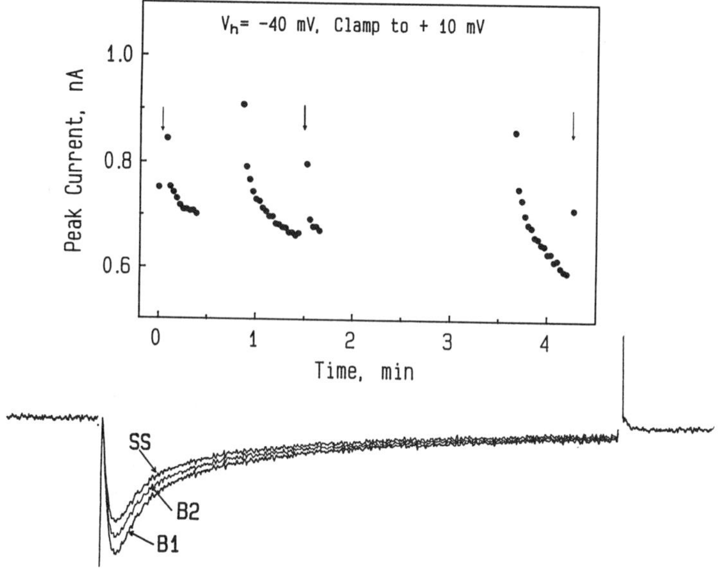

Figure 3. Ca currents recorded from the same guinea-pig myocyte as in Fig. 2 and the results are displayed in a similar manner. The right panel also includes peak I_{Ca} values around 2 min which followed the 30 sec rest from which the current traces are shown at left.

ACKNOWLEDGEMENTS

The technical assistance of Ms. Virginia Stiffel is greatly appreciated. This work was supported by grants from the USPHS (HL-30077 and HL-37124) and the California Affiliate of the American Heart Association (HL-S105). DMB is the recipient of a USPHS Research Career Development Award (HL 01526).

REFERENCES

1. D.G. Allen, B.R. Jewell and E.H. Wood, J. Physiol. Lond. 254, 1-17 (1976).
2. D.M. Bers, Am. J. Physiol 248, H366-H381 (1985).
3. J.L. Sutko and J.L. Kenyon, J. Gen. Physiol. 82, 385-404 (1983).
4. J.L. Sutko and J.T. Willerson, Circ. Res. 46, 333-343 (1980).
5. D.M. Bers, Am. J. Physiol 244, H462-H468 (1983).
6. W.R. Gibbons and H.A. Fozzard, J. Gen. Physiol. 65, 367-384 (1975).
7. J. Simurda, M. Simurdova, P. Braveny and J. Sumbera, Pflug. Arch. 362, 209-218 (1976).
8. H. Reuter, Eur. J. Cardiol. 1, 177-181 (1973).
9. S. Noble and Y. Shimoni, J. Physiol. Lond. 310, 57-75 (1981).
10. M.D. Payet, O.F. Schanne and E. Ruiz-Ceretti, J. Mol. Cell. Cardiol. 13, 207-215 (1981).
11. K.S. Lee and R.W. Tsien, J. Physiol. Lond. 354, 253-272 (1984).
12. G.A. Langer, J.S. Frank, T.L. Rich and F.B. Orner, Am. J. Physiol. 252, H314-H324 (1987).
13. G.A. Langer, Circ. Res. 57, 374-382 (1985).
14. K.S. Lee, Proc. Nat. Acad. Sci. (USA), 84, 3941-3945 (1987).
15. L.S. Miller and S.R. Houser, Biophys. J. 51, 113a.

ELECTROMECHANICAL PROPERTIES OF ISOLATED FELINE MYOCYTES

S. R. HOUSER, A. BAHINSKI, R. B. KLEIMAN, W. H. DUBELL, V. DUTHINH, H. HARTMANN, AND C. PHILIPS

Department of Physiology, Temple University School of Medicine, 3420 N. Broad Street, Philadelphia, PA 19140

INTRODUCTION

Phasic contraction of adult mammalian cardiac muscle is produced when the cytosolic calcium level is transiently elevated. Recent experiments conducted with isolated myocytes (1-3) support the idea that the sarcoplasmic reticulum (SR) is the primary source of calcium for this systolic "calcium transient". The process which produces calcium release from the SR is thought to involve calcium influx through voltage operated calcium channels, and has been termed calcium-induced calcium release (4,5). Recent studies have demonstrated the existence of more than one species of calcium channel in many cell types, including cardiac muscle (6). The T (or tiny conductance) type, activates at membrane potentials more negative than those required to activate the L type channel, which is thought to be responsible for what is usually called the slow inward current (Isi). In addition, T channels are only available for voltage dependent activation at negative (usually greater than -70 mV) resting membrane potentials (or holding potential in voltage clamp experiments) while L type channels remain fully available at membrane potentials as positive as -30 mV. Most previous experiments which have examined the relationships between membrane potential, membrane currents (usually calcium currents), and contraction (2,3) have been conducted using holding potentials near -40 mV in order to inactivate sodium channels. As a result, membrane currents which are only available for voltage dependent activation at more negative membrane potentials, such as calcium current through T type channels, have not been considered in most studies of cardiac excitation-contaction coupling. The objective of the present experiments was to determine the effects of holding potential (Vh) on the relationships between membrane currents (Im), membrane potential (Vm) and contraction in feline ventricular myocytes.

METHODS

Myocytes were isolated from hearts removed from adult cats (2-4 Kg) as described in detail previously (7). Following isolation, myocytes were placed in an experimental chamber mounted on the stage of an inverted microscope. The bathing solution contained the following (in mM); NaCl, (150); KCl, (5.4); $CaCl_2$, (2); $MgCl_2$, (1.2); Dextrose, (10); Pyruvate, (2.5); HEPES, (5); pH 7.4.

Voltage clamp experiments were conducted using low resistance (3-7 MΩ) suction pipettes in the whole cell recording mode (8). The microelectrode filling solution contained the following (in mM): KCl, (140); $MgCl_2$, (10); Na_2ATP, (5); HEPES, (5); pH 7.3. In some experiments CsCl replaced KCl in the filling solution in order to block outward

Biology of Isolated Adult Cardiac Myocytes
William A. Clark, Robert S. Decker, and Thomas K. Borg, Editors

K currents. A single microelectrode switch clamp technique was used to record both Vm and Im. In the experiments to be shown Vm was held at either -40 or -75 mV (unless otherwise stated). Vm was stepped to test potentials between -65 and +30 mV. Step duration was 500 msec. and frequency was 0.5 Hz. Data was recorded when Im (and contraction) had reached a steady state at each test potential. TTX (50 µM) was used in all experiments to block Na channels.

Myocyte shortening was recorded by projecting the cell image onto a self scanning linear photodiode array. This technique allows the position of the cell edges to be monitered every 5 msec. The output from the photodiode was processed by a digital to analog conversion circuit to produce an analog length signal. The details of this technique are described in detail in a recent publication (9).

RESULTS AND DISCUSSION

The voltage dependence of activation of Isi was not significantly different when Vh was -75 or -40 mV (Fig. 1). The threshold for activation was near -25 mV at both holding potentials. However, the magnitude of Isi was consistently smaller when Vh was -75 mV than when it was -40 mV. This probably results from the activation of overlapping transient outward currents which are available only at negative holding potentials (10).

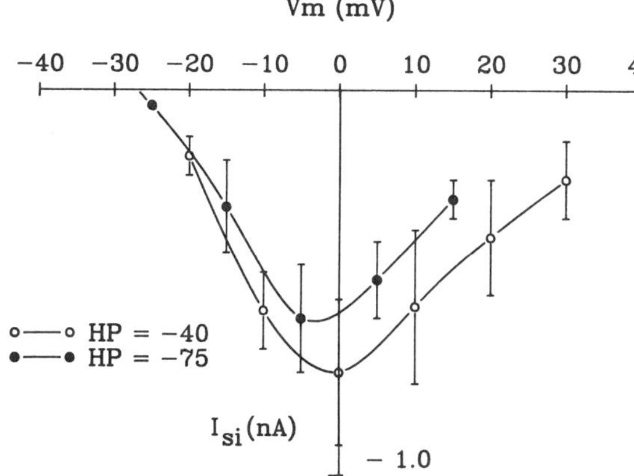

FIGURE 1 Isi is plotted versus the test potential (Vm). Vh was either -40 mV (open symbols) or -75 mV (closed symbols). Values represent the difference between the peak inward current and that at the end of the voltage step (n=4).

The voltage dependence of myocyte contraction was different at holding potentials of -40 and -75 mV. Specifically, contractions which were produced from Vh of -75 mV were consistently larger than those produced by a depolarization from Vh = -40 mV to the same test potential. The contractile threshold was also shifted to more negative levels (Fig. 2). It is important to point out that at negative holding potentials contractions could be induced by depolarizations which were subthreshold for activation of Isi.

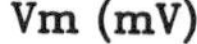

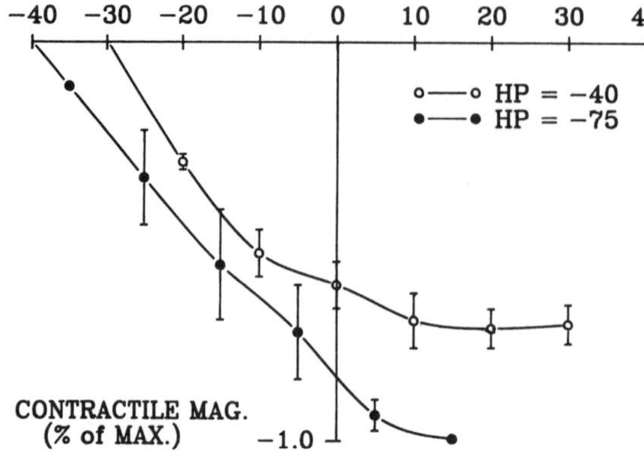

FIGURE 2 Voltage dependence of myocyte contraction. Contractions in each myocyte were normalized to the largest contraction observed in that myocyte. Values represent means +/- SEM of 4 experiments.

Specifically, depolarizations from Vh of -75 mV to Vm between -50 and -30 mV induced an inward current which was distinct from Isi (Fig 3). Contractions which occurred at potentials which were subthreshold for activation of Isi were associated with this current. This low threshold inward current activated and inactivated within 10 msec. and was not blocked by cadmium. When the calcium in the extracellular solution was eliminated, the magnitude of this current was reduced (Fig. 3B). Hyperpolarization of Vh to -100 mV, however, returned it to control levels (Fig. 3C), suggesting that the above mentioned reduction in current was related to

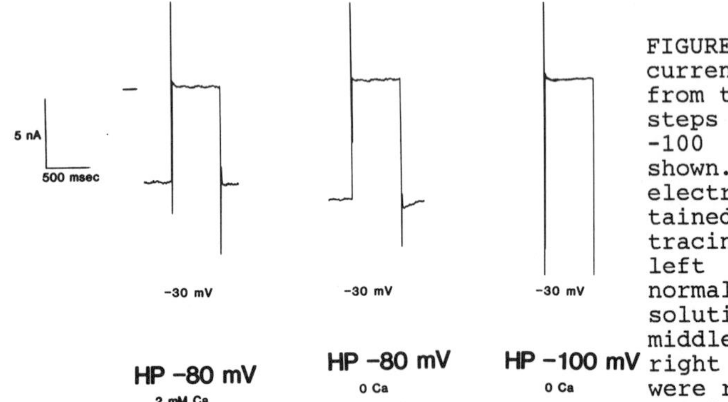

FIGURE 3 Raw current records from three voltage steps from -80 or -100 to 0 mV are shown. The microelectrode contained Cs. The tracing on the left (A) was in normal bathing solution. The middle (B) and right (C) tracings were recorded in a calcium free solution . The line by the control tracing depicts zero current level.

alteration of membrane surface charge. When the sodium in the extracellular solution was replaced with TEA, this low threshold current was eliminated (Fig. 4). Increasing the TTX concentration to 200 μM did not block this current. These results show that that the low threshold current is a TTX insensitive sodium current. The contraction that occurs in association with this current could result from 1) a small calcium influx (that we could not detect) which produces SR calcium release, 2) depolarization-induced calcium release from the SR, 3) calcium influx via Na/Ca exchange which results from subsarcolemmal sodium accumulation. The increased

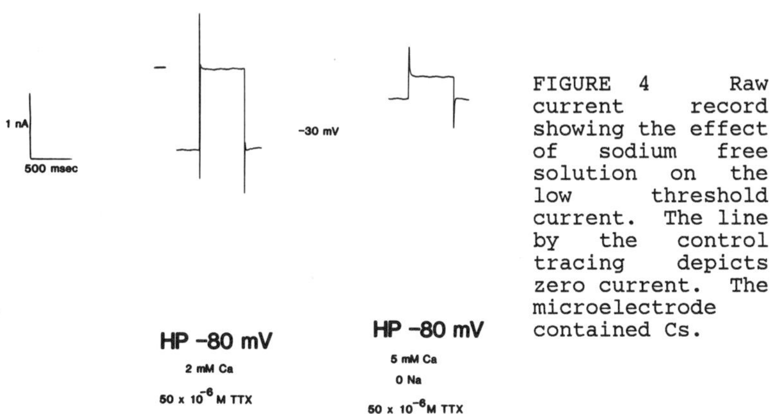

FIGURE 4 Raw current record showing the effect of sodium free solution on the low threshold current. The line by the control tracing depicts zero current. The microelectrode contained Cs.

contractions that occur at Vh of -75 mV probably occur because sodium influx is greater when depolarizing steps are made from this holding potential. This should lead to cellular calcium loading via the Na/Ca exchange mechanism.

Supported in part by NIH grants HL 33921 and HL 33648.

REFERENCES

1. D.B. Bers, Am. J. Physiol. 248, H366-H381 (1985).
2. L. Barcanes-Ruiz and W. G. Weir, Circ. Res. 61, 148-154, (1987).
3. B. London and J. W. Kreuger, J. Gen. Physiol. 88, 475-505, (1986).
4. A. Fabiato, Am J. Physiol. 245, C1-C14, (1983).
5. A. Fabiato, J. Gen. Physiol. 85, 291-320, (1985).
6. B. Nilius, P. Hess, J. B. Lansman and R. W. Tsien, Nature, 1, 443-446, (1985).
7. L. H. Silver, E. L. Hemwall, T. A. Marino, and S. R. Houser, Am. J. Physiol. 245, H891-H896, (1983).
8. O. P. Hamill, A. Marty, E. Neher, B. Sakmann, and F. J. Sigworth, Pfleugers Arch. 391, 85-100, (1981).
9. C. M. Philips, V. Duthinh, and S. R. Houser, IEEE Trans. Biomed. Eng. Vol. BME-33, 929-934, (1986).
10. I. R. Josephson, J. Sanchez-Chapula, and A. M. Brown, Circ. Res. 54, 157-162, (1984).

GLYCOLYSIS AND THE METABOLIC REGULATION OF CARDIAC ATP-SENSITIVE K^+ CHANNELS

JAMES N. WEISS AND SCOTT T. LAMP
Department of Medicine, Division of Cardiology, UCLA School of Medicine, Los Angeles, Ca. 90024-1736

INTRODUCTION

ATP-sensitive K^+ channels are activated when cytosolic ATP concentration falls below a critical level [1-4]. They have been implicated in the marked increase in K^+ efflux that occurs during ischemia, hypoxia and inhibition of glycolytic (anaerobic) or oxidative (aerobic) metabolism in heart [1-3] and in the control of insulin release by pancreatic beta islet cells [4]. In heart glycolysis may be a preferential metabolic pathway for the support of membrane functions, including K^+ balance and maintenance of action potential duration [5,6]. The purpose of the present study was to investigate whether the metabolic source of ATP is important in the regulation of cardiac ATP-sensitive K^+ channels.

METHODS

Single ventricular myocytes were isolated enzymatically from hearts of 300-400 g guinea pigs [7] and studied at room temperature with the gigaseal patch-clamp technique [8], using fire-polished patch electrodes (tip diameter 1-4 m) and a List EPC-7 patch clamp amplifier. The experimental chamber (0.5 ml) was continuously perfused throughout the experiment. The standard filling solution of the patch electrode contained (in mM): 150 KCl, 5 HEPES, pH 7.3 with KOH. The standard bath solution contained: 138-147 KCl (150 total K^+), 5 HEPES, 2 EGTA, 0.5 $CaCl_2$, 2 $MgCl_2$, pH 7.1 with KOH. Single channel recordings were made from cell-attached patches on cells permeabilized by brief exposure at one end to saponin [3] or excised (cell-free) inside-out patches [8].

Arterially perfused interventricular septa were isolated from the hearts of 2-3 kg New Zealand white rabbits [6] and perfused at 37°C through the septal branch of the left coronary artery by a peristaltic pump (flow rate of 1.75 ml/min). Standard perfusate contained (in mM): 120 NaCl, 4 KCl, 1.5 $CaCl_2$, 25 $NaHCO_3$, 0.44 Na_2HPO_4, 1 $MgCl_2$, 5.6 D-glucose, and 10 IU/l insulin, gassed with a 5% CO_2 and 95% O_2 gas mixture (pH 7.3-7.4). Tension was monitored with a tension transducer sutured to one corner of the preparation. For measurement of K^+ efflux, preparations were exposed to standard perfusate containing $^{42}K^+$ (1.75 µCuries/ml) for a loading period of >45 minutes and then washed out for at least 20 minutes before any experimental intervention. During washout venous effluent was collected for 15 seconds of each 30 second interval and analyzed for radioactivity with a gamma counter. Cpm were corrected for background and decay.

RESULTS

In cell-attached patches on cells permeabilized at one end by saponin, openings of inward rectifying K^+ channels, I_{K1}, were commonly observed as long as 2 mM ATP was present in the bath solution. The single channel conductance of I_{K1} was 39 ± 4 pS. Removal of ATP from the bath solution perfusing the cell reversibly activated ATP-sensitive K^+ channels in the membrane patch distinguishable from I_{K1} channels by their larger single channel conductance (76 ± 5 pS). Permeabilized cells were capable of generating ATP endogenously by a variety of metabolic pathways if provided with the appropriate substrates [9]. In the absence of exogenous ATP, addition of mitochondrial substrates consisting of (in mM) 2 pyruvate, 2 glutamate, 1 inorganic phosphate (P_i), and 0.5 ADP to the bath completely prevented

Biology of Isolated Adult Cardiac Myocytes
William A. Clark, Robert S. Decker, and Thomas K. Borg, Editors

ATP-sensitive K^+ channels from opening unless a mitochondrial inhibitor was present. Glycolytic substrates beyond the ATP-consuming steps of glycolysis including 2 phosphoenol pyruvate, 2 fructose-1,6-diphosphate, 1 NAD, 1 P_i and 0.5 ADP were equally effective even in the presence of a mitochondrial inhibitor. In typical permeabilized cells ATP-sensitive K^+ channels could be activated and suppressed repeatedly for as long as 45 minutes by transiently removing ATP or various substrates.

These findings demonstrated that in a state of low intrinsic ATP consumption relaxed non-beating permeabilized myocytes were capable of generating ATP via several metabolic processes. In the intact beating heart, however, many cellular processes compete for the available ATP. To simulate the high intrinsic ATP consumption of the beating heart, permeabilized myocytes were exposed to an exogenous ATP-consuming system consisting of hexokinase (HK, 10 IU/l) and 2-deoxyglucose (2-DG, 10 mM). In the presence of ATP, HK phosphorylates 2-DG to 2-DG-6-phosphate (which is nonmetabolizable), degrading ATP to ADP in the process. Fig. 1A compares the effectiveness of mitochondrial substrates (MSS) and glycolytic substrates (GSS) at closing ATP-sensitive K^+ channels in a cell-attached patch on a permeabilized myocyte in the presence of HK + 2-DG. At the beginning of the continuous trace, openings of a single I_{K1} channel were occasionally observed during exposure to standard bath solution containing MSS and HK. Removal of MSS and addition of 2-DG to the HK in the bath solution (first arrow) caused many ATP-sensitive K^+ channels to open. Re-exposure to MSS (second arrow) in the presence of both HK and 2-DG now resulted in only a partial transient suppression of ATP-sensitive K^+ channel activity, presumably because ATP generated by mitochondria was being degraded by the reaction with HK and 2-DG before it could reach the ATP-sensitive K^+ channels in the patch. However, GSS (third arrow) remained effective at supressing ATP-sensitive K^+ channels in the presence of HK + 2-DG, even after 1 μM FCCP (fourth arrow) was added to inhibit mitochondrial ATP production. Note that I_{K1} channels remained active with GSS present. The findings were reproducible. In 15 permeabilized cells the average current through ATP-sensitive K^+ channels in the patch with HK + 2-DG present fell to 81 ± 35% (SD) of the control value when MSS were added and to 34 ± 29% when GSS and FCCP were added ($p < .005$ by paired T-test). Inclusion of 2 mM creatine with MSS in 11 of these cells did not improve their effectiveness at suppressing ATP-sensitive K^+ channels. In all of these cells MSS had completely suppressed ATP-sensitive K^+ channels when HK but no 2-DG was present.

Two possible explanations for the greater effectiveness of glycolytic than mitochondrial substrates at suppressing ATP-sensitive K^+ channels when HK + 2-DG were present are that an intermediate of glycolytic metabolism might directly block the channels or increase their sensitivity to ATP, or glycolytic enzymes located in close proximity to the channels might generate a higher local ATP concentration than mitochondria. The effects of various glycolytic intermediates on ATP-sensitive K^+ channels were therefore studied in excised (cell-free) inside-out patches. In the absence of exogenous ATP none of the individual glycolytic intermediates between fructose-1,6-diphsophate and pyruvate significantly affected the average current through ATP-sensitive K^+ channels. However, in 5 of 27 inside-out patches, a combination of all the necessary substrates for the ATP-producing steps of glycolysis (involving phosphoglycerokinase and pyruvate kinase) reversibly and reproducibly suppressed ATP-sensitive K^+ channels, reducing the average current through the channels to 1.6, 3.3, 7.1, 13.6, and 64% respectively relative to the control value with 0.5 mM ADP present. In 1 of 11 inside-out patches, substrates for the second ATP-producing step alone (involving pyruvate kinase) reduced the average current through ATP-sensitive K^+ channels to zero. Fig. 1B shows an example. Replacement of ATP with 0.5 mM ADP activated multiple ATP-sensitive K^+ channels which were reversibly suppressed by glycolytic substrates (GSS*). The ability of the appropriate combination of glycolytic substrates to suppress ATP-sensitive K^+ channels in some excised patches is consistent with the hypothesis that phosphogly-

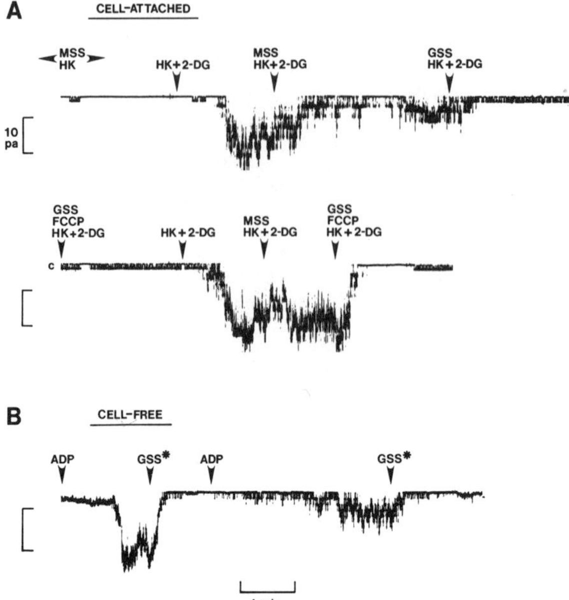

Fig. 1. A. Effects of mitochondrial (MSS) vs glycolytic substrates (GSS) on ATP-sensitive K^+ channels in a cell-attached patch on a permeabilized myocyte with hexokinase (HK) and 2-deoxyglucose (2-DG) present. Recording is continuous. Composition of MSS and GSS as described in text. B. Effect of glycolytic substrates (GSS*) on ATP-sensitive K^+ channels in an excised inside-out patch. GSS* included 2 mM glyceraldehyde-3-phosphate and phosphoenolpyruvate, 2 IU/ml glyceraldehyde-3-phosphate dehydrogenase, 1 mM NAD and K_2HPO_4, and 0.5 mM ADP. In both A and B the patch electrode potential was +40 mV throughout. Filter setting 50 Hz.

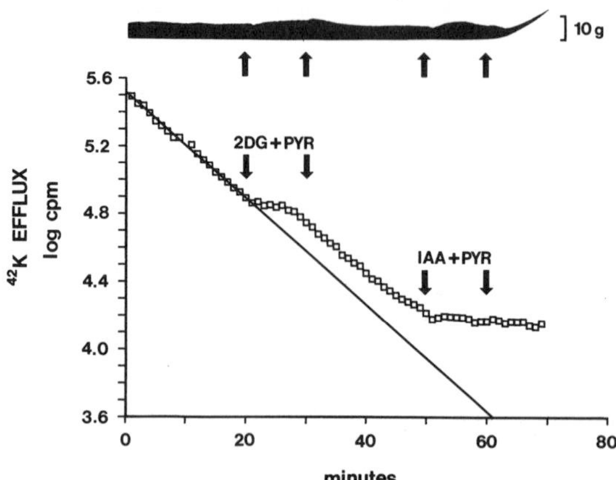

Fig. 2. Effect of selectively inhibiting glycolysis on $^{42}K^+$ washout in in an arterially perfused rabbit septum. Tension is shown above.

cerate kinase and/or pyruvate kinase are located in the sarcolemma or cytoskeleton in the immediate vicinity of K^+ channels. The ineffectiveness of the substrates in the majority of patches may be related to damage or loss of enzymes during patch excision, or to a patch geometry which did not permit ATP generated locally by glycolytic enzymes to accumulate sufficiently to suppress ATP-sensitive K^+ channel activity.

These findings suggest that under conditions of high intrinsic ATP consumption glycolysis is more effective than mitochondrial metabolism at suppressing ATP-sensitive K^+ channels in permeabilized myocytes. To investigate the relevance of these results to the intact beating heart, we examined the effects of inhibiting glycolysis on unidirectional $^{42}K^+$ efflux in isolated arterially perfused rabbit interventricular septa. Fig. 2 shows that upon replacing 5.6 mM glucose in the perfusate with 5.6 mM pyruvate (substrate for oxidative metabolism) and 5.6 mM 2-DG (to inhibit glycolysis) there was an immediate increase the rate of $^{42}K^+$ efflux. The increased rate of $^{42}K^+$ efflux did not reverse when 5.6 mM glucose was readmitted, possibly due the intracellular accumulation of 2-DG-6-phosphate. Subsequent exposure to perfusate containing 5.6 mM pyruvate and 1 mM iodoacetate (IAA) caused a further marked increase in K^+ efflux which was irreversible. Similar results were obtained in 2 other preparations. We have previously shown that total cellular levels of ATP and creatine phosphate remain normal when glycosis is selectively inhibited by these agents [6].

DISCUSSION

During myocardial ischemia, a rapid increase in K^+ efflux results in marked extracellular K^+ accumulation, predisposing the heart to lethal arrhythmias. Activation of ATP-sensitive K^+ channels has been suggested as a possible mechanism, but the threshold of [ATP] at which these channels are activated (approximately 0.2 mM in excised inside-out patches) [1] is much lower than occurs until late ischemia. Unless either the sensitivity of the channels to [ATP] is altered by sequellae of metabolic inhibition, or ATP stores are compartmentalized in myocardial cells, it seems unlikely that activation of ATP-sensitive K^+ channels could contribute to increase K^+ efflux. The single cell experiments described above indicate that ATP derived from glycolysis is more effective than ATP derived from oxidative metabolism at regulating the activity of ATP-sensitive K^+ channels in heart when the rate of cellular ATP utilization is intrinsically high. Furthermore in the intact beating ventricle $^{42}K^+$ efflux increased dramatically when glycolysis was selectively inhibited despite maintenance of normal total cellular ATP levels by oxidative metabolism. Although it is not known whether the increase in K^+ efflux was due to activation of ATP-sensitive K^+ channels, this possibility seems plausible in view of the findings in single myocytes. These results are consistent with the hypothesis that glycolysis plays a preferential role in the maintenance of membrane functions in heart [5,6].

REFERENCES

1. A. Noma, Nature 305, 147-148 (1983).
2. G. Trube and J. Hescheler, Pflugers Arch. 401, 178-184 (1984).
3. M. Kakei, A. Noma, T. Shibasaki, J. Physiol. 363, 441-462 (1985).
4. D.L. Cooke and N. Hales, Nature 311, 271-273 (1984).
5. T.F. McDonald and D.P. McLeod, J. Physiol. 229, 559-582 (1973).
6. J. Weiss and B. Hiltbrand, J. Clin. Invest. 75, 436-447 (1985).
7. R. Mitra and M. Morad, Am. J. Physiol. 249, H1056-H1060 (1986).
8. O.P. Hamill, A. Marty, E. Neher, B. Sakmann, F.J. Sigworth, Pflugers Arch. 391, 85-100 (1981).
9. J.N. Weiss, S.T. Lamp, Science, in press (1987).

Supported by NIH grants HL27845, HL36729, and Research Career Development Award HL01890, AHA grant-in-aid 83-626 and the Laubisch Endowment.

CARDIAC MYOCYTE SODIUM CHANNEL: BIOCHEMICAL EVIDENCE FOR A RECEPTOR FOR ANTIARRHYTHMIC DRUGS

Roger J. Hill, Henry J. Duff, Nancy J. Cannon and Robert S. Sheldon
Division of Cardiology, Department of Medicine, University of Calgary, Calgary, Alberta, Canada

INTRODUCTION

The antiarrhythmic action of class I antiarrhythmic drugs is thought to be mediated by their ability to slow action potential propagation via sodium channel blockade [1]. The exact mechanism by which class I agents mediate sodium channel blockade is unclear. Models based on electrophysiological data have led to the concept that the drugs bind to specific sites associated with cardiac sodium channels, thereby modulating channel function and producing electrophysiologic changes [2,3]. It is our premise that the interaction of class I antiarrhythmic drugs with the cardiac sodium channel is essentially biochemical; that is, the interaction between small ligands (drugs) and a macromolecule (the sodium channel). To test this hypothesis we wished to develop a radioligand assay which reflected the interaction of class I drugs with the cardiac sodium channel. However, no class I drug has been described with a sufficiently tight affinity for the channel to enable the use of a conventional class I antiarrhythmic agent as a radioligand. Accordingly we have exploited toxins which bind tightly to specific sites on sodium channels in order to characterize an antiarrhythmic drug receptor associated with the rat cardiomyocyte sodium channel.

Previous studies of the nerve sodium channel have revealed at least four receptor sites for neurotoxins [4]. Two sites are germane to this work. Site 2 binds alkaloid toxins such as aconitine and batrachotoxin which cause persistent activation of the channel. Site 3 binds sea anemone toxin II (ATX) which slows inactivation of the channel and synergistically enhances alkaloid toxin binding to site 2. A radiolabelled derivative of batrachotoxin, [^{3}H]Batrachotoxinin A 20α-benzoate ([^{3}H]BTXB), has been used to study the interaction of local anaesthetics with the nerve sodium channel [5,6]. Local anaesthetics bind at or near site 2 and inhibit [^{3}H]BTXB binding in a stereospecific manner at pharmacologically relevant concentrations and with the same rank order of potency *in vitro* and *in vivo*, suggesting that the pharmacologic effect of local anaesthetics is mediated by their binding site on the nerve sodium channel. The structural and functional similarities between local anaesthetics and class I antiarrhythmic drugs prompted us to examine the interactions between [^{3}H]BTXB, antiarrhythmic drugs and the sodium channel on freshly isolated rat cardiac myocytes.

METHODS

Myocyte Preparation

Cardiac myocytes were isolated by collagenase digestion from adult male Sprague-Dawley rats (200-250g) using the method of Kryski et al. [7]. This method routinely yielded about 100 mg (dry weight) of myocytes, which corresponds to 2 x 10^7 cells [8,7]. The cells were 82-92% viable rod-shaped cells which excluded Trypan Blue. The cells maintained a resting potential of -75mV to -80mV, and have been characterized by Kryski et al. [7].

Biology of Isolated Adult Cardiac Myocytes
William A. Clark, Robert S. Decker, and Thomas K. Borg, Editors

Radioligand Binding

The conditions of binding of $[^3H]$BTXB and ATX to myocytes, and subsequent filtration and radioisotope measurement have been described previously [9].

Drug Selection

Class I antiarrhythmic drugs were selected for study if they were thought to be effective in treating ventricular tachycardia, and had known therapeutic serum concentrations.

RESULTS AND DISCUSSION

Characterization of $[^3H]$Batrachotoxinin Binding to Myocytes

The synergistic binding of ATX and $[^3H]$BTXB to nerve sodium channels led to the demonstration that binding of $[^3H]$BTXB to nerve channels is demonstrable in the presence but not the absence of ATX [10]. In preliminary experiments we found that 1 μM ATX stimulated the total binding of $[^3H]$BTXB to myocytes about 2-4 fold. To determine if $[^3H]$BTXB binds to a specific site we characterized the inhibition by batrachotoxin of $[^3H]$BTXB binding. We observed that batrachotoxin inhibited ATX-stimulated $[^3H]$BTXB binding with an IC_{50} of 100 nM. A Hill plot of these data gave a Hill number of 0.91 suggesting that batrachotoxin binds to a single class of specific, saturable binding sites. Scatchard analysis of concentration dependent $[^3H]$BTXB binding indicated a single class of saturable sites with a K_D of 25-35 nM, which is similar to the K_D of $[^3H]$BTXB for the nerve sodium channel. In addition, this analysis suggested that there are 4-15 sites/μM^2 of myocytes surface area, in good agreement with estimates of sodium channel surface density from patch-clamp [11] and $[^3H]$saxitoxin [12] data. In a separate set of experiments we showed that a proportion of the $[^3H]$BTXB binding was voltage-sensitive as would be expected if binding was to a voltage-sensitive sodium channel. Thus, we conclude that the toxins bind to specific saturable sites with characteristics which indicate binding to sodium channels.

Class I Drugs Inhibit $[^3H]$BTXB Binding

We then turned to the question of whether class I antiarrhythmic drugs inhibited $[^3H]$BTXB binding in a fashion consistent with their binding to a specific receptor site on cardiac myocytes [13]. The effect of three class I drugs (O-demethylencainide, lidocaine, and procainamide) on $[^3H]$BTXB binding to myocytes is shown in Figure 1.

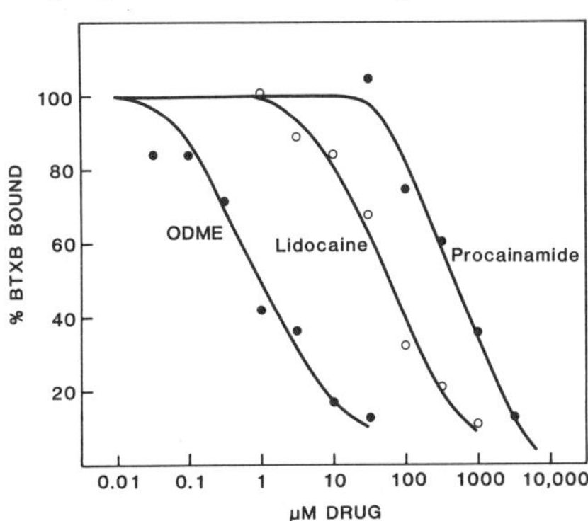

Figure 1. Effect of Type I Drugs on $[^3H]$BTXB Binding to Myocytes

The inhibition by the drugs is dose dependent and follows a sigmoid curve characteristic of ligand binding to a single class of saturable sites. Eight drugs were tested and all inhibited [^{3}H]BTXB binding with IC_{50} values ranging from 1.34 μM to 811 μM. When one compares the known therapeutic serum concentration of these drugs with their IC_{50} values obtained from this assay, there is a striking similarity over a 100-fold range of serum concentrations. The data are plotted in Figure 2 as log (IC_{50}) vs. log (serum concentration).

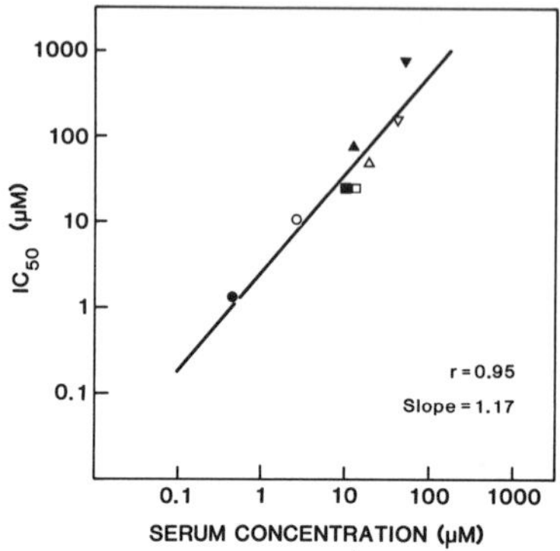

Figure 2. Correlation of IC_{50} values for inhibition of [^{3}H]BTXB binding by type I antiarrhythmic agents *in vitro* with their effective serum concentrations *in vivo*.

Linear regression analysis of the log-log plot yields a slope of 1.17 and a correlation coefficient, r, of 0.95. Thus the drugs have the same rank order of potency *in vitro* as *in vivo* suggesting that binding is relevant to clinical effect.

Another characteristic of ligand binding to a specific receptor site is the reversibility of such binding. The reversibility of lidocaine inhibition of [^{3}H]BTXB binding was determined by incubating the myocytes sequentially in two different concentrations of lidocaine and assessing whether the degree of inhibition of [^{3}H]BTXB binding was determined by the first or the final concentration of lidocaine. We observed that there was a similar amount of [^{3}H]BTXB bound in the presence of a final concentration of 39 μM lidocaine independent of whether the myocytes were first incubated with 39 μM lidocaine or 390 μM lidocaine. Thus the inhibition of [^{3}H]BTXB binding by lidocaine is reversible and lidocaine does not irreversibly alter the [^{3}H]BTXB receptor.

Finally, we examined whether antiarrhythmic drug binding to myocytes is stereospecific. Tocainide is a class I drug whose R(-) stereoisomer is a three-fold more potent antiarrhythmic agent than the S(+) isomer. We have shown that R(-) tocainide is significantly more potent than S(+) tocainide in prolonging conduction time in an *ex vivo* rabbit myocardium model [14]. This suggested that R(-) tocainide would bind more tightly to the sodium channel than S(+) tocainide, and that R(-) tocainide would more potently inhibit [^{3}H]BTXB binding than would S(+) tocainide. In these radioligand studies we found that R(-) tocainide was three times more potent than S(+) tocainide as determined by comparison of their IC_{50} values for inhibition of [^{3}H]BTXB binding. Thus the stereospecific effects of antiarrhythmic effect, conduction time and [^{3}H]BTXB binding seem to correlate.

In review, we have used a radioligand binding assay to show that class I antiarrhythmic drugs bind to specific sites on myocytes and that this binding inhibits the binding of toxins to the cardiac sodium channel. This suggests that these drugs bind to a specific site associated with the sodium channel. The characteristics of this binding suggests that it is involved in the pharmacological effect of the drugs. We anticipate that use of this method will provide molecular insights into the mechanism of action of class I antiarrhythmic drugs.

ACKNOWLEDGEMENTS

Supported by the Alberta Heart and Stroke Foundation, the Alberta Heritage Foundation for Medical Research and the Medical Research Council of Canada. Dr. Duff is an Alberta Heritage Foundation for Medical Research Scholar and Dr. Hill is a Canadian Heart Foundation Postdoctoral Fellow. We thank Mr. G. Douglas for his customary invaluable help with the manuscript.

REFERENCES

1. E. M. Vaughan Williams, Pharm. Therap. 1, 115-138 (1975).
2. L. M. Hondeghem, and B. G. Katzung, Biochim. Biophys. Acta 472, 373-398 (1977).
3. A. O. Grant, C. F. Starmer and H. C. Strauss, Circ. Res. 55, 427-439 (1984).
4. W. A. Catterall. Science (Wash. D.C.) 223, 653-661 (1984).
5. C. R. Creveling, E. T. McNeal, J. W. Daly, and G. B. Brown. Mol. Pharmacol. 23, 350-358 (1983).
6. S. W. Postma and W. A. Catterall, Mol. Pharmacol. 25, 219-227 (1984).
7. A. Kryski, K. A. Kenno and D. L. Severson, Am. J. Physiol. 248, H208-H216 (1985).
8. B. B. Farmer, M. Mancina, E. S. Williams, and M. Watanabe, Life Sci. 33, 1-18 (1983).
9. R. S. Sheldon, N. J. Cannon and H. J. Duff, Molec. Pharmac. 30, 617-623 (1986).
10. W. A. Catterall, C. S. Morrow, J. W. Daly and G. B. Brown, J. Biol. Chem. 256, 8922-8927 (1981).
11. H. A. Fozzard, C. T. January and J. C. Makielski, Circ. Res. 56, 475-485 (1985).
12. D. D. Doyle and E. Page, Circulation 70 (Suppl. II), 74 (1984).
13. R. S. Sheldon, N. J. Cannon and H. J. Duff, Circ. Res. (1987a) (In press).
14. R. S. Sheldon, N. J. Cannon and H. J. Duff, (1987b) (Submitted).

THE SINGLE VENTRICULAR MYOCYTE AS A MODEL FOR WENCKEBACH PERIODICITY

MARIO DELMAR, DONALD C MICHAELS AND JOSE JALIFE
Dept. of Pharmacology. SUNY/Health Science Center. Syracuse NY 13210.

INTRODUCTION

The term Wenckebach periodicity is applied to those patterns of cardiac impulse propagation in which successive proximal-distal (e.g. atrium-ventricle) intervals increase by decreasing increments until transmission failure occurs, whereupon temporary restitution of conductivity initiates a new cycle.

Several years ago, Rosenblueth [1, 2] analyzed the rate dependency of active propagation through the atrioventricular node and concluded that Wenckebach periodicity can not be present in a homogeneously conducting system, but it develops when an area of functional heterogeneity causes the impulse to be blocked momentarily, and to resume its journey after a delay imposed by the excitability properties of the tissue beyond the site of block.

Studies in humans [3, 4]and in isolated tissue preparations [5, 6] support this hypothesis. In particular, previous studies from our laboratory using the Purkinje fiber-sucrose gap model [5, 6] show that during repetitive stimulation, the progressive prolongation and eventual failure of proximal to distal transmission is related to discontinuous propagation imposed by the presence of inexcitable tissue separating two active fiber segments. In that model, action potentials of constant amplitude initiated in one segment stop at the junction with the inexcitable tissue (i.e. "the gap"). However, transmission to the distal segment may be accomplished as a result of electrotonic spread across that inexcitable zone. Hence, cyclic phenomena such as in Wenckebach periodicities can be adequately explained in terms of slow recovery of excitability of the distal element during diastole. As activation is delayed progressively during subsequent beats, the impulse encounters the distal cells less and less recovered until, finally, the electrotonically mediated depolarization is incapable of attaining threshold and block occurs.

In this paper, we present results from our studies on the cellular and subcellular bases of slow recovery of excitability and rate-dependent activation failure in cardiac cells. Using single, enzymatically dissociated guinea-pig ventricular myocytes as well as computer simulations, we have demonstrated that Wenckebach periodicity is a direct consequence of diastolic changes in excitability that occur normally in cardiac cells. Furthermore, we present compelling evidence that these changes in excitability can be explained for the most part by mechanisms related to the slow deactivation kinetics of the outward current i_K.

METHODS

Isolated ventricular myocytes:

Single ventricular myocytes were obtained by enzymatic dissociation of Langendorff-perfused guinea pig hearts [7]. Recordings were attempted after at least 30 minutes of starting superfusion with the normal Tyrode solution. A healthy adult ventricular myocyte was identified by its rod-like, striated appearance and either impaled with a 3M KCl microelectrode (DC resistances 20-40 mOhms; only for current clamp experiments) or attached to a patch pipette in the whole-cell configuration [8]. Signals were amplified either with a WPI MS-700 unit for current clamping, or an Axoclamp 2A amplifier (Axon Instruments), for

Biology of Isolated Adult Cardiac Myocytes
William A. Clark, Robert S. Decker, and Thomas K. Borg, Editors

voltage clamping. Power input was provided by 1 or 2 Frederick Haer p6i stimulation units. All signals were displayed on a Tektronix 5113 storage oscilloscope, and photographed with a Grass kymographic camera.

Computer simulation techniques:

Computer simulations of the delayed rectifier (i_K) current were performed using a modified version of the original equations described by Beeler and Reuter [9]. The cell is modelled as a 1 cm^2 surface with a specific membrane capacitance of 1 uF/cm^2 in parallel with a non-linear conductance. The computer programs were written in FORTRAN and run on a PDP 11/73 computer (Cyberchron Corp., Garrison, NY) equipped with 2.5 megabytes of core memory and 56 megabytes of Winchester disk storage. Graphic outputs during the computer runs were displayed on either a VT125 graphics terminal (Digital Equipment Corp.), or a Tektronix 4010 graphics terminal. Hardcopies were produced using a a Tektronix hard copy unit (Model 4631).

RESULTS

Frequency-dependent activation delay and failure can be demonstrated in normal heart cells. Figure 1A shows an example, obtained from a ventricular myocyte with a resting potential of -81 mV. Five superimposed traces are shown. Depolarizing current pulses, 40 msec in duration and 0.15 nA in strength were applied at a constant cycle length of 1000 msec. A 5:4 stimulus:response activation pattern was clearly manifest in which the stimulus:response latency increased in decreasing increments until failure occurred, reproducing very closely the typical sequence of Wenckebach periodicity described in the literature [10, 11]. Panel B shows another example. Constant current pulses (0.25 nA amplitude and 200 msec duration) were applied through the recording microelectrode at a constant cycle length (1100 msec). Under these conditions, alternations of the 3:2 and 2:1 patterns developed. Note that in both panels, failure occurred always several miliseconds after the repolarization phase of the action potential had been completed, thus suggesting the presence of post-repolarization refractoriness.

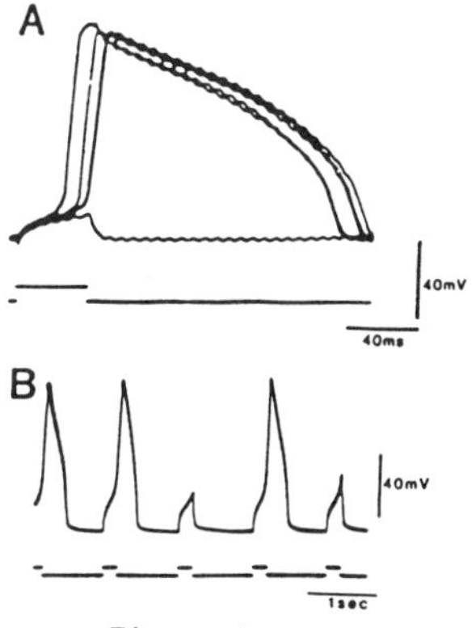

Figure 1.

Previous studies from our laboratory [5, 6, 12, 13] have shown that, as a result of post-repolarization refractoriness, the amplitude and shape of the subthreshold responses during the failed beat (see figure 1B) are dependent on the test interval. This is illustrated diagrammatically in figure 2. The top superimposed tracings represent hypothetical action potentials from a single cell, and the bottom tracing represents a stimulus monitor. At brief delays, the subthreshold depolarization conforms to the normal RC (resistance-capacitance) properties of the cell membrane whereas, at longer intervals, its amplitude increases and its shape becomes distorted. At still longer intervals, activation ensues. We have

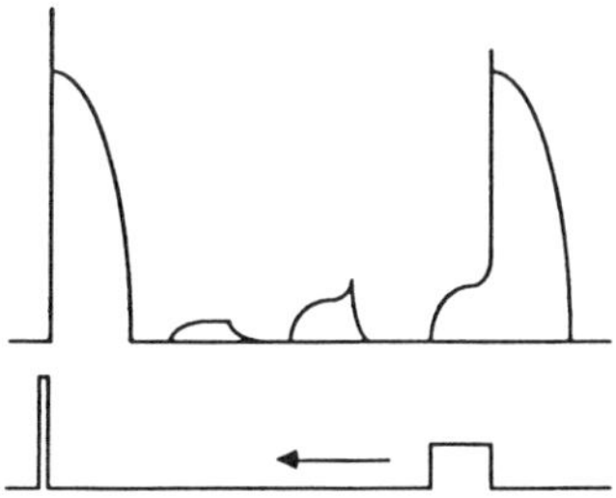

Figure 2.

studied the possible role of the delayed rectifier (i_K) current in determining the amplitude and shape of the subthreshold response at various coupling intervals. Figure 3 shows an example. In panel A we present results obtained from an isolated myocyte that was continuously superfused with 2 mM $CoCl_2$ and 30 uM of Tetrodotoxin to block the active inward currents.

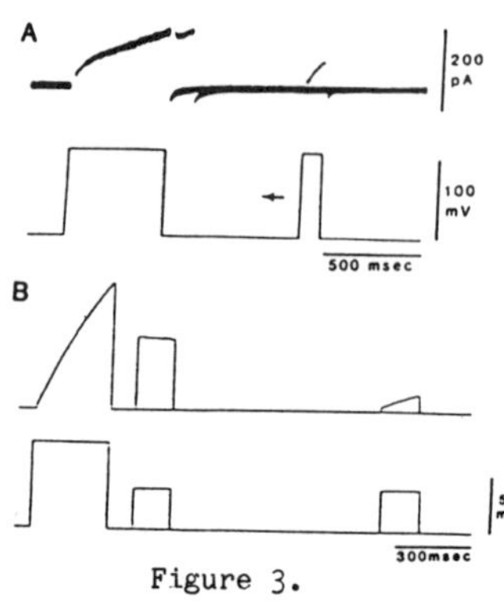

Figure 3.

Recordings were obtained with a suction pipette in a whole-cell voltage clamp configuration. The top trace shows the current records and the bottom trace, the voltage clamp protocol. From a holding potential of -90 mV, a conditioning command potential of 500 msec to +20 mV was followed by brief test pulses of 100 msec to +10 mV applied at variable coupling intervals. During the command potential, the i_K current was activated. On returning to the holding potential, only a very small tail current was recorded, as a result of the proximity of the holding potential to the equilibrium potential of i_K. On the other hand, the instantaneous responses elicited by the test pulse reflected the degree of deactivation of i_K at variable coupling intervals. For the purpose of illustration, only two intervals are shown. However, complete scans of the entire deactivation period revealed that the current relaxation follows an exponential time course, with a time constant of 384 ms. Panel B shows a computer simulation utilizing a similar protocol to that used for the experiments. In the case of the model, the voltage clamp parameters were the following: Holding potential: -77 mV; command potential, 300 msec duration, depolarization to 0 mV. Test pulses, 100 msec duration to -40 mV at variable coupling intervals. Clearly, as in the biological preparation, the instantaneous amplitude of the current elicited by the test pulse reflected the degree of deactivation of the current, which occurred in the form of a single exponential with a time constant of 370 msec.

DISCUSSION

The use of isolated ventricular myocytes provides us with a simplified, direct method for testing the role of cell excitability in the development of rate-dependent activation failure. Although we can not be absolutely certain that the physiological properties of the ventricular myocyte after the dispersion procedure are identical to those of the intact tissue, our results are in complete agreement with those previously obtained in multicellular preparations [5, 6, 12]. Furthermore, computer simulations using a modified version of the Beeler and Reuter [9] model of a single ventricular cell substantially support our experimental observations.

Since the original description of Wenckebach periodicity [14] several hypotheses have been proposed to explain its mechanism. In 1960, Paes de Carvalho and de Almeida [15] suggested that the progressive lengthening of the proximal-distal interval would indicate a "fatigue" of the conduction system, hence leading to decremental conduction. According to this hypothesis, the impulse would find a progressively increasing threshold, a decreasing space constant and a decreased amplitude and rate of rise of the action potential along its journey, leading to a gradual decay of the effectiveness of active regions to depolarize more distal tissue. This explanation, however, has not been demonstrated experimentally and, in fact, does not conform with the physiological behavior of tissues exhibiting impaired conduction [1, 2, 16]. Our experiments demonstrate that cyclic rate-dependent activation failure can be explained as a consequence of the slow process of recovery of excitability that follows each action potential. This process is intrinsic to the physiological behavior of a normally polarized cell.

Post-repolarization refractoriness is a property of the cell membrane. Hence, the isolated cell provides us with an excellent model for characterizing the ionic current changes that take place during the diastolic interval, and that may be responsible for post-repolarization refractoriness and the rate-dependent phenomena associated with it. In this paper, we have reported our results on the time course of relaxation of the delayed rectifier current i_K. These results indicate that the time and voltage dependent characteristics of i_K are such that it does not completely deactivate upon repolarization from an action potential and that, to a large extent, this process takes place during the diastolic interval. Slow deactivation of i_K probably plays a major role in determining the amplitude of the cell response to closely coupled electrotonic events in that it opposes depolarization and prevents the membrane from reaching its threshold level.

AKNOWLEDGMENTS

This work was supported by grant HL 29439 from the National Heart, Lung and Blood Institute, and was completed during Dr. Jalife's tenure of an Established Investigatorship from the American Heart Association. Dr. Delmar is the recipient of the Kenneth M. Rosen Fellowship from the North American Society of Pacing and Electrophysiology.

REFERENCES

1. A. Rosenblueth, Am. J. Physiol. 194, 171-183 (1958).
2. A. Rosenblueth, Am. J. Physiol. 194, 491-494 (1958).
3. M. Levy, P. J. Martin, H. Zieske and D. Adler, Circ Res. 34, 697-710 (1974).
4. M. B. Simson, J. F. Spear and E. N. Moore, Am. J. Cardiol. 41, 244-258 (1978).
5. J. Jalife and G. K. Moe, Circ. Res. 49, 233-347 (1981).
6. J. Jalife, PACE 6, 1106-1122 (1983).
7. G. Isenberg and U. Klochner, Pfluegers. Arch. 395, 6-18 (1982).
8. O. P. Hamill, A. Marty, E. Neher, B. Sakmann and F. J. Sigworth, Pfluegers. Arch, 391, 85-100 (1981).
9. G. W. Beeler and H. Reuter, J. Physiol. (Lond). 268, 177-210 (1982).
10. T. Lewis, Mechanism and Graphic Registration of the Heart Beat (Shaw and Sons, Ltd, London 1925).
11. A. Pick and R. Langendorf, Interpretation of Complex Arrhythmias (Lea and Febiger, Philadelphia 1979).
12. G. J. Rozanski, J. Jalife and G. K. Moe, Circ. Res. 55, 486-496 (1984).
13. M. Delmar, J. Jalife and D. C. Michaels, Biophys. J. 51, 265a (1987).
14. K. F. Wenckebach, Z. Klin. Med. 37, 475-488 (1899).
15. A. Paes de Carvalho and D. F. de Almeida, Circ. Res. 8, 801-809 (1960).
16. D. Scherf, Weiner Arch Inn Med 18, 403-416 (1929).

Current-voltage relationship of the backward-running Na/K pump in isolated cells from guinea-pig ventricle.

Anthony Bahinski and David C. Gadsby
Laboratory of Cardiac Physiology, The Rockefeller University, 1230 York Avenue, New York, New York, 10021

INTRODUCTION

Under usual physiological conditions, the Na/K pump transports more Na out of the cell than K in and so it generates an outward component of membrane current (for review see [1, 2]). Both ions are transported against their electrochemical potential gradients and the energy for this work derives from the hydrolysis of ATP. By steepening the transmembrane Na and K gradients and reducing the energy available from ATP by artificially lowering the ratio $[ATP]/([ADP]\cdot[P_i])$, it is possible to drive the Na/K pump reaction cycle backwards [3]. Under these conditions, the Na/K pump retains its Na/K>1 stoichiometry [3] and so generates an inward current, at least in squid giant axons [4,5]. The present study was designed to see whether the backward-running Na/K pump generates a measurable inward current in isolated heart cells and, if so, to determine its voltage dependence.

METHODS

Rod-shaped, quiescent cells were isolated from left ventricles of guinea-pig hearts by collagenase digestion followed by enzyme-free incubation in high [K], low [Ca] medium [6]. The myocytes were allowed to settle on the glass coverslip bottom of the recording chamber before being superfused at 34-36°C with normal Tyrode's solution containing (in mM): 145 NaCl, 5.4 KCl, 1.8 $CaCl_2$, 0.5 $MgCl_2$, 5.5 dextrose, and 5 NaHEPES (*p*H 7.4). The whole-cell version of the patch-clamp technique [7] was used with a device for changing the solution inside the pipette [8]. Giga-ohm seals were obtained using wide-tipped (~5 µm), fire-polished pipettes filled with Tyrode's solution (pipette resistance ~1MΩ) which was then exchanged [8], just before rupturing the membrane patch, for a solution designed to minimize ion channel current and Na/Ca exchange current while supporting Na/K pump activity. After equilibration of the pipette solution with the cell interior, the normal Tyrode's solution superfusing the cell was exchanged for a nominally Ca-free Tyrode's solution. To support Na/K pumping in the forward direction, the internal solution contained (in mM) 100 aspartic acid, ~80 CsOH, 34 NaOH, 10 $Tris_2ATP$, 5 K_2-creatine phosphate, 1 NaH_2PO_4, 20 TEACl, 5.5 $MgCl_2$, 5 EGTA and 5 HEPES (*p*H 7.4), while the external solution contained (in mM) 145 NaCl, 5.4 KCl, 0.3 NaH_2PO_4, 2.3 $MgCl_2$, 0.9 $BaCl_2$, 0.2 $CdCl_2$, 1 $CsCl_2$, 5.5 dextrose and 5 NaHEPES (*p*H 7.4). To drive the Na/K pump backwards, the Na-free internal solution contained (in mM) 90 aspartic acid, 140 KOH, 5 MgATP, 5 $Tris_2ADP$, 5 KH_2PO_4, 20 TEACl, 2 $MgCl_2$, 5 pyruvic acid, 10 EGTA, 5.5 dextrose and 10 HEPES (*p*H 7.4), while the external solution was K-free and contained (in mM) 150 NaCl, 2.3 $MgCl_2$, 5 $BaCl_2$, 0.5 $CdCl_2$, 5.5 dextrose and 5 NaHEPES (*p*H 7.4). The osmolarity of all solutions was 295-310 mosmol kg^{-1}. Ouabain was added from a 10^{-2} M aqueous stock solution. Strophanthidin was added from a 0.5 M stock solution in dimethyl sulfoxide (DMSO): control experiments showed that up to 0.5% DMSO (by volume) had no effect on membrane currents under the conditions of our experiments.

Current and voltage signals were low-pass filtered at 2 kHz (6 pole Bessel), digitized at 0.15-0.4 ms intervals with 12-bit resolution, either on-line or during play-back from FM tape, and then stored for later analysis by computer.

Biology of Isolated Adult Cardiac Myocytes
William A. Clark, Robert S. Decker, and Thomas K. Borg, Editors

RESULTS AND DISCUSSION

Cells were held at -40 mV to inactivate Na channels, and steady currents were measured near the end of 100-300 ms voltage-clamp steps to potentials between +60 mV and -140 mV. Under our experimental conditions, membrane current changes in response to the voltage steps were small (Figs. 1B, 2A) and virtually time-independent (Fig. 1B). The chart record in Fig. 1A illustrates changes in holding current during activation and inhibition of the Na/K pump caused by raising the pipette [Na] from 1 mM to 34 mM and then exposing the cell to 10 µM ouabain, a specific inhibitor of the Na/K pump. The representative currents in Fig. 1B were recorded during pump activation (a) and during inhibition by ouabain (b), and the ouabain-sensitive currents (c) were obtained by computer subtraction; they vary in size with membrane potential, being much smaller at -120 mV (c: lowest trace, ~50 pA) than at the holding potential, -40 mV, (c: initial current, ~150 pA).

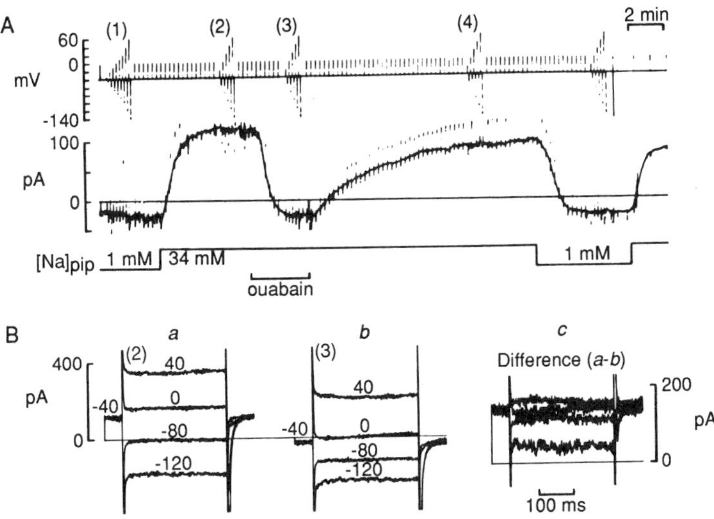

Fig. 1 Changes in whole-cell current due to activation or inhibition of the Na/K pump in a myocyte superfused with 5.4 mM K, Ca-free Tyrode's solution. **A**, upper trace, membrane potential; middle trace, whole-cell current; the lower line indicates changes in $[Na]_{pip}$ between 1 and 34 mM, and the bar beneath it marks exposure to 10 µM ouabain; the numbers above the voltage trace indicate acquisition of four sets of current-voltage data. **B**, Superimposed sample currents taken from A, just before (*a*) and during (*b*) exposure to ouabain. The pulse potential is indicated for each record; holding potential -40 mV. *c*, Superimposed difference currents obtained by computer subtraction of each record in *b* from its counterpart in *a*; pulse potentials were, from top to bottom, 0, +40, -80 and -120 mV. Reproduced from Gadsby et al (1985) [13] with permission.

This voltage dependence of outward current generated by the forward-running Na/K pump is more clearly illustrated in Fig. 2, which illustrates steady-state current-voltage relationships from the experiment in Fig.1. The lower curve in Fig. 2A is drawn through steady current levels measured with 1 mM pipette [Na] (Δ), or with 34 mM pipette [Na] in the presence of ouabain (●);

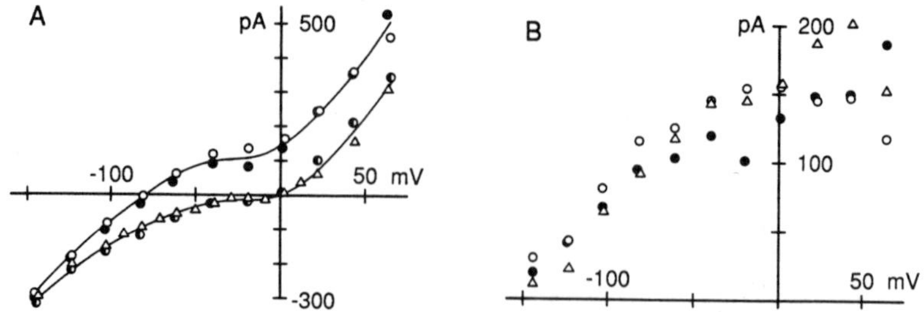

Fig. 2 Voltage dependence of current associated with Na/K pump activity, from the experiment in Fig. 1. **A**, Whole-cell currents in the presence and absence of Na/K pump activity. Ordinate, steady current levels, obtained by averaging digitized values over the final ~100 ms of each 300-ms pulse. Abscissa, membrane potential during the pulse. The data were recorded during the periods numbered in Fig. 1A: Δ (1), 1mM $[Na]_{pip}$; o (2), 34 mM $[Na]_{pip}$; ◐ (3), 34 mM $[Na]_{pip}$ during exposure to ouabain; • (4), 34 mM $[Na^+]_{pip}$ after recovery from ouabain. Arbitrary curves were fitted to the points by eye. **B**, Steady-state levels of difference currents derived by subtracting currents recorded in the absence of Na/K pump activity from those recorded, at the same voltage, in its presence. The three sets of points are: Δ, (2)-(1), current activated by raising $[Na]_{pip}$; ouabain-sensitive current on application, o, (2)-(3), and withdrawal, •, (4)-(3), of ouabain, respectively. Reproduced from Gadsby et al (1985) [13] with permission.

the upper curve is drawn through current levels obtained with the pump activated by 34 mM pipette [Na] in the absence of ouabain (o,•). The forward-running Na/K pump current-voltage relationships in Fig. 2B were determined by appropriate subtraction of the currents in Fig. 2A: triangles show Na-activated current, and open and closed circles show ouabain-sensitive currents determined, respectively, by washing on and washing off ouabain. The three sets of points all suggest that outward pump current approaches a maximal amplitude at positive potentials and declines steeply with voltage at negative potentials.

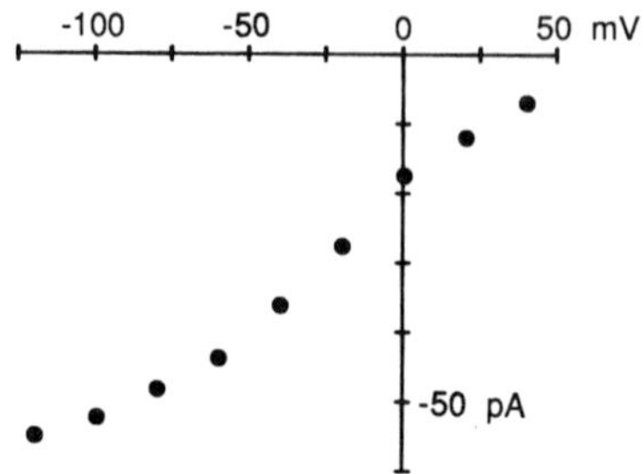

Fig. 3 Current-voltage relationship of backward-running Na/K pump in a cell exposed to zero K, 150 mM Na fluid, and dialyzed with pipette solution containing no Na, 145 mM K, 5 mM ATP, 5 mM ADP, and 5 mM P_i. Steady current was measured near the end of 100-ms voltage pulses from -40 mV. Pump current was determined by subtracting current levels in 0.5 mM strophanthidin from the average of control current levels obtained just before, and just after, the brief exposure to strophanthidin. Reproduced from Bahinski et al (1988) [14] with permission.

Fig.3 shows a steady-state pump current-voltage relationship obtained under conditions designed to reverse the Na/K pump reaction cycle. The external solution was K-free, but contained 150 mM Na, while the internal solution was Na-free, but contained 145 mM K, 5 mM ATP, 5 mM ADP, and 5mM P_i. Under those conditions, strophanthidin caused an outward shift of holding current at -40 mV, reflecting inhibition of inward pump current. The inward pump current was strongly voltage-dependent, increasing with membrane hyperpolarization from a very small size near +50 mV to an apparent maximal level near -100 mV. The steepest voltage dependence occurred between -50 mV and +25 mV under our experimental conditions, and there was no evidence of a region of negative slope conductance [cf. ref 4]. A similar voltage dependence of inward Na/K pump current has recently been reported in internally-dialyzed, voltage-clamped squid axons [5].

These experiments demonstrate that both inward and outward pump current are strongly voltage-dependent over the physiological range of membrane potentials, suggesting that the rate-limiting step of the Na/K pump reaction cycle is either voltage-dependent or is preceded by a rapid voltage-sensitive step (for review, see [9]). Na translocation has recently been shown to be voltage-dependent [10, 11, 12].

ACKNOWLEDGEMENTS

Supported by NIH grants HL 14899 and HL 36783, the AHA NYC Affiliate, and the Irma T. Hirschl Trust.

REFERENCES

1. Thomas, R.C., Physiol. Rev. 52, 563-594 (1972).
2. Glynn, I.M., in: Electrogenic Transport: Fundamental Principles and Physiological Implications, Blaustein, M.P. and Lieberman, M., eds. (Raven, New York 1984) pp.33-48.
3. Garrahan, P.J., and Glynn, I.M., J. Physiol.(Lond) 192, 237-256 (1967).
4. De Weer, P. and Rakowski, R.F., Nature 309, 450-452 (1984).
5. Rakowski, R.F., Gadsby, D.C., and De Weer, P., Biol. Bull. 173, 445 (1987).
6. Isenberg, G., and Klöckner, U., Pflügers Arch. 395, 6-18 (1982).
7. Hamill, O.P., Marty, A., Neher, E., Sakmann, B., and Sigworth, F.J., Pflügers Arch. 391, 85-100 (1981).
8. Soejima, M. and Noma, A., Pflügers Arch. 400, 424-431 (1984).
9. De Weer, P., Gadsby, D.C. and Rakowski, R.F., Ann. Rev. Physiol. 50, (1988). In press.
10. Nakao, M., and Gadsby, D.C., Nature 323, 628-630 (1986).
11. Goldshlegger, R., Karlish, S.J.D., Rephaeli, A., and Stein, W.D., J. Physiol. (Lond) 387, 331-355 (1987).
12. Borlinghaus R., Apell H-J., and Läuger P., J. Membrane Biol. 97, 161-178 (1987).
13. Gadsby, D.C., Kimura, J., and Noma, A., Nature 315, 63-65 (1985).
14. Bahinski, A., Gadsby, D.C., and Nakao, M., J. Physiol. (Lond) 390, (1988). In press.

BINDING OF OUABAIN TO ISOLATED, ADULT DOG HEART CELLS: EFFECTS ON NA+-PUMP FUNCTION AND CONTRACTILITY

L.M. PORTERFIELD, B.D. TUCKER, AND R.W. CALDWELL
Univ. of Tenn., Dept. of Pharmacology, Memphis, TN 38163

ABSTRACT

To correlate the binding characteristics and cellular actions of ouabain, we isolated left ventricular cardiac myocytes from adult mongrel dogs. These Ca^{++}-tolerant, digitalis sensitive cells were utilized to determine specific equilibrium binding of [^{3}H]ouabain and cellular Na^{+}-pump function ($^{86}Rb^{+}$-uptake) over a range of glycoside concentrations. Ouabain-induced changes in contractility were assessed using electrical field stimulation and computer-assisted analysis of microscopic images. Specific binding of ouabain occurred over a concentration range of 10^{-8} M to 10^{-5} M. Scatchard analysis revealed a curvilinear plot. A high affinity component had an estimated K_D of 1.58 X 10^{-7} M ± 0.58 M and a B_{max} of 3.06 pmoles ± 1.62/mg protein. A second, low affinity component had an estimated K_D of 4.43 X 10^{-6} ± 1.29 M and a B_{max} of 13.4 pmoles ± 0.73/mg protein. Ouabain produced dose-dependent inhibition of Na^{+}-pump activity and enhancement of contractility over a concentration range and in a manner that closely paralleled specific binding. Our data suggest the existence of two classes of binding sites for ouabain in dog heart cells, both of which appear to be associated with inhibition of the Na^{+}-pump and a positive inotropic effect.

INTRODUCTION

For over 200 years the search for the mechanism of action of digitalis has continued without the emergence of a satisfactory solution. Many aspects of myocardial cellular function have been scrutinized, in the hopes of understanding the true manner by which these agents increase the contractile state of heart muscle.

The objective of this study was to examine the characteristics of digitalis binding sites and to correlate receptor binding with physiologic responses by performing parallel experiments which assessed cellular Na^{+}-pump and contractile function. Ventricular cells from the dog were chosen as this species is particularly sensitive to cardiac glycosides [1,2,3], and the use of isolated Ca^{++}-tolerant cells allowed the direct effects of ouabain to be examined in normal ionic conditions without neuronal interference.

METHODS AND MATERIALS

The method used was a modification of that of Spanier and Weglicki [4]. Briefly, adult mongrel dogs of either sex were anesthetized with pentobarbital. The heart was exposed and the coronaries perfused *in situ* with a saline-sucrose buffer solution (Ca^{++}=0). This was followed by perfusion with buffer solution containing collagenase. The entire heart was excised and 25 g of left ventricle removed and minced. This tissue was incubated at 35°C in a closed spinning flask with buffer solution containing

Biology of Isolated Adult Cardiac Myocytes
William A. Clark, Robert S. Decker, and Thomas K. Borg, Editors

collagenase, hyaluronidase, and trypsin equilibrated with 95% O_2-5% CO_2. The cell suspensions were centrifuged and the pellets resuspended. The resuspension-centrifugation process was repeated 5 times. During this four hour process, Ca^{++} levels in the medium were progressively raised from 0.1 mM to a final conentration of 1.6 mM. The isolated Ca^{++}-tolerant myocytes were then transferred to culture flasks containing modified Joklik medium supplemented with 18% horse serum and 1.6 mM Ca^{++}.

Binding of [^{3}H]ouabain

Freshly isolated heart cells in culture medium were mixed with one concentration of [^{3}H]ouabain and 12 different concentrations of unlabeled ouabain. The cell suspension was incubated for 120 minutes, since equilibrium binding was achieved within this time frame for all ouabain concentrations utilized. The binding reaction was terminated by filtering the samples through Millipore filters (8.0 µm pore size) on a vacuum manifold. The filters were washed 3X with 5 ml of iced saline. The amount of [^{3}H]ouabain bound to cells was determined and specific binding was calculated as total binding minus nonspecific binding (that which occurred in the presence of 10^{-4} M ouabain).

Linear least square fit for Scatchard analysis was unsatisfactory. Therefore, [^{3}H]ouabain binding was analyzed by a Scatchard nonlinear least square method.

$^{86}Rb^+$-uptake

Sodium-pump activity was estimated as digitalis-sensitive $^{86}Rb^+$-uptake. Isolated heart cells in culture medium were mixed with various concentrations of ouabain and incubated for 120 minutes at 37°C. Trace $^{86}Rb^+$ was then added to the cell suspension for an additional 30 minutes (active $^{86}Rb^+$-uptake remained linear for at least 60 min.). After incubation, cells were separated and washed in a filter system as above. Specific $^{86}Rb^+$-uptake in cells retained on the filters was calculated as total minus that uptake of $^{86}Rb^+$ that occurred in the presence of 10^{-4} M ouabain.

Assessment of contractile changes in isolated cells

Culture flasks containing quiescent cardiac myocytes in culture medium were mounted on the stage of phase-contrast microscope equipped with a constant temperature chamber at 37°C. The cells were magnified using a 20 X objective and the image displayed on a TV monitor via a video camera. Cells were electrically driven at a frequency of 0.5 Hz in the field of two platinum wires at 2X threshold voltage. The concentration of ouabain was progressively increased in the culture flasks and after each contractile response had reached a steady state level, a tape recording was made of at least five consecutive contractions. The data were analyzed for change in cell length by using an image analysis system consisting of a digitizer tablet coupled with an Apple II computer.

RESULTS AND DISCUSSION

A. Binding of ouabain to dog heart cells.

Scatchard analysis was performed to determine the affinity of the ouabain for its binding site(s) and to ascertain the number of binding sites in canine isolated heart cells. The Scatchard plot for ouabain was curvilinear indicating at least two components of binding (Figure 1). The high affinity component had an estimated K_D of 1.58×10^{-7} M ± 0.58 M and a B_{max} of 3.06 pmoles ± 1.62/mg protein (n=5). The second, low affinity component had an estimated K_D of 4.43 X 10^{-6} ± 1.29 M and a B_{max} of 13.4 pmoles ± 0.73/mg protein.

Negative cooperativity was excluded as a cause of the curvilinear Scatchard plot by measurement of [^{3}H]ouabain dissociation in the presence and absence of excess unlabelled ouabain [5]. The term negative cooperativity is defined as the phenomenon of decreasing apparent affinity of the receptors as a consequence of increasing occupancy. The results of these experiments (data not shown) demonstrated that excess ligand did not accelerate the dissociation rate compared to simple dilution.

It is highly likely that the curvilinear ouabain Scatchard plots generated in this study could be explained by the existence of multiple classes of binding sites that have different, but fixed affinities.

B. Inhibition of Na^+, K^+-ATPase by ouabain.

A physiologic effect must occur after a drug binds to a specific binding site to be classified as a receptor. Therefore, in heart muscle cells from adult dogs, degree of specific binding of ouabain was correlated with inhibition of Na^+,K^+-ATPase. Ouabain inhibited the Na^+-pump over a concentration range of 10^{-9} to 10^{-5} M (figure 2). The concentration of ouabain that caused half maximal inhibition (IC_{50}) of the sodium pump was 3.7 X 10^{-8} M.

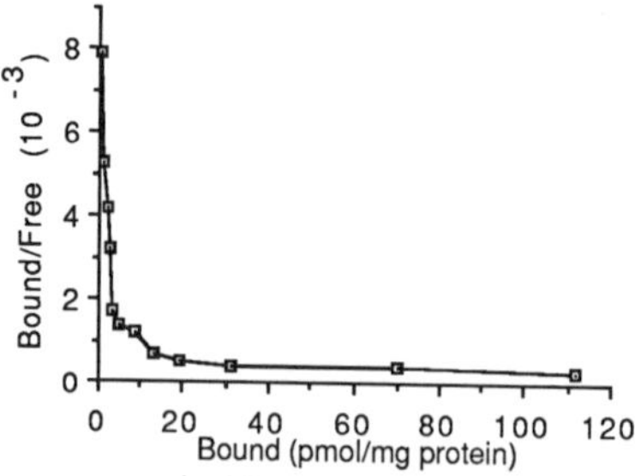

Figure 1. Example of Scatchard analysis of [^{3}H]ouabain equilibrium binding. The K_D and B_{max} of the high affinity, low capacity component were 5.3 X 10^{-8} M and 2.2 pmoles/mg protein, respectively; the values were about 3.5 X 10^{-6} M (K_D) and 6.3 pmoles/mg protein (B_{max}) for the low affinity, high capacity component.

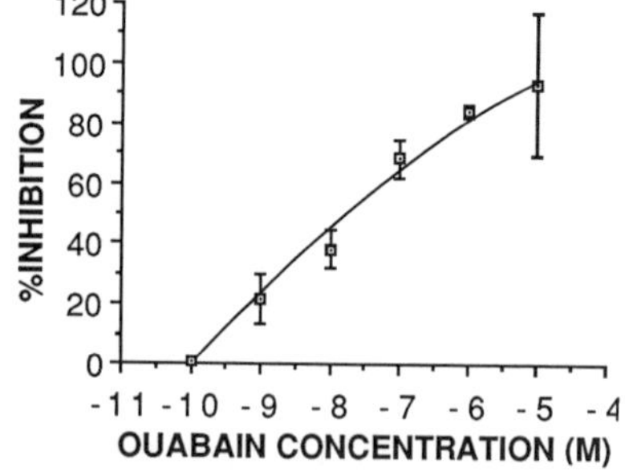

Figure 2. Inhibition of ^{86}Rb-uptake by ouabain in the presence of 5.4 mM K^+ and 1.6 mM Ca^{++} for 120 minutes. Specific $^{86}Rb^+$-uptake, indicative of Na^+-pump activity, was then determined over a 30 minute period. Values represent mean ± S.E.M. for three to eight experiments performed in duplicate.

A close relationship between the cellular binding of ouabain and inhibition of the sodium pump was evident from these experiments. All concentrations of ouabain that bound to dog heart cells, were demonstrated to inhibit the pump. The concentration producing 50% inhibition of $^{86}Rb^+$ influx was close to the K_D for the high affinity, low capacity component of binding.

C. Effect of ouabain on contractility of electrically stimulated dog heart cells.

Initial time course studies demonstrated the maximal contractility changes at any one concentration of ouabain occurred by five to ten minutes. Ouabain caused in increase in contractility in a concentration dependent manner (figure 3). Threshold and maximally inotropic concentration were 10^{-8} M and 10^{-5} M, respectively, for ouabain. Higher concentrations led to spontaneous depolarizations and cell contracture. This was most likely an indication of digitalis toxicity. Interestingly, the high affinity K_D for ouabain fell on the first phase of the contractility curve, while the low affinity K_D was located on the steeper, second portion of the curve.

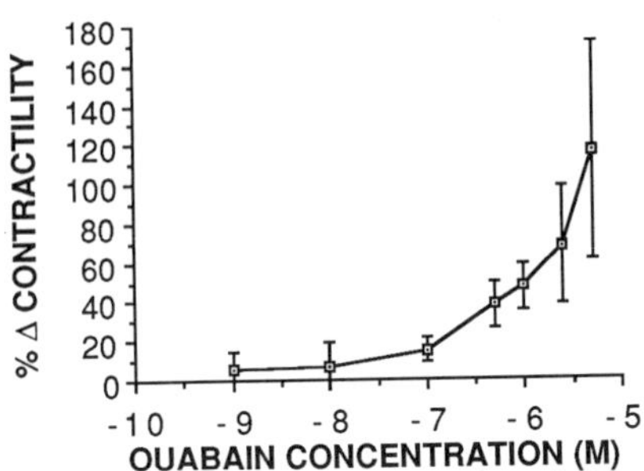

Figure 3. Effect of various concentrations of ouabain on contractility of dog heart cells. Myocytes incubated in the presence of 5.4 mM K^+ and 1.6 mM Ca^{++} were exposed to increasing concentrations of ouabain. Data points represent the mean ± S.E.M. for three to nine experiments.

SUMMARY

1. There appears to be multiple classes of ouabain binding sites in isolated, adult dog heart cells.

2. Ouabain produced concentration-dependent inhibition of Na^+-pump activity and enhancement of contractility.

3. The low and high affinity sites for ouabain binding in dog heart cells can be classified as active ouabain receptors, since their occupation is linked to the inhibition of the Na^+-pump and positive inotropic effects.

ACKNOWLEDGEMENTS

We would like to thank Drs. Arthur M. Spanier, Robert E. Kramer, Clinton B. Nash and Margaret T. Weis for their expert advice.

REFERENCES

1. T. Akera, F.S. Larsen, and T.M. Brody, J. Pharmacol. Exp. Ther. 170, 17-26 (1969).

2. T. Akera and T.M. Brody, Pharmacol. Rev. 29, 187-218 (1978).

3. T.W. Smith, E.M. Antman, P.L. Friedman, C.M. Blatt, and J.D. Marsh, Prog. Cardiovasc. Dis. 26, 495-540 (1984).

4. A.M. Spanier and W.B. Weglicki, Am. J. Physiol. 243, H448-H455 (1982).

5. P. DeMeyts, A.F. Bianco, and J. Roth, J. Biol. Chem. 251, 1877-1888 (1976).

AUTHOR INDEX

SUBJECT INDEX